CONTENTS

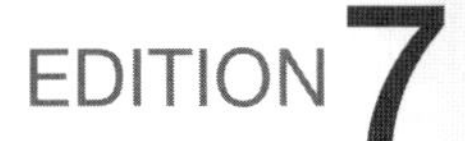

Understanding Nursing Research

Building an Evidence-Based Practice

Susan K. Grove, PhD, RN, ANP-BC, GNP-BC
Professor Emerita
College of Nursing and Health Innovation
The University of Texas at Arlington
Arlington, Texas;
Adult Nurse Practitioner
WellMed Clinic
Grand Prairie, Texas

Jennifer R. Gray, PhD, RN, FAAN
Associate Dean, College of Natural and Health Sciences
Oklahoma Christian University
Oklahoma City, Oklahoma;
Professor Emerita
College of Nursing and Health Innovation
The University of Texas at Arlington
Arlington, Texas

ELSEVIER

ELSEVIER

3251 Riverport Lane
St. Louis, Missouri 63043

UNDERSTANDING NURSING RESEARCH: BUILDING AN EVIDENCE-BASED PRACTICE, SEVENTH EDITION

ISBN: 978-0-323-53205-1

Notices

Knowledge and best practice in this field are constantly changing. As new research and experience broaden our understanding, changes in research methods, professional practices, or medical treatment may become necessary.

Practitioners and researchers must always rely on their own experience and knowledge in evaluating and using any information, methods, compounds, or experiments described herein. In using such information or methods they should be mindful of their own safety and the safety of others, including parties for whom they have a professional responsibility.

With respect to any drug or pharmaceutical products identified, readers are advised to check the most current information provided (i) on procedures featured or (ii) by the manufacturer of each product to be administered, to verify the recommended dose or formula, the method and duration of administration, and contraindications. It is the responsibility of practitioners, relying on their own experience and knowledge of their patients, to make diagnoses, to determine dosages and the best treatment for each individual patient, and to take all appropriate safety precautions.

To the fullest extent of the law, neither the Publisher nor the authors, contributors, or editors, assume any liability for any injury and/or damage to persons or property as a matter of products liability, negligence or otherwise, or from any use or operation of any methods, products, instructions, or ideas contained in the material herein.

Previous editions copyrighted 2015, 2011, 2007, 2003, 1999, and 1995.

Library of Congress Cataloging-in-Publication Control Number: 2018944739

Content Strategist: Lee Henderson
Content Development Specialist: Laurel Shea
Publishing Services Manager: Julie Eddy
Senior Project Manager: Rachel E. McMullen
Design Direction: Renee Duenow

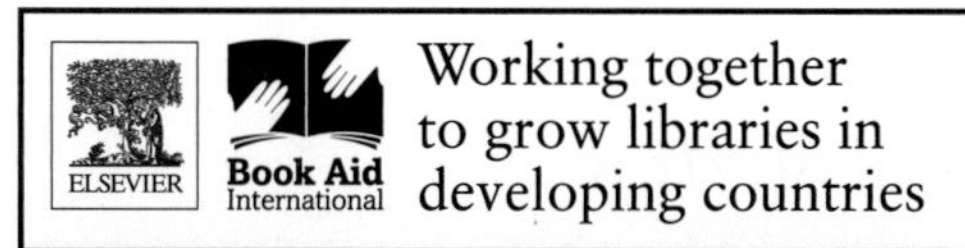

Printed in Canada
Last digit is the print number: 9 8 7 6 5 4 3 2

CONTRIBUTORS AND REVIEWERS

CONTRIBUTORS

Christy J. Bomer-Norton, PhD, RN, CNM, IBCLC
Concord, Massachusetts

Kathryn M. Daniel, PhD, MS, BSN, BA
Associate Professor
College of Nursing and Health Innovation
The University of Texas at Arlington
Arlington, Texas

REVIEWERS

Sue Ellen Bingham, PhD, RN
Professor of Nursing
Clayton State University
Morrow, Georgia

Sara L. Clutter, PhD, RN
Professor of Nursing
Waynesburg University
Waynesburg, Pennsylvania

Angela N. Cornelius, DNP, RN, CNE, CNL
Associate Professor of Nursing
Central Methodist University
Fayette, Missouri

Polly A. Hulme, PhD, CNP, RN
Professor
College of Nursing
South Dakota State University
Brookings, South Dakota

Tamara M. Kear, PhD, RN, CNS, CNN
Associate Professor of Nursing
College of Nursing
Villanova University
Villanova, Pennsylvania

Llynne C. Kiernan, DNP, MSN, RN-BC
Assistant Professor of Nursing
Norwich University School of Nursing
Northfield, Vermont

Kathleen S. Murtaugh, MSN, RN, CNA
Assistant Professor
Saint Joseph College—St. Elizabeth School of Nursing Cooperative Program
Rensselaer, Indiana

Michael Perlow, DNS, RN
Professor of Nursing
School of Nursing and Health Professions
Murray State University
Murray, Kentucky

To all nurses who change the lives of patients, families, and students
through applying the best research evidence in practice and education.
Susan and Jennifer

In memory of my beloved sister, and to my husband Jay Suggs and my daughters
Monece Appleton and Nicole Horn who have provided me love and support
during my 30 years of developing research textbooks.
Susan

To my husband Randy Gray, our children, and grandchildren
who give me space when I am writing and love me anyway.
Jennifer

PREFACE

Research is a major force in nursing, and the evidence generated from research is constantly changing practice, education, and health policy. A major goal of professional nursing and health care is the delivery of evidence-based care. By making nursing research an integral part of baccalaureate education, we hope to facilitate the movement of research into the mainstream of nursing. Our aim in developing this essentials of research text, *Understanding Nursing Research: Building an Evidence-Based Practice*, is to create excitement about research in undergraduate students. The text emphasizes the importance of baccalaureate-educated nurses being able to read, critically appraise, and synthesize research so this evidence can be used to make changes in practice. We also hope this text increases student awareness of the knowledge that has been generated through nursing research and that this knowledge is relevant to their practice. Only through research can nursing truly be recognized as a profession with documented effective outcomes for the patient, family, nurse provider, and healthcare system.

Developing a seventh edition of *Understanding Nursing Research* has provided us with an opportunity to update, clarify, and refine the essential content for an undergraduate research text. The text is designed to assist undergraduate students in overcoming the barriers they frequently encounter in understanding the language used in nursing research. The revisions in this edition are based on our own experiences with the text and input from dedicated reviewers, inquisitive students, and supportive faculty from across the country who provided us with many helpful suggestions.

Chapter 1, Introduction to Nursing Research and Its Importance in Building an Evidence-Based Practice, introduces you to nursing research, the history of research, and the significance of research evidence for nursing practice. The most relevant types of research synthesis being conducted in nursing—systematic review, meta-analysis, meta-synthesis, and mixed-methods systematic review—are described. The definition of evidence-based practice (EBP) has been updated based on current literature and EBP activities implemented in nursing. The discussion of research methodologies and their importance in generating an EBP for nursing has been updated and expanded to include mixed methods research. A discussion of the Quality and Safety Education for Nursing (QSEN) competencies and their link to research has been included to increase students' understanding of the importance in delivering quality, safe health care to patients and families.

Chapter 2, Introduction to Quantitative Research, presents the steps of the quantitative research process in a concise, clear manner and introduces students to the focus and findings of quantitative studies. Extensive, recent examples of descriptive, correlational, quasi-experimental, and experimental studies are provided, which reflect the quality of current nursing research.

Chapter 3, Introduction to Qualitative Research, describes four approaches to qualitative research and the philosophies upon which they are based. These approaches include phenomenology, grounded theory, ethnography, and exploratory-descriptive qualitative. Data collection and analysis methods specific to qualitative research are discussed. Guidelines for reading and critically appraising qualitative studies are explained using examples of published studies.

Chapter 4, Examining Ethics in Nursing Research, provides an extensive discussion of the use of ethics in research and the regulations that govern the research process, including recent changes to the Common Rule being implemented by the U.S. Department of Health and Human Services to protect human subjects. The implications of the Health Insurance Portability and Accountability Act (HIPAA) for research are described. Guidelines are provided to assist students in critically appraising the ethical discussions in published studies and to participate in the ethical review of research in clinical agencies.

Chapter 5, Examining Research Problems, Purposes, and Hypotheses, clarifies the difference between a problem and a purpose. Example problems and purpose statements are included from current qualitative and quantitative studies. Detailed critical appraisal guidelines are applied to current studies to assist students in critically appraising the problems, purposes, hypotheses, and variables in studies.

Chapter 6, Understanding and Critically Appraising the Literature Review, begins with a description of the content and quality of different types of publications that might be included in a review. Guidelines for critically appraising published literature reviews are explored with a focus on the differences in the purpose and timing of the literature review in quantitative and qualitative studies. The steps for finding appropriate sources, reading publications, and synthesizing information into a logical, cohesive review are presented.

Chapter 7, Understanding Theory and Research Frameworks, briefly describes the components of theory and the different types of theories that serve as the basis for study frameworks. The purpose of a research framework is discussed with the acknowledgement that the framework may be implicit. Guidelines for critically appraising the study framework are presented as well. The guidelines are applied to studies with frameworks derived from research findings and from different types of theories.

Chapter 8, Clarifying Quantitative Research Designs, addresses descriptive, correlational, quasi-experimental, and experimental designs and criteria for critically appraising these designs in studies. The major strengths and threats to design validity are summarized in a table and discussed related to current studies.

Chapter 9, Examining Populations and Samples in Research, provides a detailed discussion of the concepts of sampling in research. Different types of sampling methods for both qualitative and quantitative research are described. Guidelines are included for critically appraising the sampling criteria, sampling method, and sample size of quantitative and qualitative studies.

Chapter 10, Clarifying Measurement and Data Collection in Quantitative Research, has been updated to reflect current knowledge about measurement methods used in nursing research. Content has been expanded and uniquely organized to assist students in critically appraising the reliability and validity of scales; precision and accuracy of physiological measures; and the sensitivity, specificity, and likelihood ratios of diagnostic and screening tests.

Chapter 11, Understanding Statistics in Research, focuses on the theories and concepts of the statistical analysis process and the statistics conducted to describe variables, examine relationships, predict outcomes, and examine group differences in studies. Guidelines are provided for critically appraising the results and discussion sections of nursing studies. The results from current studies are critically appraised and presented as examples throughout this chapter to assist students in understanding this content.

Chapter 12, Critical Appraisal of Quantitative and Qualitative Research for Nursing Practice, was revised to include three major criteria for critically appraising quantitative and qualitative studies. These criteria are: (1) to identify the steps or elements of studies; (2) to determine the strengths and weaknesses of studies; and (3) to evaluate the credibility, trustworthiness, and meaning of studies. These criteria include questions for critically appraising quantitative and qualitative studies. This chapter also includes a current qualitative and quantitative study, and these two studies are critically appraised using the guidelines provided in this chapter.

Chapter 13, Building an Evidence-Based Nursing Practice, has been significantly updated to reflect the current trends in health care to provide evidence-based nursing practice. Detailed guidelines are provided for critically appraising the four common types of research synthesis conducted in nursing (systematic review, meta-analysis, meta-synthesis, and mixed-methods systematic review). These guidelines were used to critically appraise current research syntheses to assist students in examining the quality of published research syntheses and the potential use of research evidence in practice. The chapter includes updated models to assist nurses and agencies in moving toward EBP. Translational research is introduced as a method for promoting the use of research evidence in practice.

Chapter 14, Introduction to Additional Research Methodologies in Nursing: Mixed Methods and Outcomes Research, was significantly revised to include both mixed methods and outcomes studies. Mixed methods studies, including both quantitative and qualitative methodologies, are increasing in the nursing literature and require an expanded focus in this text. The goal of this chapter is to increase students' knowledge of the influence of mixed methods and outcomes research on nursing and health care. Content and guidelines are provided to assist students in reading and critically appraising the mixed methods and outcomes studies appearing in the nursing literature.

The seventh edition is written and organized to facilitate ease in reading, understanding, and critically appraising studies. The major strengths of the text are as follows:

- State-of-the art coverage of EBP—a topic of vital importance in nursing.
- Balanced coverage of qualitative and quantitative research methodologies.
- Introduction to mixed methods and outcomes research methodologies.
- Rich and frequent illustration of major points and concepts from the most current nursing research literature from a variety of clinical practice areas.
- A clear, concise writing style that is consistent among the chapters to facilitate student learning.
- Electronic references and websites that direct the student to an extensive array of information that is important in reading, critically appraising, and using research knowledge in practice.

This seventh edition of *Understanding Nursing Research* is appropriate for use in a variety of undergraduate research courses for both RN and pre-licensure students because it provides an introduction to quantitative, qualitative, mixed methods, and outcomes research methodologies. This text not only will assist students in reading research literature, critically appraising published studies, and summarizing research evidence to make changes in practice, but it also can serve as a valuable resource for practicing nurses in critically appraising studies and implementing research evidence in their clinical settings.

LEARNING RESOURCES TO ACCOMPANY *UNDERSTANDING NURSING RESEARCH*, 7th EDITION

The teaching and learning resources to accompany *Understanding Nursing Research* have been revised for both the instructor and student to reflect content updates to the seventh edition and to promote a maximum level of flexibility in course design and student review.

Evolve Instructor Resources

A comprehensive suite of Instructor Resources is available online at http://evolve.elsevier.com/Grove/understanding/ and consists of a Test Bank, PowerPoint slides, Image Collection, Answer Guidelines for the Appraisal Exercises provided for students, and TEACH for Nurses, which include teaching strategies and other educator resources for research and EBP courses.

Test Bank

The Test Bank consists of approximately 550 NCLEX® Examination–style questions, including approximately 10% of questions in alternate item formats. Each question is coded with the correct answer, a rationale from the textbook, and the cognitive level in the new Bloom's Taxonomy. The Test Bank is provided in ExamView and Evolve LMS formats.

PowerPoint Slides

The PowerPoint slide collection contains approximately 550 slides, including seamlessly integrated Audience Response System Questions, images, and Unfolding Case Studies. The PowerPoints have been simplified, with the Notes area of the slides featuring additional content details. Unfolding Case Studies focus on practical EBP/PICO or PICOS questions, such as a nurse on a unit needing to perform a literature search or to identify a systematic review or meta-analysis to address a practice problem. PowerPoint presentations are fully customizable.

Image Collection

The electronic Image Collection consists of all images from the text. This collection can be used in classroom or online presentations to reinforce student learning.

TEACH for Nurses

TEACH for Nurses is a robust, customizable, ready-to-use collection of chapter-by-chapter teaching strategies and educational resources that provide everything you need to create an engaging and effective course. Each chapter includes the following:

- Chapter Objectives
- Student Resources
- Instructor Resources
- Teaching Strategies
- In-Class/Online Case Study
- Nursing Curriculum Standards
  - BSN Essentials

Evolve Student Resources

The Evolve Student Resources include interactive Review Questions, a Research Article Library consisting of 10 full-text research articles, and Appraisal Exercises based on the articles in the Research Article Library.

- The interactive Review Questions (approximately 25 per chapter) aid the student in reviewing and focusing on the chapter material.
- The Research Article Library is an updated collection of 10 research articles taken from leading nursing journals.
- The Appraisal Exercises are a collection of application exercises, based on the articles in the Research Article Library, that help students learn to critically appraise and apply research findings. Answer Guidelines are provided for the instructor.

Study Guide

The companion Study Guide, written by the authors of the main text, provides both time-tested and innovative exercises for each chapter in *Understanding Nursing Research*, 7th Edition. Included for each chapter are a brief Introduction, Terms and Definitions exercises, Linking Ideas exercises, Web-Based Information and Resources exercises, and Conducting Critical Appraisals to Build an Evidence-Based Practice exercises. An integral part of the Study Guide are the appendices, which feature three published research studies that are referenced throughout the critical appraisal exercises. These three recently published nursing studies (a quantitative study, a qualitative study, and a mixed methods study) can be used in classroom or online discussions, as well as to address the Study Guide questions. The Study Guide provides exercises that target comprehension of concepts included in each chapter. Exercises—including fill-in-the-blank, matching, and multiple-choice questions—encourage students to validate their understanding of the chapter content. Critical Appraisal Activities provide students with opportunities to apply their new research knowledge to evaluate the quantitative, qualitative, and mixed methods studies provided in the back of the Study Guide in Appendices A, B, and C.

Unique to this edition are the following features: an increased emphasis on evidence-based practice, new Web-Based Activities, an increased emphasis on high-value learning activities, updated back matter for quick reference, and quick-reference printed tabs.

- Increased emphasis on EBP: This edition of the Study Guide features an expanded focus on EBP to match that of the revised textbook. This focus helps students who are new to nursing research see the value of understanding the research process and applying it to promote evidence-based nursing practice.
- Web-Based Activities: Each chapter includes a current Web-Based Activity section, to teach students to use the Internet appropriately for scholarly research and EBP.
- Increased high-value learning activities: The exercises in this study guide have been updated to promote nursing students' understanding of research methodologies, critical appraisal of studies, and use of research evidence in practice.
- Back matter was updated for quick reference: An "Answer Key" is provided for the exercises developed for each chapter. Each published study is in a separate appendix (three appendices total), which simplifies cross referencing in the body of the Study Guide.
- Quick-reference printed tabs: Quick-reference printed tabs have been added to differentiate the Answer Key and each of the book's three published studies (four tabs total), for improved navigation and usability.

ACKNOWLEDGMENTS

Developing this essentials of research text was a 2-year project, and there are many people we would like to thank. We want to extend a very special thank you to Dr. Christy Bomer-Norton for her revision of Chapter 6 focused on literature review and Chapter 12 with emphasis on critical appraisal of quantitative and qualitative studies. We also want to thank Dr. Kathryn M. Daniel for her revision of Chapter 2 focused on quantitative research. We are very fortunate that these individuals were willing to share their expertise and time in developing the seventh edition of this text.

We want to express our appreciation to faculty of our universities, The University of Texas at Arlington College of Nursing and Health Innovation and Oklahoma Christian University, for their support and encouragement. We also would like to thank other nursing faculty members across the world who are using our book to teach research and have spent valuable time to send us ideas and to identify errors in the text. Special thanks to the students who have read our book and provided honest feedback on its clarity and usefulness to them. We would also like to recognize the excellent reviews of the colleagues, listed on the previous pages, who helped us make important revisions in the text.

In conclusion, we would like to thank the people at Elsevier who helped produce this book. We thank the following individuals who have devoted extensive time to the development of this seventh edition, the instructor's ancillary materials, student study guide, and all of the web-based components. These individuals include Lee Henderson, Lisa Newton, Laurel Shea, Anne Konopka, and Hari Maniyaan. Laurel Shea has been in constant communication with us to promote the quality and consistency of the format and content in this text. It has been such a pleasure working with you.

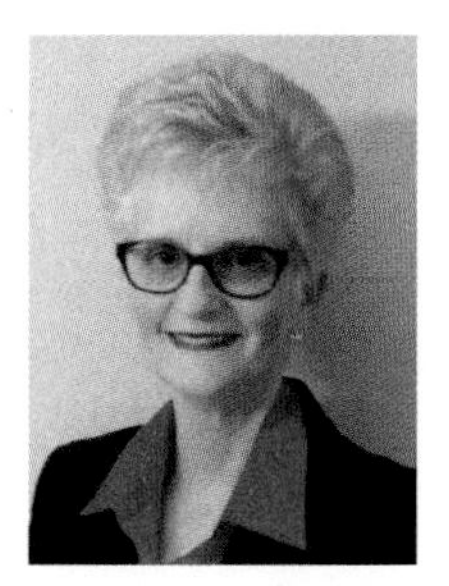

Susan K. Grove
PhD, RN, ANP-BC, GNP-BC

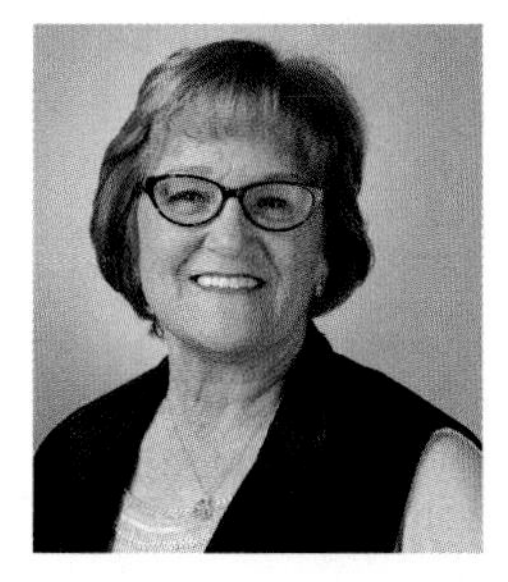

Jennifer R. Gray
PhD, RN, FAAN

CONTENTS

CHAPTER

1

Introduction to Nursing Research and Its Importance in Building an Evidence-Based Practice

Susan K. Grove

CHAPTER OVERVIEW

LEARNING OUTCOMES

After completing this chapter, you should be able to:

1. Define research, nursing research, and evidence-based practice.
2. Discuss the past and present activities influencing research in nursing.
3. Examine ways of acquiring nursing knowledge—tradition, authority, borrowing, trial and error, personal experience, role modeling, intuition, and reasoning.
4. Describe the common types of research—quantitative, qualitative, mixed methods, and outcomes—conducted to generate evidence for nursing practice.
5. Describe the purposes of research in implementing an evidence-based nursing practice.
6. Discuss your role in research as a professional nurse.
7. Describe the following strategies for synthesizing healthcare research: systematic review, meta-analysis, meta-synthesis, and mixed-methods systematic review.
8. Examine the levels of research evidence available to nurses for practice.

Welcome to the world of nursing research. You may think it strange to consider research a *world*, but it is a truly new way of experiencing reality. Entering a new world means learning a unique language, incorporating new rules, and using new experiences to learn how to interact effectively in that world. As you become a part of this new world, you will modify and expand your perceptions and methods of reasoning. For example, using research to guide your practice involves questioning, and you will be encouraged to ask such questions as these:

- What is the patient's healthcare problem?
- What nursing intervention(s) would effectively manage this problem in your practice?
- Are these interventions based on sound research evidence that enable you to select the most affective one for your patient population?
- How can you use research most effectively in promoting an evidence-based practice (EBP)?

Because research is a new world to many of you, we have developed this text to facilitate your entry into this world and your understanding of its contribution to the delivery of quality, safe nursing care. Chapter 1 clarifies the meaning of nursing research and its significance in developing an EBP for nursing. The research accomplishments in the profession over the last 170 years are discussed. The ways of acquiring knowledge in nursing are described, and the common research methodologies conducted for generating research evidence for practice are introduced. Nurses' roles in research are described based on their level of education and their contributions to the implementation of EBP. The chapter concludes with the critical elements of evidence-based nursing practice, such as strategies for synthesizing research evidence, levels of research evidence, and evidence-based guidelines.

WHAT IS NURSING RESEARCH?

The word *research* means "to search again" or "to examine carefully." More specifically, **research** is a diligent systematic inquiry or study that validates and refines existing knowledge and develops new knowledge. Diligent systematic study indicates planning, organization, and persistence. The ultimate goal of research is to develop an empirical body of knowledge for a discipline or profession, such as nursing.

Defining nursing research requires determining the relevant knowledge needed by nurses. Because nursing is a practice profession, research is essential to develop and refine knowledge that nurses can implement to improve clinical practice and promote quality outcomes (Melnyk, Gallagher-Ford, & Fineout-Overholt, 2017). Expert researchers have studied many interventions, and nurses have synthesized these studies to provide guidelines and protocols for use in practice. Practicing nurses and nursing students, like you, need to be able to read research reports and syntheses of research findings to implement evidence-based interventions in practice. For example, extensive research has been conducted to determine the most effective technique for administering medications by an intramuscular (IM) injection. This research was synthesized and used to develop evidence-based guidelines for administering IM injections to adults (Cocoman & Murray, 2008; Nicoll & Hesby, 2002; Ogston-Tuck, 2014). More recently, research has been synthesized to determine if nurses should aspirate during an IM injection procedure, which is discussed later in this chapter (Sisson, 2015; Thomas, Mraz, & Rajcan, 2016).

Nursing research is also needed to generate knowledge about nursing education, nursing administration, healthcare services, characteristics of nurses, and nursing roles. The findings from these studies influence nursing practice indirectly and add to nursing's body of empirical knowledge. Research is essential to provide quality learning experiences for nursing students. Through research, nurses can develop and refine the best methods for delivering distance nursing education and for using simulation to improve student learning. Nursing administration and health services studies are needed to improve the quality, safety, and cost-effectiveness of the healthcare delivery system. Studies of nurses and nursing roles can influence nurses' quality of care, productivity, job satisfaction, and retention. In this era of a nursing shortage, additional research is needed to determine effective ways to recruit individuals and retain them in the nursing profession. In summary, nursing research is a scientific process that validates and refines existing knowledge and generates new knowledge that directly and indirectly influences nursing practice. Nursing research is the key to building an EBP for our profession.

WHAT IS EVIDENCE-BASED PRACTICE?

The ultimate goal of nursing is an EBP that promotes quality, safe, and cost-effective outcomes for patients, families, healthcare providers, and the healthcare system (Melnyk et al., 2017; Moorhead, Johnson, Maas, & Swanson, 2013). EBP in nursing evolves from the integration of the best research evidence with our clinical expertise and our patients' circumstances and values to produce quality health outcomes (Institute of Medicine [IOM], 2001; Straus, Glasziou, Richardson, Rosenberg, & Haynes, 2011). Fig. 1.1 identifies the elements of EBP and demonstrates the major contribution of best research evidence to the delivery of this practice. The best research evidence is the empirical knowledge generated from the synthesis of quality health studies to address a clinical problem. Teams of expert researchers, healthcare professionals, and sometimes policy makers and consumers synthesize the best research evidence in different areas to develop national standardized guidelines for clinical practice. For example, a team of experts conducted, critically appraised, and synthesized research related to the chronic health problem of high blood pressure (BP) to develop an EBP guideline for practice that is discussed later in this section.

Clinical expertise is the knowledge and skills of the healthcare professional providing care. The clinical expertise of a nurse depends on his or her years of clinical experience, current knowledge of the research and clinical literature, and educational preparation. The stronger the nurse's clinical expertise, the better is her or his clinical judgment in implementing the best research evidence in practice.

EBP also incorporates the circumstances and values of a patient. Patient circumstances include the individual's clinical state, which might focus on health promotion, illness prevention, acute or chronic illness management, rehabilitation, and/or a peaceful death, and the clinical setting (e.g., hospital, clinic, home; Straus et al., 2011). In addition, a patient brings values or unique preferences, expectations, concerns, and cultural beliefs to each clinical encounter that need to be integrated

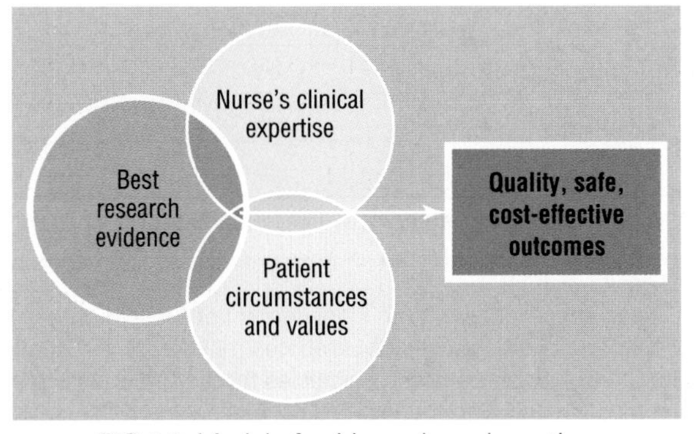

FIG 1.1 Model of evidence-based practice.

by the nurse into the care delivered. Thus EBP is the unique combination of the best research evidence being implemented by expert nurse clinicians in providing care to patients and families with specific health circumstances and values to promote quality, safe, cost-effective outcomes (see Fig. 1.1). With EBP, the patient and their family are encouraged to take an active role in the management of their health.

Evidence-Based Practice Guideline for High Blood Pressure

Research evidence from multiple studies are synthesized to develop guidelines, standards, protocols, algorithms (clinical decision trees), and/or policies to direct the implementation of a variety of nursing interventions. As noted earlier, members from the Eighth Joint National Committee (JNC 8) have developed the *2014 Evidence-Based Guideline for the Management of High Blood Pressure (BP) in Adults* (James et al., 2014, p. 507). High BP or hypertension (HTN) is diagnosed as a BP of 140/90 mm Hg or higher in adults younger than 60 years (Table 1.1). For individuals 60 years of age and older (≥60 years), the JNC 8 guideline has indicated that HTN is diagnosed as a BP of 150/90 mm Hg or higher (James et al., 2014). In contrast, the American and International Societies of Hypertension guideline has stated that HTN is diagnosed with a BP of 140/90 mm Hg or higher for persons younger than 80 years and a BP of 150/90 mm Hg or higher for those 80 years of age and older (Weber et al., 2014). Table 1.1, based on the JNC 8 guideline for high BP, also indicates that individuals 60 years of age or older who have diabetes mellitus (DM) or chronic kidney disease (CKD) have HTN if their BP is 140/90 mm Hg or higher.

As a nursing student or practicing nurse, you have a role in the management of patients with high BP. You need to know when patients have high BP based on their age and whether they have DM or CKD. Table 1.1 directs you when to report high BP readings to advance practice nurses and physicians and indicates the goals for systolic and diastolic BP readings for patients with HTN. The JNC 8 guideline recommends lifestyle modifications (LSMs) for all patients with HTN, such as a balanced diet, exercising regularly, achieving normal weight, and smoking cessation, if needed. You need to educate patients about the LSMs and monitor their success in making healthy changes

TABLE 1.1 EVIDENCED-BASED GUIDELINE FOR THE ASSESSMENT AND MANAGEMENT OF HIGH BLOOD PRESSURE IN ADULTS

HIGH BP OR HTN CLASSIFICATION				INTERVENTIONS BY REGISTERED NURSES		
AGE (yr)	HTN	SYSTOLIC BP GOAL (mm Hg)[a]	DIASTOLIC BP GOAL (mm Hg)[a]	LIFESTYLE MODIFICATION[b]	DM OR CKD[c]	PATIENT RECEIVING PHARMACOLOGIC TREATMENT
<60	≥140/90	<140 *and*	<90	Yes	No	Yes
<60	≥140/90	<140 *and*	<90	Yes	Yes	Yes
≥60	≥150/90	<150 *and*	<90	Yes	No	Yes
≥60	≥140/90	<140 *and*	<90	Yes	Yes	Yes

[a]Treatment is determined by the highest BP category, systolic or diastolic.

[b]Lifestyle modification: balanced diet, exercising regularly, achieving normal BP, and smoking cessation, if needed, should be promoted for all adults with HTN.

[c]Patients with DM or CKD need education about the management of these diseases and the link with hypertension.

BP, Blood pressure; *CKD*, chronic kidney disease; *DM*, diabetes mellitus; *HTN*, hypertension.

Data from James et al. (2014). 2014 evidence-based guidelines for the management of high blood pressure in adults: Report from the panel members appointed to the Eighth Joint National Committee (JNC 8). *Journal of the American Medical Association, 311*(5), 507–520.

in their lives. Patients with DM and CKD need education and support to assist them in managing these chronic diseases along with HTN. Patients diagnosed with HTN should be receiving pharmacological management that needs to be monitored by nurses and other healthcare providers (see Table 1.1). Many standardized, national guidelines are available through the National Guideline Clearinghouse (NGC, 2017).

Delivery of Evidence-Based Care to a Selected Patient Population With Hypertension

Fig. 1.2 provides an example of the delivery of evidence-based nursing care to adult, Hispanic women who are younger than 60 years with BP readings of 140/90 mm Hg or higher. In this example, the best research evidence identifies the following:

1. BP readings for HTN
2. Goals for systolic and diastolic BP readings <140/90
3. Education for LSMs
4. Support and education for management of DM and CKD with HTN (if appropriate)
5. Monitoring of pharmacological management (see Table 1.1; James et al., 2014).

These guidelines, developed from the best research evidence, are translated by registered nurses (RNs) and nursing students to address the circumstances and values of adult Hispanic women with HTN. These women need to manage their chronic illness in ways consistent with their cultural values. The quality, safe, and cost-effective outcomes of EBP in this example are women who monitor

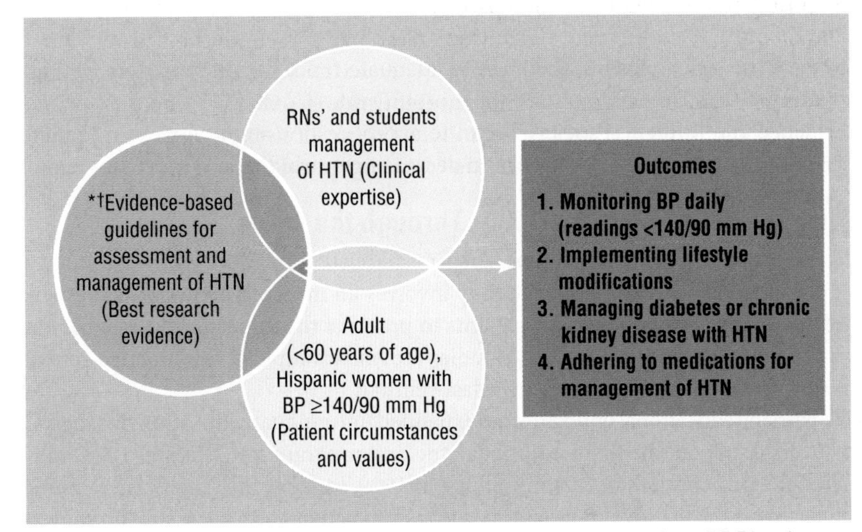

FIG 1.2 Evidence-based practice for adult Hispanic women with hypertension. *BP,* Blood pressure; *HTN,* hypertension; *RN,* registered nurse.

*James, P. A., Oparil, S., Carter, B. L., Cushman, W. C., Denison-Himmelfard, C., Handler, J., et al. (2014). 2014 evidence-based guidelines for the management of high blood pressure in adults: Report from the panel members appointed to the Eighth Joint National Committee (JNC 8). *Journal of the American Medical Association, 311*(5), 507–520.

†Weber, M. A., Schiffrin, E. L., White, W. B., Mann, S., Lindholm, L. H., Kenerson, J. G., et al. (2014). Clinical practice guidelines for the management of hypertension in the community: A statement by the American Society of Hypertension and the International Society of Hypertension. *Journal of Hypertension, 32*(1), 3–15.

their BP, determining that it is less than 140/90 mm Hg, implementing LSMs, managing DM and CKD as needed, and adhering to medication(s) prescribed for HTN.

HISTORICAL DEVELOPMENT OF RESEARCH IN NURSING

Initially, nursing research evolved slowly, from the investigations of Nightingale in the 19th century to the studies of nursing education in the 1930s and 1940s and the research of nurses and nursing roles in the 1950s and 1960s. From the 1970s to the present, an increasing number of nursing studies have focused on clinical problems, with the goal of developing an EBP for nursing. Reviewing the history of nursing research enables you to identify the accomplishments and understand the need for further research to determine the best research evidence for use in practice. Table 1.2 outlines the key historical events that have influenced the development of research in nursing.

Florence Nightingale

Nightingale (1859) is recognized as the first nurse researcher, with her initial studies focused on the importance of a healthy environment in promoting patients' physical and mental well-being. She studied ventilation, cleanliness, purity of water, and diet to determine their influence on patients' health (Herbert, 1981). Nightingale is also noted for her data collection and statistical analyses, especially during the Crimean War. She studied soldiers' morbidity and mortality rates and the factors influencing them and presented her results in tables and pie charts. Nightingale was the first woman elected to the Royal Statistical Society based on her research and statistical expertise (Oakley, 2010).

Nightingale's research enabled her to instigate attitudinal, organizational, and social changes. She changed the attitudes of the military and society about the care of the sick. The military began to view the sick as having the right to adequate food, suitable quarters, and appropriate medical treatment, which greatly reduced the mortality rate (Cook, 1913). Because of Nightingale's research evidence and influence, society began to accept responsibility for testing public water, improving sanitation, preventing starvation, and decreasing morbidity and mortality rates (Palmer, 1977).

Nursing Research in the 1900s Through the 1970s

The *American Journal of Nursing* was first published in 1900, with case studies appearing in this journal late in the 1920s. A **case study** involves an in-depth analysis and systematic description of one patient or group of similar patients to promote the understanding of healthcare interventions, problems, and/or situations. Case studies are one example of the practice-related research that has been conducted in nursing over the last century.

Nursing educational opportunities expanded into graduate education. Teachers College at Columbia University offered the first educational doctoral program for nurses in 1923, and Yale University offered the first master's degree in nursing in 1929. In 1950, the American Nurses Association (ANA) initiated a 5-year study on nursing functions and activities. In 1959, the findings from this study were used to develop statements on functions, standards, and qualifications for professional nurses. During that time, clinical research began expanding as nursing specialty groups, such as those in community health, psychiatric-mental health, medical-surgical, pediatrics, and obstetrics, developed standards of care. The research conducted by the ANA and specialty groups provided the basis for the nursing practice standards that currently guide professional practice (Gortner & Nahm, 1977).

In the 1950s and 1960s, nursing schools began introducing research and the steps of the research process at the baccalaureate level, and Master of Science in Nursing (MSN) level nurses were provided a background for conducting small replication studies. In 1953, the Institute for Research and Service in Nursing Education was established at Teachers College of Columbia University and began providing research experiences for doctoral students (Gortner & Nahm, 1977). The increase in

TABLE 1.2 HISTORICAL EVENTS INFLUENCING RESEARCH IN NURSING

YEAR	EVENT
1850	Florence Nightingale recognized as first nurse researcher
1900	*American Journal of Nursing*
1923	First educational doctoral program for nurses, Teachers College, Columbia University
1929	First Master's in Nursing Degree at Yale University
1932	Association of Collegiate Schools of Nursing formed to promote conduct of research
1950	American Nurses Association (ANA) study of nursing functions and activities
1952	First research journal in nursing, *Nursing Research*
1955	American Nurses Foundation established to fund nursing research
1957	Southern Regional Educational Board, Western Interstate Commission on Higher Education, Midwestern Nursing Research Society, and New England Board of Higher Education developed to support and disseminate nursing research
1965	ANA sponsored first nursing research conferences
1970	ANA Commission on Nursing Research established
1972	Cochrane published *Effectiveness and Efficiency*, introducing concepts relevant to evidence-based practice (EBP)
1973	First Nursing Diagnosis Conference held, becoming the North American Nursing Diagnosis Association (NANDA)
1976	*Stetler-Marram Model for Application of Research Findings to Practice* published
1980s–1990s	Methodologies developed to determine "best evidence" for practice by Sackett and colleagues
1982–1983	*Conduct and Utilization of Research in Nursing Project* published
1983	*Annual Review of Nursing Research*
1985	National Center for Nursing Research (NCNR) established
1989	Agency for Health Care Policy and Research established
1990	American Nurses Credentialing Center implemented the Magnet Hospital Designation Program for Excellence in Nursing Services
1992	*Healthy People* was initiated by the federal government; Cochrane Center established
1993	NCNR renamed the National Institute of Nursing Research (NINR); Cochrane Collaboration initiated providing systematic reviews and EBP guidelines
1999	AHCPR renamed Agency for Healthcare Research and Quality (AHRQ).
2001	Stetler revised model Steps of Research Utilization to Facilitate EBP; Institute of Medicine report *Crossing the Quality Chasm: A New Health System for the 21st Century*
2002	The Joint Commission revised accreditation policies for hospitals supporting EBP; NANDA became international—NANDA-I
2005	Quality and Safety Education for Nurses initiated
2006	American Association of Colleges of Nursing (AACN) statement on nursing research
2016	NINR mission statement and strategic plan updated
2017	AACN leading initiatives of research and data management; AHRQ current mission and funding priorities; *Healthy People 2020* topics and objectives; NINR current research funding and other activities to promote research in nursing

research activities prompted the publication of the first research journal, *Nursing Research,* in 1952, which is still one of the strongest research journals today. The American Nurses Foundation was established in 1955 to fund nursing research projects. The Southern Regional Educational Board, Western Interstate Commission on Higher Education, Midwestern Nursing Research Society, and New England Board of Higher Education were formed in 1957 and have an important role today in supporting and disseminating nursing research across the United States.

In the 1960s, an increasing number of clinical studies focused on quality care and the development of criteria to measure patient outcomes. Intensive care units were developed, which promoted the investigation of nursing interventions, staffing patterns, and cost-effectiveness of care (Gortner & Nahm, 1977). Another research journal, the *International Journal of Nursing Studies,* was published in 1963. In 1965, the ANA sponsored the first of a series of nursing research conferences to promote the communication of research findings and the use of these findings in clinical practice.

In the late 1960s and 1970s, nurses developed models, conceptual frameworks, and theories to guide nursing practice. These nursing theorists generated propositions that required testing, which provided direction for nursing research. In 1978, Chinn became the editor of a new journal, *Advances in Nursing Science,* which published nursing theorists' work and related research. In 1970, the ANA Commission on Nursing Research was formed to expand the conduct of research. The commission influenced the development of federal guidelines for research with human subjects and sponsored research programs nationally and internationally (See, 1977).

The communication of research findings to clinical nurses was a major issue in the 1970s. Sigma Theta Tau International, the Honor Society for Nursing, sponsored national and international research conferences, and chapters of this organization sponsored many local conferences to communicate research findings. This organization and its chapters are still very involved in facilitating, funding, and communicating research. Stetler and Marram developed the first model in nursing to promote the application of research findings to practice in 1976. *Research in Nursing & Health* was first published in 1978, and the *Western Journal of Nursing Research* was published in 1979 to expand the communication of research.

In the late 1970s, Professor Archie Cochrane originated the concept of EBP and advocated for the provision of health care based on research to improve its quality. To facilitate the use of research evidence in practice, the Cochrane Center was established in 1992 and the Cochrane Collaboration in 1993. The Cochrane Collaboration and Library house numerous resources to promote EBP, such as systematic reviews of research and evidence-based guidelines for practice (see the Cochrane Collaboration, http://www.cochrane.org).

The nursing process became the focus of many studies in the 1970s, with investigations of assessment techniques, nursing diagnoses classification, goal-setting methods, and specific nursing interventions. The first Nursing Diagnosis Conference, held in 1973, evolved into the North American Nursing Diagnosis Association (NANDA). In 2002, NANDA expanded internationally, known as NANDA-I. NANDA-I supports research activities focused on identifying appropriate diagnoses for nursing and generating an effective diagnostic process. NANDA's journal, *Nursing Diagnosis,* was published in 1990 and was later renamed the *International Journal of Nursing Terminologies and Classifications.* Details on NANDA-I can be found on their website (http://www.nanda.org).

Nursing Research in the 1980s and 1990s

The conduct of clinical research was the focus of the 1980s, and clinical journals began publishing more studies. One new research journal was published in 1987, *Scholarly Inquiry for Nursing Practice,* and two in 1988, *Applied Nursing Research* and *Nursing Science Quarterly.* Although the body of empirical knowledge generated through clinical research increased rapidly in the 1980s, little of this knowledge was used in practice. During 1982 and 1983, the studies from a federally funded project, Conduct and Utilization of Research in Nursing, were published to facilitate the use of research to improve practice (Horsley, Crane, Crabtree, & Wood, 1983).

In 1983, the first volume of the *Annual Review of Nursing Research* was published (Werley & Fitzpatrick, 1983). These volumes include experts' reviews of research organized into four areas: nursing practice, nursing care delivery, nursing education, and the nursing profession. Publication of the *Annual Review of Nursing Research* continues today, with leading expert nurse scientists providing summaries of research in their areas of expertise. These summaries of current research knowledge encourage the use of research findings in practice and provide direction for future research. These increased clinical nursing studies led to the publication of *Clinical Nursing Research* in 1992.

Qualitative research was introduced in nursing in the late 1970s; the first studies appeared in nursing journals in the 1980s. Qualitative research explored the holistic nature of people and phenomena, discovering meaning and gaining new insights into issues relevant to nursing. The number of qualitative researchers and studies expanded greatly in the 1990s, with qualitative studies appearing in most of the nursing research and clinical journals. In 1994, a journal focused on disseminating qualitative research, *Qualitative Health Research,* was first published.

Another priority of the 1980s was to obtain increased funding for nursing research. Most of the federal funds in the 1980s were designated for medical studies involving the diagnosis and treatment of diseases. However, the ANA achieved a major political victory for nursing research with the creation of the National Center for Nursing Research (NCNR) in 1985. The purpose of this center was to support the conduct and dissemination of knowledge developed through basic and clinical nursing research, training, and other programs in patient care research (Bauknecht, 1985). The NCNR became the National Institute of Nursing Research (NINR) in 1993 to increase the status of nursing research and obtain more funding for studies.

Outcomes research emerged in the late 1980s and 1990s as an important methodology for documenting the effectiveness of healthcare services. This effectiveness research evolved from the quality assessment and quality assurance functions that originated with the professional standards review organizations in 1972. In 1989, the Agency for Healthcare Policy and Research (AHCPR) was established to facilitate the conduct of outcomes research (Rettig, 1991). AHCPR also had an active role in communicating research findings to healthcare practitioners and was responsible for publishing the first clinical practice guidelines. These guidelines included a synthesis of the best research evidence, with directives for nursing and medical practice developed by healthcare experts in various areas. The Healthcare Research and Quality Act of 1999 reauthorized the AHCPR, changing its name to the Agency for Healthcare Research and Quality (AHRQ). This significant change positioned the AHRQ as a scientific partner with the public and private sectors to improve the quality and safety of patient care.

Building on the process of research utilization, physicians, nurses, and other healthcare professionals focused on the development of EBP for health care during the 1990s. A research group led by Dr. David Sackett developed explicit research methodologies to determine the "best evidence" for practice. David Eddy first used the term *evidence-based* in 1990, with the focus on providing EBP for medicine (Straus et al., 2011). EBP grew in importance for nursing in 1990 when the American Nurses Credentialing Center implemented the Magnet Hospital Designation Program for Excellence in Nursing Services. A hospital's designation of Magnet status ensures that the nurses are involved in research activities and the delivery of evidence-based care to patients.

The emphasis on EBP encouraged nurses to conduct more randomized controlled trials (RCTs) and quasi-experimental studies to test the effectiveness of nursing interventions.

Nursing Research in the 21st Century

The vision for nursing research in the 21st century includes conducting quality studies using a variety of methodologies, synthesizing the study findings into the best research evidence, and using this research evidence to guide practice (Brown, 2018; Melnyk & Fineout-Overholt, 2015; Melnyk et al., 2017). In 2002, The Joint Commission, responsible for accrediting healthcare organizations, revised the accreditation policies for hospitals to support the implementation of evidence-based health care (The Joint Commission, 2017). To expand EBP in clinical agencies, Stetler (2001) revised the Research Utilization to Facilitate EBP Model (see Chapter 13 for a description of this model). The focus on EBP in nursing was supported with the initiation of the *Worldviews on Evidence-Based Nursing* journal in 2004.

The American Association of Colleges of Nursing (AACN, 2006) presented their position statement on nursing research to provide future directions for the discipline. To ensure an effective research enterprise in nursing, the discipline must:

1. Create a research culture.
2. Provide high-quality educational programs (e.g., baccalaureate, master's, practice-focused doctorate, research-focused doctorate, postdoctorate) to prepare a workforce of nurse scientists.
3. Develop a sound research infrastructure.
4. Obtain sufficient funding for essential research.

The focus of healthcare research and funding has expanded from the treatment of illness to include health promotion and illness prevention. *Healthy People 2000* and *Healthy People 2010* documents have increased the visibility of health promotion goals and research. *Healthy People 2020* topics and objects can be reviewed on the US Department of Health and Human Services (2017) website. Some of the topics include adolescent health, blood disorders and blood safety, dementias (including Alzheimer disease), early and middle childhood, genomics, global health, healthcare–associated infections, lesbian, gay, bisexual, and transgender health, older adults, emergency preparedness in times of disaster, sleep health, and social determinants of health. Over the next decade, nurse researchers will have a major role in the development of interventions to promote health and prevent illness in individuals and families.

The AHRQ (2017) is the lead agency supporting research designed to improve the quality of health care, reduce its cost, improve patient safety, decrease medical errors, and broaden access to essential services. AHRQ conducts and sponsors research that provides evidence-based information on healthcare outcomes, quality, cost, use, and access. This research information is needed to promote effective healthcare decision making by patients, clinicians, health system executives, and policy makers.

The current mission of the NINR (National Institute of Nursing Research, 2017) is to "promote and improve the health of individuals, families, communities, and populations. The Institute supports and conducts clinical and basic research and research training on health and illness across the lifespan to build the scientific foundation for clinical practice, prevent disease and disability, manage and eliminate symptoms caused by illness, and improve palliative and end-of-life care." The NINR has been seeking expanded funding for nursing research and is encouraging a variety of methodologies to be used to generate essential knowledge for nursing practice. The NINR website (http://ninr.nih.gov) provides the most current information on the institute's research funding opportunities and supported studies. The strategic plan for the NINR was updated in 2016 and is available online.

Linking Quality and Safety Education for Nursing Competencies and Nursing Research

In 2001, the IOM published a report that emphasized the importance of quality and safety in the delivery of health care. Based on this report, six competency areas were identified as essential for nursing education to ensure that students were able to deliver quality, safe care. Specific competencies were identified for the following six areas: patient-centered care, teamwork and collaboration, EBP, quality improvement, safety, and informatics. The Quality and Safety Education for Nurses (QSEN) initiative identified the requisite knowledge, skills, and attitude statements for each of the competencies for prelicensure and graduate education.

The QSEN Institute website (http://qsen.org) features teaching strategies and resources to facilitate the accomplishments of the QSEN competencies in nursing educational programs. The most current competencies for the prelicensure educational programs can be found online at http://qsen.org/competencies/pre-licensure-ksas/ (QSEN, 2017; Sherwood & Barnsteiner, 2017). The EBP competency is defined as "integrating the best current evidence with clinical expertise and patient/family preferences and values for delivery of optimal health care" (QSEN, 2017). You, as an undergraduate nursing student, need to be skilled in the critical appraisal of studies, use of appropriate research evidence in practice, adherence to institutional review board guidelines, and appropriate data collection. Your faculty will implement strategies to improve your learning experiences and outcomes based on these QSEN competencies (Barnsteiner et al., 2013). Your expanded knowledge of research is necessary to attain EBP and the QSEN competencies.

ACQUIRING KNOWLEDGE IN NURSING

Knowledge is essential information that is acquired in a variety of ways and is expected to be an accurate reflection of reality that is used to direct a person's actions (Kaplan, 1964). During your nursing education, you acquire an extensive amount of knowledge from your classroom and clinical experiences. You learn to synthesize, incorporate, and apply this knowledge so that you can practice as a nurse. Nursing has historically acquired knowledge through traditions, authority, borrowing, trial and error, personal experience, role modeling, intuition, and reasoning. This section introduces these different ways of acquiring knowledge and their link to research knowledge or evidence.

Traditions

Traditions include "truths" or beliefs based on customs and trends. Nursing traditions from the past have been transferred to the present by role modeling and communication, both written and oral. Traditions continue to influence the practice of nursing today. For example, some of the policy and procedure manuals in hospitals contain traditional ideas. Traditions can positively influence nursing practice because they were developed from effective past experiences. However, traditions also can narrow and limit the knowledge sought for nursing practice. For example, nursing units are frequently organized according to set rules or traditions that may not be efficient or effective. Often, these traditions are neither questioned nor changed because they have existed for years and are frequently supported by those with power and authority. Nursing's body of knowledge needs to be more research-based than traditional if nurses are to have a powerful impact on patient outcomes.

Authority

An authority is a person with expertise and power who is able to influence opinion and behavior. A person is given authority because it is thought that she or he knows more in a given area than others. Knowledge acquired from an authority is illustrated when one person credits another as the source of information. Nurses who publish articles and books or develop theories are frequently considered authorities. Students usually view their instructors as authorities, and clinical nursing experts are considered authorities within the clinical practice setting. Nurses with authority must be careful to teach and practice based on research evidence because they are influencing the actions of others.

Borrowing

Some nursing leaders have described part of nursing's knowledge as information borrowed from disciplines such as medicine, sociology, psychology, physiology, and education (McMurrey, 1982). Borrowing in nursing involves the appropriation and use of knowledge from other fields or disciplines to guide nursing practice. Nursing has borrowed in two ways. For years, some nurses have taken information from other disciplines and applied it directly to nursing practice. This information was not integrated within the unique focus of nursing. For example, some nurses have used the medical model to guide their nursing practice, thus focusing on the diagnosis and treatment of disease. This type of borrowing continues today as nurses use advances in technology to become highly specialized and focused on the detection and treatment of disease. The second way of borrowing, which is more useful in nursing, involves integrating information from other disciplines within the focus of nursing. For example, nurses borrow knowledge from other disciplines such as psychology and sociology as the basis for therapeutic communication. They integrate this psychosocial knowledge in their holistic care of patients and families who are experiencing acute and chronic illnesses.

Trial and Error

Trial and error, an approach with unknown outcomes, is used in situations of uncertainty in which other sources of knowledge are unavailable. Because each patient responds uniquely to a situation, nursing practice involves a degree of uncertainty. Thus nurses must use some degree of trial and error in providing nursing care to patients based on research evidence. The unknown is the responses of individual patients and families to specific nursing interventions. However, this trial and error approach frequently involves no formal documentation of effective and ineffective nursing actions. With this strategy, knowledge is gained from experience but often it is not shared with others, resulting in continued implementation of some ineffective interventions.

Personal Experience

Personal experience involves gaining knowledge by being personally involved in an event, situation, or circumstance. Personal experience enables you to gain skills and expertise by providing care to patients and families in clinical settings. Learning through personal experience enables you to cluster ideas into a meaningful whole. For example, you may read about giving an IM injection or be told how to give an injection in a classroom setting, but you do not know how to give an injection until you observe other nurses giving injections to patients and actually give several injections yourself.

The amount of personal experience affects the complexity of a nurse's knowledge base. Benner (1984) conducted a phenomenological qualitative study to identify the levels of experience in the development of clinical knowledge and expertise for nursing practice. She identified the following phases for developing expertise: (1) novice; (2) advanced beginner; (3) competent; (4) proficient; and (5) expert. Novice nurses have no personal experience in the work they are to perform, but have some preconceptions and expectations about clinical practice that they have learned during their education. These preconceptions and expectations are challenged, refined, confirmed, or refuted by personal experience in a clinical setting. The advanced beginner nurse has just enough experience to recognize and intervene in recurrent situations. For example, the advanced beginner is able to recognize and intervene in managing patient pain. Competent nurses are able to generate plans and achieve long-range goals because of years of personal experience. The competent nurse also can use her or his personal knowledge to take conscious and deliberate actions that are efficient and organized. From a more complex knowledge base, the proficient nurse views the patient as a whole and as a member of a family and community. The proficient nurse recognizes that each patient and family responds differently to illness and health and can make adjustments based on the patient's and family's responses. The expert nurse has an extensive background of experience and is able to intervene skillfully in a situation. Personal experience increases the ability of the expert nurse to grasp a situation intuitively, with accuracy and speed. In other words, expert nurses can skillfully and seamlessly integrate personal experience and research evidence in their responses to patients' changing circumstances.

Benner's phenomenological qualitative research (1984) has provided an increased understanding of how knowledge is acquired through personal experience. As you gain clinical experience during your educational program and after you graduate, you will note your movement through these different levels of clinical expertise and ability to use research evidence in practice.

Role Modeling

When you acquire knowledge through **role modeling,** you are learning by imitating the behaviors of an expert. In nursing, role modeling enables the novice nurse to learn through observing and interacting with highly competent, expert nurses. Role models include admired teachers, expert clinicians, researchers, and those who inspire others through their example. An intense form of role modeling is **mentorship,** in which the expert nurse serves as a teacher, sponsor, guide, and counselor for the novice nurse. The knowledge gained through personal experience is greatly enhanced by a quality relationship with a role model or mentor. Many new graduates enter clinical agency internships or residency programs so that they may receive mentoring from expert nurses during their first few months of employment. During internships, expert nurses need to role model evidence-based nursing practice.

Intuition

Intuition is an insight into or understanding of a situation or event as a whole that a person usually cannot explain logically. Because intuition is a type of knowing that seems to come unbidden, nurses often describe it as a "gut feeling" or "hunch." Because intuition cannot easily be explained scientifically, some people are uncomfortable with it and even think that it does not exist. What they do not understand is that intuition is not the lack of knowing; rather, it is a result of deep knowledge (Benner, 1984). This deep knowledge is incorporated so completely into the subconscious of intuitive people that they find it difficult to explain what and how they know and express it in a logical manner. Some nurses can intuitively recognize when a patient is experiencing a health crisis, such as having a stroke. Using this intuitive knowledge, these nurses can assess the patient's condition, intervene, and contact the provider as needed for medical intervention.

Reasoning

Reasoning is the processing and organizing of ideas to reach conclusions. Through reasoning, people are able to make sense of their thoughts, experiences, and research evidence

(Gray, Grove, & Sutherland, 2017). Through reasoning, nurses recognize that more evidence is needed for making changes in practice, which provides direction for future research.

Using logical thinking, you may orally present an argument, in which each part is linked to reach a logical conclusion. The science of logic includes inductive and deductive reasoning. **Inductive reasoning** moves from the specific to the general; particular instances are observed and then combined into a larger whole or a general statement (Chinn & Kramer, 2015). An example of inductive reasoning follows.

PARTICULAR INSTANCES

A headache is an altered level of health that is stressful.

A terminal illness is an altered level of health that is stressful.

GENERAL STATEMENT

Therefore it can be induced that all altered levels of health are stressful. Inductive reasoning is involved in synthesizing the findings of multiple studies to draw conclusions about best practices. Later in this chapter, you will find formal ways that inductive reasoning is applied to develop EBP.

Deductive reasoning moves from the general to the specific or from a general premise to a particular situation or conclusion (Chinn & Kramer, 2015). A general premise may be a **proposition,** which is a statement from a theory describing a proposed relationship between two or more concepts (see Chapter 7). An example of deductive reasoning follows.

PROPOSITIONS

All humans experience loss.

All adolescents are humans.

CONCLUSION

Therefore it can be deduced that all adolescents experience loss.

In this example, deductive reasoning is used to move from the two general propositions about humans and adolescents to the conclusion that "All adolescents experience loss." However, the conclusions generated from deductive reasoning are valid only if they are based on valid propositions. Research is a means to test and confirm or refute a proposition so that valid propositions can be used as a basis for reasoning in nursing practice.

ACQUIRING KNOWLEDGE THROUGH NURSING RESEARCH

The research knowledge needed for practice is specific and holistic, as well as process-oriented and outcomes-focused. Thus a variety of research methods are needed to generate this knowledge. This section introduces quantitative, qualitative, mixed methods, and outcomes research methods that are commonly conducted to generate empirical knowledge for nursing practice (Box 1.1). These research methods are essential to generate evidence for the following goals of the nursing profession (AACN, 2017; NINR, 2016):

- Promoting an understanding of patients' and families' experiences with health and illness (a common focus of qualitative research).
- Testing the effectiveness of nursing interventions in promoting individuals' and families' health (a common focus of quantitative research).
- Combining quantitative and qualitative methods to expand the understanding of complex health problems, behaviors, and situations (a common focus of mixed methods research).
- Examining the outcomes of care to determine the quality, safety, and cost-effectiveness of nursing care within the healthcare system (a common focus of outcomes research).

BOX 1.1 CLASSIFICATION OF RESEARCH METHODS FOR THIS TEXT

Types of Quantitative Research
Descriptive research
Correlational research
Quasi-experimental research
Experimental research

Types of Qualitative Research
Phenomenological research
Grounded theory research
Ethnographic research
Exploratory-descriptive qualitative research

Mixed Methods Research

Outcomes Research

Introduction to Quantitative and Qualitative Research

Quantitative and qualitative research methods complement each other because they generate different types of knowledge that are useful in nursing practice. Familiarity with these two types of research will help you identify, understand, and critically appraise these studies. Quantitative and qualitative research methodologies have some similarities; both require researcher expertise, involve rigor in conducing the studies, and generate scientific knowledge for nursing practice. Some of the differences between the two methodologies are presented in Table 1.3.

Most of the studies conducted in nursing included quantitative research methods, which are considered the traditional scientific method. **Quantitative research** is a formal, objective, systematic process in which numerical data are used to obtain information about the world. The quantitative approach toward scientific inquiry emerged from a branch of philosophy called *logical positivism*, which

TABLE 1.3 CHARACTERISTICS OF QUANTITATIVE AND QUALITATIVE RESEARCH METHODS

CHARACTERISTIC	QUANTITATIVE RESEARCH	QUALITATIVE RESEARCH
Philosophic origin	Logical positivism	Naturalistic, interpretive, humanistic
Basis of knowing	Cause and effect relationships	Meaning, discovery, understanding
Theoretical focus	Tests theory	Develops theory and frameworks
Researcher involvement	Objective	Shared interpretation
Common methods of measurement	Scales, questionnaires, and physiological measures	Unstructured interviews, observations, focus groups
Data	Numbers	Words
Analysis	Statistical analysis	Text-based analysis
Findings	Description variables, relationships among variables, and effectiveness of interventions; generalization	Unique, dynamic, focused on understanding of phenomena and facilitating theory development

operates on strict rules of logic, truth, laws, and predictions. Quantitative researchers hold the position that "truth" is absolute and that a single reality can be defined by careful measurement. To find truth, the researcher must be objective, which means that values, feelings, and personal perceptions should not enter into the measurement of reality. Quantitative research is conducted to test theory by describing variables (descriptive research), examining relationships among variables (correlational research), and determining cause and effect interactions between variables (quasi-experimental and experimental research; Shadish, Cook, & Campbell, 2002). The methods of measurement commonly used in quantitative research include scales, questionnaires, and physiological measures (see Table 1.3). The data collected are numbers that are analyzed with statistical techniques to determine results (Grove & Cipher, 2017). Quantitative researchers strive to extend their findings beyond the situation studied. With extensive research in an area, findings might be generalized to different populations and settings. Chapter 2 describes the types of quantitative research and the quantitative research process.

Qualitative research is a systematic subjective approach used to describe life experiences and situations and give them meaning (Creswell & Poth, 2018). The philosophic base of qualitative research is interpretive, humanistic, and naturalistic and is concerned with understanding the meaning of social interactions and shared interpretations by those involved (see Table 1.3). Qualitative researchers believe that truth is complex and dynamic and can be found only by studying people as they interact with and in their sociohistorical settings (Creswell, 2014). Because human emotions are difficult to quantify (assign a numerical value to), qualitative research seems to be a more effective method of investigating emotional responses and personal experiences than quantitative research. Data in qualitative research take the form of words, which are collected through interviews, observations, and focus groups and analyzed for meaning. Qualitative research findings are unique, dynamic, focused on understanding, and facilitate theory development. A variety of qualitative studies are conducted to generate findings. Chapter 3 describes the types of qualitative research presented in this text.

Types of Quantitative and Qualitative Research

Several types of quantitative and qualitative research have been conducted to generate nursing knowledge for practice. These types of research can be classified in a variety of ways. The classification system for this text is presented in Box 1.1 and includes the most common types of quantitative and qualitative research conducted in nursing. The quantitative research methods are classified into four categories: descriptive, correlational, quasi-experimental, and experimental (Gray et al., 2017; Shadish et al., 2002).

- Descriptive research explores new areas of research and describes situations as they exist in the world.
- Correlational research examines relationships and is conducted to develop and refine explanatory knowledge for nursing practice.
- Quasi-experimental and experimental studies determine the effectiveness of nursing interventions in predicting and controlling the outcomes desired for patients and families.

The qualitative research methods included in this text are phenomenological, grounded theory, ethnographic research, and exploratory-descriptive (see Box 1.1).

- Phenomenological research is an inductive holistic approach used to describe an experience as it is lived by individuals, such as the lived experience of losing a child.
- Grounded theory research is an inductive research technique used to formulate, test, and refine a theory about a particular phenomenon (Charmaz, 2014). Grounded theory research initially was described by Glaser and Strauss (1967) in their development of a theory about grieving.

- Ethnographic research was developed by the discipline of anthropology for investigating cultures through an in-depth study of the members of the culture. Health practices vary among cultures, and these practices need to be recognized when delivering care to patients and families (Creswell & Poth, 2018; Marshall & Rossman, 2016).
- Exploratory-descriptive qualitative research is conducted to address an issue or problem in need of a solution and/or understanding. Qualitative nurse researchers use this methodology to explore a problem area using varied qualitative techniques, with the intent of describing the topic of interest and promoting understanding.

Introduction to Mixed Methods Research

Mixed methods research is an approach to inquiry that combines quantitative and qualitative research methods in a single study. The research purpose and questions are stated to address both the quantitative and qualitative elements of the study. Researchers might have a stronger focus on either a quantitative or qualitative research method based on the purpose of their study. Mixed methods studies usually involve the collection of both qualitative and quantitative data and the analysis of both forms of data (Creswell, 2014). The data are analyzed and integrated as directed by the study design. Sometimes quantitative and qualitative research methods are implemented concurrently or consecutively based on the knowledge to be generated. For example, researchers might examine the effectiveness of an intervention using a quasi-experimental design, and then conduct qualitative research to obtain an understanding of the patients' perceptions of the intervention. The different strategies for combining qualitative and quantitative research methods in mixed methods studies are described in Chapter 14.

Introduction to Outcomes Research

The spiraling costs of health care have generated many questions about the quality, safety, and effectiveness of healthcare services and patient outcomes related to these services. Consumers want to know what services they are purchasing and whether these services will improve their health. Healthcare policy makers want to know whether the care is cost-effective and of high quality. These concerns have promoted the conduct of outcomes research, which focuses on examining the results of care and determining the changes in health status for the patient and family. Some essential areas that require investigation through outcomes research include the following: (1) patient responses to nursing and medical interventions; (2) functional maintenance or improvement of physical, mental, and social functioning for the patient; (3) financial outcomes achieved with the provision of healthcare services; and (4) patient satisfaction with health outcomes, care received, and healthcare providers.

Nurses are actively involved in identifying nurse-sensitive outcomes and conducting outcomes studies. "A nursing-sensitive outcome is an individual, family, or community state, behavior, or perception that is measured along a continuum in response to nursing intervention(s)" (Moorhead et al., 2013, p. 2). The Nursing Outcomes Classification (NOC) was developed to standardize terminology for nursing-sensitive outcomes, and is to be used across nursing specialties and in a variety of practice settings to capture changes in patient status after an intervention. NOC contains 490 outcomes that have been developed over the last 20 years (Moorhead et al., 2013). Some of the outcomes include exercise participation, self-management: asthma, and knowledge: weight management. Nursing outcomes research determines the quality, safety, and cost-effectiveness of nursing care and provides a basis for improving that care in the future. Chapter 14 includes a discussion of outcomes research.

These different types of research methods (see Box 1.1) provide information important to nurses in implementing an EBP.

PURPOSES OF RESEARCH FOR IMPLEMENTING AN EVIDENCE-BASED NURSING PRACTICE

Nurses need a solid research base as a foundation for implementing selected nursing interventions and documenting their effectiveness in treating particular patient health problems. Effective interventions promote positive patient and family outcomes. The research evidence needed in clinical practice includes studies focused on the description, explanation, prediction, and control of phenomena.

Description

Description involves identifying and understanding the nature of nursing phenomena and, sometimes, the relationships among them (Chinn & Kramer, 2015). Through research, nurses describe what exists in nursing practice and discover new information. Descriptive research is also used to promote understanding of situations and classify information for use in the discipline. Some examples of clinically important research evidence that have been developed from research focused on description include the following:

- Identification of the hope phenomenon and its dimensions or characteristics.
- Identification and classification of nursing diagnoses.
- Description of the responses of individuals to a variety of health conditions and aging.
- Determination of the incidence of a disease locally (e.g., West Nile virus in Dallas, Texas), nationally, and internationally (e.g., Zika virus in the United States and other countries).

An example of research conducted for the purpose of description was a qualitative study by Koehn, Ebright, and Draucker (2016, p. 567) "to explore nurses' decision-making processes regarding reporting errors." They found that:

"Making an error is a complex dynamic process often situated in the context of a high-stress working environment. The nurses' most salient response to making an error was learning from the error so it would not happen again. Making an error is typically a highly distressing experience for nurses, and lack of institutional follow-up and support exacerbate this distress" (Koehn et al., 2016, p. 572).

Koehn and colleagues (2016) provided a unique dynamic description of nurses' experiences after making a medical error. They recommended that future studies focus on developing strategies to facilitate reporting of errors and improving the learning and coping of nurses in the aftermath of an error. Research focused on identification and description is essential groundwork for studies to provide explanations, predictions, and control of nursing phenomena in practice.

Explanation

An **explanation** clarifies the relationships among phenomena and identifies possible reasons why certain events occur. Research focused on explanation provides the following types of evidence essential for practice:

- Understanding which factors are related to and the full nature of caring for a newborn in the family.
- Examining the relationships among the assessment data and a nursing diagnosis.
- Determining the relationships among health risks, health behaviors, and health status.

For example, Newland, Lunsford, and Flach (2017) studied "the interaction of fatigue, physical activity, and health-related quality of life [HRQOL] in adults with multiple sclerosis (MS) and cardiovascular disease (CVD)." They found "the complex and interconnected nature of fatigue, which adversely impacts physical activity and HRQOL, is challenging for adults with MS and CVD in the community. Nurses and other healthcare team members may underestimate and/or poorly understand the need for adults with MS and CVD to engage in physical activity to improve HRQOL as part of self-management regimen" (Newland et al., 2017, p. 52). Future studies focused on interventions to manage fatigue, increase physical activity, and promote HRQOL have the potential to improve adults' self-management of their chronic illnesses.

Prediction

Through **prediction,** one can estimate the probability of a specific outcome in a given situation (Chinn & Kramer, 2015). However, predicting an outcome does not necessarily enable one to modify or control the outcome. It is through prediction that the risk of illness or injury is identified and linked to possible screening methods to identify and prevent health problems. Knowledge generated from research focused on prediction is essential for EBP and includes the following:

- Prediction of the risk for a disease or injury in different populations.
- Prediction of behaviors that promote health and prevent illness.
- Prediction of the nursing care required based on a patient's circumstances and values.

Lee, Faucett, Gillen, Krause, and Landry (2013) conducted a quantitative study to examine the factors that were perceived by critical care nurses (CCNs) to predict the risk of musculoskeletal (MSK) injury from work. They found that a greater physical workload, greater job strain, more frequent patient-handling tasks, and lack of a lifting team or devices were predictive of the CCNs' perceptions of risk of MSK injury. They concluded that "Improving the physical and psychosocial work environment may make nursing jobs safer, reduce the risk of MSK injury, and improve nurses' perceptions of job safety" (Lee et al., 2013, p. 43).

This predictive study isolated independent variables—physical workload, job strain, patient-handling tasks, and lack of lifting devices or teams—that were predictive of MSK injuries in CCNs. The variables identified in predictive studies require additional research to ensure that their manipulation or control results in quality outcomes for patients, healthcare professionals, and healthcare agencies.

Control

If one can predict the outcome of a situation, the next step is to control or manipulate the situation to produce the desired outcome. In health care, **control** is the ability to write a prescription to produce the desired results. Using the best research evidence, nurses could prescribe specific interventions to meet the needs of patients and their families (Melnyk et al., 2017; Straus et al., 2011). The results of multiple studies in the following areas have enabled nurses to deliver care that increases control over the outcomes desired for practice:

- Testing the effectiveness of interventions to improve the health status of individuals and families.
- Synthesis of research for development into EBP guidelines.
- Determining the effectiveness of EBP guidelines in your clinical agency.

As discussed earlier, extensive studies have been conducted with regard to the safe administration of IM injections and synthesized into EBP guidelines. The EBP guideline for IM injections includes the following: (1) the appropriate needle size and length to use for administering different types of medications; (2) the safest injection site (ventrogluteal) for many medications; and (3) the best injection technique to deliver a medication, minimize patient discomfort, and prevent physical damage (Cocoman & Murray, 2008; Nicoll & Hesby, 2002; Ogston-Tuck, 2014). Research has continued regarding aspiration during an IM injection with Sisson (2015) recommending no aspiration and Thomas et al. (2016) recommending aspiration. Thus RNs should use a decision-making process to determine whether to aspirate or not based on the situation. Using the evidence-based knowledge for administering IM injections helps control the following outcomes: (1) adequate administration of medication to promote patient health; (2) minimal patient discomfort; and (3) no physical damage to the patient. However, Greenway (2014) has recently reviewed the literature and found that many nurses were using traditional knowledge rather than EBP guidelines when giving IM injections. EBP guidelines significantly improve the quality of IM injections and decrease the incidence of pain and muscle and sciatic nerve damage (Stringer, 2010).

Broadly, the nursing profession is accountable to society for providing quality, safe, and cost-effective care for patients and families. The extensive number of clinical studies conducted in the last 50 years has greatly expanded the scientific knowledge available to you for describing, explaining, predicting, and controlling phenomena within your nursing practice.

UNDERSTANDING YOUR ROLE IN NURSING RESEARCH

Generating an empirical knowledge base for implementation in practice requires the participation of all nurses in a variety of research activities. Some nurses are developers of research and conduct studies to generate and refine the knowledge needed for nursing practice. Others are consumers of research and use research evidence to improve their nursing practice. The AACN (2006, 2017) and ANA (2010) have published statements about the roles of nurses in research. No matter their education or position, all nurses have roles in research; some ideas about those roles are presented in Table 1.4. The research role that a nurse assumes usually expands with his or her advanced education, clinical expertise, and career path. Nurses with a Bachelor of Science in Nursing (BSN) degree

TABLE 1.4 NURSES' PARTICIPATION IN RESEARCH AT VARIOUS LEVELS OF EDUCATION

NURSES' EDUCATIONAL PREPARATION	RESEARCH EXPECTATIONS AND COMPETENCIES
Bachelor of Science in Nursing (BSN)	Read and critically appraise studies; use best research evidence in practice with guidance; assist with problem identification and data collection
Master of Science in Nursing (MSN)	Critically appraise and synthesize studies to develop and revise protocols, algorithms, and policies for practice. Implement best research evidence in practice; collaborate in research projects and provide clinical expertise for research
Doctor of Nursing Practice (DNP)	Participate in evidence-based guideline development; develop, implement, evaluate, and revise as needed protocols, policies, and evidence-based guidelines in practice; conduct clinical studies, usually in collaboration with other nurse researchers
Doctor of Philosophy (PhD) in Nursing	Major role, such as primary investigator, in conducting research and contributing to the empirical knowledge generated in a selected area of study; obtain funding for research; coordinate research teams of BSN, MSN, and DNP nurses
Postdoctorate	Implement a funded program of research; lead and/or participate in nursing and interdisciplinary research teams; identified as experts in their areas of research; mentor PhD-prepared researchers

have knowledge of the research process and skills in reading and critically appraising studies. They assist with the implementation of evidence-based guidelines, protocols, algorithms, and policies in practice (Melnyk et al., 2017). In addition, these nurses might provide valuable assistance in identifying research problems and collecting data for studies. The QSEN (2017) competencies identify such knowledge and skills as being essential for prelicensure students.

Nurses with an MSN have undergone the educational preparation to critically appraise and synthesize findings from studies to revise or develop protocols, algorithms, or policies for use in practice. They also have the ability to identify and critically appraise the quality of evidence-based guidelines developed by national organizations. Advanced practice nurses (APNs)—nurse practitioners, clinical nurse specialists, nurse anesthetists, and nurse midwives—and nurse administrators have the ability to lead healthcare teams in making essential changes in nursing practice and in the healthcare system based on current research evidence. Some MSN-prepared nurses conduct studies but usually do so in collaboration with other nurse scientists (see Table 1.4).

The doctoral degrees in nursing can have a practice-focus (doctor of nursing practice [DNP]) or research-focus (doctor of philosophy [PhD]). Nurses with DNPs are educated to have the highest level of clinical expertise, with the ability to translate scientific knowledge for use in practice. Many APNs are obtaining a DNP degree to expand their knowledge base. The DNP-prepared nurses have advanced research and leadership knowledge to develop, implement, evaluate, and revise evidence-based guidelines, protocols, algorithms, and policies for practice (Butts & Rich, 2015). In addition, DNP-prepared nurses have the expertise to conduct and/or collaborate with clinical studies.

PhD-prepared nurses assume a major role in the conduct of research and the generation of nursing knowledge in a selected area of interest. These nurse scientists often coordinate research teams that include DNP-, MSN-, and BSN-prepared nurses to facilitate the conduct of rigorous studies in a variety of healthcare agencies and universities. Nurses with postdoctoral education have the expertise to develop highly funded programs of research. They lead interdisciplinary teams of researchers and sometimes conduct studies in multiple settings. These scientists often are identified as experts in selected areas of research and provide mentoring for new PhD-prepared researchers (see Table 1.4).

DETERMINING THE BEST RESEARCH EVIDENCE FOR PRACTICE

EBP involves the use of the best research evidence to support clinical decisions in practice. Best research evidence was previously defined as a summary of the highest quality, current, empirical knowledge in a specific area of health care that has been developed from a synthesis of quality studies in that area. As a nurse, you make numerous clinical decisions each day that affect the health outcomes of your patients. By using the best research evidence available, you can make quality clinical decisions that will improve patients' and families' health outcomes. This section focuses on expanding your understanding of best research evidence for practice by providing the following: (1) a description of the strategies used to synthesize research evidence; (2) a model of the levels of research evidence available; and (3) a link of the best research evidence to evidence-based guidelines for practice.

Strategies Used to Synthesize Research Evidence

The synthesis of study findings is a complex, highly structured process that is best conducted by at least two people or even a team of researchers and healthcare providers. Various types of research synthesis are conducted based on the quality, number, and types of research evidence available. Research evidence in nursing is usually synthesized by the following processes: (1) systematic

TABLE 1.5 PROCESSES USED TO SYNTHESIZE RESEARCH EVIDENCE

SYNTHESIS PROCESS	PURPOSE OF SYNTHESIS	TYPES OF RESEARCH INCLUDED IN THE SYNTHESIS (SAMPLING FRAME)	ANALYSIS FOR ACHIEVING SYNTHESIS
Systematic review	Systematically identify, select, critically appraise, and synthesize research evidence to address a particular problem or question in practice	Quantitative studies with similar methodology, such as randomized controlled trials and meta-analyses focused on a practice problem	Narrative and statistical
Meta-analysis	Pooling of the results from several previous studies using statistical analysis to determine the effect of an intervention or the strength of relationships	Quantitative studies with similar methodology, such as quasi-experimental and experimental studies focused on the effect of an intervention or correlational studies focused on relationships	Statistical
Meta-synthesis	Systematic compilation and integration of qualitative studies to expand understanding and develop a unique interpretation of the studies' findings in a selected health-related area	Original qualitative studies and summaries of qualitative studies	Narrative
Mixed-methods systematic review	Synthesis of the findings from independent studies conducted with a variety of methods—quantitative, qualitative, and mixed—to determine the current knowledge in an area	Variety of quantitative, qualitative, and mixed methods studies	Narrative and sometimes statistical

Based on content from Barnett-Page, E., & Thomas, J. (2009). Methods for the synthesis of qualitative research: A critical review. *BMC Medical Research Methodology, 9*, 59; Cooper, H. (2017). *Research synthesis and meta-analysis: A step-by-step approach* (5th ed.). Los Angeles, CA: Sage; Creswell, J. W. (2014). *Research design: Qualitative, quantitative and mixed methods approaches* (4th ed.). Thousand Oaks, CA: Sage; Finfgeld-Connett, D. (2010). Generalizability and transferability of meta-synthesis research findings. *Journal of Advanced Nursing, 66*(2), 246–254; Gray, J. R., Grove, S. K., & Sutherland, S. (2017). *Burns and Grove's the practice of nursing research: Appraisal, synthesis, and generation of evidence* (8th ed.). St. Louis, MO: Elsevier; Higgins, J. P. T., & Green, S. (2008). *Cochrane handbook for systematic reviews of interventions.* West Sussex, England: Wiley-Blackwell and The Cochrane Collaboration; Sandelowski, M., & Barroso, J. (2007). *Handbook for synthesizing qualitative research.* New York, NY: Springer; Whittemore, R., Chao, A., Jang, M., Minges, K. E., & Park, C. (2014). Methods for knowledge synthesis: An overview. *Heart & Lung, 43*(5), 453–461.

review; (2) meta-analysis; (3) meta-synthesis; and (4) mixed-methods systematic review. Depending on the quantity and strength of the research findings available, nurses and healthcare professionals use one or more of these four synthesis processes to determine the current best research evidence in an area. Table 1.5 identifies the common processes used in research synthesis, the purpose of each synthesis process, the types of research included in the synthesis (sampling frame), and the analytical techniques used to achieve the synthesis of research evidence (Cooper, 2017; Higgins & Green, 2008; Sandelowski & Barroso, 2007; Whittemore, Chao, Jang, Minges, & Park, 2014).

A **systematic review** is a structured, comprehensive synthesis of the research literature to determine the best research evidence available to address a healthcare question. A systematic review involves identifying, locating, appraising, and synthesizing quality research evidence for expert clinicians to use to promote an EBP (Gray et al., 2017; Higgins & Green, 2008; Melnyk & Fineout-Overholt, 2015). Teams of expert researchers, clinicians, and sometimes students conduct these reviews to determine the current best knowledge for use in practice. Systematic reviews are also used in the development of national and international standardized guidelines for managing health problems such as acute pain, high BP, and depression. Standardized guidelines are made available online, published in articles and books, and presented at conferences and professional meetings. The process for critically appraising systematic reviews is discussed in Chapter 13.

A **meta-analysis** is conducted to combine or pool the results from previous quantitative studies into a single statistical analysis that provides strong evidence about an intervention's effectiveness (Andrel, Keith, & Leiby, 2009; Cooper, 2017). Because qualitative studies do not produce statistical findings, they cannot be included in a meta-analysis. Some of the strongest evidence for using an intervention in practice is generated from a meta-analysis of multiple, controlled quasi-experimental and experimental studies. In addition, a meta-analysis can be performed on correlational studies to determine the type (positive or negative) and strength of relationships among selected variables (Grove & Cipher, 2017). Many systematic reviews conducted to generate evidence-based guidelines include meta-analyses (see Chapter 13).

Qualitative research synthesis is the process and product of systematically reviewing and formally integrating the findings from qualitative studies (Sandelowski & Barroso, 2007). The process for synthesizing qualitative research is still evolving, and a variety of synthesis methods have appeared in the literature (Barnett-Page & Thomas, 2009; Finfgeld-Connett, 2010). In this text, the concept of meta-synthesis is used to describe the process for synthesizing qualitative research. **Meta-synthesis** is defined as the systematic compilation and integration of qualitative study results to expand understanding and develop a unique interpretation of study findings in a selected area. The focus is on interpretation rather than on combining study results, as with quantitative research synthesis. Chapter 13 provides more details on meta-synthesis.

Over the last 10 years, nurse researchers have conducted mixed methods studies that include quantitative and qualitative research methods (Creswell, 2014). In addition, determining the current research evidence in an area might require synthesizing quantitative and qualitative studies. Higgins and Green (2008) have referred to this synthesis of quantitative, qualitative, and mixed methods studies as a **mixed-methods systematic review** (see Table 1.5). Mixed-methods systematic reviews might include a variety of study designs, such as qualitative research and quasi-experimental, correlational, and/or descriptive studies (Creswell, 2014). Some researchers have conducted syntheses of quantitative and qualitative studies, termed *integrative reviews of research*. The value of these reviews depends on the standards used to conduct them (see Chapter 13).

Levels of Research Evidence

Experimental quantitative studies, such as RCTs, provide the strongest research evidence (see Chapter 8). Also, the replication or repeating of studies with a similar methodology increases the strength of the research evidence generated. The levels of research evidence are presented in a pyramid (Fig. 1.3) that shows a continuum, with the highest quality of research evidence at the top end and the weakest research evidence at the base (Brown, 2018; Melnyk et al., 2017). The systematic research reviews and meta-analyses of high-quality quasi-experimental and experimental studies provide the strongest or best research evidence for use by clinicians in practice. Meta-analyses of correlational, quasi-experimental, experimental, and outcomes studies also provide very strong research

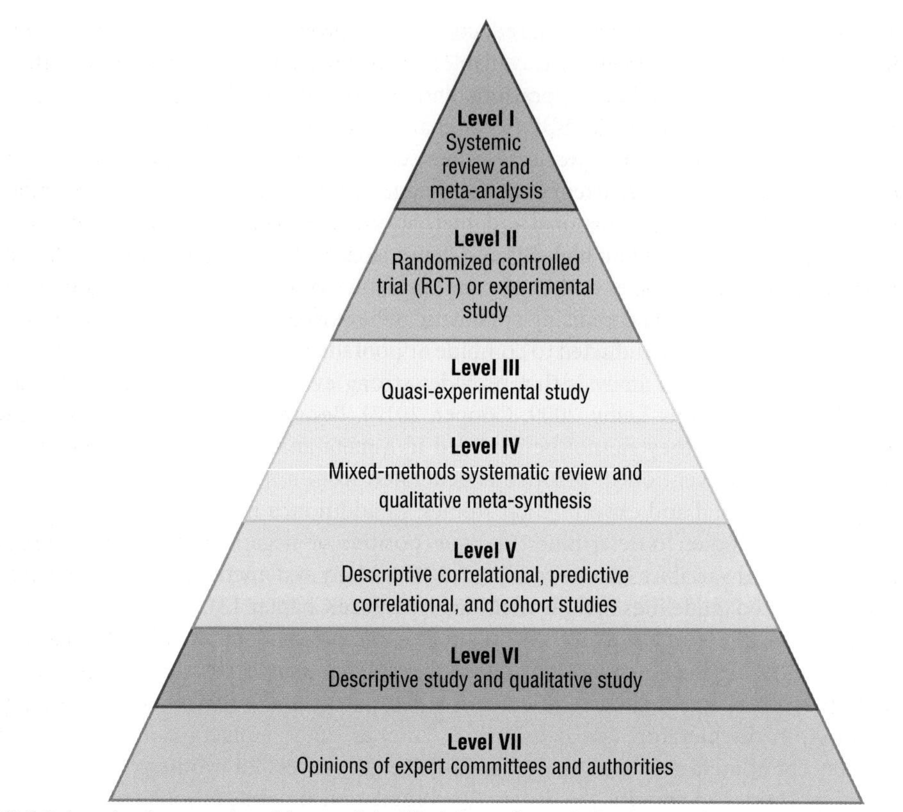

FIG 1.3 Levels of research evidence. (Modified from Gray, J. R., Grove, S. K., & Sutherland, S. [2017]. *Burns and Grove's the practice of nursing research: Appraisal, synthesis, and generation of evidence* [8th ed.]. St. Louis, MO: Elsevier).

evidence for managing practice problems. Mixed-methods systematic reviews and meta-syntheses provide quality syntheses of quantitative, qualitative, and/or mixed methods studies. The evidence from individual correlational, predictive correlational, and cohort studies provides direction for future research but is not ready for use in practice. Descriptive and qualitative studies often provide initial knowledge, which serves as a basis for generating correlational, quasi-experimental, experimental, and outcomes studies (see Fig. 1.3). The base of the pyramid includes the weakest evidence, which is generated from opinions of expert committees and authorities.

When making a decision in your clinical practice, be sure to base that decision on the best research evidence available. The levels of research evidence identified in Fig. 1.3 will help you determine the quality of the evidence that is available. The best research evidence generated from systematic reviews, meta-analyses, meta-syntheses, and mixed-methods systematic reviews is used to develop standardized evidence-based guidelines for use in practice.

Introduction to Evidence-Based Guidelines

Evidence-based guidelines are rigorous and explicit clinical guidelines that have been developed based on the best research evidence available in that area. These guidelines are usually developed by a team or panel of expert clinicians (e.g., nurses, physicians, pharmacists), researchers, and sometimes consumers, policy makers, and economists. The expert panel works to achieve consensus on the content of the guideline to provide clinicians with the best information for making clinical decisions in practice. There has been a dramatic growth in the production of evidence-based guidelines to assist healthcare providers in building an EBP and improving healthcare outcomes for patients, families, providers, and healthcare agencies.

Every year, new guidelines are developed, and some of the existing guidelines are revised based on new research evidence. These guidelines have become the **gold standard** (standard of excellence) for patient care, and nurses and other healthcare providers are highly encouraged to incorporate these standardized guidelines into their practice. Many of these evidence-based guidelines have been made available online by national and international government agencies, professional organizations, and centers of excellence. The most important source for evidence-based guidelines in the United States is the National Guideline Clearinghouse (NGC, 2017), initiated in 1998 by the AHRQ. The NGC started with 200 guidelines and has expanded to more than 2000 evidence-based guidelines. When selecting a guideline for practice, ensure that the guideline was developed by a credible agency or organization and that the reference list reflects the synthesis of an extensive number of studies.

In summary, Chapter 13 provides you with direction for critically appraising the quality of evidence-based guidelines and implementing them in your practice. Chapters 2 through 12 were developed to expand your understanding of the quantitative and qualitative research processes so you will be able to critically appraise these types of studies. A **critical appraisal of research** involves the careful examination of all aspects of a study to judge its strengths, limitations, meaning, and significance. Chapter 14 provides an introduction to outcomes and mixed methods research. We think that you will find that nursing research is an exciting adventure that holds much promise for the future practice of nursing.

KEY POINTS

- Research is defined as diligent systematic inquiry to validate and refine existing knowledge and develop new knowledge.
- Nursing research is defined as a scientific process that validates and refines existing knowledge and generates new knowledge that directly and indirectly influences nursing practice.
- EBP is the conscientious integration of best research evidence with clinical expertise and patient circumstances and values in the delivery of quality, safe, and cost-effective health care.
- Florence Nightingale was the first nurse researcher who developed empirical knowledge to improve nursing practice in the 19th century.
- The conduct of clinical research continues to be a major focus in the 21st century, with the goal of developing an EBP for nursing.
- Knowledge is acquired in nursing in a variety of ways, including tradition, authority, borrowing, trial and error, personal experience, role modeling, intuition, reasoning and, most importantly, research.
- Quantitative research is a formal, objective, and systematic process using numerical data to obtain information about the world. This research method is used to describe, examine relationships, and determine cause and effect.
- Qualitative research is a unique, dynamic, and subjective approach used to describe life experiences and give them meaning. Knowledge generated from qualitative research will provide meaning and understanding of life experiences, situations, events, and cultures.
- Mixed methods research is an approach to inquiry that combines quantitative and qualitative research methods in a single study.

- Outcomes research focuses on examining the end results of care and determining the changes needed to improve the health status for the patient and the quality of the healthcare system.
- The purposes of research in nursing include description, explanation, prediction, and control of phenomena in practice.
- Nurses with a BSN, MSN, doctoral degree (DNP, PhD), and postdoctorate education have clearly designated roles in research based on the breadth and depth of the research knowledge gained during their educational programs and their clinical and research experiences.
- Research evidence in nursing is synthesized using the following processes: (1) systematic review; (2) meta-analysis; (3) meta-synthesis; and (4) mixed-methods systematic review.
- A systematic review is a structured comprehensive synthesis of quantitative studies in a particular healthcare area to determine the best research evidence available for clinicians to use to promote an EBP.
- Meta-analysis is a type of study that statistically combines or pools the results from previous studies into a single quantitative analysis to provide one of the highest levels of evidence for an intervention's efficacy.
- Meta-synthesis involves the systematic compilation and integration of qualitative studies in an area to expand understanding and develop a unique interpretation of the findings.
- A mixed-methods systematic review is the synthesis of findings from individual studies conducted with a variety of methods—quantitative, qualitative, and mixed methods—to determine the current knowledge in an area.
- The levels of research evidence are a continuum, with the highest quality of research evidence at the top of the pyramid and the weakest research evidence at its base (see Fig. 1.3). Systematic research reviews and meta-analyses of quality experimental studies provide the best research evidence for practice.
- Evidence-based guidelines are rigorous and explicit clinical guidelines that have been developed based on the best research evidence available in a particular area.

REFERENCES

Agency for Healthcare Research and Quality (AHRQ), (2017). *Research tools and data*. Rockville, MD: Author. Retrieved November 8, 2017, from http://www.ahrq.gov/research/index.html.

American Association of Colleges of Nursing (AACN), (2006). *AACN position statement on nursing research*. Washington, DC: AACN. Retrieved February 20, 2017, from http://www.aacn.nche.edu/publications/position/nursing-research.

American Association of Colleges of Nursing (AACN), (2017). *News & information: Research and data center*. Washington, DC: Author. Retrieved November 10, 2017, from http://www.aacnnursing.org/news-information/research-data.

American Nurses Association (ANA), (2010). *Nursing: Scope and standards of practice* (2nd ed.). Washington, DC: Author.

Andrel, J. A., Keith, S. W., & Leiby, B. E. (2009). Meta-analysis: A brief introduction. *Clinical and Translational Science*, *2*(5), 374–378.

Barnett-Page, E., & Thomas, J. (2009). Methods for the synthesis of qualitative research: A critical review. *BMC Medical Research Methodology*, *9*, 59. https://doi.org/10.1186/147-2288-9-59.

Barnsteiner, J., Disch, J., Johnson, J., McGuinn, K., Chappell, K., & Swartwout, E. (2013). Diffusing QSEN competencies across schools of nursing: The AACN/RWJF faculty development institutes. *Journal of Professional Nursing*, *29*(2), 68–74.

Bauknecht, V. L. (1985). Capital commentary: NIH bill passes, includes nursing research center. *American Nurse*, *17*(10), 2.

Benner, P. (1984). *From novice to expert: Excellence and power in clinical nursing practice*. Menlo Park, CA: Addison-Wesley.

Brown, S. J. (2018). *Evidence-based nursing: The research-practice connection* (4th ed.). Sudbury, MA: Jones & Bartlett.

Butts, J. B., & Rich, K. L. (2015). *Philosophies and theories for advanced nursing practice*. Burlington, MA: Jones & Bartlett Learning.

Charmaz, K. (2014). *Constructing grounded theory* (2nd ed.). Los Angeles, CA: Sage.

Chinn, P. L., & Kramer, M. K. (2015). *Knowledge development in nursing: Theory and process* (9th ed.). St. Louis, MO: Mosby Elsevier.

Cocoman, A., & Murray, J. (2008). Intramuscular injections: A review of best practice for mental health nurses. *Journal of Psychiatric and Mental Health Nursing, 15*(5), 424–434.

Cook, E. (1913). *The life of Florence Nightingale:* (Vol. 1). London, England: Macmillan.

Cooper, H. (2017). *Research synthesis and meta-analysis: A step-by-step approach* (5th ed.). Los Angeles, CA: Sage.

Creswell, J. W. (2014). *Research design: Qualitative, quantitative and mixed methods approaches* (4th ed.). Thousand Oaks, CA: Sage.

Creswell, J. W., & Poth, C. N. (2018). *Qualitative inquiry & research design: Choosing among five approaches* (4th ed.). Thousand Oaks, CA: Sage.

Finfgeld-Connett, D. (2010). Generalizability and transferability of meta-synthesis research findings. *Journal of Advanced Nursing, 66*(2), 246–254.

Glaser, B. G., & Strauss, A. L. (1967). *The discovery of grounded theory: Strategies for qualitative research*. Chicago, IL: Aldine.

Gortner, S. R., & Nahm, H. (1977). An overview of nursing research in the United States. *Nursing Research, 26*(1), 10–33.

Greenway, K. (2014). Rituals in nursing: Intramuscular injections. *Journal of Clinical Nursing, 23*(23/24), 3583–3588.

Gray, J. R., Grove, S. K., & Sutherland, S. (2017). *Burns and Grove's the practice of nursing research: Appraisal, synthesis, and generation of evidence* (8th ed.). St. Louis, MO: Elsevier.

Grove, S. K., & Cipher, D. J. (2017). *Statistics for nursing research: A workbook for evidence-based practice* (2nd ed.). St. Louis, MO: Elsevier.

Herbert, R. G. (1981). *Florence Nightingale: Saint, reformer or rebel?* Malabar, FL: Robert E. Krieger.

Higgins, J. P. T., & Green, S. (2008). *Cochrane handbook for systematic reviews of interventions*. West Sussex, England: Wiley-Blackwell and The Cochrane Collaboration.

Horsley, J. A., Crane, J., Crabtree, M. K., & Wood, D. J. (1983). Using research to improve nursing practice: A guide. *CURN project*. New York, NY: Grune & Stratton.

Institute of Medicine. (2001). *Crossing the quality chasm: A new health system for the 21st century*. Washington, DC: National Academy Press.

James, P. A., Oparil, S., Carter, B. L., Cushman, W. C., Denison-Himmelfard, C., Handler, J., et al. (2014). 2014 evidence-based guidelines for the management of high blood pressure in adults: Report from the panel members appointed to the Eighth Joint National Committee (JNC 8). *Journal of the American Medical Association, 311*(5), 507–520.

Kaplan, A. (1964). *The conduct of inquiry; Methodology for behavioral science*. San Francisco, CA: Chandler.

Koehn, A. R., Ebright, P. R., & Draucker, C. B. (2016). Nurses' experiences with errors in nursing. *Nursing Outlook, 64*(6), 566–574.

Lee, S., Faucett, J., Gillen, M., Krause, N., & Landry, L. (2013). Risk perception of musculoskeletal injury among critical care nurses. *Nursing Research, 62*(1), 36–44.

Marshall, C., & Rossman, G. B. (2016). *Designing qualitative research* (6th ed.). Thousand Oaks, CA: Sage.

McMurrey, P. H. (1982). Toward a unique knowledge base in nursing. *Image, 14*(1), 12–15.

Melnyk, B. M., & Fineout-Overholt, E. (2015). *Evidence-based practice in nursing and healthcare: A guide to best practice* (3rd ed.). Philadelphia, PA: Lippincott, Williams, & Wilkins.

Melnyk, B. M., Gallagher-Ford, E., Fineout-Overholt, E. (2017). *Implementing evidence-based practice competencies in healthcare: A practical guide for improving quality, safety, & outcomes*. Indianapolis, IN: Sigma Theta Tau International.

Moorhead, S., Johnson, M., Maas, M. L., & Swanson, E. (2013). *Nursing outcomes classification (NOC): Measurement of health outcomes* (5th ed.). St. Louis, MO: Elsevier.

National Guideline Clearinghouse (2017). *AHRQ's national guideline clearinghouse: Public resource for summaries of evidence-based clinical practice guidelines*. Retrieved March 3, 2017, from https://www.guideline.gov/.

National Institute of Nursing Research (2016). *The NINR Strategic Plan: Advancing science, improving lives*. Retrieved February 20, 2017, from https://www.ninr.nih.gov/sites/www.ninr.nih.gov/files/NINR_StratPlan2016_reduced.pdf.

National Institute of Nursing Research, (2017). *About the NINR*. Retrieved November 10, 2017, from https://www.ninr.nih.gov/aboutninr.

Newland, P. K., Lunsford, V., & Flach, A. (2017). The interaction of fatigue, physical activity, and health-related quality of life in adults with multiple sclerosis (MS) and cardiovascular disease (CVD). *Applied Nursing Research, 33*(1), 49–53.

Nicoll, L. H., & Hesby, A. (2002). Intramuscular injections: An integrative research review and guideline for evidence-based practice. *Applied Nursing Research, 16*(2), 149–162.

Nightingale, F. (1859). *Notes on nursing: What it is, and what it is not*. Philadelphia, PA: Lippincott.

Oakley, K. (2010). Nursing by the numbers. *Occupational Health, 62*(4), 28–29.

Ogston-Tuck, S. (2014). Intramuscular injection technique: An evidence-based approach. *Nursing Standard, 29*(4), 52–59.

Palmer, I. S. (1977). Florence Nightingale: Reformer, reactionary, researcher. *Nursing Research, 26*(2), 84–89.

Quality, Safety Education for Nurses (QSEN), (2017). *Pre-licensure knowledge, skills, and attitudes (KSAs)*. Retrieved October 31, 2017, from http://qsen.org/competencies/pre-licensure-ksas/.

Rettig, R. (1991). History, development, and importance to nursing of outcomes research. *Journal of Nursing Quality Assurance, 5*(2), 13–17.

Sandelowski, M., & Barroso, J. (2007). *Handbook for synthesizing qualitative research*. New York, NY: Springer.

See, E. M. (1977). The ANA and research in nursing. *Nursing Research, 26*(3), 165–171.

Shadish, W. R., Cook, T. D., & Campbell, D. T. (2002). *Experimental and quasi-experimental designs for generalized causal inference*. Chicago, IL: Rand McNally.

Sherwood, G., & Barnsteiner, J. (2017). *Quality and safety in nursing: A competency approach to improving outcomes* (2nd ed.). Ames, IA: Wiley-Blackwell.

Sisson, H. (2015). Aspirating during the intramuscular injections procedure: A systematic literature review. *Journal of Clinical Nursing, 24*(17/18), 2368–2375.

Stetler, C. B. (2001). Updating the Stetler model of research utilization to facilitate evidence-based practice. *Nursing Outlook, 49*(6), 272–279.

Straus, S. E., Glasziou, P., Richardson, W. S., Rosenberg, W., & Haynes, R. B. (2011). *Evidence-based medicine: How to practice and teach EBM* (5th ed.). Edinburgh: Churchill Livingstone Elsevier.

Stringer, P. M. (2010). Sciatic nerve injury from intramuscular injections: A persistent and global problem. *International Journal of Clinical Practice, 64*(11), 1573–1579.

The Joint Commission (2017). *About The Joint Commission*. Retrieved March 7, 2017, from https://www.jointcommission.org.

Thomas, C. M., Mraz, M., & Rajcan, L. (2016). Blood aspiration during IM injection. *Clinical Nursing Research, 25*(5), 549–559.

US Department of Health and Human Services (US DHHS) (2017). *Healthy people 2020: Topics and objectives*. Retrieved November 10, 2017, from https://www.healthypeople.gov/2020/topics-objectives.

Weber, M. A., Schiffrin, E. L., White, W. B., Mann, S., Lindholm, L. H., Kenerson, J. G., et al. (2014). Clinical practice guidelines for the management of hypertension in the community: A statement by the American Society of Hypertension and the International Society of Hypertension. *Journal of Hypertension, 32*(1), 3–15.

Werley, H. H., & Fitzpatrick, J. J. (1983). *Annual review of nursing research* (Vol. 1). New York, NY: Springer.

Whittemore, R., Chao, A., Jang, M., Minges, K. E., & Park, C. (2014). Methods for knowledge synthesis: An overview. *Heart & Lung, 43*(5), 453–461.

Because of funding changes, the Agency for Healthcare Research and Quality (AHRQ) National Guideline Clearinghouse website was scheduled for decommissioning as of July 16, 2018. For more information, go to https://www.ahrq.gov/.

CHAPTER

2

Introduction to Quantitative Research

Kathryn M. Daniel

CHAPTER OVERVIEW

LEARNING OUTCOMES

After completing this chapter, you should be able to:

1. Define terms relevant to the quantitative research process—*basic research, applied research, rigor,* and *control.*
2. Compare and contrast the problem-solving process, nursing process, and research process.
3. Identify the steps of the quantitative research process in descriptive, correlational, quasi-experimental, and experimental published studies.
4. Read quantitative research reports.
5. Conduct initial critical appraisals of quantitative research reports.

What do you think of when you hear the word *research*? Frequently, the idea of experimentation or study comes to mind. Typical features of an experiment include randomizing subjects into groups, collecting data, and conducting statistical analyses. You may think of researchers conducting a study to determine the effectiveness of an intervention, such as determining the effectiveness of a walking exercise program on the body mass index (BMI) of patients with type 2 diabetes. These ideas are associated with quantitative research, which includes specific steps that are detailed in study reports. Critically appraising quantitative studies requires learning new terms, understanding the quantitative research process, and applying a variety of analytical skills.

This chapter provides an introduction to quantitative research to assist you in reading and understanding quantitative research reports. Relevant terms are defined, and the problem-solving and nursing processes are presented to provide a background for understanding the quantitative research process. The steps of the quantitative research process are introduced, and a descriptive correlational study is presented as an example to promote understanding of the process. Critical thinking skills needed for reading research reports and guidelines for conducting an initial critical appraisal of these reports are also provided. The chapter concludes with the identification of the steps of the research process from a quasi-experimental study, with an initial critical appraisal of this study.

WHAT IS QUANTITATIVE RESEARCH?

Quantitative research is a formal, objective, rigorous, and systematic process for generating numerical information about the world. Quantitative research is conducted to describe new situations, events, or concepts, examine relationships among variables, and determine the effectiveness of interventions on selected health outcomes. Some examples include the following:

1. Describing the spread of flu cases each season and their potential influence on local, national, and global health (descriptive study).
2. Examining the relationships among the variables, such as minutes watching television per week, minutes playing video games per week, and BMI of a school-age child (correlational study).
3. Determining the effectiveness of a fall prevention program on the fall rate of hospitalized older patients (quasi-experimental study).

The classic experimental designs to test the effectiveness of treatments were originated by Sir Ronald Fisher (1935). He is noted for adding structure to the steps of the quantitative research process with ideas such as the hypothesis, research design, and statistical analysis. Fisher's studies provided the groundwork for what is now known as experimental research.

Throughout the years, a number of other quantitative approaches have been developed. Campbell and Stanley (1963) developed quasi-experimental approaches to study the effects of treatments under less controlled conditions. Karl Pearson (Porter, 2004) developed statistical approaches for examining relationships among variables, which were used in analyzing data from correlational studies. The fields of sociology, education, and psychology are noted for their development and expansion of strategies for conducting descriptive research. A broad range of quantitative research approaches is needed to develop the empirical knowledge for building evidence-based practice (EBP) in nursing (Melnyk, Gallagher-Ford, & Fineout-Overholt, 2017). EBP was introduced in Chapter 1 and detailed in Chapter 13 of this text. EBP is essential for promoting quality and safe outcomes for patients and families, nursing education, and the healthcare system (Straus, Glasziou, Richardson, Rosenberg, & Haynes, 2011). Understanding the quantitative research process is essential for meeting the Quality and Safety Education for Nurses (QSEN, 2017) competencies for undergraduate nursing students, which are focused on patient-centered care, teamwork and collaboration, EBP, quality improvement, safety, and informatics (Sherwood & Barnsteiner, 2017). This section introduces you to the different types of quantitative research and provides definitions of terms relevant to the quantitative research process.

Types of Quantitative Research

The four common types of quantitative research included in this text are presented in Fig. 2.1. The type of quantitative research conducted is influenced by current knowledge about a research problem. When little knowledge is available, descriptive studies are conducted that provide a basis for correlational research. Descriptive and correlational studies are conducted frequently to provide a basis for the more highly controlled quasi-experimental and experimental studies (see Fig. 2.1).

Descriptive Research

Descriptive research is the exploration and description of phenomena in real-life situations. It provides an accurate account of characteristics of particular individuals, situations, or groups using numbers (Kerlinger & Lee, 2000). Descriptive studies are usually conducted with large numbers of subjects or study participants, in natural settings, with no manipulation of the situation. Through descriptive studies, researchers discover new meaning, describe what exists, determine

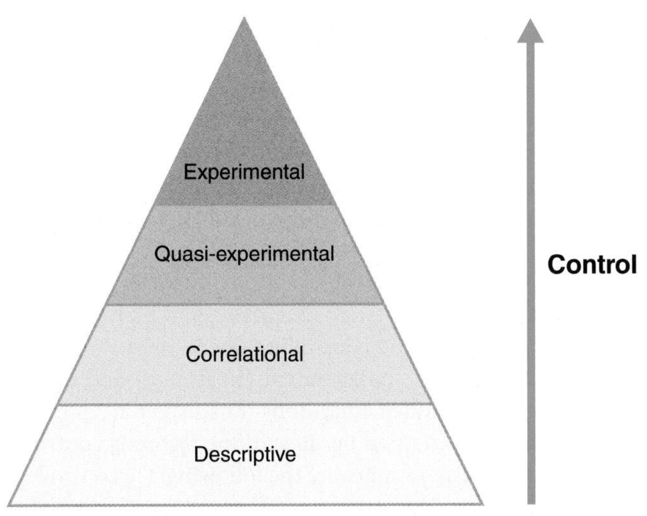

FIG 2.1 Types of quantitative research conducted in nursing.

the frequency with which something occurs, and categorize information in real-world settings. The outcomes of descriptive research include the identification and description of concepts, identification of possible relationships among concepts, and development of hypotheses that provide a basis for future quantitative research.

Correlational Research

Correlational research involves the systematic investigation of relationships between or among variables. When conducting this type of study, researchers measure selected variables in a sample and then use correlational statistics to determine the relationships among the study variables. Using correlational analysis, the researcher is able to determine the degree or strength and type (positive or negative) of a relationship between two variables. The strength of a relationship varies, ranging from −1 (perfect negative correlation) to +1 (perfect positive correlation), with 0 indicating no relationship (Grove & Cipher, 2017).

A positive relationship indicates that the variables vary together; that is, both variables increase or decrease together. For example, research has shown that the more minutes people exercise each week, the greater their bone density. A negative relationship indicates that the variables vary in opposite directions; thus as one variable increases, the other will decrease. For example, research has shown as the number of smoking pack-years (number of years smoked multiplied by the number of packs smoked per day) increases, people's life spans decrease. The primary intent of correlational studies is to explain the nature of relationships in the real world, not to determine cause and effect. However, the relationships identified with correlational studies are the means for generating hypotheses to guide quasi-experimental and experimental studies that do focus on examining cause and effect relationships (see Fig. 2.1).

Quasi-Experimental Research

The purpose of quasi-experimental research is to examine causal relationships or determine the effect of one variable on another. These studies involve implementing an intervention and examining the effects of this intervention using selected methods of measurement (Shadish, Cook, & Campbell, 2002). For example, an intervention of a swimming exercise program might be implemented to improve the balance and muscle strength of older women with osteoarthritis.

Quasi-experimental studies differ from experimental studies by the level of control achieved by the researchers. Quasi-experimental studies have less control over the implementation of the intervention, management of the setting, and/or selection of study participants than experimental studies. When studying human behavior, especially in clinical settings, researchers frequently are unable to select the participants randomly or control certain variables related to the intervention or setting. As a result, nurse researchers conduct more quasi-experimental studies than experimental studies. Control is discussed in more detail later in this chapter.

Experimental Research

Experimental research is an objective, systematic, and highly controlled investigation conducted for the purposes of predicting and controlling phenomena in nursing practice. In an experimental study, causality between the independent (treatment) and dependent (outcome) variables is examined under highly controlled conditions (Shadish et al., 2002). Experimental research is the most powerful quantitative method because of the rigorous control of variables. The three main characteristics of experimental studies are the following: (1) controlled manipulation of at least one treatment variable (independent variable); (2) exposure of some of the study participants to the treatment (experimental group) and no exposure of the remaining participants (control group); and (3) random assignment of participants to the control or experimental group. The degree of control achieved in experimental studies varies according to the population studied, variables examined, and environment of the study. Randomly selecting participants and conducting the study in a laboratory or research facility strengthen the control in a study.

Liao, Chung, and Chen (2017) examined the effects of regular elastic band exercises on the production of free radicals and antioxidant enzymes in older adults. Regular exercise has many benefits for all persons, including older adults. However, it is unknown if high-intensity, rapid, short-term exercise can increase free radicals and antioxidant enzymes, which are associated with chronic disease and other generalized effects of aging. A total of 22 older adults were recruited from a community center and randomly assigned to the intervention or control group. Those in the intervention group exercised regularly in a class with elastic bands; those in the control group continued their usual daily routines. All participants provided blood specimens 30 minutes before the intervention and 1 hour after the exercise classes were completed. To answer the study question, the researchers compared levels of thiobarbituric acid and glutathione peroxidase between the intervention and control groups.

The study participants were randomized into the intervention or control group, which increased study control and reduced the potential for errors in the study results. Participants were excluded from the study if they had conditions that might influence the study outcomes. For example, persons with dementia, those taking antioxidant vitamin supplements, or those who smoked were all excluded from participation in the study because these factors could affect their levels of thiobarbituric acid and glutathione peroxidase. The study intervention was structured and implemented consistently to the experimental group. Based on the strength of this study's design, Liao and colleagues (2017) were able to say with confidence that elastic band exercise does not increase the generation of free radicals and antioxidant enzyme activities and has promise as a beneficial exercise activity for older adults.

Defining Terms Relevant to Quantitative Research

Understanding quantitative research requires comprehension of the following important terms—*basic research, applied research, rigor,* and *control.* These terms are defined in the following sections, with examples provided from quantitative studies.

Basic Research

Basic research is sometimes referred to as pure research or even bench research. It includes scientific investigations conducted for the pursuit of knowledge for its own sake or for the pleasure of learning and finding truth. Basic researchers seek new knowledge about health phenomena, with the hope of establishing general scientific principles that often require applied research for use in practice. Basic nursing research might include laboratory investigations with animals or humans to promote further understanding of physiological functioning, genetic and inheritable disorders, and pathological processes. The National Institute of Nursing Research (NINR, 2016) is supportive of and provides funding for basic or bench research. These studies might focus on increasing our understanding of oxygenation, immune system disorders, eating and exercise patterns, sleeping disorders, and pain and comfort status.

You might conduct an initial critical appraisal of quantitative studies by identifying whether basic or applied research was conducted. For example, Wacker and colleagues (2016) conducted a study to expand understanding of the cellular and muscle pathology involved in hypophosphatemic osteomalacia (rickets). Researchers have found that human patients with rickets commonly experience muscle weakness, which further compound their chronic bone pathology. Wacker et al. (2016) conducted a basic experimental study of this process using mice that have similar muscle and bone pathophysiology.

The Wacker and colleagues' (2016) study demonstrates the importance of laboratory research to increase our understanding of the effects of treatments on cellular pathological processes. Bench research using animals is often conducted to provide an increased understanding of the genetics of health problems and establish a basis for further human research in this area. A major force in genetic research is the National Human Genome Research Institute (NHGRI, 2017), which plans and conducts a broad program of laboratory research to increase our understanding of human genetic makeup, genetics of diseases, and potential gene therapy. Basic research provides a basis for conducting applied "clinical research to translate genomic and genetic research into a greater understanding of human genetic disease, and to develop better methods for the detection, prevention, and treatment of heritable and genetic disorders" (NHGRI, 2017).

Applied Research

Applied research is also called practical research, which includes scientific investigations conducted to generate knowledge that will directly influence or improve clinical practice. The purpose of applied research is to solve problems, make decisions, and/or predict or control outcomes in real-life practice situations. The findings from applied studies can also be invaluable to policy makers as a basis for making changes to address health and social problems. Many of the studies conducted in nursing are applied studies because researchers have chosen to focus on clinical problems and the testing of nursing interventions to improve patient outcomes. Applied research also is used to test theory and validate its usefulness in clinical practice (Gray, Grove, & Sutherland, 2017). Researchers often examine the new knowledge discovered through basic research for its usefulness in practice by applied research, making these approaches complementary.

Finch, Griffin, and Pacala (2017) conducted an applied study to determine the effectiveness of an ambient assisted living technology intervention in reducing healthcare resource utilization. This intervention consisted of passive remote patient monitoring of older adults combined with the proactive intervention of a case manager whenever deviation from baseline behavior was detected. Study participants were independently determined to be nursing home eligible. Although participants were not randomized into groups, the study design was strengthened by including a historical control group, intervention group, and group that declined the intervention. The intervention lasted for 12 months, and the researchers measured the insurance claims made by the study participants during this time period. Even though the findings were not statistically significant, the intervention group used substantially less custodial care, had fewer emergency department visits and inpatient hospitalizations, and lower emergency room costs than the historical control group or the nonintervention group.

The findings of Finch and colleagues (2017) support further investment into passive technologies to preserve the safety and health of frail older adults. These findings, combined with the findings of additional studies in this area, have the potential to generate important knowledge for the delivery of evidence-based care to frail older adults living in the community. Applied studies with extensive rigor and control provide strong research evidence for practice.

Rigor in Quantitative Research

Rigor is the striving for excellence in research, which requires discipline, adherence to detail, precision, and accuracy. A rigorously conducted quantitative study has precise measuring tools, a representative sample, and a tightly controlled study design. Critically appraising the rigor of a study involves examining the reasoning used in conducting the study. Logical reasoning, including deductive and inductive reasoning (see Chapter 1), is essential to the development of quantitative studies (Chinn & Kramer, 2015). The research process, discussed later in this chapter, includes specific steps that are rigorously developed with meticulous detail and are logically linked in descriptive, correlational, quasi-experimental, and experimental studies.

Another aspect of rigor is **precision,** which encompasses accuracy, detail, and order. Precision is evident in the concise statement of the research purpose and detailed development of the study design. However, the most explicit example of precision is the measurement or quantification of the study variables (Waltz, Strickland, & Lenz, 2017). For example, a researcher might use a cardiac monitor to measure and record the heart rate of subjects in a database during an exercise program, rather than palpating a radial pulse for 30 seconds and recording it on a data collection sheet. Precision is essential for transparency in research so that other investigators know as explicitly as possible the exact steps and elements that make up a study. Precision allows for replication and for variation, which is necessary for other scientists to validate or extend the findings.

Control in Quantitative Research

Control involves the imposing of rules by researchers to decrease the possibility of error, thereby increasing the probability that the study's findings are an accurate reflection of reality. The rules used to achieve control in research are referred to as **design**. Quantitative studies include various degrees of control, ranging from uncontrolled to highly controlled, depending on the type of study. Table 2.1 provides examples of quantitative studies discussed in this chapter and the level of control achieved in them. Descriptive and correlational studies are rigorously conducted but are often designed with minimal researcher control because no intervention is implemented and study participants are examined as they exist in their natural setting, such as home, work, school, or healthcare clinic (see Fig. 2.1).

Quasi-experimental studies focus on determining the effectiveness of an intervention in producing a desired outcome in a partially controlled setting. These studies are conducted with more control of extraneous variables, selection of participants and settings, and implementation of the intervention (Shadish et al., 2002; see Table 2.1). However, experimental studies are the most highly controlled type of quantitative research conducted to examine the effect of interventions on dependent variables. Experimental studies often are conducted on participants in experimental units in healthcare agencies or on animals in laboratory settings. For example, Wacker and

TABLE 2.1 CONTROL IN QUANTITATIVE RESEARCH

TYPE OF QUANTITATIVE RESEARCH	EXAMPLE STUDIES	RESEARCHER CONTROL OF INTERVENTION AND EXTRANEOUS VARIABLES	RESEARCH SETTING
Descriptive and correlational	Moon et al. (2017)	No intervention; limited or no control of extraneous variables	Natural or partially controlled setting
Quasi-experimental	George et al. (2017)	Controlled intervention; rigorous control of extraneous variables	Partially controlled setting
Experimental	Liao et al. (2017)	Highly controlled intervention and extraneous variables	Research unit or laboratory setting

Data from Moon, H., Rote, S., & Beaty, J. A. (2017). Caregiving setting and Baby Boomer caregiver stress processes: Findings from the National Study of Caregiving (NSOC). *Geriatric Nursing, 38*(1), 57–62; George, L. E., Locasto, L. W., Pyo, K. A., & Cline, T. W. (2017). Effect of the dedicated education unit on nursing student self-efficacy: A quasi-experimental research study. *Nurse Education in Practice, 23*(1), 48–53; Liao, L. Y., Chung, W. S., & Chen, K. M. (2017). Free radicals and antioxidant enzymes in older adults after regular senior elastic band exercising: An experimental randomized controlled pilot study. *Journal of Advanced Nursing, 73*(1), 108–111.

BOX 2.1 ELEMENTS CONTROLLED IN QUANTITATIVE RESEARCH

- Extraneous variables
- Selection of setting(s)
- Sampling process
- Assignment of study participants to groups
- Development and implementation of the study intervention

colleagues (2016) studied mice to understand the effects of hypophosphatemic osteomalacia on skeletal muscle. The most common elements controlled in quantitative studies are presented in Box 2.1.

Extraneous Variables

Through control, the researcher can reduce the influence of extraneous variables. Extraneous variables exist in all studies and can interfere with obtaining a clear understanding of the relationships among the study variables. For example, if a study focused on the effect of relaxation therapy on the perception of incisional pain, the researchers would have to control the extraneous variables, such as the type of surgical incision and time, amount, and type of pain medication administered after surgery, to prevent their influence on the patient's perception of pain. Selecting only patients with abdominal incisions who are hospitalized and receiving only one type of pain medication intravenously after surgery would control some of these extraneous variables.

Research Settings

The setting is the location in which a study is conducted. There are three common settings for conducting research—natural, partially controlled, and highly controlled (see Table 2.1). A natural setting, or field setting, is an uncontrolled real-life situation or environment. Conducting a study in a natural setting means that the researcher does not manipulate or change the environment for the study. Descriptive and correlational studies often are conducted in natural settings. A partially controlled setting is an environment that the researcher has manipulated or modified in some way. An increasing number of nursing studies are conducted in partially controlled settings to limit the effects of extraneous variables on the study outcomes. A highly controlled setting is an artificially constructed environment developed for the sole purpose of conducting research. Laboratories, research centers, and test units in universities or healthcare agencies are highly controlled settings in which bench and experimental studies often are conducted. Multiple settings with increased control of extraneous variables usually provide more accurate and credible findings in quantitative studies.

Sampling and Assignment of Participants to Groups

Sampling is a process of selecting participants who are representative of the population being studied. Random sampling usually provides a sample that is representative of a population because each member of the population is selected independently and has an equal chance, or probability, of being included in the study. In quantitative research, random and nonrandom samples are used. A randomly selected sample is very difficult to obtain in nursing research, so quantitative studies often are conducted with nonrandom samples. To increase the control and rigor of a study and decrease the potential for **bias** (slanting of findings away from what is true or accurate), the participants who are initially selected with a nonrandom sampling method are often randomly assigned to the intervention or control group in quasi-experimental and experimental studies. For example, Liao and colleagues (2017) initially obtained their sample of older adults using a nonrandom convenience sampling method. However, the study design was strengthened by the random assignment of these older adults to receive the elastic band exercise intervention (experimental group) or continued their usual activity (comparison group).

Study Interventions

Quasi-experimental and experimental studies examine the effect of an independent variable or intervention on a dependent variable or outcome. More intervention studies are being conducted in nursing to establish an EBP for nursing. Controlling the development and implementation of a study intervention increases the validity of the study design (see Chapter 8) and credibility of the findings. A study intervention needs to be: (1) clearly and precisely developed; (2) consistently implemented; and (3) examined for effectiveness through quality measurement of the dependent variables. The detailed development of a quality intervention and the consistent implementation of this intervention are known as *intervention fidelity* (Eymard & Altmiller, 2016; Murphy & Gutman, 2012).

PROBLEM-SOLVING AND NURSING PROCESSES: BASIS FOR UNDERSTANDING THE QUANTITATIVE RESEARCH PROCESS

Research is a process that is similar in some ways to other processes. Therefore the background acquired early in nursing education in problem solving, and the nursing process also is useful in research. A **process** includes a purpose, series of actions, and goal. The purpose provides direction for the implementation of a series of actions to achieve an identified goal or outcome. The specific steps of the process can be revised and re-implemented to reach the endpoint or goal. Table 2.2 links the steps of the problem-solving process, nursing process, and research process. Relating the research process to the problem-solving and nursing processes may be helpful in understanding the steps of the quantitative research process.

TABLE 2.2 COMPARISON OF THE PROBLEM-SOLVING PROCESS, NURSING PROCESS, AND RESEARCH PROCESS

PROBLEM-SOLVING PROCESS	NURSING PROCESS	RESEARCH PROCESS
Data collection	**Assessment** Data collection (objective and subjective data) Data interpretation	**Knowledge of nursing world** Clinical experiences Literature review
Problem definition	**Nursing diagnosis**	**Problem and purpose identification**
Plan Setting goals Identifying solutions	**Plan** Setting goals Planning interventions	**Methodology** Design Sample Measurement methods Data collection Data analysis
Implementation	**Implementation**	**Implementation**
Evaluation and revision	**Evaluation and modification**	**Outcomes, communication, and synthesis of study findings to promote evidence-based nursing practice**

Comparing Problem-Solving With the Nursing Process

The problem-solving process involves: (1) systematic collection of data to identify a problem, difficulty, or dilemma; (2) determination of goals related to the problem; (3) identification of possible approaches or solutions to achieve those goals (plan); (4) implementation of the selected solutions; and (5) evaluation of goal achievement (Chinn & Kramer, 2015). Problem solving frequently is used in daily activities and nursing practice. For example, you use problem solving when you select your clothing, decide where to live, or turn a patient with a fractured hip.

The nursing process is a subset of the problem-solving process. The steps of the nursing process are assessment, diagnosis, plan, implementation, evaluation, and modification (see Table 2.2). Assessment involves the collection and interpretation of subjective data (health history) and objective data (physical examination) for the development of nursing diagnoses. These diagnoses guide the remaining steps of the nursing process, just as the step of identifying the problem directs the remaining steps of the problem-solving process. The planning step in the nursing process is the same as in the problem-solving process. Both processes involve implementation (putting the plan into action) and evaluation (determining the effectiveness of the process). If the process is ineffective, nurses need to review all steps and revise (modify) them as necessary to achieve quality outcomes for the patient and family. Nurses implement the nursing process until the diagnoses are resolved, and the identified goals are achieved.

Comparing the Nursing Process With the Research Process

The nursing process and research process have important similarities and differences. The two processes are similar because they both involve abstract critical thinking and complex reasoning. These processes help identify new information, discover relationships, and make predictions about phenomena. In both processes, information is gathered, observations are made, problems are identified, plans are developed (methodology), and actions are taken (data collection and analysis).

Both processes are reviewed for effectiveness and efficiency—the nursing process is evaluated, and outcomes are determined in the research process (see Table 2.2). Implementing the two processes expands and refines the user's knowledge. With this growth in knowledge and critical thinking, the user can implement increasingly complex nursing processes and studies.

Knowledge of the nursing process will assist you in understanding the research process. However, the research process is more complex than the nursing process and involves the rigorous application of a variety of research methods (Creswell, 2014). The research process also has a broader focus than that of the nursing process, in which the nurse focuses on a specific patient and family. During the quantitative research process, the researcher focuses on large groups of individuals, such as a population of patients with hypertension. In addition, researchers must be knowledgeable about the world of nursing to identify problems that require study. This knowledge comes from clinical and other personal experiences and by conducting a review of relevant literature (see Chapter 6).

The theoretical underpinnings of the research process are much stronger than those of the nursing process. All steps of the research process are logically linked to each other, as well as to the theoretical foundations of the study (see Chapter 7). The conduct of research requires greater precision, rigor, and control than those that are needed in the implementation of the nursing process. The outcomes from research frequently are shared with a large number of nurses and other healthcare professionals through presentations and publications. In addition, the outcomes from several studies can be synthesized to provide sound evidence for nursing practice (Melnyk et al., 2017).

IDENTIFYING THE STEPS OF THE QUANTITATIVE RESEARCH PROCESS

The quantitative research process involves conceptualizing a research project, planning and implementing that project, and communicating the findings. Fig. 2.2 identifies the steps of the quantitative research process that are usually included in a research report. The figure illustrates the logical flow of the process as one step builds progressively on another. The research process is depicted in a circle because there is a flow back and forth as the different steps of a study are developed and implemented. The steps of the quantitative research process are briefly introduced here; Chapters 4 to 11 discuss them in more detail. The descriptive correlational study conducted by Moon, Rote, and Beaty (2017) on the relationships of caregiver (CG) stress processes among baby boomer caregivers and caregiving setting is used as an example to introduce the steps of the quantitative research process.

Research Problem and Purpose

A research problem is an area of concern in which there is a gap in the knowledge needed for nursing practice. The problem statement in a study usually identifies an area of concern for a particular population that requires investigation. Research is then conducted to generate essential knowledge that addresses the practice concern, with the ultimate goal of developing sound research evidence for nursing practice (Brown, 2018; Melnyk et al., 2017). The research problem is usually broad and could provide the basis for several studies. The research purpose is generated from the problem and identifies the specific focus or goal of the study. The focus of a quantitative study might be to identify, describe, or explain a situation, predict a solution to a situation, or control a situation to produce positive outcomes in practice. The purpose includes the variables, population, and often the setting for the study (see Chapter 5).

Moon and colleagues (2017) identified their research topic as CG stress that has the potential to affect millions of aging baby boomers as they reach retirement age. These aging baby boomers are dealing with caregiving responsibilities related to their own aging parents at the same time that they are dealing with their own aging issues. The focus of this study is to examine the relationships among variables important to the CG stress processes of baby boomers. The study problem and purpose are presented in Research Example 2.1.

RESEARCH EXAMPLE 2.1

Problem and Purpose

Research Study Excerpt

Research Problem

Over 46 million people in the United States [U.S.] are 65 years or older, and major driver of the rapidly aging population is the Baby Boomer generation (born between 1946 and 1964)… By 2040, when all Baby Boomers are over the age of 65, the older population will constitute over 20% of the general U.S. population… Many of the boomers' care recipients are 85 years and older and while the majority of elders receiving care assistance live in the community, 13% reside in institutional settings… A better understanding of boomer CGs' emotional well-being and physical health will be beneficial not only to care providers but also to family CGs themselves, to increase awareness both of their health and the areas to improve their well-being. (Moon et al., 2017, pp. 57–58)

Research Purpose

The aim of this study was to provide a comprehensive understanding of how the caregiving setting relates to caregiving experience among Baby Boomer caregivers (CGs). (Moon et al., 2017, pp. 57)

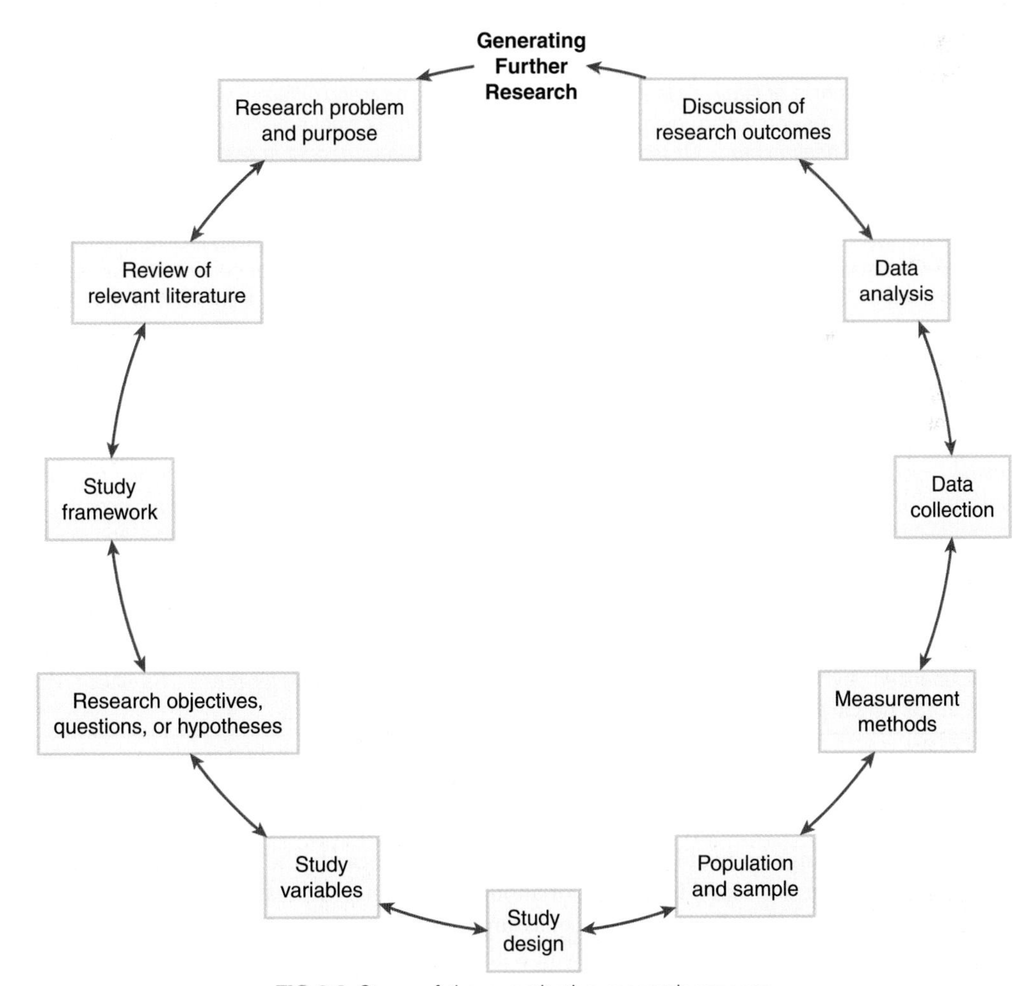

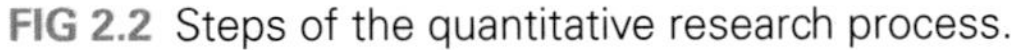

FIG 2.2 Steps of the quantitative research process.

Review of Relevant Literature

Researchers conduct a review of relevant literature to generate a picture of what is known and not known about a particular problem and to document why a study needs to be conducted. Relevant literature includes only those sources that are pertinent to or highly important in providing the in-depth knowledge needed to study a selected problem (Aveyard, 2014). Often, the literature review section concludes with a summary paragraph that indicates the current knowledge of a problem area and identifies the additional research that is needed to generate essential evidence for practice (see Chapter 6).

Moon et al. (2017) presented a review of literature with relevant studies that provided a basis for their study purpose and methods section. Key aspects of this review are presented in Research Example 2.2.

RESEARCH EXAMPLE 2.2

Review of Literature

Research Study Excerpt

The expectation that CGs will not experience distress or burden after an older family member is placed in a long-term care facility is a myth… Studies suggest that family CGs to older adults in residential care settings, despite obtaining relief from direct-care tasks… report continuing distress post-institutionalization, including depression, sadness, loss, guilt, and, potentially, family conflict… This risk for distress likely results from the continued involvement… of family CGs after placement, albeit in new and different ways: visiting, interacting with staff and relatives, providing instrumental assistance such as transportation, and making decisions about finances and health care… Of the available studies on CGs to people in residential care, most have focused on nursing homes (NHs) and changes in the role of the family CG following institutionalization.

Of the few studies on the topic, research shows that dementia CGs providing care in the community report greater work-related strain than dementia CGs providing care in assisted living facilities, and that CGs to patients in assisted living facilities report higher burden than dementia CGs to patients in nursing homes (NH)… In addition, one study suggests that CGs may continue to feel guilt at least 10 months after their elderly family member has been admitted to a NH or residential care home (Kolanowski et al., 2012), indicating a risk for depression and other negative health outcomes. Less attention has been paid to the predictors of burden and well-being of family CGs to people living in non-NH residential care settings including assisted living facilities, care homes, and continuing care retirement homes… Non-NH residential care settings tend to house residents with less disability and have less intensive supervision, allowing CGs to older adults living in these facilities more frequent visits and involvement with instrumental care tasks… While the majority of institutional care is provided in nursing home settings, in recent years there has been an increase in the use of non-NH settings,… especially as the Baby Boom generation meets the needs of work and family life.

In particular, Baby Boomer CGs… experience multiple care demands. For instance, unlike previous generations, Boomers can expect to spend 40 years simultaneously working and providing personal care and financial assistance for their children, aging parents, older siblings, spouses and/or their spouses' children, and themselves… Institutional care providers still face the challenges of understanding family CGs' needs and experiences, and may find it difficult to devise appropriate interventions for these CGs (Wethington & Burgio, 2015). (Moon et al., 2017, pp. 57–58)

Study Framework

A framework is the abstract theoretical basis for a study that enables the researcher to link the findings to nursing's body of knowledge. In quantitative research, the framework is a testable theory that has been developed in nursing or another discipline, such as psychology, physiology, pathology, or sociology. A theory consists of assumptions, an integrated set of defined concepts, and relational statements that present a view of a phenomenon and can be used to describe, explain, predict, or control the phenomenon (Chinn & Kramer, 2015). Assumptions are statements that are taken for granted or are considered true, even though they have not been scientifically tested, and provide a basis for the phenomenon described by the theory. A concept is a term that abstractly names and describes an object or phenomenon, providing it with a separate identity and meaning.

The relational statements in theories identify the links between two or more concepts that are tested in research. In quantitative studies, researchers test selected relational statements of the theory, but usually not the entire theory. A study framework can be expressed as a map or a diagram of the relationships that provide the basis for a study and is described in the research report, or the framework can be presented in a narrative format (see Chapter 7).

Moon et al. (2017) based their study framework on CG stress and coping model (Haley, Levine, Brown, & Bartolucci, 1987) and presented their framework within the narrative of the text, described in Research Example 2.3.

RESEARCH EXAMPLE 2.3

Framework

Research Study Excerpt

Predictors of caregiver well-being include primary stressors, which include both (a) objective indicators of the caregiving recipient's (CRs) cognitive and physical health status, and (b) subjective indicators of CG overload. Stressors within the caregiving domain influence secondary role strains on family cohesion and finances, and intrapsychic strains, including self-esteem and loss of self. A key component of this framework is the role of background and resources, which are influential at every stage of the caregiving stress process. We do not have all of the proposed factors from the CG stress process model in our data set. However, we do have variables for the key primary stressors and objective indicators of CR health (i.e., AD [Alzheimer's disease] or other dementia) as well as indicators for disability, such as needing help with daily activities and whether there was a regular schedule for care provision. We also included indicators for secondary strains, such as financial difficulties and relationship quality, resources (including informal support) and the emotional well-being and self-rated general health of CGs. (Moon et al., 2017, p. 58)

Research Objectives, Questions, or Hypotheses

Investigators formulate research objectives (or aims), questions, or hypotheses to bridge the gap between the more abstractly stated research problem and purpose and the study design and plan for data collection and analysis. Objectives, questions, and hypotheses are narrower in focus than the purpose and often specify only one or two research variables. They also identify the relationship between the variables and indicate the population to be studied. Some descriptive studies include only a research purpose, whereas others include a purpose and objectives or questions to direct the study. Some correlational studies include a purpose and specific questions or hypotheses. Quasi-experimental and experimental studies need to include hypotheses to direct the conduct of the studies and the interpretation of findings (Gray et al., 2017; see Chapter 5).

Moon and colleagues (2017) posed two research questions, identified in Research Example 2.4.

RESEARCH EXAMPLE 2.4

Research Questions

Research Study Excerpt

1. *Are there differences in primary stressor, secondary stressors, resources, and outcomes between CGs of older adults in non-NH residential care settings and those of Baby Boomer CGs for older adults in the community?...*
2. *Are there differences in factors associated with the CGs' emotional well-being and self-perceived health status, based on CG setting (non-NH residential care or community)?* (Moon et al., 2017, p. 58)

Study Variables

The research purpose and objectives, questions, or hypotheses identify the variables to be examined in a study. **Variables** are concepts at various levels of abstraction that are measured, manipulated, or controlled in a study. More concrete concepts, such as temperature, weight, or blood pressure, are referred to as variables in a study. More abstract concepts, such as creativity, empathy, or social support, sometimes are referred to as research concepts.

Researchers operationalize the variables or concepts in a study by identifying conceptual and operational definitions. A **conceptual definition** provides a variable or concept with theoretical meaning (Gray et al., 2017), and it comes from a theorist's definition of the concept or is developed through concept analysis. The conceptual definitions of variables provide a link from selected concepts in the study framework to the study variables. Researchers develop an **operational definition** so that the variable can be measured or an intervention implemented in a study (see Chapter 5). The knowledge gained from studying the variable will increase understanding of the theoretical concept from the study framework that the variable represents.

Moon and colleagues (2017) clearly identified the following study variables in their research purpose and questions: primary stressors, secondary stressors, resources, CG background and health, and outcomes of emotional well-being and self-rated general health. Clear conceptual definitions were provided for the two variables of primary stressors and secondary stressors from the conceptual framework. The conceptual and operational definitions for primary and secondary stressors are provided as an example in Research Example 2.5.

RESEARCH EXAMPLE 2.5

Variables

Research Study Excerpts

Primary Stressors

Conceptual Definition

Primary stressors included the CRs' dementia status, level of care provided by CG, and whether care was provided on a regular schedule. (Moon et al., 2017, p. 58)

Operational Definition

We defined the CR's dementia status using either report by National Health & Aging Trends Study (NHATS) participants or by proxy (if a doctor told the CR that he/she had dementia or AD). We created a level of care activities variable based on the sum of the responses to the five NSOC [National Study of Caregiving] questions related to helping with: 1) chores, 2) shopping, 3) personal care, 4) getting around home, and 5) transportation. Response categories ranged from 1 = rarely to 4 = every day. Higher scores indicated higher level of involvement in helping with daily activities. We also created a variable for whether care was provided on a regular schedule or not (0 = varied, 1 = regular schedule). (Moon et al., 2017, p. 58)

Secondary Stressors

Conceptual Definition

Secondary stressors included perceived financial difficulty and relationship quality between the CG and the CR. (Moon et al., 2017, p. 58)

Operational Definition

Respondents were asked if providing care for the CR was financially difficult (1 = yes, 0 = no). We defined the quality of the CG's relationship with the older adult as the sum of four questions (how much CG enjoys being with the CR, how much CR appreciates CG, how much CR argues with CG, and how much CR gets on CG nerves)... Higher scores indicated a better relationship. (Moon et al., 2017, p. 58)

Study Design

Research design is a blueprint for the conduct of a study that maximizes control over factors that could interfere with the study's desired outcome. The type of design directs the selection of a population, procedures for sampling, methods of measurement, and plans for data collection and analysis. The choice of research design depends on what is known and not known about the research problem, the researcher's expertise, the purpose of the study, and the intent to generalize the findings. Sometimes the design of a study indicates that a pilot study was conducted. A **pilot study** is often a smaller version of a proposed study, and researchers frequently conduct these to refine the study sampling process, intervention, or measurement of variables (Hertzog, 2008).

Designs have been developed to meet unique research needs as they emerge; thus a variety of descriptive, correlational, quasi-experimental, and experimental designs have been generated over time. In descriptive and correlational studies, no treatment is administered, so the purposes of these study designs include improving the precision of measurement, describing what exists, and clarifying relationships that provide a basis for quasi-experimental and experimental studies. Quasi-experimental and experimental study designs usually involve intervention and control groups and focus on achieving high levels of control, as well as precision in measurement (see Table 2.1). A study's design usually is in the methodology section of a research report. Chapter 8 presents a variety of designs that are frequently implemented in quantitative studies.

Moon and colleagues (2017) did not identify the design of their study. However, the study purpose and research questions indicate that a descriptive correlational study was conducted with a simple descriptive design and predictive correlational design. The descriptive part of the design provided a basis for describing and comparing the study variables of primary stressors, secondary stressors, resources, CG background and health, and outcomes of CG emotional and general physical health (see Research Example 2.1). The predictive correlation part of the design focused on examining the relationships among the study variables and the use of primary and secondary stressors, resources, and background of the CR to predict emotional and general physical health of baby boomer CGs (see Research Example 2.2).

Population and Sample

The **population** is all elements (individuals, objects, or substances) that meet certain criteria for inclusion in a study. A **sample** is a subset of the population selected for a particular study, and the members of a sample are the participants. Sampling was introduced earlier in this chapter, and Chapter 9 provides a background for critically appraising populations, samples, and settings in research reports.

Moon et al. (2017) used an existing database that included the variables they wished to study in the population of baby boomer CGs. They provided a detailed description of the source of their study sample. For this study, they examined only a subset of the original data, which included those participants who were identified as a family CG according to specific sampling criteria. The sample characteristics were presented in a table and described in the article narrative. Research Example 2.6 includes a discussion of the sample for this study.

RESEARCH EXAMPLE 2.6

Population and Sample

Research Study Excerpt

This study was based on secondary data of the NSOC [National Study of Caregiving], which is a sample of 2007 informal CGs identified by Medicare beneficiaries aged 65 and older who participated in the 2011 National Health and Aging Trends study (NHATS), a nationally representative study that collects data from older adults on an annual basis. The NSOC collects information on how the CG helps the older respondent in the NHATS with everyday activities along with information on the CG's own health, family, and income... We excluded those CGs who were not born between 1946 and 1964 (n = 994). The NSOC includes all eligible CGs for whom the NHATS respondents provided contact information. To identify the primary CG for a given CR, we counted the number of CGs interviewed per older adult. If an older adult had one CG, we used his/her information. For older adults with multiple CGs, we identified the primary CG as the one who performed the most caregiving duties... Thus, our analyses included only those CGs (N = 782) who provided the most care to an older adult living in a community or in a non-NH [nursing home] residential care setting. (Moon et al., 2017, p. 58)

Measurement Methods

Measurement is the process of "assigning numbers to objects (or events or situations) in accord with some rule" (Kaplan, 1964, p. 177). A component of measurement is instrumentation, which is the application of specific rules to the development of a measurement method or instrument (Waltz et al., 2017). An instrument is selected to measure a specific variable in a study. The numerical data generated with an instrument may be at the nominal, ordinal, interval, or ratio level of measurement. The level of measurement, with nominal being the lowest form of measurement and ratio being the highest, determines the type of statistical analysis that can be performed on the data. Chapter 10 introduces you to the concept of measurement, describes different types of measurement methods, and provides direction to appraise measurement techniques in studies critically.

Moon and coworkers (2017) measured primary and secondary stressors using CG survey answers found in the NSOC. (These instruments were mentioned earlier in the operational definition of primary and secondary stressors.) Research Example 2.7 identifies the scales and questionnaires used to measure the other study variables. The researchers provided quality descriptions of the measurement methods used in their study and indicated that these methods were commonly used in other studies and found to be reliable (consistent measurement) and valid (accurate in measuring a variable).

RESEARCH EXAMPLE 2.7

Measurement Methods

Research Study Excerpts

Resources

We defined informal support as the sum of three questions about the existence of supportive friends and family and ability to call on support networks (response options include 1 = yes, 0 = no). (Moon et al., 2017, pp. 58–59)

CG Background and Health

The background characteristics included CG's age, gender (0 = male, 1 = female) and education (0 = high school or less, 1 = some college or more). The NSOC participants were asked about whether they had any of ten chronic conditions... We defined pain through a single NSOC item (whether the participant was bothered by pain) (0 = no, 1 = yes). (Moon et al., 2017, pp. 58–59)

Outcomes

We estimated that the CG's emotional well-being as the sum of 7 questions (each with a 4-level response ranging from 1 = 'not at all' to 4 = 'nearly every day'). Higher scores indicated a better self-perceived emotional well-being. We categorized the CGs overall self-rated general health into five levels, from poor (1) to excellent (5). (Moon et al., 2017, pp. 58–59)

Data Collection

Data collection is the precise systematic gathering of information relevant to the research purpose or the specific objectives, questions, or hypotheses of a study. To collect data, the researcher must obtain permission from the setting or agency in which the study will be conducted. Researchers must also obtain consent from all study participants to indicate their willingness to be in the study. Frequently, the researcher asks the study participants to sign a consent form, which describes the study, promises them confidentiality, and indicates that they can withdraw from the study at any time. The research report should document permission from an agency to conduct a study and consent of the study participants (see Chapter 4).

During data collection, investigators use a variety of techniques for measuring study variables, such as observations, interviews, questionnaires, scales, and biological measures. In an increasing number of studies, nurses are measuring physiological and pathological variables using high-technology equipment. Researchers collect and systematically record data on each study participant, organizing the data in a way that facilitates computer entry (see Chapter 10). Data collection is usually described in the methodology section of a research report under the subheading of "Procedures."

Moon and colleagues (2017) covered their data collection process in Research Example 2.8 regarding procedures.

RESEARCH EXAMPLE 2.8

Data Collection

Research Study Excerpt

The NSOC collects information on how the CG helps the older respondent in the NHATS with everyday activities along with information on the CG's own health, family, and income... None NHATS respondents in NSOC lived in nursing homes (among 2007 NHATS respondents in NSOC, they lived [in] either the community (n = 1786) or non-NH residential care settings (assisted living, care homes, and continuing care retirement homes, n = 221). We excluded those CGs who were not born between 1946 and 1964 (n = 994). The NSOC includes all eligible CGs... for whom the NHATS respondents provided contact information. To identify the primary CG for a given CR, we counted the number of CGs interviewed per older adult. If an older adult had one CG, we used his/her information. For older adults with multiple CGs, we identified the primary CG as the one who performed the most caregiving duties (based on hours per day) and used his/her information (n = 180), eliminating the secondary CGs (n = 231). Thus our analyses included only those CGs (N= 782) who provided the most care to an older adult living in [a] community or in a non-NH residential care setting. (Moon et al., 2017, p. 58)

Data Analysis

Data analysis reduces, organizes, and gives meaning to the data. Analysis techniques conducted in quantitative research include descriptive and inferential analyses (see Chapter 11; Grove & Cipher, 2017) and some sophisticated, advanced analysis techniques. Investigators base their choice of analysis techniques primarily on the research objectives, questions, or hypotheses and level of measurement achieved by the measurement methods. Often, research reports indicate the analysis techniques that were used in the study, and this content is covered before the study results. You can find the outcomes of the data analysis process in the results section of the research report; this section is best organized by the research objectives, questions, or hypotheses of the study.

Moon and colleagues (2017) identified the analysis techniques conducted on their study data in Research Example 2.9. The study results were presented in tables and described in the narrative.

RESEARCH EXAMPLE 2.9

Data Analysis

Research Study Excerpts

We used two-tailed independent t-tests and chi-square tests to assess the differences in characteristics between Baby Boomer CGs of older adults in community and in non-NH residential care settings. (Moon et al., 2017, p. 59)

Results

...Baby Boomer CGs of older adults in non-NH residential care settings reported a lower level of providing help with daily activities including transportation ($t(774) = 8.85$, $p < .001$); a better relationship quality with the CRs ($t(766 = -2.03$, $p < .001$); a better physical health ($t(558) = -4.054$, $p < .001$); and a better emotional well-being ($t(762) = -2.055$, $p < .05$). Moreover, Baby Boomer CGs of older adults in non-NH residential care settings reported a higher level of informal support ($t(733) = -2.035$, $p < .05$). There were also significant differences in providing care on a regular basis ($\chi^2(1, N = 777) = 13.4$, $p < .001$) and financial difficulties ($\chi^2(1, N = 779) = 12.589$, $p < .001$). (Moon et al., 2017, p. 59)

Moon and colleagues (2017) also conducted regression analyses to predict emotional well-being and perceived general health between the two groups. Regression analysis is a common technique used in nursing studies for making predictions (see Chapter 11).

Discussion of Research Outcomes

The results obtained from data analyses require interpretation to be meaningful. **Interpretation of research outcomes** involves examining the results from data analysis, identifying study limitations, exploring the significance of the findings, forming conclusions, generalizing the findings, considering the implications for nursing, and suggesting further studies. The study outcomes are usually presented in the discussion section of the research report. **Limitations** are restrictions in a study methodology and/or framework that may decrease the credibility and generalizability of the findings. A **generalization** is the extension of the conclusions made based on the research findings from the sample studied to a larger population. The study conclusions provide a basis for the implications of the findings for practice and identify areas for further research (see Chapter 11). Study outcomes are usually presented in the discussion section of the research report. Moon and associates (2017) provided the following discussion of their study outcomes in Research Example 2.10.

RESEARCH EXAMPLE 2.10

Discussion

Research Study Excerpts

While extensive research has focused on the experience of CGs of older adults residing in the community, fewer studies have paid attention to CGs of older adults in institutions, especially in non-NH residential care facilities such as assisted living, board and care home, non-NH home parts of a continuing care retirement community. In light of this our purpose was to provide a comprehensive understanding of the demographics, the prevalence of chronic illness, perceived mood, feelings, and other caregiving experiences of Baby Boomer CGs of older adults in non-NH care settings. Our results contribute to the body of caregiving research in several ways. We address the gap in literature on Baby Boomer CGs, present results using national data and highlight important differences in the caregiving experience between Baby Boomer CGs of older adults in non-NH residential care settings and in the community.

Our findings show the importance of CG background factors, especially gender, income, and educational attainment. Boomer CGs to older adults residing in the community (vs. non-NH residential care) tend to report lower household incomes and educational levels; however educational attainment was associated with health and well-being for both groups. Financial resources and strain are also related to the health status of Baby Boomer CGs regardless of care setting. Overall, more supports and interventions should focus on the needs of low income CGs and their families who have less financial resources to address the complex needs of CRs. In addition, the majority of CGs in the study are women providing care for women. The results show that placement in a non-NH residential care facility is related to better emotional well-being of women than men and institutionalization may help to offset the strain of addressing multiple work and family needs for women boomer CGs. (Moon et al., 2017, pp. 60–61)

Limitations and Suggestions for Further Study

There are some limitations to our findings. First, we used a cross-sectional design [where all participants in a study are evaluated at the same point in time], which limits the ability to test for any changes over time in relationships among stressors, outcomes, and resources. Longitudinal investigations of individuals with dementia may be particularly informative when change is examined during critical periods or transition points (e.g., moving to other facilities, CR's behavioral or cognitive functional changes). It may be possible to understand how stressors, outcomes, and resources change over time in CGs of older adults in non-NH residential care settings as well as CGs of older adults in community. Second, this study is based on a secondary data analysis. We focused on CGs who spent longer time on caregiving provision among multiple caregivers per older adult. Stress and well-being of secondary caregivers is an important avenue for future research... We also focused only on those CG primary stressors directly related to caregiving. Information was not available on the impact on CG's emotional well-being and general health of their relationship with facility staff or their satisfaction with the facility... Future studies should include this information in their analyses of the effects of stressors on well-being and self-perceived health. (Moon et al., 2017, p. 61)

Conclusions and Implications for Nursing Practice

Our findings contribute to current knowledge in several ways. Boomer CGs who continue to provide care for their loved ones in non-NH residential care settings should become more informed about the ways in which non-NH residential care settings provided care affects the caregiving experience. Our findings on the experience of Baby Boomer CGs of older adults in non-NH residential care settings and those of older adults in a community increase our understanding of the caregiving experience for the Baby Boomer cohort of CGs. In particular, we provide evidence that residential care for CRs might be helpful for not only the CGs' physical health but also their emotional well-being. Our results also contribute critical information on risk factors for boomer CGs of older adults in non-NH residential care settings and those of older adults living in the community. Finally, we have provided information useful to care providers in identifying the needs of boomer CGs, especially boomer CGs of older adults in non-NH residential care settings. (Moon et al., 2017, p. 61)

READING RESEARCH REPORTS

Understanding the steps of the research process and learning new terms related to those steps will assist you in reading research reports. A **research report** summarizes the major elements of a study and identifies the contributions of that study to nursing knowledge. Research reports are presented at professional meetings and conferences and are published online and in print journals and books. These reports often are difficult for nursing students and new graduates to read and to apply the knowledge in practice. Maybe you have had difficulty locating research articles or understanding the content of these articles. We would like to help you overcome some of these barriers and assist you in understanding the research literature by (1) identifying sources that publish research reports; (2) describing the content of a research report; and (3) providing tips for reading the research literature.

Sources of Research Reports

The most common sources for nursing research reports are professional journals. Research reports are the major focus of multiple nursing research journals, which were identified in Chapter 1. Two journals in particular, *Applied Nursing Research* and *Clinical Nursing Research*, focus on communicating research findings to practicing nurses. The journal *Worldviews on Evidence-Based Nursing* focuses on innovative ideas for using evidence to improve patient care globally.

Many of the nursing clinical specialty journals also place a high priority on publishing research findings. A few of the clinical journals with high publications of studies include the following: *Geriatric Nursing, Oncology Nursing Forum, Journal of Pediatric Nursing, Heart & Lung,* and *Nephrology Nursing.* More than 100 nursing journals are published in the United States, and most of them include research articles. The findings from many studies are now communicated through the Internet as journals are placed online; selected websites include those presenting the most current healthcare research (see Chapter 6).

Content of Research Reports

At this point, you may be overwhelmed by the seeming complexity of a research report. You will find it easier to read and comprehend these reports if you understand each of the component parts. A research report often includes six parts: (1) abstract, (2) introduction, (3) methods, (4) results, (5) discussion, and (6) references. These parts are described in this section, and the study by Chan, Yates, and McCarthy (2016) that examined fatigue self-management behaviors in patients with advanced cancer is presented as an example.

Abstract Section

The report usually begins with an **abstract,** which is a clear concise summary of a study. Abstracts range from 100 to 250 words and usually include the study purpose, design, setting, sample size, major results, and conclusions. The American Psychological Association (APA, 2010) has provided guidance for developing quality abstracts. Researchers hope that their abstracts will convey the findings from their study concisely and capture your attention so that you will read the entire report. Usually, four major content sections of a research report follow the abstract: introduction, methods, results, and discussion. Box 2.2 outlines the content covered in each of these sections; Chan and colleagues (2016) developed the following clear, concise abstract in Research Example 2.11, which conveys the critical information about their quasi-experimental study and includes the study's clinical relevance.

RESEARCH EXAMPLE 2.11

Abstract

Research Study Excerpt

Purpose

To explore the fatigue self-management behaviors and factors associated with effectiveness of these behaviors in patients with advanced cancer.

Design

Prospective longitudinal interviewer-administered survey.

Methods

Patients were surveyed on three occasions: at baseline, four weeks, and eight weeks.

Findings

The participants reported moderate levels of fatigue at baseline and maintained moderate levels at four and eight weeks. On average, participants consistently used about nine behaviors at each time point. Factors significantly associated with higher levels of perceived effectiveness of fatigue self-management behaviors were higher self-efficacy, higher educational level, and lower levels of depressive symptoms.

Conclusions

The findings of this study demonstrate that patients with cancer, even those with advanced disease, still want and are able to use a number of behaviors to control their fatigue. Self-management interventions that aim to enhance self-efficacy and address any concurrent depressive symptoms have the potential to reduce fatigue severity.

Implications for Nursing

Nurses are well positioned to play a key role in supporting patients in their fatigue self-management. (Chan et al., 2016, p. 762)

BOX 2.2 MAJOR SECTIONS OF A RESEARCH REPORT

Introduction

- Statement of the problem, with background and significance
- Statement of the purpose
- Brief literature review
- Identification of the framework
- Identification of the research objectives, questions, or hypotheses (if applicable)

Methods

- Identification of the research design
- Description of the intervention (if applicable)
- Description of the sample and setting
- Description of the methods of measurement
- Discussion of the data collection process

Results

- Description of the data analysis procedures
- Presentation of results in tables, figures, or narrative organized by the purpose(s) and/or objectives, questions, or hypotheses

Discussion

- Discussion of major findings
- Identification of the limitations
- Presentation of conclusions
- Implications of the findings for nursing practice
- Recommendations for further research

Introduction Section

The introduction section of a research report identifies the nature and scope of the problem being investigated and provides a case for the conduct of the study. You should be able to identify the significance of conducting the study. Chan and colleagues (2016) identified cancer-related fatigue as a distressing symptom that occurs in approximately three-fourths of all cancer patients. Fatigue is debilitating and reduces the quality of life of these patients. The knowledge of the pathophysiology and causes of fatigue have improved, but the management of cancer-related fatigue has not. The purpose of this study addressed this area of concern.

Depending on the type of research report, the literature review and framework may be in separate sections or part of the introduction. The literature review documents the current knowledge of the problem, including what is known and not known, and provides a basis for the study purpose. For example, Chan et al. (2016) synthesized studies in the background section of their report. The literature review focused on the areas of pharmacological and nonpharmacological strategies to manage fatigue, such as sleep hygiene, conserving energy, and exercise.

A research report should include a framework, but only about half of the published studies identify one. Chan and colleagues (2016) clearly identified the self and family management framework proposed by Grey, Knafl, and McCorkle (2006) to guide their study of fatigue and self-management behaviors. This framework is reflective of and consistent with Bandura's (1977) self-efficacy theory. The relationships in the framework provide a basis for the formulation of hypotheses to be tested in quasi-experimental and experimental studies.

Investigators often end the introduction by identifying the objectives, questions, or hypotheses that they used to direct the study. Because this is a descriptive correlational study, Chan et al. (2016, p. 763) posed the following questions at the end of their literature review:

- "What are the management strategies that patients choose to use (i.e., patient preferences)?
- How effective are these strategies from the perspective of the patient?
- What are the factors associated with the effectiveness of these strategies?"

Methods Section

The methods section of a research report describes how the study was conducted and usually includes the study design, intervention (if appropriate), sample, setting, measurement methods, and data collection process (see Box 2.2). This section of the report needs to be presented in enough detail so that readers can critically appraise the adequacy of the study methods to produce credible findings.

Chan and colleagues (2016) provided extensive coverage of their study methodology. The design was clearly identified as a prospective longitudinal, interviewer-administered survey. The sample, setting, and survey tools were detailed, including the schedule for surveying the participants. Institutional approval for the conduct of this study and the consent of the participants were also discussed.

Results Section

The results section includes the outcomes from the statistical analyses and their significance. The researchers identify the statistical analyses conducted to address the purpose or each objective, question, or hypothesis and present the results in tables, figures, or narrative of the report (see Box 2.2; Grove & Cipher, 2017). Focusing more on the summary of the study results and their significance than on the statistical values can help reduce the confusion that may be caused by the numbers.

Chan and colleagues' (2016) results section included a description of the sample, and sample characteristics were presented in a table. The study results were organized by the study variables of fatigue severity, fatigue frequency, and the effectiveness and self-efficacy of self-management behaviors. The researchers extended their analysis to include predictive factors of perceived effectiveness of self-management behaviors.

Discussion Section

The discussion section ties together the other sections of the research report and gives them meaning. This section includes the major findings, limitations of the study, conclusions drawn from the findings, implications of the findings for nursing, and suggestions for further research (see Box 2.2).

Chan and associates (2016) discussed their findings in detail and compared and contrasted them with the findings of previous studies. They also presented their study limitations; all the participants had known metastatic cancer, but were fairly robust and had a high performance status at the beginning of the study while they were concurrently receiving chemotherapy. A portion of study participants were lost to follow-up over the course of the study because they became too ill and could no longer participate. Known risk factors for fatigue in cancer patients—anemia, cachexia, weight loss, and certain chemotherapeutic agents—were not measured because of patient burden and the exploratory nature of the study. The tool used for data collection was developed for this study by the authors, so it had no known reliability and validity.

The conclusions drawn from a research project can be useful in at least three different ways. First, you can implement the intervention tested in a study with your patients to improve their care and promote a positive health outcome. Second, reading research reports might change your view of a patient's situation or provide greater insight into the situation. Finally, studies heighten your awareness of the problems experienced by patients and assist you in assessing and working toward solutions for these problems. Chan et al. (2016) provided relevant conclusions, implications for practice, and suggestions for further study that were highlighted in the study abstract.

References Section

The reference section or list includes the studies, theories, and methodology resources that provided a basis for the conduct of the study. These sources provide an opportunity to read about the research problem in greater depth. We strongly encourage you to read Chan and colleagues' (2016) article to identify the sections of a research report and examine the content in each of these sections. They detailed a rigorously conducted descriptive correlational study, provided findings that are supportive of previous research, and identified conclusions that provide sound evidence to direct the care of cancer patients with fatigue.

Tips for Reading Research Reports

When you start reading research reports, you may be overwhelmed by the new terms and complex information presented. We hope that you will not be discouraged but will see the challenge of examining new knowledge generated through research. You probably will need to read the report slowly two or three times. You can also use the glossary at the end of this book to review the definitions of unfamiliar terms. We recommend that you read the abstract first and then the discussion section of the report. This approach will enable you to determine the relevance of the findings to you personally and to your practice. Initially, your focus should be on research reports that you believe can provide relevant information for your practice.

Reading a research report requires the use of a variety of critical thinking skills, such as skimming, comprehending, and analyzing, to facilitate an understanding of the study (Wilkinson, 2012). **Skimming a research report** involves quickly reviewing the source to gain a broad overview of the content. Try this approach. First, familiarize yourself with the title, and check the author's name. Next, scan the abstract or introduction and discussion sections. Knowing the findings of the study will provide you with a standard for evaluating the rest of the article. Then read the major headings and perhaps one or two sentences under each heading. Finally, reexamine the conclusions and implications for practice from the study. Skimming enables you to make a preliminary judgment about the value of a source and whether to read the report in depth.

Comprehending a research report requires that the entire study be read carefully. During this reading, focus on understanding major concepts and the logical flow of ideas within the study. You may wish to highlight information about the researchers, such as their education, current positions, and any funding they received for the study. As you read the study, steps of the research process might also be highlighted. Record any notes in the margin so that you can easily identify the problem, purpose, framework, major variables, study design, treatment, sample, measurement methods, data collection process, analysis techniques, results, and study outcomes. Also, record any creative ideas or questions that you have in the margin of the report.

We encourage you to highlight the parts of the article that you do not understand, and ask your instructor or other nurse researchers for clarification. Your greatest difficulty in reading the research report probably will be in understanding the statistical analyses (see Chapter 11). Basically, you must identify the particular statistics used, results from each statistical analysis, and meaning of the results. Statistical analyses describe variables, examine relationships among variables, and/or determine differences among groups. The study purpose or specific objectives, questions, or hypotheses indicate whether the focus is on description, relationships, or differences (Grove & Cipher, 2017). Therefore you need to link each analysis technique to its results and then to the study purpose or objectives, questions, or hypotheses presented in the study.

The final reading skill, **analyzing a research report,** involves determining the value of the report's content. Break the content of the report into parts, and examine the parts in depth for accuracy, completeness, uniqueness of information, and organization. Note whether the steps of the research process build logically on each other or whether steps are missing or incomplete. Examine the discussion section of the report to determine whether the researchers have provided a critical argument for using the study findings in practice. Using the skills of skimming, comprehending, and analyzing while reading research reports will increase your comfort with studies, allow you to become an informed consumer of research, and expand your knowledge for making changes in practice. These skills for reading research reports are essential for conducting a comprehensive critical appraisal of a study.

PRACTICE READING A QUASI-EXPERIMENTAL STUDY

Knowing the sections of the research report—Introduction, Methods, Results, and Discussion (see Box 2.2)—provides a basis for reading research reports of quantitative studies. You can apply the critical thinking skills of skimming, comprehending, and analysis to your reading of the quasi-experimental study provided here. Being able to read research reports and identify the steps of the research process (see Fig. 2.2) should enable you to conduct an initial critical appraisal of a report. Throughout this text, you'll find boxes, entitled "Critical Appraisal Guidelines," which provide questions that you will want to consider in your critical appraisal of various research elements or steps. This chapter concludes with initial critical appraisals of a quasi-experimental study using the guidelines provided.

The purpose of quasi-experimental research is to examine cause and effect relationships among selected independent and dependent variables. Researchers conduct quasi-experimental studies in nursing to determine the effects of nursing interventions (independent variables) on patient outcomes (dependent variables; Shadish et al., 2002). George, Locasto, Pyo, and Cline (2017) conducted a quasi-experimental study to compare nurse student outcomes from a dedicated education unit model with a traditional clinical education model. The steps for this study are illustrated in Research Example 2.12, with brief excerpts from the research report.

RESEARCH EXAMPLE 2.12

Steps of the Research Process in a Quasi-Experimental Study

Research Study Excerpts

1. Introduction

Research Problem

There is growing awareness that current clinical education models may not provide the most effective learning experiences for pre-licensure nursing students... Nurse educators and their clinical partners have been challenged to improve the quality and capacity of clinical education. In 2010, several landmark publications provided support for the transformation in nursing education. The first was 'Educating Nurses: A Call for Radical Transformation' (Benner et al., 2010) and another was 'The Future of Nursing: Leading Change, Advancing Health' (IOM [Institute of Medicine], 2010)... The development of Dedicated Education Units (DEUs) can be linked to the call for transformation of nursing education. Although several models of DEUs are currently in use, most DEUs have a central concept that a more comprehensive collaboration between the nurse educator, staff nurse, and student provides the optimal clinical learning environment. (George et al., 2017, p. 49)

Research Purpose

The purpose of this quantitative, quasi-experimental study was to compare student outcomes from the traditional clinical education (TEU) model with those from the DEU model. (George et al., 2017, p. 48)

Literature Review

The literature review in the study by George et al. (2017) included relevant and current studies that summarized what is known and not known about the impact of DEUs on students' self-efficacy. The sources were current; and publication dates ranged from 1999 to 2014, with most of the studies published in the last 5 years. The study was accepted for publication on February 10, 2017 and published in the March 2017 issue. George et al. (2017, p. 48) summarized the current knowledge about the effect of DEUs on nursing student self-efficacy by stating that "Although the DEU has shown initial promise related to satisfaction with the teaching/learning environment, limited studies have examined student outcomes related to DEU participation beyond student satisfaction."

Framework

George and colleagues (2017) used the Bandura self-efficacy theory to explain the concepts and relationships involved in their study.

Self-efficacy is considered an important outcome of nursing education because nurses with high self-efficacy have been linked to the following abilities: setting appropriate goals, trying different strategies, persevering to complete a task, and making an easier transition from student to nursing professional. (George et al., 2017, p. 50)

Hypothesis Testing

The researchers stated the null hypothesis:

there will be no difference in the self-efficacy scores of students who participate in a DEU clinical education model when compared with those students who participate in a TEU model. (George et al., 2017, p 49)

Continued

RESEARCH EXAMPLE 2.12—cont'd

Variables

The independent variable was the DEU, and the dependent variable was student self-efficacy scores. Only the DEU and self-efficacy scores were defined with conceptual and operational definitions. The conceptual definitions were derived from the study framework, and the operational definitions were derived from the methods section of this study.

Independent Variable: Dedicated Education Unit

Conceptual Definition: "In the DEU, staff nurses and nurse educators form a partnership that combines the expertise of both with a focus on using evidence-based clinical and educational practices to create the most effective clinical learning environment for the student" (George et al., 2017, p. 48).

Operational Definition: The DEU implemented in this study is based on the University of Portland's model and involves a "comprehensive collaboration between the nurse educator, staff nurse, and student to provide an optimal clinical learning environment" (George et al., 2017, p. 49).

Dependent Variable: Self-Efficacy

Conceptual Definition: Self-efficacy is a reflection of the students' belief that they are able to carry out a course of action that will produce the desired results. Nurses with high self-efficacy have been linked to the achievement of desirable skills and abilities in professional nursing.

Operational Definition: Self-efficacy was measured using the 10-item Adapted Self-Efficacy Scale (ASE).

2. Methods

Design

The design was a convenience sample, two-group, pretest/posttest quasi-experimental design. Students who consented to participate in the study were assigned to the intervention group DEUs or the control group TEUs. Both groups completed the ASE before and after completion of their clinical rotations.

Sample

A convenience sample of nursing students enrolled in a 4-year baccalaureate program was recruited. Students were not randomly assigned to DEU or TEU, but the department's clinical placement policy was followed, allowing for student preferences when possible. After clinical assignments had been made, information about the study was presented to all students, and informed consent was obtained. The sample included 193 students (58 in the DEU group and 132 in the TEU group), who completed both the preclinical and postclinical education ASE.

Intervention

The intervention in this study was the DEU. In a DEU,

> *staff nurses and nurse educators form a partnership that combines the expertise of both with a focus on using evidence based clinical and educational practices to create the most effective clinical learning environment for the student. In the DEU model, a student is typically partnered with a staff nurse who takes on the role of Clinical Instructor. Academic educator, called the Clinical Faculty coordinator, partner with the clinical instructor and the student to link classroom concepts with the practicum activities and provide guidance for the educational process.* (George et al., 2017, p. 48)

Measurement

Preclinical and postclinical self-efficacy scores were measured using the 10-item ASE scale. The ASE scale was adapted from the General Self-Efficacy Scale developed by Schwarzer and Jerusalem (1995), with permission to include only essential items and content related to undergraduate clinical education. The items on the ASE scale are presented in the George et al. article (2017, p. 51). The reliability values for this scale pretests and posttests were strong, indicating high reliability for this adapted scale.

Data Collection

The participants' demographic information was collected after the students signed the informed consent. The ASE scale was administered before attending any clinical and after all clinical had been completed.

3. Results

All study participants were assessed for self-efficacy at the start of the study, and no significant difference was found between the students in the DEU versus the TEU group. However, after the completion of the clinical rotation, the students in the DEU group, who received the intervention, had significantly higher self-efficacy scores than those in the TEU group.

4. Discussion

The study findings support the notion that students who are placed in a DEU will experience a greater benefit in terms of increased self-efficacy when compared with students who are placed in a traditional clinical site. The study findings suggest that students benefit most when faculty and clinical nursing staff work together to promote the self-efficacy of nursing students in a dedicated educational unit. Of particular importance is the development of self-efficacy among students, because this trait has been shown to be associated with persons more likely to take on challenging tasks, work harder to accomplish those tasks, and persist longer in the face of opposition (Gore, 2006). These qualities are important to foster in novice nursing students.

Limitations of this study are those common to many studies examining teaching methodologies. The study was conducted at a single school, even though there were multiple DEUs within the potential clinical sites to which the students could be assigned. Students were not randomly assigned to a DEU or TEU and did have the opportunity to self-select a unit for their clinical experience based on other factors, such as geographic convenience. Future studies could focus on overcoming the limitations of this study (lack of randomization, single school) to strengthen and test the findings in a broader population, thus moving these findings toward generalizable knowledge that could be applied to other schools and programs.

CRITICAL APPRAISAL GUIDELINES

Quantitative Research

The following questions are important in conducting an initial critical appraisal of a quantitative research report:

1. What type of quantitative study was conducted—descriptive, correlational, quasi-experimental, or experimental?
2. Can you identify the following sections in the research report—Introduction, Methods, Results, and Discussion—as identified in Box 2.2?
3. Were the steps of the study clearly identified? Fig. 2.2 identifies the steps of the quantitative research process.
4. Were any of the steps of the research process missing?

When we examine the example research report provided as an example, George et al. (2017) explicitly identified their study as quasi-experimental. There were two groups of study participants (nursing students) who were very similar. One group of students was exposed to the intervention of the study (DEU), and the other group of students was exposed to a traditional clinical education experience (TEU). Within the body of the report, there are clearly identified portions of the manuscript, which describe the introduction, methods, results, and conclusions of their study. The introduction section in this manuscript includes a section on the background and significance of the problem that is being studied and brief literature reviews related to both the idea of a dedicated education unit and self-efficacy. The authors discussed their results in detail thoroughly, as well as the methods and statistical analyses. Although their prognostications about future research and broader implications of their finding were circumspect and modest, no steps of the research process were missed.

KEY POINTS

- Quantitative research is the traditional research approach in nursing; it includes descriptive, correlational, quasi-experimental, and experimental types of studies.
- Basic, or bench, research is a scientific investigation that involves the pursuit of knowledge for knowledge's sake or for the pleasure of learning and finding truth.
- Applied, or practical, research is a scientific investigation conducted to generate knowledge that will directly influence or improve clinical practice.
- Conducting quantitative research requires rigor and control.
- A comparison of the problem-solving process, nursing process, and research process shows the similarities and differences in these processes and provides a basis for understanding the research process.
- The quantitative research process involves conceptualizing a research project, planning and implementing that project, and communicating the findings. The steps of the quantitative research process have been briefly introduced in this chapter.
- The research problem is an area of concern in which there is a gap in the knowledge needed for nursing practice. The research purpose is generated from the problem and identifies the specific goal or focus of the study.
- The review of relevant literature is conducted to generate a picture of what is known and not known about a particular problem and provides a rationale for why the study needs to be conducted.
- The study framework is the theoretical basis for a study that guides the development of the study and enables the researcher to link the findings to nursing's body of knowledge.
- Research objectives, questions, and/or hypotheses are formulated to bridge the gap between the more abstractly stated research problem and purpose and the study design and plan for data collection and analysis.
- Study variables are concepts at various levels of abstraction that are measured, manipulated, or controlled in a study.
- Research design is a blueprint for conducting a study that maximizes control over factors that could interfere with the study's desired outcomes.
- The population is all the elements that meet certain criteria for inclusion in a study. A sample is a subset of the population that is selected for a particular study; the members of a sample are the subjects or study participants.
- Measurement is the process of assigning numerical values to objects, events, or situations in accord with some rule. Methods of measurement are identified to measure each of the variables in a study.
- The data collection process involves the precise and systematic gathering of information relevant to the research purpose or the objectives, questions, or hypotheses of a study.
- Data analyses are conducted to reduce, organize, and give meaning to the data and address the research purpose and/or objectives, questions, or hypotheses.
- Research outcomes include the findings, limitations, generalization of findings, conclusions, implications for nursing, and suggestions for further research.

- The content of a research report includes six parts—abstract, introduction, methods, results, discussion, and references.
- Reading research reports involves skimming, comprehending, and analyzing the report.
- The guidelines for conducting an initial critical appraisal of a quantitative study are provided.
- The steps of a quasi-experimental study are identified, followed by an initial critical appraisal of this study.

REFERENCES

American Psychological Association (APA). (2010). *Publication manual of the American Psychological Association* (6th ed.). Washington, DC: APA.

Aveyard, H. (2014). *Doing a literature review in health and social care: A practical guide* (3rd ed.). New York, NY: McGraw Hill Education Open University Press.

Bandura, A. (1977). Self-efficacy: Toward a unifying theory of behavioral change. *Psychological Review, 84*(2), 191–215.

Benner, P., Sutphen, M., Leonard, V., & Day, I. (2010). *Educating nurses: A call for radical transformation.* San Francisco, CA: Jossey-Bass.

Brown, S. J. (2018). *Evidence-based nursing: The research-practice connection* (4th ed.). Sudbury, MA: Jones & Bartlett.

Campbell, D. T., & Stanley, J. C. (1963). *Experimental and quasi-experimental designs for research.* Chicago, IL: Rand McNally.

Chan, R. J., Yates, P., & McCarthy, A. L. (2016). Fatigue self-management behaviors in patients with advanced cancer: A prospective longitudinal survey. *Oncology Nursing Forum, 43*(6), 762–771.

Chinn, P. L., & Kramer, M. K. (2015). *Knowledge development in nursing: Theory and process* (9th ed.). St. Louis, MO: Elsevier Mosby.

Creswell, J. W. (2014). *Research design: Qualitative, quantitative, and mixed methods approaches* (4th ed.). Thousand Oaks, CA: Sage.

Eymard, A. S., & Altmiller, G. (2016). Teaching nursing students the importance of treatment fidelity in intervention research: Students as interventionists. *Journal of Nursing Education, 55*(5), 288–291.

Finch, M., Griffin, K., & Pacala, J. T. (2017). Reduced healthcare use and apparent savings with passive home monitoring technology: A pilot study. *Journal of the American Geriatrics Society*, https://doi.org/10.1111/jgs.14892.

Fisher, R. A. (1935). *The designs of experiments. New York.* NY: Hafner.

George, L. E., Locasto, L. W., Pyo, K. A., & Cline, T. W. (2017). Effect of the dedicated education unit on nursing student self-efficacy: A quasi-experimental research study. *Nurse Education in Practice, 23*(1), 48–53.

Gore, P. A., Jr. (2006). Academic self-efficacy as a predictor of college outcomes: Two incremental validity studies. *Journal of Career Assessment, 14*(1), 92–115.

Gray, J. R., Grove, S. K., & Sutherland, S. (2017). *The practice of nursing research: Appraisal, synthesis, and generation of evidence* (8th ed.). St. Louis, MO: Elsevier.

Grey, M., Knafl, K., & McCorkle, R. (2006). A framework for the study of self- and family management of chronic conditions. *Nursing Outlook, 54*(5), 278–286.

Grove, S. K., & Cipher, D. J. (2017). *Statistics for nursing research: A workbook for evidence-based practice* (2nd ed.). St. Louis, MO: Elsevier.

Haley, W. E., Levine, E. G., Brown, S. L., & Bartolucci, A. A. (1987). Stress, appraisal, coping, and social support as predictors of adaptational outcome among dementia caregivers. *Psychology and Aging, 2*(4), 323.

Hertzog, M. A. (2008). Considerations in determining sample size for pilot studies. *Research in Nursing & Health, 31*(2), 180–191.

Institute of Medicine (IOM) (2010). *The future of nursing: Leading change, advancing health.* Washington, DC: The National Academies Press.

Kaplan, A. (1964). *The conduct of inquiry: Methodology for behavioral science.* San Francisco, CA: Chandler.

Kerlinger, F. N., & Lee, H. B. (2000). *Foundations of behavioral research* (4th ed.). Fort Worth, TX: Harcourt.

Kolanowski, A., Bossen, A., Hill, N., Guzman-Velez, E., & Litaker, M. (2012). Factors associated with sustained attention during an activity intervention in persons with dementia. *Dementia and Geriatric Cognitive Disorders, 33*(4), 233–239.

Liao, L. Y., Chung, W. S., & Chen, K. M. (2017). Free radicals and antioxidant enzymes in older adults after regular senior elastic band exercising: An experimental randomized controlled pilot study. *Journal of Advanced Nursing, 73*(1), 108–111.

Melnyk, B. M., Gallagher-Ford, E., & Fineout-Overholt, E. (2017). *Implementing evidence-based practice competencies in healthcare: A practical guide for improving quality, safety, & outcomes*. Indianapolis, IN: Sigma Theta Tau International.

Moon, H., Rote, S., & Beaty, J. A. (2017). Caregiving setting and Baby Boomer caregiver stress processes: Findings from the National Study of Caregiving (NSOC). *Geriatric Nursing, 38*(1), 57–62.

Murphy, S. L., & Gutman, S. A. (2012). Intervention fidelity: A necessary aspect of intervention effectiveness studies. *American Journal of Occupational Therapy, 66*(4), 387–388.

National Human Genome Research Institute (NHGRI). (2017). *An overview of the division of intramural research*. Retrieved May 26, 2017, from http://www.genome.gov/10001634.

National Institute of Nursing Research (NINR). (2016). *The NINR Strategic Plan: Advancing science, improving lives*. Retrieved February 20, 2017, from https://www.ninr.nih.gov/sites/www.ninr.nih.gov/files/NINR_StratPlan2016_reduced.pdf.

Porter, T. M. (2004). *Karl Pearson: The scientific life in a statistical age*. Oxfordshire, United Kingdom: Princeton University Press.

Quality and Safety Education for Nurses (QSEN). (2017). *Pre-licensure knowledge, skills, and attitudes (KSAs)*. Retrieved January 16, 2018, from http://qsen.org/competencies/pre-licensure-ksas/.

Schwarzer, R., & Jerusalem, M. (1995). Generalized self-efficacy scale. In J. Weinman, S. Wright, & M. Johnson (Eds.), *Measures in health psychology: A user's portfolio, causal and control beliefs* (pp. 35–37). Windsor, UK: NFER-NELSON.

Shadish, W. R., Cook, T. D., & Campbell, D. T. (2002). *Experimental and quasi-experimental designs for generalized causal inference*. Chicago, IL: Rand McNally.

Sherwood, G., & Barnsteiner, J. (2017). *Quality and safety in nursing: A competency approach to improving outcomes* (2nd ed.). Ames, IA: Wiley-Blackwell.

Straus, S. E., Glasziou, P., Richardson, W. S., Rosenberg, W., & Haynes, R. B. (2011). *Evidence-based medicine: How to practice and teach EBM* (5th ed.). Edinburgh: Churchill Livingstone Elsevier.

Wacker, M. J., Touchberry, C. D., Silswal, N., Brotto, L., Elmore, C. J., Bonewald, L. F., et al. (2016). Skeletal muscle, but not cardiovascular function, is altered in a mouse model of autosomal recessive hypophosphatemic rickets. *Frontiers in Physiology, 7*, 173. https://doi.org/10.3389/fphys.2016.00173.

Waltz, C. F., Strickland, O. L., & Lenz, E. R. (2017). *Measurement in nursing and health research* (5th ed.). New York, NY: Springer Publishing Company.

Wethington, E., & Burgio, L. D. (2015). Translational research on caregiving: Missing links in the translation process. In E. Wethington, & L. D. Burgio (Eds.), *Family caregiving in the new normal*, (pp. 193–210). https://doi.org/10.1016/b978-0-12-417046-9.00011-8.

Wilkinson, J. M. (2012). *Nursing process and critical thinking* (5th ed.). Upper Saddle River, NJ: Pearson.

Because of funding changes, the Agency for Healthcare Research and Quality (AHRQ) National Guideline Clearinghouse website was scheduled for decommissioning as of July 16, 2018. For more information, go to https://www.ahrq.gov/.

CHAPTER

3

Introduction to Qualitative Research

Jennifer R. Gray

CHAPTER OVERVIEW

LEARNING OUTCOMES

After completing this chapter, you should be able to:

1. Identify the steps of the qualitative research process.
2. Describe four qualitative research designs—phenomenological research, grounded theory research, ethnography, and exploratory-descriptive qualitative research—and their intended outcomes.
3. Identify differences in sampling, recruitment, data collection, and data analysis for quantitative and qualitative research.
4. Describe strategies used by qualitative researchers to increase the credibility and transferability of their findings.
5. Critically appraise qualitative studies for application to practice.

Qualitative research is a systematic approach used to describe experiences and situations from the perspective of persons in the situation. The researcher analyzes the words of the participant(s), finds meaning in the words, and provides a description of the experience that promotes deeper understanding of the experience (Creswell & Poth, 2018). Because caring about people and wanting to help them are core nursing values, you may find qualitative research valuable for the insights it provides into the lives and circumstances of your patients. Qualitative research can generate rich descriptions of the experiences of patients and families that increase nurses' understanding of the best ways to intervene and be supportive (Powers, 2015). As a result, qualitative findings make a distinct contribution to evidence-based practice (Hall & Roussel, 2017).

This chapter includes the elements of the qualitative research process and presents an overview of four qualitative designs commonly conducted in nursing: phenomenological research, grounded theory research, ethnographic research, and exploratory-descriptive qualitative research.

An example of each type of study is described. You are introduced to some of the more common methods used to collect, analyze, and interpret qualitative data. This content provides a background for you to use in reading and comprehending published qualitative studies, critically appraising qualitative studies, and applying study findings to your practice.

IDENTIFYING THE STEPS OF THE QUALITATIVE RESEARCH PROCESS

Qualitative research is conducted in natural settings to learn about a topic from the perspectives of the participants. The researcher is the key research instrument, collecting and analyzing textual and experiential data (Creswell & Poth, 2018). Other characteristics of qualitative research include multiple sources of data, emergent designs, and reflexivity. Box 3.1 displays several characteristics of qualitative research.

The **qualitative research process** follows the same general steps as the quantitative research process, but is based on different philosophical values and assumptions (Table 3.1). Qualitative researchers value unique individual perceptions and perspectives in understanding the meaning of a phenomenon to those who have experienced it. Instead of seeking information about a well-defined problem from a group (sample) to generalize to a larger group (population), as in quantitative research, qualitative researchers seek information about a less defined research problem by obtaining multiple individual perspectives to develop a deeper understanding of the phenomenon. The steps of the qualitative research process are interconnected, with each one being influenced by the previous step and affecting subsequent steps.

The research problem is a gap in knowledge. The patient or practice concerns that can best be addressed by qualitative research are those about which very little is known. Even for problems that have been studied, what may be missing is the perspective of those affected. Creswell and Poth (2018, p. 52) note that qualitative research problems are "emotion-laden, close to people, and practical." For example, Weyant, Clukey, Roberts, and Henderson (2017) conducted a qualitative study on the use of restraints in intensive care. As they interviewed patients who had been restrained while they were mechanically ventilated and interviewed their family members, the researchers asked the participants to identify actions of the nurses that were seen as helpful. The researchers identified the gap in knowledge to be the lack of published literature on "the perceptions of patients undergoing mechanical ventilation and their families who spend time in the intensive care unit" (Weyant et al., 2017, p. 112). The study purpose was to "explore perceptions of nurses' caring behaviors among intubated patients and their family members" (Weyant et al., 2017, p. 111). The purpose should be and was congruent with the research problem.

BOX 3.1 CHARACTERISTICS OF QUALITATIVE RESEARCH

Natural setting
Context dependent
Researcher as instrument
Multiple sources of data
Inductive and deductive analysis
Reflexivity
Focuses on participants' perspective
Emergent and evolving design
Holistic, complex description

Adapted from Creswell, J., & Poth, C. (2018). *Qualitative inquiry and research design: Choosing among five approaches* (4th ed.). Thousand Oaks, CA: Sage, p. 45.

TABLE 3.1 SIMILARITIES AND DIFFERENCES IN THE QUANTITATIVE AND QUALITATIVE RESEARCH PROCESSES

QUANTITATIVE RESEARCH PROCESS	QUALITATIVE RESEARCH PROCESS
Identify a Research Problem	
Building on previous knowledge, a gap in knowledge is identified.	Little may be known about the topic; qualitative approach used to explore and describe.
Formulate the Research Purpose	
Should be congruent with the research problem.	Should be congruent with the research problem.
Identify the Study Methodology	
Selected quantitative methodology should be implied in the purpose.	Selected type of qualitative study should be implied in the purpose.
Review the Literature	
Extensive review should be conducted to ensure that questions and/or hypotheses reflect what is known and not known.	Limited review of the literature; extent will vary depending on qualitative design; researcher does not want to be biased by the literature.
Describe the Theoretical Framework	
Researcher may or may not make the framework explicit.	Researcher may use a philosophy instead of a framework or may not select a framework to remain open to participants' perspectives.
State the Research Objectives, Questions, Hypotheses, and Procedures	
The researcher may use any of these; when possible, she or he will state hypotheses based on what is known. Questions or hypotheses are set before data collection.	Researcher will use research objectives or questions. Hypotheses are not consistent with qualitative methods. Questions may evolve over the course of the study.
Define variables, conceptually and operationally.	No comparable step in qualitative research.
Specify procedures consistent with the study design. These may include a controlled setting and an intervention.	Specify how data will be collected (interview, observation, focus groups) in a natural setting; no intervention. Procedures may evolve.
Recruit a large sample of predetermined size.	Recruit purposive, network, and theoretical sampling methods, the size of which will not be predetermined. Size will depend on when saturation of the data occurs.
Collect numerical data.	Collect textual, verbal, visual, and sensory data.
Analyze data according to predetermined statistical analyses.	Analyze data using flexible and iterative steps of spending extended periods of time reading and processing the data.
Determine results and prepare tables and/or figures.	Determine results, which will vary according to qualitative approach (e.g., ethnography—a description of a culture; grounded theory—an emerging framework).
Present Results	
Concisely state outcomes of statistical analyses. Tables and figures may be used with limited narrative.	Provide a narrative of patterns or themes identified. Participant quotes from interviews or focus groups to support results may be used.
Discuss Findings	
Compare findings with previous research findings.	Compare findings with previous research findings.
Identify limitations.	Identify limitations.
State implications of the findings, including future research needed on the topic	State implications of the findings, including future research needed on the topic.

The next three steps in the qualitative research process—identifying a study design, reviewing the literature, and selecting a theoretical framework—are the same as they are in quantitative research, but with some modification (see Table 3.1). Researchers make decisions about the study design early in the process of developing a study. When the study purpose is written, the researcher has selected the design based on structuring the study in a way that allows the research gap to be addressed. Research designs for qualitative studies are more open and flexible than the designs used for quantitative study. The methods of a qualitative study may evolve over the course of the study (Creswell & Poth, 2018). Qualitative researchers view the step of reviewing the literature cautiously because they want to remain open to the insider's perspective. As a result, qualitative researchers may review the literature to identify the research problem, but may delay further literature review until after the data are collected. The type and extent of the early literature review may vary, depending on the research design being used (see Chapter 6).

Selecting a theoretical framework may or may not occur. For example, in grounded theory studies, the qualitative researcher is seeking to describe the social processes at work in an experience for the purpose of developing a beginning theory (Charmaz, 2014). Researchers using grounded theory methods usually do not select a theoretical framework. In other types of studies, such as exploratory-descriptive qualitative studies and ethnographic studies, researchers may select a theoretical framework to give structure to the study. Weyant et al. (2017) identified their study as phenomenological, which indicates the philosophical foundation. They did not, however, specify a theoretical framework, which is common for phenomenological studies. The literature review was very limited. However, what was reported in the article may not have represented all the literature that the researchers reviewed before the study. Some journals have page limits for articles, and researchers may summarize the literature to have adequate space in the article for the findings.

Determining the research objectives, questions, or hypotheses is the next step in the research process. Qualitative researchers may use objectives or questions to provide direction to the collection of the data (Creswell & Poth, 2018). Weyant et al. (2017, p. 112) identified their questions to be "How do family members of intubated and restrained patients in a cardiac intensive care unit perceive the care received from nurses? What do they identify as caring or not caring behaviors?"

Qualitative and quantitative research differ a great deal in the methods, results, and discussion sections of the research reports. The data collected by quantitative researchers for each variable will be numerical; in contrast, qualitative researchers collect data in the form of text and images, so identifying variables and defining them are inappropriate (see Table 3.1). The data collection methods should be consistent with the research problem and study purpose, a condition described by Creswell and Poth (2018) as **methodological congruence**. The data collection methods may evolve as the study progresses. For example, you may start with four broad interview questions. As you collect and analyze data, you identify a potential theme and add a question about the emerging theme to subsequent interviews. Weyant et al. (2017) described their methods that included transcribing the interviews they conducted with the previously ventilated patients and their families and analyzing the text of the transcript to identify caring behaviors.

The sampling step in the research process occurs in both quantitative and qualitative studies, but the characteristics of a quality sample for each type of research are different. Quantitative researchers ideally are able to recruit a large random sample so that the findings can be generalized to the target population. By conducting a power analysis, the researchers can determine the minimum sample size for a quantitative study. Because qualitative researchers want to understand the identified research problem from the perspective of the participants, they deliberately recruit fewer participants but ensure that each one has experience with the research topic or is living or working in a specific culture. Sample size may vary according to the study's qualitative method.

Phenomenological studies may need 10 or fewer participants if the topic is narrow and the participants provide adequate data (Creswell & Poth, 2018). Grounded theory studies may require more than 30 participants to ensure that adequate detail is available to develop a robust theory (Bolderston, 2012). Typically, sampling occurs until **saturation** is reached (Creswell & Poth, 2018), defined as when additional participants or data sources do not provide new information. Each participant provides rich data that allows the researcher to identify the participants' perspective and meaning of the phenomenon. Weyant et al. (2017, p. 112) reported that "data were collected until saturation of common themes was reached." They interviewed 14 patients and 8 family members. There is more information on sampling later in this chapter.

Data analysis occurs in both quantitative and qualitative studies. For quantitative studies, the numerical data are analyzed using formulas and statistical equations calculated by a computer program. The analysis of qualitative data is non-statistical, meaning that hypotheses are not tested in qualitative studies. In qualitative studies, the researcher's mind is the "program" that analyzes the data, notices patterns, identifies themes, and allows the meaning of the data to emerge. The researcher's mind inductively finds common elements and then thinks deductively, going back to the data to find more evidence to support the common element (Creswell & Poth, 2018). A computer program may be used during the data analysis process to keep a record of themes that the researcher finds and the decisions made during the study. Weyant et al. (2017) provided a list of interview questions for their study of caring behaviors as perceived by mechanically ventilated patients and provided a very brief description of how data were analyzed. "...any personal identifying information was removed and code letters were used to protect confidentiality. Data were collected until saturation of common themes was reached. Data were analyzed by using NVivo 9 qualitative research software (QSR International) (Weyant et al., 2017, p. 112).

For both types of research, the results of the study are presented in the research report. The presentation of quantitative results will be the outcomes of the statistical analysis, whereas the qualitative results are presented as rich descriptions, themes, or an emerging theory. In quantitative reports, numbers and statistical results are concisely presented. For qualitative studies, the results section may be very long because the researcher presents a theme and supports the theme with one or more quotes from the participants (see Table 3.1).

In the Weyant et al. (2017) study, five types of nursing behaviors were perceived as caring by patients who had been mechanically ventilated, and by their families. The caring behaviors included providing information, providing reassurance, demonstrating proficiency, being present, and giving guidance in a soothing tone of voice (Weyant et al., 2017). For each of these, the researchers provided quotes and exemplars from their interviews with patients and families.

The remaining steps of the research process are the same. During the step of interpreting the findings, the researchers compare what they found with what others have found and previously published in the literature (see Table 3.1). For example, Weyant et al. (2017) noted two other researchers who had found similar caring behaviors.

Quantitative and qualitative researchers identify study limitations and then discuss whether the findings can be generalized or applied to other groups. Generalizability is a desired outcome for quantitative studies when the sample is representative of the target populations. Applicability of the findings to similar individuals or transferability is the desired outcome for qualitative studies. The researchers also make recommendations for practice, when appropriate, and for future studies. The recommendations for future studies may include studies that would be designed to overcome the current study's limitations, expand the sample to other groups, or refine the data collected. In a few sentences, Weyant et al. (2017) stated the limitations, the extent of transferability, and recommendations for future studies in the following quote. "This study was conducted at 1 facility and in 1 kind of critical care setting.

Thus the transferability of the results is limited...future research is recommended at various institutions in critical care settings. Expansion on the findings of this study are needed to further build a body of knowledge related to caring behaviors in intensive care units" (p. 116).

QUALITATIVE RESEARCH APPROACHES

Phenomena are the conscious awareness of experiences that comprise the lives of humans (van Manen, 2017). An experience is considered unique to the individual, time, and context and qualitative researchers seek to describe a phenomenon from the perspective of the persons who have had the experience being studied (Cypress, 2015). Qualitative researchers recognize that people experience life from different perspectives because a person's thoughts, words, and actions are influenced by the past and present, as well as by the physical, psychological, and social contexts of the behavior or experience (Hoggan, Mälkki, & Finnegan, 2017). The findings from a qualitative study lead to an understanding of a phenomenon in a particular situation and are not generalized in the same way as a quantitative study. The **rigor** or strength of a qualitative study is the extent to which the identified meanings represent the perspectives of the participants accurately. Rigorous qualitative methods can facilitate the researcher to maintain an open perspective on the phenomenon.

Each of the four qualitative approaches is based on a philosophical orientation that influences the interpretation of the data. For each approach, whether phenomenology, grounded theory, ethnography, or exploratory-descriptive qualitative research, it is critical to understand the philosophy on which the method is based. Each approach is discussed in relation to its philosophical orientation and intended outcome. A study is provided to illustrate each qualitative research approach. Deciding which qualitative approach to use depends on the research question and purpose of the study (Creswell & Poth, 2018). Each of the studies will be critically appraised using the following guidelines for identifying and understanding the qualitative approaches.

CRITICAL APPRAISAL GUIDELINES

Qualitative Studies

1. What type of qualitative study was conducted: phenomenology, grounded theory, ethnography, or exploratory-descriptive qualitative research?
2. Was the outcome of the study as presented in the research report appropriate for the type of qualitative study conducted?
   a. Phenomenology—rich description of lived experience
   b. Grounded theory—theoretical description of social processes
   c. Ethnography—description of a culture, whether race/ethnic or an organization
   d. Exploratory-descriptive qualitative research—problem-solving answer to the research question
3. Can you identify the following sections in the research report: Introduction, Methods, Results, and Discussion?
4. Were the steps of the study clearly identified? Table 3.1 identifies the steps of the qualitative research process.
5. Were any of the steps of the research process missing?

Phenomenological Research

Philosophical Orientation

Phenomenology refers to both a philosophy and group of research methods congruent with the philosophy that guides the study of experiences or phenomena (Tuohy, Cooney, Dowling, Murphy,

& Sixmith, 2013). Phenomenologists view the person as integrated with the environment. The world shapes the person, and the person shapes the world. The broad research question that phenomenologists ask is, "What is this lived experience like?" (van Manen, 2017, p. 776). Through a phenomenological study, the researcher collects data from persons who have had the experience and seeks to create a composite of the essence of experience (Creswell & Poth, 2018).

Phenomenologists differ in their philosophical beliefs. Nursing phenomenological researchers usually base their study design on Husserl or Heidegger, two early philosophers in phenomenology. Each of these philosophical perspectives supports a specific type of phenomenological research.

Husserl's focus was on the phenomenon itself. The aim of the research is to "capture experience in its...essence, without interpreting, explaining, or theorizing" (van Manen, 2017, p. 775). The meaning-laden statements are analyzed to discover the structure within the phenomenon. Husserl's philosophy supports **descriptive phenomenological research,** whose purpose is to describe experiences as they are lived or, in phenomenological terms, to capture the "lived experience" of study participants. To describe lived experiences, according to Husserl, researchers must **bracket** or set aside their own biases and preconceptions to describe the phenomenon in a naïve way (Dowling & Cooney, 2012).

Heidegger argued that it was impossible to set aside one's preconceptions and understand the world naïvely. He believed that phenomenological researchers describe how participants have interpreted or given meaning to their experiences (Converse, 2012). The researchers then analyze the participants' interpretations of the experience, looking for the hidden meaning (Dowling & Cooney, 2012). **Interpretative phenomenological research,** consistent with Heidegger's philosophy, involves analyzing the data and presenting a rich word picture of the phenomenon, as interpreted by the researcher.

Hermeneutics is one type of interpretative phenomenological research method that is congruent with Heidegger's philosophical perspective and is being used by nurse researchers (Dowling & Cooney, 2012). Hermeneutics involves textual analysis that begins with a naïve reading of the texts (Flood, 2010). To read a text naïvely, the researcher consciously remains open to the participant's viewpoint. Transcripts of interviews and published documents are the texts analyzed by nurse researchers. From these naïve readings, the researcher identifies subthemes and themes that are examined in light of the study's research questions. As the text, themes, and relevant literature are integrated, a description of the phenomenon as interpreted is produced.

Phenomenology's Outcome

The purpose of phenomenological research is to provide a thorough description of a lived experience. Some researchers write a detailed rich description or an exemplar of the experience. Sometimes, the participants will have widely varying perspectives on the phenomena, and the researcher may develop two or more detailed descriptions of the lived experience.

A severe burn may radically change the course of an individual's life and affect all aspects of health. Abrams, Ogletree, Ratnapradipa, and Neumeister (2016) interviewed eight participants about the experience of surviving a major burn in their phenomenological study. Previous studies had explored specific long-term effects of burns such as psychological adjustment and vocational re-entry, but there was a lack of knowledge about how the interrelated aspects of health and stage in life affected survivors' postburn health. A phenomenological approach to the research problem allowed the participants to share their lived experiences of being a burn survivor. Excerpts of the study and related discussion are provided in Research Example 3.1.

RESEARCH EXAMPLE 3.1

Phenomenological Study

Research Study Excerpt

Introduction: *The individual implications of major burns are likely to affect the full spectrum of patients' physical, emotional, psychological, social, environmental, spiritual and vocational health. Yet, not all of the post-burn health implications are inevitably negative. Utilizing a qualitative approach, this heuristic phenomenological study explores the experiences and perceptions of early (ages 18–35) and midlife (ages 36–64) adults...*

Methods: *Participants were interviewed using semi-structured interview questions... Interview recordings were transcribed verbatim then coded line by line...Qualitative content analysis rendered three emergent health-related categories and associated themes that represented shared meanings within the participant sample. The category of "Physical Health" reflected the theme physical limitations, pain and sensitivity to temperature. Within the category of "Intellectual Health" were themes of insight, goal setting and self-efficacy, optimism and humor and within "Emotional Health" were the themes empathy and gratitude...*

Conclusions: *By exploring subjective experiences and perceptions of health shared through dialog with experienced burned persons, there are opportunities to develop a more complete picture of how holistic health may be affected by major burns that in turn could support future long-term rehabilitative trajectories of early and midlife adult burn patients.* (Abrams et al., 2016, p. 152)

The study purpose was to "explore the phenomenon of major burns on early and midlife adult survivors' holistic health" (Abrams et al., 2016, p. 153). Purposive sampling was used to recruit participants who met the inclusion criteria of an English-speaking individual, age 18–64 years, and survivor of a burn that covered a minimum of 20% of the total body surface area. Participants were sought who had been "discharged after their initial burn hospitalization at least 12 months prior to study interviews" (Abrams et al., 2016, p. 153). The researchers identified their study as a heuristic phenomenological study. According to the article, the label of 'heuristic' was added to acknowledge and incorporate the personal experience of the primary investigator, who was also a burn survivor.

As primary investigator, my interests in the positive and negative long-term bio-psycho-social implications of burns and resiliency of burn survivors have developed over a lifetime. Having sustained major burns as a child, I have lived my life with obvious burn scars and grafts on my face and upper extremities...there was early recognition by participants that I had personal experience with major burns. (Abrams et al., 2016, p. 159)

The data were collected through interviews at locations selected by the eight participants. Each participant was asked to identify a person who had been actively involved in the aftermath and recovery from the burn to provide corroborating information (network sampling; see Chapter 9). A total of 12 interviews (eight participants and four family members) were conducted that lasted 45 to 60 minutes. The verbatim transcripts of the interviews were mailed to the participants, who checked for accuracy of the transcripts. Additional data included the reflective journal entries of the primary investigator and the observations written following each interview. Data were coded and analyzed from the survivors' transcripts, with the family members' transcripts used for support.

The researchers increased the trustworthiness of their findings by "engaging family members as corroborating sources and member checking interview transcripts to triangulate data, as well as third-party review of categories and themes to support study findings" (Abrams et al., 2016, p. 160). **Triangulation** means that the researchers use at least two different perspectives to converge into a unique perspective on the topic. In this article, Abrams et al. (2016) combined and compared input from the participant and family member interviews, as well as the input from peers. Abrams et al. also noted the potential for bias because of the primary investigator being a burn survivor, but emphasized the benefit of "a level of candor and honesty...found between peers with a shared traumatic experience" (p. 160).

Content analysis revealed three categories of shared meanings. The researchers highlighted how the participants used humor to help others be more comfortable in social situations. Humor allowed the burn survivors to talk about their "burns without making others uncomfortable and/or being rejected" (Abrams et al., 2016, p. 157). Emotional health was revealed in the empathy and gratitude expressed by the participants.

The participants noted that they had experienced personal growth, became more sensitive to the difficulties of others, and developed empathy. Gratitude was described as being felt toward "family, community members, providers, and rescue personnel, with each group holding a place in participants' stories of survival" (Abrams et al., 2016, p. 160).

The findings were descriptions of the "lived experiences of challenge, adaptation, resilience and hope as participants worked to regain their health-based equilibrium following major burns" (Abrams et al., 2016, p. 158). The researchers provided a summary of the study findings, with implications for postburn care.

Critical Appraisal

Abrams et al. (2016) conducted an interpretative phenomenological study. The outcome, a thematic description of the lived experience of postburn health, was consistent with the qualitative approach used for the study. The key sections of the research report were clearly identified. As is common in phenomenological studies, a theoretical framework was not identified because the study was guided by the philosophy of phenomenology. The researchers did refer to Erikson's stages of development and indicated that the person's stage of development was introduced to different developmental challenges postburn. The literature review was integrated into the introduction, instead of being identified as a separate step of the research process. All other steps of the research process were clearly identified. The researchers acknowledged differences among the participants, with some demonstrating more self-efficacy and resilience than others. They also identified areas for future studies, such as functional and psychosocial aftereffects of burns and the impact of geographic location and availability of community resources on adaptation.

Grounded Theory Research

Grounded theory research is an inductive technique that emerged from the discipline of sociology. The term *grounded* means the theory developed from the research; in other words, the theory is grounded in the real world based on data provided by participants. Most scholars base the grounded theory methodology on symbolic interaction theory. George Herbert Mead (Mead, 1934), a social psychologist, developed symbolic interaction theory that explores how people define reality and how their beliefs are related to their actions. Reality is created by attaching meanings to situations. Meaning is expressed in symbols such as words, religious objects, patterns of behavior, and clothing. These symbolic meanings are the basis for actions and interactions. However, symbolic meanings are different for each individual, and we cannot completely know the symbolic meanings for another individual. In social life, meanings are shared by groups and are communicated to new members through socialization processes. Group life is based on consensus and shared meanings. Interaction may lead to redefining a meaning or constructing new meanings. The grounded theory researcher seeks to understand the interaction between self and group from the perspective of those involved and, from that understanding, develop a theory of the interaction or social processes (Creswell & Poth, 2018).

Grounded theory has been used most frequently to study areas in which little previous research has been conducted and to gain a new viewpoint in familiar areas of research. Through their interviews to understand the perspectives of persons who were dying, Glaser and Strauss (1967) developed grounded theory research as a method and published a book describing it as a qualitative method. Nurses were attracted to the method because of its applicability to the life experiences of persons with health problems and its potential for developing explanations of human behavior (Wuerst, 2012). Nurse researchers continue to use grounded theory methods to study a wide range of topics, such as living with the choice of resettlement from the perspective of Iraqi refugees (Davenport, 2017), multidisciplinary rehabilitation for patients with fibromyalgia (Rasmussen, Amris, & Rydahl-Hanson, 2017), and how nurses in pediatric palliative care deal with their own emotions (Erikson & Davies, 2017).

Intended Outcome

Fully developed grounded theory studies result in theoretical frameworks with relational statements between concepts. Some grounded theorists provide a diagram displaying the interactions among the social processes that were identified. Others describe the concepts and relationships through a narrative description.

Medical errors have been found to be the third leading cause of death in the United States (Makary & Daniel, 2016). Unfortunately, nurses were responsible for some of these errors. Koehn, Ebright, and Draucker (2016) developed a grounded theory from interviews with nurses who had made an error in patient care. Their study identified stages through which nurses moved as they realized an error had been made and began to deal with the consequences. Research Example 3.2 is a description of their study.

RESEARCH EXAMPLE 3.2

Grounded Theory Study

Research Study Excerpt

A better understanding of nurses' decision-making regarding error reporting and workplace factors that influence their decisions can inform the development of strategies to improve the frequency and accuracy of error reporting by nurses. The purpose of study, therefore, was to explore nurses' decision-making processes regarding reporting errors.... Licensed RNs [registered nurses] who worked in an adult intensive care unit (ICU) as direct patient caregivers comprised the study sample. ICUs were chosen because high rates of errors are reported on nursing units that provide acute care for critically ill patients... Data collection and analysis progressed simultaneously. Procedures outlined by Charmaz (2014) were used to analyze the data. These procedures are based on a strategy referred to as constant comparison analysis, which is a process whereby data are compared within and across narratives and increasingly abstract theoretical renderings of the data are generated... The label "Being Off-Kilter" was chosen for the first stage because the errors made by participants often occurred in the context of working conditions that were challenging or that flustered them in some way... The label "Living the Error" was chosen for the second stage because of the consuming and personal nature of these error experiences. Most of the participants told vivid and detailed stories about making an error and described the intense emotions that surrounded the experience... The label "Reporting or Telling About the Error" was chosen for the third stage because it reflects the varied ways in which the error became known to others in the workplace. All the participants discussed whether, when, and how they revealed the error to others... The label "Living the Aftermath" was chosen for the fourth stage because the participants were often plagued by memories of the error even after it was resolved and were determined not to have it happen again... The label "Lurking in Your Mind" was chosen for the final stage because most participants believed that their memories of making an error would never go away or even dampen. The participants were convinced that these memories would "stick with" them throughout their careers and continue to influence their practice. (Koehn et al., 2016, pp. 567–570)

Koehn et al. (2016) began their study by observing nurses in eight intensive care units. By being present with the nurses, they found opportunities to talk to nurses about the study and obtain contact information from those who seemed interested. The 30 interviews that resulted from their recruitment occurred in a private location that the researcher and nurse found acceptable. The approach was that errors were a universal experience of nurses (Koehn et al., 2016).

As noted in the excerpt, constant comparison was the data analysis approach that was used. The researchers compared and combined initial codes during the focused coding stage. In the axial coding stage of analysis, Koehn and colleagues proposed relationships among the focused codes, integrated them into a tentative framework, and developed a diagram with the concepts and relationships among them. They named the tentative theory "Learning Lessons from the Error" and the process of learning from the error occurred in five stages (Fig. 1).

The nurses described the lessons learned that would help them prevent a similar error in the future. The benefits they had gained from learning "painful personal lessons" were "not shared with other nurses working in the same environments," which could have resulted in system improvements (Koehn et al., 2016, p. 570).

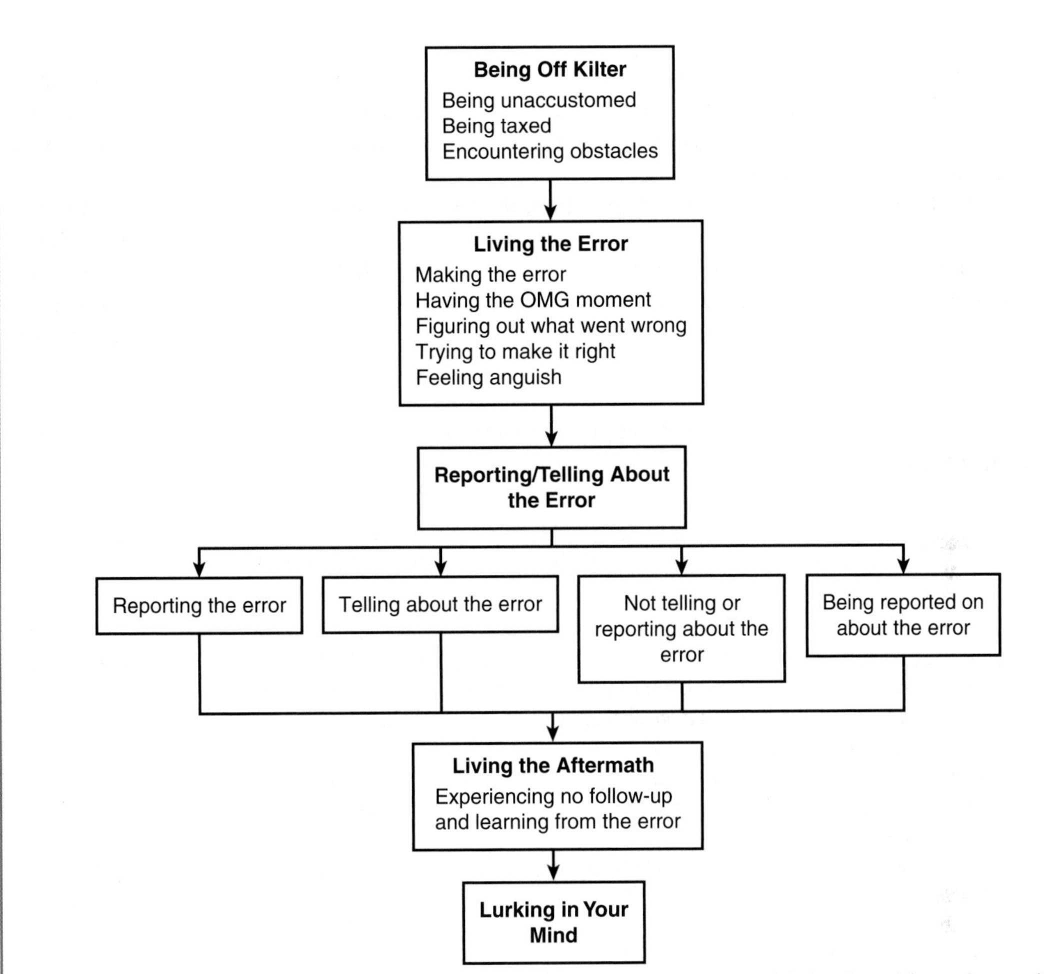

FIG 1 Learning lessons from error. This figure illustrates the theoretical model developed from the study by Koehn et al. (Redrawn from Koehn, A., Ebright, P., & Draucker, C. [2016]. Nurses' experiences with errors in nursing. *Nursing Outlook, 64*[6], 566–574.) *OMG*, Oh my God.

The richness of the findings and the diagram of the stages and relationships among them provide the background around which an institution could consider ways to decrease the complexity of the work environment and enhance its error follow-up to provide more psychological and emotional support to nurses after errors occur.

Critical Appraisal

Koehn et al. (2016) identified their study as being a grounded theory study. They conducted an adequate number of interviews because they had rich data, which they analyzed using a structured framework. The intended outcome, a theoretical description of social processes, was achieved, and the stages of living with a nursing error were diagrammed in a figure. Each component of the research report was clearly identifiable. Appropriately, Koehn et al. (2016) did not identify a theoretical framework because they were developing a theory "grounded" in the social processes experienced by nurses after an error. The robust literature review was included in the introduction of the article. The other steps of the research process were all included in the report. The well-designed grounded theory study provided robust findings with clinical significance.

Ethnographic Research

Ethnographic research was developed by anthropologists as a method to study how cultures develop and are maintained over time (Marshall & Rossman, 2016). Through immersion in the culture, anthropologists study a group of people who share a culture and their origins, past ways of living, and ways of surviving through time (Creswell & Poth, 2018). The term *ethnography* can also be applied to the product of the investigation, the written description of the study of the culture (Morgan-Trimmer & Wood, 2016). Early ethnography researchers studied primitive, foreign, or remote cultures. Such studies enabled the researcher who spent 1 year or longer in another culture to acquire new perspectives about a specific people, including their ways of living, believing, and adapting to changing environmental circumstances. This reflects the emic approach, one of studying behaviors from within the culture that recognizes the uniqueness of the individual (Morgan-Trimmer & Wood, 2016). The emic view from inside the culture is the typical goal of ethnography but may be alternated with the etic approach. The etic approach is to view the culture as a naïve outsider and analyze its elements as a researcher. Morgan-Trimmer and Wood (2016) have argued for using both approaches to achieve the goals of ethnography.

The philosophical perspective of ethnographic research is based in anthropology and recognizes that culture is material and nonmaterial. Material culture consists of all created or constructed aspects of culture, such as buildings used for cultural events, symbols of the culture, family traditions, networks of social relations, and the beliefs reflected in social and political institutions. Symbolic meaning, social customs, and beliefs—components of the nonmaterial culture—may be apparent in a different culture only over time, but are essential elements of cultures. Cultures also have ideals that people hold as desirable, even though they do not always live up to these standards. Anthropologists and nurse ethnographers seek to discover the multiple parts of a culture and determine how these parts are interrelated. A picture of the culture as a whole becomes clearer.

Nurses may not observe a culture over months or years, but may observe an organizational culture for a shorter time to learn about "the shared experiences of a more confined, predetermined phenomenon" (Rashid, Caine, & Goez, 2015, p. 3). This type of study is called a focused ethnography (Savage, 2006). Observations shorter than months or years are appropriate when the research question is narrower, and the scope of the study is limited to a specific place or organization. However, Morse (2016, p. 875) reminds researchers that "good ethnography takes *time*."

The nurse who increased the visibility of ethnography in nursing was Madeline Leininger, a nurse who earned her doctoral degree in anthropology. The fieldwork for her degree was a year that she spent in Papua New Guinea. From this experience, she developed the Sunshine Model of Transcultural Nursing Care, which identifies aspects of culture to consider when communicating with patients and families of another culture (Leininger, 1988). Nurses use Leininger's theory of transcultural nursing (Leininger, 2002) in practice by assessing multiple aspects of the patient, family, and their environment, including religion, societal norms, economic status, country of origin, ethnic subgroup, and beliefs about illness and healing. This theory has led to an ethnographic research strategy for nursing, termed *ethnonursing research.* Ethnonursing research "focuses mainly on observing and documenting interactions with people [and] how these daily life conditions and patterns are influencing human care, health, and nursing care practices" (Leininger, 1985, p. 238). However, a number of nurse anthropologists not associated with the ethnonursing orientation are also providing important contributions to nursing's body of knowledge (Roper & Shapiro, 2000).

The ethnographic researcher must become very familiar with the culture being studied by observing the culture, actively participating in it, and interviewing members of the culture. Even for focused ethnographies, the researcher must become immersed in the culture being studied.

Being immersed involves being in the culture and gaining increasing familiarity with aspects of the culture, such as language, sociocultural norms, traditions, and other social dimensions, including family, communication patterns (verbal and nonverbal), religion, work patterns, and expression of emotion. Through immersion, the ethnographic researcher becomes increasingly accepted into the culture. Although ethnographic researchers must be actively involved in the culture they are studying, they must avoid "going native," which would interfere with data collection and analysis. In going native, the researcher becomes a part of the culture and loses her or his ability to observe clearly (Creswell & Poth, 2018).

Intended Outcome

The ethnographer prepares a written report based on the analysis of the culture. Traditional ethnographies are often book-length and exceed what can be published in a professional journal. Focused ethnographies are more likely to be published in a nursing journal. Similar to a focused ethnography in that the study has a narrower focus, nurses have used critical ethnography, a method that focuses on the socioecological and political factors within a culture (Sanon, Spigner, & McCullagh, 2016). Depending on the specific method chosen and the initial research question, the researcher may propose strategies to increase the cultural acceptability of a health intervention, encourage health promotion behaviors, or improve the quality of care that is being delivered in an organization.

A neonatal intensive care unit (NICU) is a technology-dependent environment with vulnerable babies and parents. Based on the findings of her previous studies, Cricco-Lizza (2016) conducted a focused ethnography in an NICU to better understand the barriers and supports for infant feeding methods (Research Example 3.3).

RESEARCH EXAMPLE 3.3

Ethnographic Study

Research Study Excerpt

Purpose: *The purpose is to examine the infant feeding beliefs and day-to-day feeding practices of NICU nurses with the goal of identifying ways to improve breastfeeding promotion... Breastfeeding beliefs do not occur in a vacuum, and a broad scale approach is important to explore the context of infant feeding in the NICU...*

Sample: *There were 250 nurses employed in this NICU... In this study, 114 general informants were selected at the bedside based on their varied interactions during infant feeding and nursing care... 18 key informants who were selected from the group of 114 general informants. They were identified during participant observation as being knowledgeable and articulate about varied infant feeding beliefs and practices and agreed to in-depth follow-up...*

Data Collection: *Fieldwork in the NICU was conducted during 1 or 2 hour sessions on varying days, times, and shifts over a 14 month period... The nurse researcher role varied from observation to informal interviewing during the 128 participant observation sessions in this study... They were observed/informally interviewed an average of 3.5 times each with a range of 1 to 24 throughout the study. These data were documented in detailed field notes immediately after each session and pseudonyms were used to protect confidentiality.... There was a formal, 1-hour, tape-recorded interview with each of the 18 key informants... The field notes from observations, the transcripts from interviews, and regularly composed analytic memos were entered into the QSR NUD*IST computer software program.... Data analyses were conducted alongside data collection in a spiral fashion. Questions raised during analyses were then explored in greater depth in the next interview or observation...*

Continued

RESEARCH EXAMPLE 3.3—cont'd

Findings: *The findings of this study reflect the infant feeding beliefs and day-to-day practices of nurses in a well staffed, high acuity NICU…*

Conclusions: *Novel strategies are needed to overcome challenges to breastfeeding promotion in the NICU. Vulnerable NICU babies and mothers need their nurses to be clinically prepared to support, promote, and protect breastfeeding at the bedside. The nurses in this study identified that they felt anxious, frustrated, or embarrassed with the challenges of breastfeeding in the NICU. This research demonstrates that both the emotional and educational needs of the NICU staff nurses must be addressed before they can feel competent and comfortable with the promotion and support of breastfeeding.* (Cricco-Lizza, 2016, pp. e92–e97)

Cricco-Lizza (2016, p. e92) identified the gap in knowledge as the need to have a "more nuanced understanding of the NICU feeding culture." As noted, the primary methods in the ethnography were participant observation, informal interviews, formal interviews, and detailed field notes (Cricco-Lizza, 2016). The credibility of the finding was strengthened by the use of multiple methods, triangulation across methods, prolonged engagement, member checking, and peer review at the researcher's university during data analysis.

Three major themes with subcomponents emerged from the data as indicators of the environment of the NICU and the beliefs and behaviors of the nurses. These findings are provided in Box 3.2. The NICU nurses described the advantages of breastfeeding to be "intellectual, nutritional, digestive, anti-infective, and anti-allergenic benefits for babies, along with bonding and empowerment for mothers" (Cricco-Lizza, 2016, p. e93). The nurses' beliefs about the challenges of breastfeeding were difficult to overcome and included "vulnerable babies, anxious mothers, and discomfort of staff, along with the lack of privacy in the NICU environment" (p. e94). The logistics of day-to-day practices of breastfeeding in the NICU resulted in other challenges. Supporting a mother to breastfeed or preparing breast milk to give in a bottle were more time-consuming than simply giving a bottle of formula. Formula feeding was viewed as safe, convenient, and more acceptable to adolescent mothers. Breastfeeding was seen as risky in situations when mothers were taking medications. The last theme described the differences in the beliefs of NICU nurses who had had a positive personal experience with breastfeeding or who had received continuing education about the benefits of breastfeeding compared with nurses without these experiences or education. The nurses with positive experiences or education were strong advocates for breastfeeding and were willing to invest time and energy in helping mothers breastfeed their babies in the NICU.

BOX 3.2 THEMES AND SUBTHEMES FROM AN ETHNOGRAPHY OF INFANT FEEDING IN A NEONATAL INTENSIVE CARE UNIT

Theme 1. The nurses identified health benefits of breastfeeding, but spoke in greater detail and with more emotion about day-to-day challenges of breastfeeding in the NICU.

- Beliefs about health benefits of breastfeeding
- Beliefs about challenges of breastfeeding in the NICU
- Day-to-day practice challenges of breastfeeding in the NICU

Theme 2. Formula feeding evoked less emotion, and most nurses viewed it as safe and convenient.

Theme 3. Despite infant feeding challenges in the NICU, nurses who had breastfeeding continuing education and/or some positive experiences with breastfeeding identified evidence-based breastfeeding benefits for mothers and babies, emphasized the health-based differences between breast milk and formula, and were more committed to working through difficulties with breastfeeding.

From Cricco-Lizza, R. (2016). Infant feeding beliefs and day-to-day feeding practices of NICU nurses. *Journal of Pediatric Nursing, 31*(2), e93–e94.

NICU, Neonatal intensive care unit.

Critical Appraisal

Cricco-Lizza (2016) provided a strong example of a rigorous ethnography. The strengths of the study were the detailed information provided in the report about the methods and the immersion of the researcher in the culture over time. The researcher noted one limitation as being the generous staffing of the high-intensity NICU that was the setting of the study. Future research needs to be focused on NICUs with lower acuity and possibly fewer staff. The conclusion of the ethnography was that "novel strategies are needed to overcome the challenges to breastfeeding promotion in the NICU" (Cricco-Lizza, 2016, p. e97). These strategies, to be effective, must address the "emotional and educational needs of the NICU staff nurses" to help them be "more competent and comfortable with the promotion and support of breastfeeding" (Cricco-Lizza, 2016, p. e97).

Cricco-Lizza (2016) conducted a focused ethnography of a specific aspect of infant care in a single setting. She achieved the desired outcome of ethnography by providing a thorough description of the culture of an NICU that affected infant feeding. She provided details about the number and type of interviews and observations that supported her conclusions. Each section of the research report was clearly identified, and the report was well organized. Although no theoretical framework was identified, the researcher's previous studies on the topic provided findings and conceptual statements that guided the approach and methods of this study. The literature review was integrated into the introduction. All steps of the research process were addressed.

Exploratory-Descriptive Qualitative Research

Some reports of qualitative studies do not include mention of a specific design or approach, such as phenomenology or grounded theory. The researchers may have described their studies as being naturalistic inquiry, descriptive, or just qualitative. For example, Fallatah and Edge (2015) conducted a descriptive qualitative study to "to describe the experience of family members who provide social support to their relative with rheumatoid arthritis (RA), and explore the forms of support that they require" (p. 180).

Researchers design exploratory-descriptive qualitative studies to obtain information needed to develop a program or intervention for a specific group of patients. Usually, the researchers are exploring a new topic or describing a situation, so we have chosen to label these studies as **exploratory-descriptive qualitative research** (Gray, Grove, & Sutherland, 2017). Studies consistent with this approach are not a specific type of research; rather, they are studies conducted for a specific purpose that do not fit into another of the categories (Sandelowski, 2000, 2010).

Exploratory-descriptive qualitative studies are developed to provide information and insight into clinical or practice problems. Qualitative studies are often developed to address problems in practice when a fresh approach is needed, especially problems that require the patient's or family's perspectives to be appropriately addressed. The philosophical orientation of exploratory-descriptive qualitative research may vary, depending on the purpose of the study, but often the researcher has a pragmatic orientation (McCready, 2010). The pragmatic researcher is in search of useful information and practical solutions (Creswell & Poth, 2018) and designs studies to understand what works (Houghton, Hunter, & Meskell, 2012).

Intended Outcome

A well-designed, exploratory-descriptive qualitative study answers the research question. The purpose of the study is achieved, and the researchers have the information that they need to address the situation or patient concern that was the focus of the study. The findings of the study are applied to the practice problem that instigated the inquiry. In the Fallatah and Edge (2015) study, the family members had adjusted their own lives to provide support to their spouse or parent. Rarely had the family members "received comprehensive health information from the healthcare provider" (Fallatah & Edge, 2015, p. 184). The clinical implications were that the family members caring for a relative with RA needed social support that encompassed informational, emotional, and instrumental support to achieve balance and cope with the chronic illness. Some exploratory-descriptive qualitative studies deal with less emotional topics and with facts upon which to develop interventions. Hatzfeld, Nelson, Waters, and Jennings (2016) developed a study that did the latter on the topic of combat readiness.

Combat readiness of enlisted personnel can be compromised by their physical health. Hatzfeld et al. (2016) conducted an exploratory-descriptive qualitative study because of concerns about obesity and cardiovascular risk and their impact on combat readiness. Cardiac problems were the most common reason for critical care transport for noninjury reasons in deployed settings (Hatzfeld et al., 2016). An exploratory-descriptive qualitative approach was appropriate due to the limited research that had been done on the topic. Research Example 3.4 provides information about the study and a critical appraisal of the study's strengths and weaknesses.

RESEARCH EXAMPLE 3.4

Exploratory-Descriptive Qualitative Study

Research Study Excerpt

The USAF [United States Air Force] has developed a comprehensive fitness program with specific responsibilities for commanders at all levels and USAF medical units... Because of the importance of fitness and health within the USAF, the primary aim of this study was to identify factors that influence the lifestyle health behaviors of USAF active duty military members. A secondary aim of this analysis was to compare these factors to the elements of the Health Promotion Model (HPM).... A qualitative descriptive design (Sandelowski, 2000, 2010) was used to guide the identification of factors that influence the lifestyle health behaviors of active duty military members in the USAF... The ultimate goal of this study was to use the participants' perspectives to develop the foundation of a lifestyle modification program appropriate for the USAF population.... The two inclusion criteria for participation were (a) currently serving as an active duty member of the USAF and (b) having experienced an assignment to more than one military base... Maximum variation purposeful sampling was used to enroll participants to achieve heterogeneity and variation related to the primary dimension of interest... Along with a short demographic form developed specifically for this study, data were collected via face-to-face interviews in a neutral place away from the participants' work sites. The principal investigator conducted all of the interviews using semistructured interview questions... The codes were grouped into themes; the themes were reviewed and confirmed by the entire research team. Differences of opinion were few; these were discussed until agreement was achieved about the interpretations. The team discussions provided a diversity of input that contributed to the validity of the themes. Subsequently, the research team compared the final themes to the main elements of the HPM to identify factors that influenced health behaviors among active duty USAF members and to see how the findings fit the existing HPM model. (Hatzfeld et al., 2016, pp. 441–443)

To generate descriptions of a wide range of experiences, the researchers used maximum variation purposeful sampling to achieve heterogeneity related to hypertension (present or absent), race and ethnicity, age, and officer or enlisted status. This sampling method involves finding participants who differ on the characteristics identified. The recruitment involved a series of e-mails, word of mouth, and snowball recruitment and continued until 24 participants had been enrolled in the study.

The methods were rigorous, and the data analysis was done by a diverse team comprised of active and retired military and academic researchers. An audit trail was maintained. An **audit trail** is the record of the actions taken related to data organization and the decisions that were made during analysis and interpretation (Miles, Huberman, & Saldaña, 2014). An audit trail allows readers to have increased confidence in the transparency of the study. When the research team had differences of opinions about coding and themes, they discussed the data and possible meanings until a consensus was reached (Hatzfeld et al., 2016).

The participants defined health as being the "presence of exercise, proper eating, sufficient sleep, and a spiritual connection and the absence of smoking, excessive stress, and excessive alcohol and caffeine consumption (Hatzfeld et al., 2016, p. 443). Three factors were identified that contributed to decisions about their health behaviors. The first factor, the USAF culture, encompassed the positive and negative aspects of achieving the required fitness score. Mandatory physical training several times a week was identified as a part of the culture, along with the effect of officers on the health of the unit. Leaders were seen as role models of healthy behaviors, but also increased the stress level of the soldiers in their unit when punitive actions were taken. USAF culture also included the stresses of deployment, reintegration, assignment to a new duty station, and temporary assignments that contributed to unhealthy food choices and the use of tobacco and alcohol (Hatzfeld et al., 2016).

The second factor, "Who I am," involved the influence of childhood experiences related to diet and exercise, as well as personal awareness as an adult of preferences for certain types of food and exercise (Hatzfeld et al., 2016). Other personal characteristics included in this factor were the individual life circumstances of each person such as child care arrangements, needs of other family members, and comfort level in the gym or other workout locations.

"What works for me" was the third factor identified by Hatzfeld et al. (2016). The participants described figuring out the types of exercise that they preferred and how to incorporate it into their schedule. Food choices and sleep patterns also reflected a deliberate process of trying different approaches to identify those that worked in their personal circumstances. Some participants, however, expressed frustration and hopelessness about being unable to find what worked for them.

The second study aim was to compare the findings with the HPM (Pender, Murdaugh, & Parsons, 2011). Although the theory's concepts of personal factors and situational influences were partially reflected in the findings, Hatzfeld et al. (2016) concluded their findings were not congruent with the HPM.

Because the study was conducted consistently with standards of rigor for qualitative studies, Hatzfeld et al. (2016, p. 447) proposed that "the findings from this study offer a useful framework for military nurses and leaders as they seek appropriate interventions to more specifically reduce cardiovascular risk behaviors... nurses can best promote health among military members by integrating their personal history ("who I am") and preferences ("what works for me")" into individualized plans to implement and maintain healthy lifestyle behaviors over time.

Critical Appraisal

Hatzfeld et al. (2016) conducted an exploratory-descriptive qualitative approach to address a specific health concern among USAF personnel. They noted that strategies to reduce cardiac risks would need to incorporate the individual preferences and logistics of officers and enlisted persons to be effective. In this way, the researchers achieved the desired outcome of exploratory-descriptive qualitative studies, which was to provide information to guide a solution to a problem. The sections of the research report were identified, and the steps of the research process were incorporated into the report. The researchers identified the HPM as the study framework, but concluded that the concepts of the model were not consistent with the findings of the study.

SAMPLING AND RECRUITMENT

The methods used in conducting qualitative studies are different from methods used in quantitative studies. The unique methods of qualitative researchers are described here in some detail to enhance your understanding of qualitative research. The methods section includes how data are collected, managed, and analyzed. The methods used to ensure rigor in qualitative research also are explored. Each aspect of the methods will include guidelines for critically appraising that aspect of the study. The first section discusses how participants are selected for qualitative studies and the relationship between the researcher and participant.

Selection of Participants

Individuals in qualitative studies are referred to as participants because the researcher and participants carry out the study cooperatively. Sampling in qualitative research is purposeful. The researcher recruits participants because of their particular knowledge, experience, or views related to the study (Munhall, 2012). Additional sampling methods, such as network and theoretical, are used based on the focus of the study (see Chapter 9). For some studies, such as the study conducted by Hatzfeld et al. (2016), recruiting participants who are heterogeneous provides a wider range of experiences. Heterogeneous samples, in which participants have different characteristics, are used frequently for grounded theory studies to support the development of a theory (Creswell & Poth, 2018). For other studies, participants may have similar characteristics (a homogeneous sample) because the central focus of the study is the phenomena.

Researcher–Participant Relationships

One of the important differences between quantitative and qualitative research lies in the degree of involvement of the researcher with the participants of the study. This involvement, considered to be a source of bias in quantitative research, is thought by qualitative researchers to be a critical element of the research process. The nature of the researcher–participant relationship has an impact on the collection and interpretation of data (Maxwell, 2014). The researcher creates a respectful relationship with each participant, which includes being honest and open about the purpose and methods of the study. The researcher's aims and means of achieving the aims need to be negotiated with the participants and honor their perspectives and values (Creswell & Poth, 2018; Gray et al., 2017; Maxwell, 2014; Munhall, 2012). In various degrees, the researcher influences the people being studied and, in turn, is influenced by them. Thus the researcher must have their support and confidence to complete the research. The researcher's personality is a key factor in qualitative research. Skills in empathy and intuition are cultivated; the researcher must become closely involved in the participant's experience to interpret the data. It is necessary for researchers to be open to the perceptions of the participants, rather than to attach their own meaning to the experience.

Researcher–participant relationships in qualitative studies may be brief when data collection occurs once in an interview or a focus group. Phenomenology and grounded theory studies may involve one or two interviews, although researcher–participant relationships may extend over time when the study design involves repeated interviews to study a lived experience or process over time.

Ethnographic studies require special attention to the researcher–participant relationship. The ethnographic researcher observes behavior, communication, and patterns within groups in specific cultures. The researcher may form close bonds with participants who are key informants, persons with extensive knowledge and influence in a culture. The relationships between the researcher and participants can become complex, especially in ethnography studies in which the researcher lives for an extended time in the culture being studied.

? CRITICAL APPRAISAL GUIDELINES

Selection of Participants and the Researcher–Participant Relationship

1. Did the researchers identify the specific type of sampling that was used, such as purposive, network, or theoretical sampling?
2. Were the participants' characteristics and life experiences appropriate to the qualitative approach?
3. Was the number of participants adequate to fulfill the purpose of the study?
4. Were the length and depth of the researcher–participant relationships in the study appropriate to the study approach and study purpose?

In Koehn et al.'s (2016) grounded theory study of nursing errors, discussed previously in this chapter, the researchers recognized that nurses might be embarrassed or afraid to talk about the errors they had made. In Research Example 3.5, you will see that the researchers invested time in developing relationships with the potential participants to overcome this resistance.

RESEARCH EXAMPLE 3.5

Researcher–Participant Relationship

Research Study Excerpt

Licensed RNs who worked in an adult intensive care unit (ICU) as direct patient caregivers comprise the study sample... Following approval from each unit manager, the researcher spent time on each unit to observe and be present with the nurses. During these visits, the researcher initiated discussions regarding the study, provided details for those who appeared interested in participating, and collected contact information from those who agreed to be interviewed. (Koehn et al., 2016, pp. 567–568)

Critical Appraisal

The participants' characteristics, experiences, and number were appropriate for the study approach and adequate to fulfill the study's purpose. Koehn et al. (2016) used a convenience sample (study participants were available at the right time and place to take part in the study), but spent time in each ICU to increase the likelihood that nurses would feel safe being in the study. The time spent in the ICUs provided a foundation for a researcher–participant relationship that concluded with an interview that lasted 40 to 60 minutes on the sensitive topic of errors in clinical practice. The depth and completeness of the grounded theory that was developed by the researchers indicate that the sampling and relationships of the study met the standards of rigor for qualitative studies.

DATA COLLECTION METHODS

The data in most qualitative research studies are "the participant's thoughts, ideas, and perceptions" (Bolderston, 2012, p. 68). The most common data collection methods used in the types of qualitative studies discussed in this chapter are interviewing participants, conducting focus groups, observing participants, and examining documents and media materials. Creswell and Poth (2018) have noted that the use of audiovisual data and media is growing. Media encompasses photographs, recordings, and artifacts. These methods, as they are used in qualitative studies, are described in the following sections in some detail; examples from the literature are provided. Guidelines for critically appraising each type of qualitative data collection are provided, along with a brief critical appraisal of that method.

Interviews

Differences exist between interviews conducted for a qualitative study and those conducted for a quantitative study. In quantitative studies, the researcher structures interviews to collect participants' responses to questionnaires or surveys (see Chapter 10). Interviews in qualitative studies range from **semistructured interviews** (fixed set of questions, no fixed responses) to **unstructured interviews** (open-ended questions, with probes; Bolderston, 2012). **Probes** are queries made by the researcher to obtain more information from the participant about a particular interview question.

For unstructured interviews, also called **open-ended interviews,** the initial statement or question may be "Tell me about a time that you received bad news about a diagnostic test" or "After your diagnosis, how did you learn about diabetes?" Although the researcher defines the focus of the interview, there may be no fixed sequence of questions. The questions addressed in interviews tend to change as the researcher gains insights from previous interviews and observations. Respondents are allowed, and even encouraged, to raise important issues that the researcher may not have addressed.

The researcher's goal is to obtain an authentic insight into the participant's experiences (Creswell & Poth, 2018). Although data may be collected in a single interview, dialogue between researcher and participant may continue at intervals across weeks or months and provide rich data for analysis. Use of recurring interviews allows the researcher to explore an evolving process (Munhall, 2012) and allows the researcher–participant relationship to develop. As the relationship develops and trust grows, the participant may reveal the emotional and value-laden aspects of the process more freely.

The purpose of the interview may vary, depending on the type of qualitative approach. Interviews in a phenomenology study may have one main question, with follow-up questions used as needed to elicit the participant's perspective on the phenomenon. Interviews in grounded theory studies are similar in that only one or two questions may be asked, but the follow-up questions will focus on the social processes of the phenomenon. Interviewing in ethnography studies may be used to obtain information and explanations about aspects of the culture that the researcher has noted while observing the culture. In an exploratory-descriptive qualitative study, the interviewer may ask more structured questions to achieve the purpose of the study.

Some strategies used to record information from interviews include writing notes during the interview, writing detailed notes immediately after the interview, and recording the interview. Video may be recorded, as well as audio. For example, Cricco-Lizza (2016), in her focused ethnography on breastfeeding in the NICU, audio-recorded the formal interviews she conducted with key informants. Following an interview, the recording was transcribed to create a written document for data analysis. Although she did not note who did the transcribing, she described checking the recording line for line to ensure accuracy. In her exploratory-descriptive qualitative study of USAF personnel's health behaviors, Hatzfeld et al. (2016) also recorded interviews but used a professional transcriptionist to prepare the written document of the recordings.

Interviews should be arranged for a time and private place convenient for the participant. Interviews may be held in the participant's home, clinic office, public library meeting room, or restaurant. Ideally, the location for an interview is distraction-free (Creswell & Poth, 2018) and a place where both the researcher and participant feel safe. Meeting in a clinic, for example, may not be appropriate if the interview involves describing the care being received. A person living with an infection caused by the human immunodeficiency virus may not want to be interviewed in a place where he or she might be seen by friends or family. You also want a place that is quiet enough to allow for effective audio recording.

CRITICAL APPRAISAL GUIDELINES

Interviews

1. Do the interview questions address concerns expressed in the research problem?
2. Are the interview questions relevant for the research purpose and objectives or questions?
3. Were the interviews adequate in length and number to address the research purpose or answer the research question?

In her ethnographic study of infant feeding in the NICU, Cricco-Lizza (2016) described interviews as one of the methods of data collection she used, as depicted in Research Example 3.6.

RESEARCH EXAMPLE 3.6

Interviews

Research Study Excerpt

The 114 general informants described their beliefs and their day-to-day work in the unit. They were observed/informally interviewed an average of 3.5 times each with a range of 1 to 24 throughout the study. These data were documented in detailed field notes immediately after each session and pseudonyms were used to protect confidentiality... There was a formal, 1-hour, tape-recorded interview with each of the 18 key informants. These interviews were conducted in a private room near the NICU at specific times chosen by these nurses. They were assured of the confidentiality of their responses to open-ended questions about breastfeeding, formula feeding, and the nature of their nursing care. The nurses were asked to describe their work days and their specific responsibilities for infant feeding. In addition, the nurses were also asked for further explanation about issues that might have arisen during participant observation sessions.... (Cricco-Lizza, 2016, p. e93)

Critical Appraisal

Cricco-Lizza (2016) provided adequate detail to critically appraise the interviews used in the study as one of the data collection methods. The outcome of the study provided evidence that the interview questions addressed the concerns expressed in the research problem and were relevant to the purpose and research questions. The number of key informant interviews was supplemented by 128 informal interviews done while Cricco-Lizza was observing in the NICU. The number and length of the interviews were more than adequate to address the research question and fulfill the study's purpose.

Focus Groups

Focus groups were designed to obtain the participants' perceptions of a specific topic in a permissive and nonthreatening setting. One of the assumptions underlying the use of focus groups is that group dynamics can help people express and clarify their views in ways that are less likely to occur in a one to one interview. The group may give a sense of safety in numbers to those wary of researchers or those who are anxious. The recommended size of a focus group is five to eight participants. Larger focus groups are sometimes used but may be more difficult to moderate. Because larger focus groups have more voices to hear, transcribing the recording can be challenging. All participants should have the opportunity to speak, which may be more difficult to achieve with a larger number. Focus groups are sometimes called group interviews (Bolderston, 2012), so the principles of interviewing such as responding in a nonjudgmental way are still applicable.

Focus groups are conducted by a **moderator or facilitator,** who may or may not be the researcher. Researchers may elicit the help of moderators who share common characteristics with the participants. An example would be the urban researcher who hires a health professional who grew up in a rural farming community to moderate a focus group on preventing agricultural injuries. Moderators or focus group leaders should be thoroughly trained and understand the importance of following the procedures or script developed by the researcher.

The entire interaction is audio-recorded and, in some cases, video-recorded. In addition to the recordings, members of the research team may serve as observers to take notes of the proceedings. Ideally, a focus group should be conducted in a natural setting, but a natural setting can pose challenges. It is important for the researcher to have visited the room or location of the proposed focus group to ensure that the participants' confidentiality can be maintained and that outside noise is minimal to allow the focus group communication to be audio- or video-recorded. Confidentiality and comfort may result in richer dialogue and data.

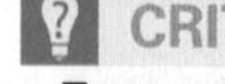

CRITICAL APPRAISAL GUIDELINES

Focus Groups

1. Were the size, composition, and length of the focus group adequate to promote group interaction and to produce robust data?
2. Were questions used during the focus group relevant to the study's research purpose and objectives or questions (Gray et al., 2017; Maxwell, 2014)?

Research Example 3.7 provides an example of a study in which focus groups were used for data collection. Culture and community are key factors in determining the effectiveness of interventions when the interventions were created for another population. Brunk, Taylor, Clark, Williams, and Cox (2017) identified a comprehensive intervention of education and support to improve outcomes of type 2 diabetes (T2D). They used focus groups to evaluate the intervention.

RESEARCH EXAMPLE 3.7

Focus Groups

Research Study Excerpt

In the context of diverse patient care environments where there might be cultural discord between the health care providers and the patients, patient-centered care has to be culturally and linguistically responsive… The aim of this project was to explore the feasibility of adapting a patient-centered lifestyle modification program for the self-management of type 2 diabetes (T2D) to a Hispanic population with low health literacy… data were gathered through focus group sessions regarding the cultural applicability of the lifestyle modification program…This descriptive qualitative study used a phenomenological approach.

Data Collection. *Data were collected through the four 2-hour class and focus group sessions, each of which was recorded digitally… Following a short break a group discussion was facilitated using leading questions such as "From your perspective, what was most helpful about today's session?"*

The researcher brought to this qualitative project not only her experiences growing up in a Spanish-speaking country but also a 29-year history of working with diverse Hispanic populations in Chicago. Member checking was accomplished, in part, by the group facilitator reviewing with the group members the previous week's feedback to ensure that what she had understood from their discussion was indeed what information the group members had intended to convey. Credibility was enhanced through working closely with the second author, meeting with her every week to review progress, the transcripts, and key themes that were emerging. (Brunk et al., 2017, pp. 187–188, 192)

Nine patients who met the inclusion criteria of being Hispanic, possessing low literacy skills, and being diagnosed with T2D or a family member of a person with diabetes were in this focus group. The setting was a rural health center. The recruited participants received and evaluated the intervention (Brunk et al., 2017). The research report included the focus group number (four), length (2 hours), and composition (eight patients and one family member). Although the researchers described the focus groups as being 2 hours long, the focus groups comprised only the latter part of each 2-hour session.

The researchers noted that some portions of the focus group recordings were unintelligible due to multiple participants speaking at the same time. The recordings were "transcribed and translated into English, and reviewed for accuracy by the translation service" (Brunk et al., 2017, p. 189). The data were analyzed and the themes were identified that addressed the research problem. "…participants shared feedback clustered around four themes: information and knowledge about T2D, motivation and barriers to changing behaviors, experiences with new self-management behaviors, and personal responsibility for disease management" (Brunk et al., 2017, p. 190).

Critical Appraisal

The study results based on the focus group data were appropriate for the research problem and study purpose. The study was strengthened by the strategies used to increase the rigor of the study. Limitations were the small number of participants and the lack of information about the focus groups. The use of focus groups could have been strengthened by explicitly describing the length of the focus group portion of the sessions and the proportion of data that was lost due to the unintelligible sections of the recordings.

Observation

Observation is a fundamental method of gathering data for qualitative studies, especially ethnography studies. The aim is to gather first-hand information in a naturally occurring situation. The researcher assumes the role of a learner to answer the question, "What is going on here?" The activities being observed may be automatic or routine for the participants, who may be unaware of some of their actions. The researcher looks carefully at the focus of the study, notices people and objects in the environment, and listens for what is said and unsaid. The researcher focuses on the details, including discrete events and the process of activities. Unexpected events occurring during routine activities may be significant and are carefully noted. As in any observation process, the qualitative researcher will attend to some aspects of the situation while disregarding others, depending on the focus of the study.

The researcher also needs to determine the observer role that will allow the research purpose and question to be addressed. The observer role is on a continuum from being a complete participant to being a complete observer (Creswell & Poth, 2018). The latter is more likely to be achieved when you are collecting the data from a video recording of the events unfolding. More often, the observer role is a mixture of participant and observer.

In studies that use observation, notes taken during or shortly after observations are called field notes. Waiting until the observation is over allows the researcher to focus entirely on the observational experience to avoid missing something meaningful, but that may result in not all pertinent data being recorded. You may want to create a checklist or an outline of key events you want to capture. Another useful strategy is to videotape the events, so that careful observations and detailed notes can be taken at a later time. Collecting data from a video recording allows you to be a complete observer in that the actors in the situation are unaware that you are observing them. From a human rights perspective, however, the actors have to have given consent to be in a study and be aware that video recordings are being made.

? CRITICAL APPRAISAL GUIDELINES

Observation

1. Were observations conducted at times and for long enough periods to collect rich data that allow for a thorough description of the culture, setting, or process of interest (Wolf, 2012)?
2. Did the researcher make field notes or journal entries (Creswell, 2014; Miles et al., 2014)?

For the ethnographic study of infant feeding in the NICU, Cricco-Lizza (2016) used observation as another source of data, described in Research Example 3.8.

RESEARCH EXAMPLE 3.8

Observation

Research Study Excerpt

Fieldwork in the NICU was conducted during 1 or 2 hour sessions on varying days, times, and shifts over a 14 month period… The nurses were observed during their interactions with babies, families, nurses, and other staff throughout the varied activities in the unit… The nurse researcher role varied from observation to informal interviewing during the 128 participant observation sessions in this study. These informal interviews were open ended and related to the immediate circumstances of NICU care. The 114 general informants described their beliefs and their day-to-day work in the unit. They were observed/informally interviewed an average of 3.5 times each with a range of 1 to 24 throughout the study. These data were documented in detailed field notes immediately after each session, and pseudonyms were used to protect confidentiality. (Cricco-Lizza, 2016, pp. e92–e93)

Critical Appraisal

The details provided by Cricco-Lizza (2016) supported the rigor of her observations in the number of observations, the duration of the study, and the number of different nurses observed. The observations were more than adequate to collect rich data and thoroughly describe infant feeding within the NICU culture. She maintained detailed field notes that became an important source of data in determining the findings of the study.

Examination of Documents and Media

In qualitative studies, documents as textual data can be considered a rich source of data. For example, in the NICU ethnography about breastfeeding, Cricco-Lizza (2016) could have reviewed policies and procedures related to infant feeding for the hospital as an additional source of data. Other sources of preexisting text are clinical notes in electronic health records, policy manuals, annual reports of an organization, and newspaper articles. Textual data are more likely to be used in ethnography studies. Other texts may be created for the purpose of the study. For example, the researcher may ask participants to write about a particular topic. In some cases, these written narratives may be solicited by mail or e-mail rather than in person. Text provided by participants may be a component of a larger study using a variety of sources of data.

Media may be photographs or recordings that the researcher makes during observations or online communication. Photovoice, a specific use of media in qualitative studies, involves participants taking photographs related to the research topic as a source of data. One nursing research team has used online materials as a source of data for several studies. For 10 years, Im and colleagues have conducted studies of female cancer survivors and multicultural midlife women using online forums as sources of data. One example was a secondary analysis of online data collected for a larger study (Im et al., 2013). Four online forums were created for the study, each one for a specific race or ethnic group. They identified common themes across the forums, as well as noting differences. The qualitative data collected have supported the development of an appropriate intervention to promote physical activity among Asian American breast cancer survivors (Chee et al., 2017).

CRITICAL APPRAISAL GUIDELINES

Examining Documents and Media as Data

1. Were the documents or media materials created specifically for the study?
2. For materials not created for the study, were their authenticity and authorship confirmed?
3. For materials created for the study, were the human rights of the participants protected by informed consent and confidentiality?
4. Were the data from these sources used to address the study purpose or answer the research question in a meaningful way?

Postma, Peterson, Vega, Ramon, and Cortez (2014) conducted a study of the environmental health risks of Latina youth in agricultural communities. Middle school students and *promotores*, or community health promoters, were the participants. The *promotores* were bilingual in English and Spanish and were established in the community as cultural liaisons between migrant communities and the health system (Postma et al., 2014). Photographs, one of several sources of data in the study, were collected in two rounds. Research Example 3.9 describes the document and media examination performed in this study.

RESEARCH EXAMPLE 3.9

Examination of Documents and Media

Research Study Excerpt

Participants had the option to use a disposable camera or their own digital or cell phone cameras. In each round, participants were asked to photograph 24–27 images representing people, places, and things that conveyed their perspectives on problems and strengths related to "children, health, and the environment." Film was sorted with each participant receiving a hard copy of their photographs. The second copy was collected as data. (Postma et al., 2014, p. 510)

The photographs alone were revealing, but Postma et al. (2014) also conducted sessions with the participants and asked each participant to select two or three significant photographs to share with the group. The participants "contextualized the photograph by telling stories about the picture through a facilitated process" (Postma et al., 2014, p. 511). The sessions were audio-recorded as another source of data. One of the problem themes was the lack of structured activities for the youth and subsequent lack of adult supervision and prevalence of gang activity. Another theme was poverty and stress, also described as "boiling points." The boiling points of poverty and stress were of concern because youths often used drugs and alcohol to relieve the pressure. The last problem theme was the benefits and detriments of agricultural work. Some of the detriments were the use of pesticides and unsafe ladders used for picking fruit from trees (Postma et al., 2014). The primary benefit of agricultural work was job creation that allowed the families to support themselves. The focus of the final session was identifying actions that could be taken in the community to improve the health of children.

Critical Appraisal

The photographs used as a data source in the Postma et al. (2014) study were created for the study. The research report included information about how the participants were trained to obtain permission and signed consents from people who would be identifiable in their photographs. The participants were given a copy of their own photographs to keep. The photographs were used for the images they contained, but also as a valuable stimulus for collecting stories and the perspectives of the participants. In this way, photovoice was rigorously and appropriately used in the study of children's environmental health risks (Postma et al., 2014).

DATA MANAGEMENT AND ANALYSIS

The limitations on the length of manuscripts for peer-reviewed journals may prevent the researchers from reporting details of the processes of data analysis and management. However, having a general understanding of this part of the process will allow you to critically appraise published studies and provide the background needed to evaluate study proposals being considered by your facility or institutional review board.

Transcribing Interviews

The most commonly used textual data in qualitative studies are **transcripts** of recorded interviews and focus groups. Transcription is at the heart of the qualitative research process, because a "verbatim transcript captures participants' own words, language, and expressions" and allows the researcher to "decode behavior, processes, and cultural meanings attached to people's perspectives" (Hennink & Weber, 2013, p. 700). Transcripts from such recordings can result in copious data for analysis. In a study report, researchers should describe how data were recorded during the interview, focus group, or observations, and the strategies that were used to ensure the accuracy of the transcriptions (Miles et al., 2014). Typically, transcripts are prepared by typing everything in the recording word for word of what the person said, including audible noises, such as laughing, coughing, or hesitating. Computer programs are now available that are voice-activated and can produce a written record of the recording. Even when computer software or a professional transcriptionist is used, the researcher will ensure accuracy by reading and correcting the transcript while listening to the recording.

Data Organization

Qualitative data analysis occurs concurrently with data collection and requires planning because qualitative studies generate a large amount of data. When qualitative researchers prepare to conduct a study, their plan includes multiple locations where data will be stored. Frequently, one of the locations is an online service or electronic network. The amount of data may be copious because a 1-hour interview may result in electronic (computer) files for the transcript, field notes, journaling related to codes or analysis, and a demographic form. Experienced researchers develop a standard way to name files before data collection begins. For example, the file name could include the name or pseudonym of the interviewee, the date the file was created, and what it is (i.e., transcript or field note). Other files may be generated from meetings of a research team or consultation with an expert about challenges that may arise during data collection. The researchers keep a record of how files are named and where they are stored, preventing wasted time looking for files during analysis, interpretation, and dissemination (Miles et al., 2014).

Nurse researchers are increasingly using computer-assisted qualitative data analysis software (CAQDAS) programs (Creswell & Poth, 2018). The researcher reads the transcripts, identifies codes, and groups similar codes into themes. The computer software does not do the analysis but can record decisions that are made. Other benefits of CAQDAS are the automatic creation of an audit trail, ease of retrieving text with the same code, maintenance of an organized storage file system, development of visual representations of the analyzed data, linkage of memos and journals to the text or code, and ability to share analysis with fellow researchers (Creswell & Poth, 2018). Disadvantages of using CAQDAS are the time invested in selecting and learning the software, perceived distancing from the data, and specific challenges with the selected software (Creswell & Poth, 2018).

Data Analysis

Data analysis is a rigorous process. Because published qualitative studies may not contain the methodology in detail, many professionals believe that qualitative research is a free-wheeling process, with little structure. Creativity and deep thought may produce innovative codes or ways to analyze the data, but the process requires discipline to develop data analysis plans consistent with the specific philosophical method of the study. For example, researchers conducting grounded theory studies use the constant comparative process by comparing concepts and themes identified through the analysis with those identified in subsequent data. In grounded theory, the analysis begins with the first participant interview, so that ideas from that participant can be integrated into questions and probes in subsequent interviews. In phenomenology, this immersion in the data is referred to as **dwelling with the data**. This phrase is used to indicate that the researcher spent considerable time reading and reflecting on the data.

Codes and Coding

Coding is the process of reading the data, breaking text down into subparts, and giving a label to that part of the text. These labels provide a way for the researcher to begin to identify patterns in the data because sections of text that were coded in the same way can be compared for similarities and differences (Miles et al., 2014). A code is a symbol or abbreviation used to classify words or phrases in the data. Codes may be handwritten on a printed transcript. In a word-processing program or CAQDAS, you code by highlighting a section of text and making a comment in the margin or sidebar. Codes may result in themes, processes, or exemplars of the phenomenon being studied. For example, in a qualitative study of medication adherence, participants mentioned clocks, schedules, and hours when doses were due that the researcher coded as "time." An exploratory-descriptive qualitative study about pain experiences of surgical patients may result in a taxonomy of types of pain, activities that resulted in pain, and types of pain relief strategies.

Themes and Interpretation

Themes emerge as codes are combined into more abstract phrases or terms. Sometimes there are several layers of themes, with each layer being another level of abstraction above the initial codes. Making links between these themes and the original data may become more difficult as the themes become more abstract. The clarity of the links between the codes and themes is essential in maintaining the rigor of the study, and CAQDAS will provide these linkages automatically. However, it is the researcher who must remain rigorous in creating the links from the themes back to codes and from the codes to the original data. If you are critically appraising a qualitative study that uses themes, identify the themes, assess whether the researcher provided appropriate participant quotes to support the themes, and determine whether the themes seem sufficient and adequate for the study. During **interpretation,** the researcher places the findings in a larger context and may link different themes or factors in the findings to each other. The researcher is answering the question, "What do the findings mean?" Interpretation may focus on the usefulness of the findings for clinical practice or may move toward theorizing.

? CRITICAL APPRAISAL GUIDELINES

Data Management, Analysis, and Interpretation

1. Were the data analysis and interpretation processes consistent with the philosophical orientation, research problem, research question, and purpose of the study?
2. Did the researchers describe how they recorded decisions made during analysis and interpretation?
3. Did the researchers link the codes and themes used with exemplar quotations?
4. Were the data analysis and interpretation logical and congruent with the study method?
5. Did the researchers provide adequate description of the data analysis and interpretation processes?

Koehn et al. (2016) conducted a grounded theory study of nurses' experiences with errors, described earlier in this chapter. The researchers provided adequate information to critically appraise their data analysis, management, and interpretation, as depicted in Research Example 3.10.

RESEARCH EXAMPLE 3.10

Data Management, Analysis, and Interpretation

Research Study Excerpt

All participants signed an informed consent document labeled with an anonymous identification number linking data collected during the interview and any subsequent memos about the interview... Data collection and analysis progressed simultaneously. Procedures outlined by Charmaz (2014) were used to analyze the data.... Initial coding was conducted by the first author, and focused and axial coding were completed by the full research team through processes of discussion and consensus. Memos were used to document all analytic decisions... The findings of this study add to [the] literature by describing the experience of making a medical error as a complex and nuanced process... how making an error affects nurses over the course of their careers, even years after it occurred... how institutional procedures and practices regarding error reporting influences nurses' experiences... suggest that organizational strategies are needed not only to encourage nurses to report errors but to support nurses when they make an error. (Koehn et al., 2016, pp. 568, 571–572)

Critical Appraisal

Data analysis and interpretation in the Koehn et al. (2016) study were appropriate for the study approach, research questions, and study purpose. They used memos to document all analysis decisions. They used direct quotations from the nurses to support each theme that emerged from the data and explicitly linked codes and themes. Koehn et al. (2016) provided a strong example of how the data for their study were analyzed and interpreted. The research report included short direct quotes from the participants to support the themes. Koehn et al. (2016) clearly linked their findings to the literature and delineated the contributions of the study to nursing knowledge. They provided less information about data organization, but the thoroughness and clarity of the report are indicators that the data were carefully managed.

RIGOR IN QUALITATIVE RESEARCH

Scientific rigor is valued because the findings of rigorous studies are seen as being more credible and of greater worth. Studies are critically appraised as a means of judging rigor. Rigor is defined differently for qualitative research because the desired outcome is different from the desired outcome for quantitative research (Gray et al., 2017). Rigor is assessed in relation to the detail built into the design of the qualitative study, carefulness of data collection, and thoroughness of analysis. When the "purposes, questions, and methods of research are interconnected and interrelated," and the researcher describes the study as a "cohesive whole," the study has methodological congruence (Creswell & Poth, 2018, p. 50). The fit between these key elements of a study (purpose, questions, methods) are important for quantitative and qualitative research, but has special significance in qualitative research because of the evolving nature of studies.

Qualitative researchers are expected to maintain an open mind and allow the meaning to be revealed, even if the meaning is not what was anticipated (Munhall, 2012). The qualitative researcher is expected to provide sufficient information in the published report so that the reader can critically appraise the dependability and confirmability of the study (Petty, Thomson, & Stew, 2012). An audit trail is one way that a researcher can assure a reader that the methods of the study were implemented appropriately. Studies that are dependable and confirmable can be said to have truth, value, or credibility. The findings of a qualitative study cannot be generalized but may be applied "in other contexts or with other participants" (Petty et al., 2012, p. 382). The extent to which the findings of a qualitative study are dependable, confirmable, credible, and transferable is the degree of rigor of the study. Chapter 12 has more information about how to determine whether a study is dependable, confirmable, credible, and transferable.

KEY POINTS

- Qualitative research is a systematic approach used to collect textual data related to the phenomenon the study addresses.
- Qualitative data are words and images, instead of numbers.
- Qualitative data are analyzed to allow the participants' perspectives and the multiple realities of the persons experiencing a phenomenon to emerge.
- Rigor in qualitative research requires critically appraising the study for congruence with the philosophical perspective; appropriateness of the collection, analysis, and interpretation of data; maintenance of an audit trail; and logic of the findings evident in the research report.
- A phenomenological researcher examines an experience and provides interpretations that enhance the meaning while staying true to the perspective of those who have lived the experience.
- Grounded theory researchers explore underlying social processes through the symbols of language, religion, relationships, and clothing and describe the deeper meaning of an event as a theoretical framework.
- Ethnographic researchers observe and interview people within a culture to understand the environment, people, power relations, and communication patterns of a work setting, community, or ethnic group.
- Exploratory-descriptive qualitative studies are conducted to provide information that will promote understanding of an experience from the perspective of the persons living the experience and possibly solve a problem.
- Data collection in qualitative studies occurs in the context of the relationship between the participant and researcher.
- Data in qualitative studies are collected through interviews, focus groups, observation, and examination of documents and media materials.
- Data management, analysis, and interpretation require clear procedures to ensure methodological rigor and credibility of the findings.

REFERENCES

Abrams, T., Ogletree, R., Ratnapradipa, D., & Neumeister, M. (2016). Adult survivors' lived experience of burns and post-burn health: A qualitative analysis. *Burns*, *42*(1), 152–162.

Bolderston, A. (2012). Conducting a research interview. *Journal of Medical Imaging and Radiation Sciences*, *43*(1), 66–76.

Brunk, D., Taylor, A., Clark, M., Williams, I., & Cox, D. (2017). A culturally appropriate self-management program for Hispanic adults with Type 2 diabetes and low health literacy skills. *Journal of Transcultural Nursing*, *28*(2), 187–194.

Charmaz, K. (2014). *Constructing grounded theory.* London, England. Sage.

Chee, W., Lee, Y., Im, E. O., Chee, E., Tsai, H., Nishigaki, M., et al. (2017). A culturally tailored Internet cancer support group for Asian American breast cancer survivors: A randomized controlled pilot intervention study. *Journal of Telemedicine & Telecare*, *23*(6), 618–626.

Converse, M. (2012). Philosophy of phenomenology: How understanding aids research. *Nurse Researcher*, *20*(1), 28–32.

Creswell, J. (2014). *Research design: Qualitative, quantitative, and mixed methods approaches* (4th ed.). Thousand Oaks, CA: Sage.

Creswell, J., & Poth, C. (2018) *Qualitative inquiry and research design: Choosing among five approaches* (4th ed.). Thousand Oaks, CA: Sage.

Cricco-Lizza, R. (2016). Infant feeding beliefs and day-to-day feeding practices of NICU nurses. *Journal of Pediatric Nursing, 31*(2), e91–e98.

Cypress, B. (2015). Qualitative research: The "what," "why," "who," and "how"!. *Dimensions of Critical Care Nursing, 34*(6), 356–361.

Davenport, L. (2017). Living with the choice: A grounded theory of Iraqi refugee resettlement to the U.S. *Issues in Mental Health Nursing, 38*(4), 352–360.

Dowling, M., & Cooney, A. (2012). Research approaches related to phenomenology: Negotiating a complex landscape. *Nurse Researcher, 20*(2), 21–27.

Erikson, A., & Davies, B. (2017). Maintaining integrity: How nurses navigate the boundaries in pediatric palliative care. *Journal of Pediatric Nursing, 35*(1), 42–49.

Fallatah, F., & Edge, D. (2015). Social support needs of families: The context of rheumatoid arthritis. *Applied Nursing Research, 28*(2), 180–185.

Flood, A. (2010). Understanding phenomenology. *Nurse Researcher, 17*(2), 2–7.

Glaser, B. G., & Strauss, A. (1967). *The discovery of grounded theory: Strategies for qualitative research.* Chicago, IL: Aldine.

Gray, J., Grove, S. K., & Sutherland, S. (2017). *The practice of nursing research: Appraisal, synthesis, and generation of evidence* (8th ed.). St. Louis, MO: Elsevier Saunders.

Hall, H., & Roussel, L. (2017). Critical appraisal of research-based evidence. In H. Hall & L. Roussel (Eds.), *Evidence-based practice: An integrative approach to research, administration, and practice* (2nd ed.) (pp. 125–143). Burlington, MA: Jones & Bartlett.

Hatzfeld, J., Nelson, M., Waters, C., & Jennings, M. (2016). Factors influencing health behaviors among active duty Air Force personnel. *Nursing Outlook, 64*(5), 440–449.

Hennink, M., & Weber, M. (2013). Quality issues of court reporters and transcriptionists for qualitative research. *Qualitative Health Research, 23*(5), 700–710.

Hoggan, C., Mälkki, K., & Finnegan, F. (2017). Developing the theory of perspective transformation: Continuity, intersubjectivity, and emancipatory praxis. *Adult Education Quarterly, 67*(1), 48–64.

Houghton, C., Hunter, A., & Meskell, P. (2012). Linking aims, paradigm and method in nursing research. *Nurse Researcher, 20*(2), 34–39.

Im, E. O., Ko, H., Hwang, H., Chee, W., Stuifbergen, A., Walker, L., & Brown, A. (2013). Racial/ethnic differences in midlife women's attitudes toward physical activity. *Journal of Midwifery & Women's Health, 58*(4), 440–450.

Koehn, A., Ebright, P., & Draucker, C. (2016). Nurses' experiences with errors in nursing. *Nursing Outlook, 64*(6), 566–574.

Leininger, M. M. (Ed.), (1985). *Qualitative research methods.* Orlando, FA: Grune and Stratton.

Leininger, M. M. (1988). Leininger's theory of nursing: Cultural care diversity and universality. *Nursing Science Quarterly, 1*(4), 152–160.

Leininger, M. M. (2002). Culture care theory: A major contribution to advance transcultural nursing knowledge and practices. *Journal of Transcultural Nursing, 13*(3), 189–192.

Makary, M., & Daniel, M. (2016). Medical error: The third leading cause of death in the US. *British Medical Journal [BMJ], 353*, i2139. Retrieved June 18, 2017, from http://www.bmj.com/content/353/bmj.i2139.

Marshall, C., & Rossman, G. B. (2016). *Designing qualitative research* (6th ed.). Los Angeles, CA: Sage.

Maxwell, J. (2014). *Qualitative research design: An interactive approach* (3rd ed.). Thousand Oaks, CA: Sage.

McCready, J. (2010). Jamesian pragmatism: A framework for working toward unified diversity in nursing knowledge development. *Nursing Philosophy, 11*(3), 191–203.

Mead, G. H. (1934). *Mind, self and society.* Chicago, IL: University of Chicago Press.

Miles, M., Huberman, A., & Saldaña, J. (2014). *Qualitative data analysis: A methods sourcebook* (3rd ed.). Thousand Oaks, CA: Sage.

Morgan-Trimmer, S., & Wood, F. (2016). Ethnographic methods for process evaluations of complex health behavior interventions. *Trials, 17,* Article 232. Retrieved June 19, 2017, from https://trialsjournal.biomedcentral.com/articles/10.1186/s13063-016-1340-2.

Morse, J. (2016). Underlying ethnography. *Qualitative Health Research, 26*(7), 875–876.

Munhall, P. L. (Ed.), (2012). *Nursing research: A qualitative perspective.* (5th ed.) Sudbury, MA: Jones & Bartlett.

Pender, N., Murdaugh, C., & Parsons, M. (2011). *Health promotion in nursing practice.* Upper Saddle River, NJ: Pearson Education.

Petty, N., Thomson, O., & Stew, G. (2012). Ready for a paradigm shift? Part 2: Introducing qualitative research methodologies and methods. *Manual Therapy, 17*(5), 378–384.

Postma, J., Peterson, J., Vega, M., Ramon, C., & Cortez, G. (2014). Latina youths' perceptions of environmental health risks in an agricultural community. *Public Health Nursing, 31*(6), 508–516.

Powers, B. (2015). Generating evidence through qualitative research. In B. M. Melnyk & E. Fineout-Overholt (Eds.), *Evidence-based practice in nursing & healthcare: A guide to best practice.* (3rd ed.) (pp. 476–489). Philadelphia, PA: Wolters Kluwer.

Rashid, M., Caine, V., & Goez, H. (2015). The encounters and challenges of ethnography as a methodology in health research. In *International Journal of Qualitative Methods.* Retrieved June 19, 2017, from http://journals.sagepub.com/doi/abs/10.1177/1609406915621421.

Rasmussen, M., Amris, K., & Ryadahl-Hansen, S. (2017). How can group-based multidisciplinary rehabilitation for patients with fibromyalgia influence patients' self-efficacy and ability to cope with their illness: A grounded theory approach. *Journal of Clinical Nursing, 26*(7-8), 931–945.

Roper, J. M., & Shapiro, J. (2000). *Ethnography in nursing research.* Thousand Oaks, CA: Sage.

Sandelowski, M. (2000). Whatever happened to qualitative description? *Research in Nursing & Health, 23*(4), 334–340.

Sandelowski, M. (2010). What's in a name? Qualitative description revisited. *Research in Nursing & Health, 33*(1), 77–84.

Sanon, M. A., Spigner, C., & McCullagh, M. (2016). Transnationalism and hypertension self-management among Haitian immigrants. *Journal of Transcultural Nursing, 27*(2), 147–156.

Savage, J. (2006). Ethnographic evidence: The value of applied ethnography in healthcare. *Journal of Research in Nursing, 11*(5), 383–395.

Tuohy, D., Cooney, A., Dowling, M., Murphy, K., & Sixmith, J. (2013). An overview of interpretive phenomenology as a research methodology. *Nurse Researcher, 20*(6), 17–20.

van Manen, M. (2017). But is it phenomenology? *Qualitative Health Research, 27*(6), 775–779.

Weyant, R., Clukey, L., Roberts, M., & Henderson, A. (2017). Show your stuff and watch your tone: Nurses' caring behaviors. *American Journal of Critical Care, 26*(2), 111–117.

Wolf, M. (2012). Ethnography: The method. In P. L. Munhall (Ed.), *Nursing research: A qualitative perspective.* (5th ed.) (pp. 285–338). Sudbury, MA: Jones & Bartlett.

Wuerst, J. (2012). Grounded theory: The method. In P. L. Munhall (Ed.), *Nursing research: A qualitative perspective.* (5th ed.) (pp. 225–256). Sudbury, MA: Jones & Bartlett.

Because of funding changes, the Agency for Healthcare Research and Quality (AHRQ) National Guideline Clearinghouse website was scheduled for decommissioning as of July 16, 2018. For more information, go to https://www.ahrq.gov/.

CHAPTER

4

Examining Ethics in Nursing Research

Jennifer R. Gray

CHAPTER OVERVIEW

LEARNING OUTCOMES

After completing this chapter, you should be able to:

1. Describe the role of the bachelor of science in nursing (BSN)-prepared nurse in ensuring ethical research.
2. Identify the historical events influencing the development of ethical codes and regulations for nursing and biomedical research.
3. Describe the ethical principles and human rights that require protection in research.
4. Identify the essential elements of the informed consent process in research.
5. Describe the levels of review that an institutional review board (IRB) may use in reviewing a study.
6. Describe the current issues in ethical research surrounding genomics research, use of animals in studies, and research misconduct.
7. Critically appraise ethical sections in research reports, with emphasis on IRB and informed consent processes.

Ethical research is essential for generating credible and trustworthy knowledge for evidence-based practice (EBP), but what does ethical conduct of research involve? The understanding of the ethical conduct of research developed, unfortunately, as the scientific community and the public were confronted with examples of unethical studies. Unethical studies that violate subjects' rights have been implemented in the United States since biomedical research began. As these studies came to light, national codes and regulations were developed to promote the ethical conduct of research. These codes and regulations dramatically reduced the number of unethical studies but, unfortunately, ethical violations and research misconduct persist today.

As a BSN-prepared nurse, you will need to be able to critically appraise the ethical aspects of published studies and of research conducted in clinical agencies. The methods section of most published studies includes information about the ethical selection of study participants and their treatment during data collection. IRBs in universities and clinical agencies have been organized to examine the ethical aspects of studies before they are conducted. You may have the opportunity to be a member of an IRB and participate in the review of research for conduct in clinical agencies.

To provide you with a background for examining ethical aspects of studies, this chapter describes the ethical codes and regulations that currently guide the conduct of biomedical and behavioral research. The following elements of ethical research are detailed: (1) protecting human rights during research; (2) understanding informed consent; (3) understanding institutional review of research; and (4) critically appraising the ethical aspects of a study. The chapter concludes with a discussion of current ethical issues surrounding genomics research, the use of animals in research, and research misconduct.

UNETHICAL RESEARCH: 1930s THROUGH THE 1980s

Four experimental projects have been highly publicized for their unethical treatment of human subjects: the Nazi medical experiments, the Tuskegee Syphilis Study, the Willowbrook Study, and the Jewish Chronic Disease Hospital Study (Berger, 1990; Levine, 1986). Nurses were involved in implementing these studies, although the primary researchers were physicians. These unethical studies demonstrate the importance of ethical conduct for nurses when they review or participate in research (Fry, Veatch, & Taylor, 2011). These studies also influenced the formulation of ethical codes and regulations that continue to direct the conduct of research today.

Nazi Medical Experiments

From 1933 to 1945, the Third Reich in Europe was engaged in atrocious and unethical medical activities, including research. Medical experiments were conducted on prisoners of war and persons considered to be valueless, such as Jews confined in concentration camps. The experiments involved exposing subjects to high altitudes, freezing temperatures, poisons, infections, untested drugs, and surgery without anesthesia. The Nazi experiments violated numerous rights of the research subjects, such as unjust selection of subjects, involuntary participation, and permanent damage, including death. Because these studies were poorly conceived and conducted, this research was not only unethical but also generated little, if any, useful scientific knowledge (Berger, 1990; Steinfels & Levine, 1976).

Tuskegee Syphilis Study

In 1932, the US Public Health Service initiated a study of the natural history of syphilis in black men in the small rural town of Tuskegee, Alabama (Rothman, 1982). Many of the subjects were not informed about the purpose and procedures of the research. Some were unaware that they were subjects in a study. By 1936, evidence was clearly available that the men with syphilis had developed more complications than the men in the control group. Ten years later the death rate among those with syphilis was twice as high as it was for the control group. The subjects were examined periodically but were not treated for syphilis, even when penicillin was determined to be an effective treatment for the disease in the 1940s. Information about an effective treatment for syphilis was withheld from the subjects, and deliberate steps were taken to deprive them of treatment (Brandt, 1978).

Published reports of the Tuskegee Syphilis Study started appearing in 1936, and additional papers were published every 4 to 6 years. No effort was made to stop the study; in fact, in 1969, the Centers for Disease Control reviewed the study and decided that it should continue. The study continued for a total of 40 years. In 1972, an account of the study in the *Washington Star* sparked public outrage; only then did the US Department of Health, Education, and Welfare (DHEW) stop the study. The study was investigated and found to be ethically unjustified (Brandt, 1978).

Willowbrook Study

From the mid-1950s to the early 1970s, Dr. Saul Krugman conducted research on hepatitis at Willowbrook, an institution for the mentally retarded in Staten Island, New York (Rothman, 1982). The subjects were children who were deliberately infected with the hepatitis virus. During the 20-year study, Willowbrook closed its doors to new inmates because of overcrowding. However, the research ward continued to admit new inmates. Parents could only admit their children if they were willing to give permission for their child to be in the study.

From the late 1950s to the early 1970s, Krugman's research team published several articles describing the study protocol and its findings. In 1966, Beecher cited the Willowbrook Study in the *New England Journal of Medicine* as an example of unethical research. The investigators defended injecting the children with the hepatitis virus because they believed that most of the children would acquire the infection shortly after being admitted to the institution. They also stressed the benefits the subjects received, which were a cleaner environment, better supervision, and a higher nurse-to-patient ratio on the research ward (Rothman, 1982). Despite the controversy, this unethical study continued until the early 1970s.

Jewish Chronic Disease Hospital Study

Another highly publicized unethical study was conducted at the Jewish Chronic Disease Hospital in New York in the 1960s. The purpose of this study was to determine patients' rejection responses to live cancer cells. A suspension containing live cancer cells that had been generated from human cancer tissue was injected into 22 patients (Levine, 1986). The researchers did not inform these patients that they were taking part in a study. The subjects also did not know the injections that they received were live cancer cells. This lack of disclosure violated their rights to self-determination and protection from harm. In addition, the study was never presented for review to the research committee of the Jewish Chronic Disease Hospital, and the physicians caring for the patients were unaware that the study was being conducted.

The physician directing the research was an employee of the Sloan-Kettering Institute for Cancer Research; there was no indication that this institution had conducted a review of the research project (Hershey & Miller, 1976). This unethical study was conducted without the informed consent of the subjects and institutional review and had the potential to injure, disable, or cause the death of the human subjects. Once the public became aware of the study, it was immediately stopped, and steps were taken to ensure proper care for the patients exposed to the cancer cells. Precautions were put into place to ensure that all future proposed research conducted in the agency was properly reviewed and approved.

ETHICAL STANDARDS FOR RESEARCH

Out of the history of unethical research has emerged international standards and US standards and laws that delineate ethical research involving human subjects. The first was developed in the aftermath of World War II.

International Standards

Ethical principles for research were first articulated following the Nuremberg Tribunals of German war crimes. Those involved in the Nazi experiments were brought to trial before the Nuremberg Tribunals, and their unethical research received international attention. In 1949, after the trial ended, the **Nuremberg Code** was released (Eastwood, 2015). Box 4.1 presents the key tenets of the Nuremberg Code. The code includes guidelines that should help you evaluate

BOX 4.1 THE NUREMBERG CODE: CHARACTERISTICS OF ETHICAL STUDIES

Rationale for Study
- Conducted when necessary knowledge cannot be gained any other way
- Based on the results of previous studies, including animal experimentation and knowledge of natural history of disease
- Designed to yield results that are needed by society
- Anticipated results justify conducting the study

Rights of Human Subjects
- Voluntary consent
- May withdraw at any time with no penalty

Risk Avoidance
- No unnecessary physical or mental suffering and injury
- Study terminated if the risk of harm increases

Resources
- Adequate resources to protect subjects

Adapted from US Government Printing Office. (1949). *Nuremberg Code.* https://history.nih.gov/research/downloads/nuremberg.pdf.

the consent process, protection of subjects from harm, and balance of benefits and risks in a study (Office of NIH History, 1949).

The Nuremberg Code provided the basis for the development of the **Declaration of Helsinki,** which was adopted in 1964. A major focus of the declaration was clarifying the differences between therapeutic research and nontherapeutic research. **Therapeutic research** provides patients with an opportunity to receive an experimental treatment that might have beneficial results. **Nontherapeutic research** is conducted to generate knowledge for science; the results may help future patients but are not expected to benefit those acting as research participants. Researchers are responsible for protecting the health, privacy, and dignity of human subjects and for selecting important study topics concerning the risks and burdens for subjects. The World Medical Association (WMA, 2013) has initiated and published the most recent revision of the Declaration.

Standards in the United States

In the United States, the first major ethical guide was the **Belmont Report,** written by the National Commission for the Protection of Human Subjects of Biomedical and Behavioral Research (1979). The commission was formed in response to the public outcry when the Tuskegee Syphilis Study was exposed. The Belmont Report identified ethical principles to guide selecting subjects, informing them of the risks and benefits of a study and documenting their consent. The report also detailed differences between therapeutic and nontherapeutic research and the application of research findings in the practice of medicine (National Commission, 1979).

President Obama issued an executive order creating the Presidential Commission for the Study of Bioethical Issues, a diverse group of national leaders to advise government leaders on emerging ethical and social issues as a result of scientific advances. The Commission was active from 2009 to 2017 and issued recommendations related to genomics, neuroscience, and protecting human subjects. The reports and other documents from their work are archived as educational resources related to bioethics (https://bioethicsarchive.georgetown.edu/pcsbi/node/851.html).

Federal Regulations for the Protection of Human Subjects

Following the Belmont Report, federal regulations to protect human research subjects were developed and continue to be updated as needed, most recently in 2017. The regulations are part of the *Code of Federal Regulations* (CFR). Each US department involved in human research has a chapter in the CFR that guides research funded by the department. Because of the similarities among the chapters, the CFR is called the **Common Rule**. The goals of the recent revision were to enhance protection of human subjects and reduce the administrative burden of regulating research in healthcare organizations and universities (Menikoff, Kaneshiro, & Pritchard, 2017). The final version of the revised rule was published in the *Federal Register* in January 2017 and was scheduled to be effective starting January 2018 (US Department of Health and Human Services [DHHS], 2017a).

The Common Rule includes requirements related to the content of an informed consent document, processes for obtaining informed consent, maintaining an IRB, and implementing special precautions for studies with vulnerable populations (Fig. 4.1). **Vulnerable populations** are defined as persons who are susceptible to undue influence or coercion, such as children, prisoners, and persons who are economically or educationally disadvantaged (DHHS, 2017a). Persons who have impaired decision making were also identified as being vulnerable. This might include persons with Alzheimer disease, traumatic brain injury, and those born with intellectual limitations.

During your clinical practice, you may facilitate obtaining patient consent to participate in clinical trials related to new drugs and medical devices. The US Food and Drug Administration (FDA) is responsible for managing the elements of the Common Rule that involve testing drugs, medical devices, biological products, dietary supplements, and electronic products for human use (FDA, 2015). To summarize, the Common Rule, including the FDA regulations, provide guidelines for federally and privately funded research to protect subjects, ensure their privacy, and maintain the confidentiality of the information obtained through research. Box 4.2 compares the regulations applicable to research on human subjects.

In 2003, another law was finalized that affected research, the **Health Insurance Portability and Accountability Act** (HIPAA; Public Law 104.191, 1996). First introduced in 1996, HIPAA has become known as the Privacy Rule and focuses on protecting electronic storage and transfer of patient information generated through providing clinical care. The Privacy Rule defined **protected health information** (PHI) as data generated and collected for research that can be linked to an individual person. With the recent revision of the Common Rule, the relationship between it and HIPAA is less clear than it was. Some experts have suggested that privacy rules will be integrated

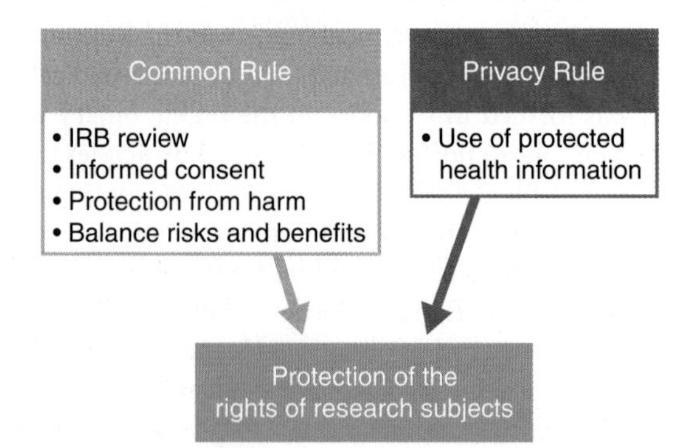

FIG 4.1 Functions of federal research guidelines. *IRB*, Institutional review board.

BOX 4.2 CLARIFICATION OF FEDERAL REGULATIONS RELATED TO HUMAN SUBJECTS RESEARCH

Regulation: Health Insurance Portability and Accountability Act (HIPAA) (Privacy Rule)
- **Key phrase:** Protected health information
- **Objective:** Privacy protections for most individually identifiable protected health information by establishing conditions for its use and disclosure by certain healthcare providers, health plans, and healthcare clearinghouses
- **Applicability:** HIPAA-defined covered entities, regardless of the source of funding; broader application than research

Regulation: US Department of Health and Human Services (DHHS) Protection of Human Subjects Regulations[a] (Common Rule)
- **Key phrase:** Human subjects research
- **Objective:** Protect the rights and welfare of human subjects involved in research conducted or supported by DHHS
- **Applicability:** Human subjects' research conducted or supported by DHHS; application has been extended to all human subjects' research, with or without funding

Regulation: US Food and Drug Administration (FDA) Protection of Human Subjects Regulations[b]
- **Key phrase:** Medications and medical devices
- **Objective:** Protect the rights, safety, and welfare of subjects involved in clinical investigations regulated by the FDA
- **Applicability:** Applies to research involving products regulated by the FDA. Federal support is not necessary for FDA regulations to be applicable. When research subject to FDA jurisdiction is federally funded, both the DHHS Protection of Human Subjects Regulations and FDA Protection of Human Subjects Regulations apply.

[a]US Department of Health and Human Services (DHHS). (2017a). Final revisions to the Common Rule: Protection of human subjects. Code of Federal Regulations, Title 45, Part 46. Retrieved March 11, 2017, from https://www.hhs.gov/ohrp/regulations-and-policy/regulations/finalized-revisions-common-rule/index.html.
[b]US Food and Drug Administration (FDA). (2015). *FDA fundamentals.* Retrieved March 5, 2017, from https://www.fda.gov/AboutFDA/Transparency/Basics/ucm192695.htm.

into the Common Rule. Fig. 4.1 provides a diagram of the current roles of the Common Rule and Privacy Rule. The rules, identified in the boxes at the top of the figure, have different foci but are united in the goal of protecting the rights of human subjects (bottom of the figure).

PROTECTING HUMAN SUBJECTS

Protecting the people who participate in research requires more than standards and laws. A responsible researcher must be guided by ethical principles that support the rights of research subjects.

Application of Ethical Principles

The previous examples of unethical research highlight the need for standards to protect research subjects. Within the published standards and laws, three **ethical principles** guide ethical research: respect for persons, beneficence, and justice (Fig. 4.2). The **principle of respect for persons** indicates that people should be treated as autonomous agents, with the right to choose whether or not to participate in research and to withdraw from a study. In the figure, the principle is linked to autonomy. Below the circle with autonomy are three ways that autonomy is applied in a study. Those with diminished autonomy, such as children, people who are terminally or mentally ill, and prisoners, are entitled to additional protection. Subjects from vulnerable populations may also need safeguards enacted to ensure that the principle of respect of persons is protected.

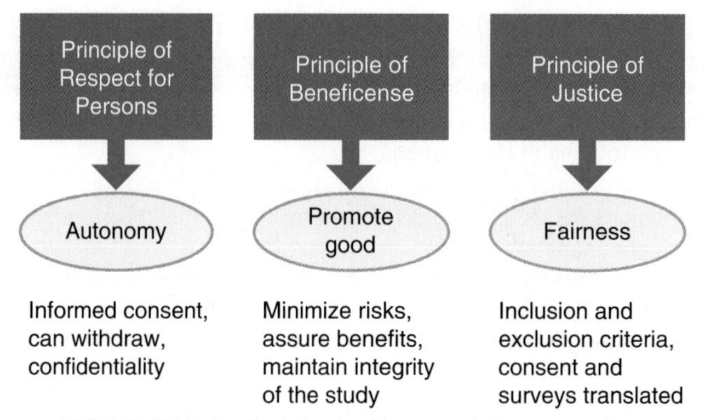

FIG 4.2 Ethical principles and human rights protection.

The **principle of beneficence** encourages the researcher to do good and "above all, do no harm." This principle is the foundation for analyzing the benefits and risks of a specific study. In Fig. 4.2, the principle is linked to the circle labeled "promote good." Researchers guided by this principle seek to reduce the risks and ensure that the subjects receive the benefits. A specific example is an intervention study in which enhanced diabetic education improves glucose control in the treatment group. At the end of the study, a researcher guided by beneficence would provide the intervention for the subjects in the control group. Beneficence also involves maintaining the integrity of the study and disseminating the findings so that maximum scientific benefit can be gained from the study. Findings of poorly designed and implemented studies have no benefit to the subjects and the wider population.

The **principle of justice** states that human subjects have a right to fair treatment, which includes access to the potential benefits of a study and not overexposure to its risks. Fig. 4.2 displays the principle of justice leading to fairness. Maintaining justice in research means that inclusion and exclusion criteria (see Chapter 9) for subjects in studies must have scientific and/or logical explanations.

In summary, the diagram in Fig. 4.2 shows how respect for persons is the basis for autonomy, beneficence results in promoting good through research, and justice supports fairness. Although ethical principles can be abstract, each can be applied as specific procedures during a study, as shown in the figure.

Consistent with the ethical principles, nurses who critically appraise published studies, review research for conduct in their agencies, or assist with data collection for a study, have an obligation to determine whether the rights of the research participants have been protected. The human rights that require protection in research are the rights to the following: (1) self-determination; (2) privacy; (3) anonymity and confidentiality; (4) protection from discomfort and harm; and (5) fair selection and treatment. The American Nurses Association (ANA) Code of Ethics for Nurses (2015) reiterates these rights and provides nurses with guidelines for ethical conduct in nursing practice and research. This code focuses on protecting the rights of patients and research participants.

Right to Self-Determination

The right to self-determination is based on the ethical principle of respect for persons, and it indicates that humans are capable of controlling their own destiny. People should be given **autonomy,** which means having the freedom to conduct their lives as they choose, without external controls. Researchers protect the autonomy of subjects when they are provided information about a study and allowed to choose whether or not to participate. In addition, a subject who consents and begins a study is allowed to withdraw from the study at any time, without penalty (DHHS, 2017a). The culture of the subjects is one factor that must be considered in treating persons autonomously because autonomy has different interpretations and implications in varying cultures (Roberts, Jadalla, Jones-Oyefeso, Winslow, & Taylor, 2017). Nurses are considered educationally prepared to advocate for potential research subjects of different backgrounds because of nursing's knowledge of cultural values related to autonomy and decision making (Halkoaho, Pietila, Ebbesen, Karki, & Kangasniemi, 2016). Potential subjects may be more open to consenting to a study when the recruiter is a member of their culture, or more open to discussing a study with a researcher who shares their culture. Roberts et al. (2017) have found that research in another country requires involvement of members of the culture in the development of the study to ensure that the study questions, methods, and approach to recruitment are acceptable to the community. Roberts and colleagues (2017) had conducted research in five countries and compared their experiences.

A subject's right to self-determination can be violated through the use of coercion, covert data collection, and deception. **Coercion** occurs when one person intentionally presents an overt threat of harm or an excessive reward to another to obtain compliance. Some subjects are coerced (forced) to participate in research because they fear harm or discomfort if they do not participate. For example, some patients, when asked by their healthcare provider to participate in a study, may fear that their medical and nursing care will be negatively affected if they do not agree to be research participants. Others are coerced to participate in studies because they believe that they cannot refuse the excessive rewards offered, such as large sums of money, special privileges, or access to experimental treatments. The Willowbrook study occurred in a facility that was overcrowded, and the only available admission to the hospital was to the research unit (Rothman, 1982). Parents felt coerced to admit their children for care, despite having concerns about the research being conducted.

With **covert data collection,** subjects are unaware that research data are being collected (Reynolds, 1979). For example, during the Jewish Chronic Disease Hospital Study, most of the patients and their physicians were unaware of the study. The subjects were informed that they were receiving an injection of cells, but the word *cancer* was omitted (Beecher, 1966).

The use of **deception,** the actual misinforming of subjects for research purposes, can also violate a subject's right to self-determination. A classic example of deception is seen in the Milgram study (1963), in which the subjects thought they were administering electric shocks to another person, but the person was really a professional actor who pretended to feel the shocks. Deception should be used only when absolutely necessary to study topics with a potential to make significant contributions to science (Boynton, Portnoy, & Johnson, 2013). To be acceptable, the use of deception should not be expected to cause any long-lasting harm. Also, the researchers should explain the deception to the subjects as soon as possible. Based on the revision of the Common Rule, deception may only be used ethically in a study when the researcher informs potential subjects that they will be unaware of or deliberately misguided about the true purpose of the study, and they agree to participate despite this condition (DHHS, 2017a).

Persons With Diminished Autonomy and Research. Persons have **diminished autonomy** when they have impaired decision making due to medications, mental illness, or mental capacity. Depending on the cause, diminished autonomy may be temporary or permanent. Persons with diminished autonomy require additional protection of their right to self-determination because of their decreased ability to give informed consent. In addition, they are vulnerable to coercion and deception.

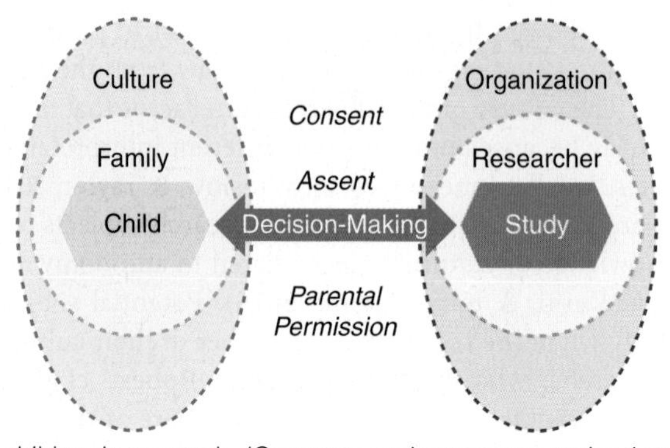

FIG 4.3 Participation of children in research. (Concepts and processes revised and redrawn from Oulton, K., Gibson, F., Sell, D., Williams, A., Pratt, L., & Wray, J. [2016]. Assent for children's participation in research: Why it matters and making it meaningful. *Child: Care, Health and Development, 42*[4], 588–592.)

Children may be considered to have diminished autonomy because of their emotional immaturity and cognitive development. Parents or guardians are the legal representative of the child and may, on a child's behalf, give **permission to participate in research**. Researchers not only obtain parental consent, but they also must solicit **assent to participate in research** from the child (Antal et al., 2017). Assent means that the child has agreed to participate in the study (Oulton et al., 2016). Determining the appropriate age at which to involve the child in decisions about participating in research is complex.

Fig. 4.3 is a simplified view of the factors that affect the methods used to obtain parental permission—also called parental consent—and pediatric assent. The figure displays the child, family, and culture as one social system interacting with another social system comprised of the study, researcher, and organization in which the research is being conducted. In the model, the inner circle labeled as "child" represents the communication and comprehension of the child (see Fig. 4.3). The child's ability to listen or absorb information through media affects the comprehension of the child. The interaction of biological age, intellectual development, degree of consciousness, and psychological and emotional maturity affect the child's communication and comprehension (Oulton et al., 2016). The "family" surrounds the child in the model, representing the parent's or guardian's perceptions of the child's decision-making ability. The outer ring is the role of children in the family's culture and the extent to which children are allowed to participate in decision making. The relationships between parents and between the parents and child directly affect how decisions will be made in the family system about participation in research (Oulton et al., 2016).

The other side of the model displays the "study" in the center, with the "researcher" surrounding the study (see Fig. 4.3). The study label represents the research methods that are planned, including the invasiveness of any procedures and the length of the study. The researcher, which may be a team of researchers, are characterized by their experience with research and with working with children and the tools and training they have received.

The study and researcher are surrounded by the "organization." The purpose of the organization (clinical care, treatment, or both), as well as the culture of the community and of the organization, influences the study and the researcher (Oulton et al., 2016).

The arrow between the two systems represents the decision-making process related to the child's participation in the study. When the decision is affirmative, the process will culminate in a combination of assent, consent, or parental permission documents (see Fig. 4.3). Oulton et al. (2016)

have argued that, with the exception of infants and toddlers, children can and should be involved in the process of giving assent or consent.

In 2003, Congress passed a bill called the Pediatric Research Equity Act (PREA) to motivate drug manufacturers to include pediatric subjects in drug trials and provide pediatric dosing when new drugs are released for use. Physicians have voiced concerns that pediatric drug research lags far behind adult studies and could result in harm, or at least loss of potential benefits for children (Bourgeosis & Hwang, 2017). Cancer drugs were not included in PREA, and a bill was introduced in Congress in 2016 called the Research to Accelerate Cures and Equity Act (RACE for Children Act). The bill was not passed but, if enacted, it would have included cancer drugs in PREA and stopped waivers that many drug manufacturers have used to delay or not comply with PREA (Kids v Cancer, 2017).

Because of the challenges of perceived risks with pediatric research, obtaining assent, and documenting consent, the research base for EBP with children and adolescents is limited. As a result, additional studies are needed with children and adolescents as subjects. Published studies need to indicate clearly that the child gave either assent or consent and the parents or guardians gave their permission before data were collected.

Right to Privacy

Privacy is the freedom people have to determine the time, extent, and general circumstances under which their private information will be shared with or withheld from others. Private information includes a person's attitudes, beliefs, behaviors, opinions, and records. The research subject's privacy is protected if the subject is informed, consents to participate in a study, and voluntarily shares private information with a researcher. An **invasion of privacy** occurs when private information is shared without a person's knowledge or against his or her will. A research report often will indicate that the subject's privacy was protected and may include the details of how this was accomplished. Trimble, Nava, and McFarlane (2013) conducted a study of intimate partner violence among women with human immunodeficiency virus (HIV) infection, a population for whom confidentiality was extremely important. The researchers noted in the report that their efforts to "safeguard the privacy of personal health information by maintaining all files related to the study under lock and key... to further protect privacy, unique identification numbers instead of names were used on all data-collection forms" (Trimble et al., 2013, p. 333).

The HIPAA Privacy Rule expanded the protection of a person's privacy—specifically, his or her protected, individually identifiable health information. According to the Common Rule, **identifiable private information** (IPI) is "private information for which the identity of the subject is or may be readily ascertained by the investigator or associated with the information" (DHHS, 2017b, Section 102). According to the HIPAA Privacy Rule, identifiable information is protected if related to a person's past or current health condition, the care received by healthcare providers, and payment for health care received. The relationships between these definitions and other aspects of the revised Common Rule and HIPAA related to research are not completely developed because the revision provides researchers expanded access to PHI to identify potential study participants. In addition, the revised Common Rule created a new type of consent called **broad consent,** through which a potential subject gives researchers permission to store, maintain, and use IPI for other studies (DHHS, 2017a). Broad consent does require that researchers protect confidentiality of the identity of the subjects. In addition, broad consent applies to identifiable biospecimens collected for other studies or clinical care. Box 4.3 lists the key points required for broad consent.

BOX 4.3 COMPONENTS OF BROAD CONSENT

Description

Researcher may store, maintain, and use for future studies identifiable private information and identifiable biospecimens.

General Requirements

Similar to informed consent (see Box 4.4); broad consent will include:

- Potential risks and benefits
- Confidentiality related to subject's identity
- Voluntary participation
- Right to withdraw at any time

In addition, broad consent will include:

- Use of biospecimens for commercial profit
- If profits occur, subjects will receive a share
- Whether analysis of the specimen will include whole genome sequencing
- Types of research for which data may be used
- Sufficient information for a reasonable person to make a decision about participation
- Length of time data will be kept, which may be indefinite
- Statement subjects not to be informed about specific studies being conducted
- Results not to be shared with subjects unless clinically relevant
- Contact information to use in getting answers to questions

Right to Anonymity and Confidentiality

On the basis of the right to privacy, the research subject has the right to anonymity and the right to assume that the data collected will be kept confidential. Complete **anonymity** exists when the researcher cannot link a subject's identity with her or his individual responses (Gray, Grove, & Sutherland, 2017). In most studies, researchers know the identity of their subjects, and they promise the subjects that their identity will be kept anonymous from others and that the research data will be kept confidential. **Confidentiality** is the researcher's safe management of information or data shared by a subject to ensure that the data are kept private from others. The researcher agrees not to share the subjects' information without their authorization. Confidentiality is grounded in two premises (ANA, 2015):

1. Because individuals own their personal information, they may share personal information to the extent that they wish and with whom they wish.
2. Accepting personal information comes with an obligation to maintain confidentiality, an obligation that is even greater for researchers and nurses.

A **breach of confidentiality** can occur when a researcher, by accident or direct action, allows an unauthorized person to gain access to the raw data of a study. Confidentiality also can be breached in reporting or publishing a study if a participant's identity is accidentally revealed, violating his or her right to anonymity. In quantitative studies, results are presented for subgroups or groups, and a breach of confidentiality is less likely to occur. In qualitative studies, however, a breach of confidentiality is more likely because the researcher gathers data from fewer study participants and reports long quotes made by those participants. In addition, qualitative researchers and participants often have relationships in which detailed stories of the participants' lives are shared, requiring careful management of study data to ensure confidentiality (Marshall & Rossman, 2016, Munhall, 2012). Breaches of confidentiality are especially harmful to participants when factors such as their religious preferences, sexual practices, income, racial prejudices, drug use, or child abuse are shared. Participants' confidentiality should be maintained during data collection, analysis, and reporting (Gray et al., 2017). Research findings, whether quantitative, qualitative, or mixed methods, should be reported so that a participant or group of participants cannot be identified by their responses.

Right to Protection From Discomfort and Harm

The right to protection from discomfort and harm in a study is based on the ethical principle of beneficence, which states that one should do good and, above all, do no harm. According to this principle, members of society must take an active role in preventing discomfort and harm and promoting good in the world around them (ANA, 2015; Levine, 1986). In research, **discomfort and harm** can be physical, emotional, social, or economic or any combination of these four types (Weijer, 2000).

Studies range from no anticipated discomfort and harm to a high risk of discomfort and harm. Research designs that involve a review of medical records, student files, or secondary analysis of de-identified data collected for another study have no anticipated discomfort and harm. When there is no or minimal interaction between the researcher and subject, the study will usually be considered exempt when reviewed by an IRB.

Studies that cause temporary discomfort are described as minimal risk studies, in which the discomfort is similar to what the subject would encounter in his or her daily life and is temporary, ending when the study is complete (DHHS, 2017a). Subjects in a minimal risk study may complete questionnaires or participate in interviews. Physical discomfort in minimal risk studies may include fatigue, headache, or muscle tension. Anxiety or embarrassment might result from answering questions on sensitive topics. The only economic harm may be the costs of travel to the study site.

Most clinical nursing studies examining the effect of a treatment involve minimal risk. For example, a study examining the effects of exercise on the blood glucose levels of diabetic subjects may involve the subjects testing their blood glucose level one extra time per day. Physical discomfort or harm may be associated with obtaining the blood or participating in the prescribed exercise. To avoid economic harm, the researcher may reimburse the subject for the cost of the additional testing supplies. The diabetic subjects encounter similar discomforts in their daily lives. The discomfort of an extra finger stick will cease when the study ends.

Discomfort and harm during some studies may go beyond the minimal level and involve unusual levels of temporary discomfort. In studies with unusual levels of temporary discomfort, the subjects may experience discomfort during and after the study. Unusual levels of temporary discomfort might be experienced during a study in which subjects have been confined to bed for 3 days to explore associations between immobility and muscle weakness. Muscle weaknesses may continue after the study until the subject is fully recovered.

Unusual levels of discomfort or harm may occur when subjects experience failure, extreme fear, or threats to their identity as part of a study. Qualitative researchers may ask questions that cause participants to relive a life crisis, such as being diagnosed with colon cancer or losing a spouse. Reliving these experiences or acting in an unnatural way involves unusual levels of temporary discomfort. In studies with unusual levels of discomfort or harm, the researcher will describe the exclusion criteria for the sample in the IRB protocol. The exclusion criteria are developed to prevent recruitment of subjects who are at higher risk for long-term discomfort or harm. In the study involving being confined to bed, persons with pulmonary disease would be excluded due to their higher risk for pneumonia. A potential participant for a qualitative study related to recovery following a sexual assault might be excluded if he or she were currently receiving counseling from a licensed professional. The research team would also indicate in the IRB protocol and subsequent research report the ways in which they assessed participants' discomfort and the resources they made available.

Studies in which there is the risk of permanent damage will undergo additional scrutiny by the IRB. The rationale for doing the study must establish reasons why the knowledge from the study cannot be gained in another way and what will be done to prevent or minimize damage. Biomedical studies involving new medications and devices are more likely to cause permanent damage than studies that nurses more typically initiate. Some topics investigated by nurses have the potential to cause permanent damage to subjects, emotionally and socially. Studies examining sensitive information, such as sexual behavior, child abuse, HIV/AIDS status, or drug use, can be very risky for subjects. These studies have the potential to cause permanent damage to a subject's personality or reputation. There also are potential economic risks, such as those resulting from a decrease in job performance or loss of employment.

The Nazi medical experiments and the Tuskegee Syphilis Study are examples of studies in which the subjects had a certainty of experiencing permanent damage. Conducting research that has a certainty of causing permanent damage to study subjects is highly questionable, regardless of the benefits that will be gained. Frequently, the benefits gained from such a study are experienced not by the research participants, but by others in society. Studies causing permanent damage to subjects violate the principles of the Nuremberg Code and should not be conducted (see Box 4.1).

Right to Fair Selection and Treatment

The right to fair selection and treatment is based on the ethical principle of justice. According to this principle, people must be treated fairly and receive what they are owed or treated in a way that is equitable to the treatment of other persons in the same situation. The research report needs to indicate that the selection of subjects and their treatment during the study were fair.

Injustices in subject selection have resulted from social, cultural, racial, and sexual biases. For many years, research was conducted on categories of people who were deemed as less valuable, such as those living in poverty, prisoners, slaves, and persons of a minority race or ethnicity. Researchers often treated these subjects without regard for harm or discomfort, sacrificing their protection for the sake of scientific or personal gain (Doody & Noonan, 2016).

Another concern with subject selection is that some researchers select subjects because they like them and want them to receive the benefits of a study. Other researchers have been swayed by power or money to ensure that certain patients become subjects so that they can receive potentially beneficial treatments. Random selection of subjects can eliminate some of the researchers' biases that may influence subject selection and strengthens the design of the study (see Chapter 9).

Each study must include a consent form describing the researcher's role and subject's participation in the study (DHHS, 2017a). A consent form is actually an agreement between the subject and researcher about what each will do during the study. While conducting the study, the researcher must treat subjects fairly and respect that agreement. For example, the activities or procedures that subjects are to perform should not be changed without the IRB's approval. The benefits promised to the subjects should be provided and distributed without regard for age, race, or socioeconomic level.

The research report needs to indicate that the selection and treatment of the subjects were fair. Inclusion criteria should reflect the research problem and study purpose. For example, the statement of the research problem might be the few studies identifying the work-related stresses of registered nurses (RNs) in acute care in the early years of their career. The purpose of study was to explore the lived experience of work-related stress among acute care RNs in the first 5 years after graduation. The inclusion criteria would be RNs employed in acute care for at least 1 year and less than 6 years. As discussed, exclusion criteria should be justified to protect potential subjects who are at higher risk for harms or to avoid the unintentional influence of a participant's characteristics on the study results. An exclusion criterion might be nurses who were working at more than one hospital or pursuing an advanced degree. Either of these conditions might influence the stress experienced at work.

The responsible researcher designs the study to minimize discomfort and the risk of harm for potential subjects, as well as protect their rights to self-determination, privacy, confidentiality, and fair selection and treatment. Details are usually not provided in the research report about how each of these was accomplished, but should indicate the basic measures taken, such as keeping data confidential by assigning code numbers to subjects' materials. The guidelines that follow will assist you in critically appraising a study to ensure the protection of human rights, with the exception of obtaining informed consent from persons vulnerable to undue influence or coercion. The informed consent aspects of protecting the human right of self-determination will be addressed in the next set of critical appraisal questions.

CRITICAL APPRAISAL GUIDELINES

Protection of Human Rights

1. Were the subjects' right to privacy protected and confidentiality of research data maintained during data collection, analysis, and reporting?
2. Was the subject's identifiable protected health information protected in compliance with the Common Rule and Privacy Rule (DHHS, 2017a)?
3. Was subject selection conducted fairly? Were the subjects treated equitably?
4. What aspects of the study could have been uncomfortable or harmful, if any? If so, what measures were in place to diminish discomfort and the potential for harm (DHHS, 2017a)?

Williams, Turner-Henson, Langhinrichsen-Rohling, and Azuero (2017) conducted a predictive correlational study of the relationships among stressful life events, perceived stress, bullying, cortisol levels, and depression in a sample of ninth graders. After completing five instruments, students were guided to collect saliva twice on the same day. The data were analyzed to determine relationships among the selected variables. The research excerpt in Research Example 4.1 includes the ethical aspects of the study related to privacy and fairness.

RESEARCH EXAMPLE 4.1

Protection of Human Rights

Research Study Excerpt

Eligibility requirements included: (1) 9th grade students aged 14–16 years; (2) agreeing to participate (signed assent); (3) capable of understanding, speaking, and responding in English; (4) capable of following instructions for collecting saliva; and (5) having parental consent. Exclusion criteria included: (1) non-English speaking; (2) unable to complete instruments; (3) self-report of pregnancy, clinical depression, bipolar disorder, and Cushing or Addison disease; (4) self-report of taking medications that would affect cortisol levels (e.g., oral contraceptives, oral or inhaled corticosteroids for asthma); and (5) physical illness with resulting self-report of elevated temperature… At the completion of the study, each participant was provided with… information about mental health counselors who are available at low or no cost… Pubertal status was measured with the Pubertal Development Scale… This self-report scale provides an estimate of pubertal status specific to gender. Adolescents are classified into five categories including pre, early, mid, late, or post pubertal status, determined by adding the points assigned to questions for males (body hair growth, voice change, and facial hair growth) and females (body hair growth, breast development, and menarche)…. (Williams et al., 2017, pp. 25–26)

Continued

RESEARCH EXAMPLE 4.1—cont'd

Critical Appraisal

Among the strengths of the study was that the inclusion criteria were congruent with the research problem and study purpose. The exclusion criteria were reasonable also, such as excluding students with specific diseases that affected the production of corticosteroids that would have affected cortisol levels. The study was designed so that subjects could be treated fairly and equitably. The researchers noted that subjects were provided information about mental health services, indicating their recognition of potential discomfort and/or harm that could result from thinking about stress, bullying, and depression.

The ethical aspects of the study that received less attention were the rights to privacy and confidentiality. There was no information in the research report about how the subjects' rights to privacy and confidentiality were protected during data collection and analysis. The report also did not have any information about how identifiable private information was protected. However, all results were presented for the sample as a group so that individuals could not be identified. The instruments for the study also included questions about puberty and sexual orientation as covariates, but the researchers did not indicate that adolescents might be uncomfortable providing this information. Some of the data were obtained in a computer laboratory at the school, and it is not clear the extent of the privacy provided students as they completed the instruments. More information about potential discomfort and harm would have been helpful in determining the potential risks of the study. The results of the study will be discussed later in the chapter.

UNDERSTANDING INFORMED CONSENT

What is informed consent? **Informed consent** is providing information to a potential subject and the opportunity to participate in the study. The process does not end with the subject's signature on a document agreeing to be in a study (Farmer & Lundy, 2017). The researcher, guided by the principle of beneficence and committed to protection of the right to self-determination, describes the study and what subjects will be asked to do. A potential subject's decision about whether to participate is the consenting part of the process. Researchers need to be knowledgeable of the culture of potential subjects. For example, collectivist cultures may view individual informed consent as inappropriate and want involvement of other family members. They may be willing to share data with the researcher, but expect ownership of the data to be retained by the subjects (Roberts et al., 2017).

If the risks and benefits of participating change during the study, the researcher maintains trust by sharing that information with subjects. Subjects provide ongoing consent by continuing to participate in the study, with the assurance that they can withdraw at any time.

Four Elements of Informed Consent

Informed consent is incomplete or unethical unless four elements are incorporated (Fig. 4.4). The researcher must *disclose* essential information about the study to potential subjects in a way that can be understood. The second element is the extent to which the potential subject *comprehends* the information. The final elements are the *competence* of the potential subject and the person's *voluntary agreement* to take part in the study.

Disclosure

The revision to the Common Rule changed the focus of the consent process from sharing every possible detail of a study to providing the information that a reasonable person would need to make a decision about participation (DHHS, 2017a). Box 4.4 contains the characteristics of informed consent. HIPAA authorization and broad consent for future use of research specimens, discussed earlier in the chapter, may be included in the consent for a study or may be separate.

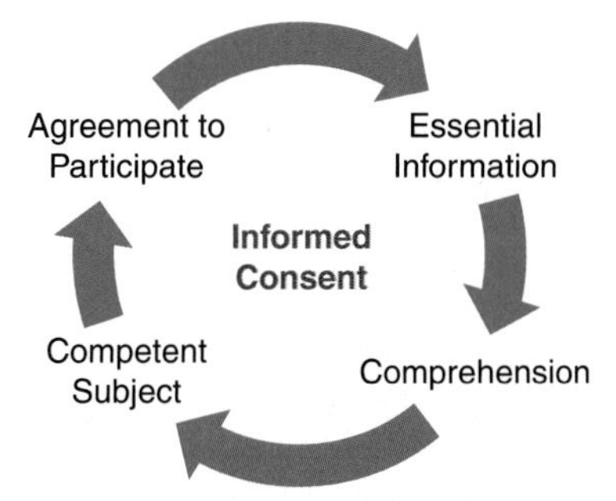

FIG 4.4 Required elements of consent.

BOX 4.4 COMPONENTS OF INFORMED CONSENT

Description

Voluntary agreement of a competent subject to participate in a study after comprehending knowledge to assess the benefits and risks.

General Requirements

- **Comprehendible**
  - Circumstances provide opportunity to discuss and make a deliberate decision without pressure
  - Language that is understandable
  - Presented not as unrelated facts, but in a way that is meaningful
- **Cautious**
  - Subject does not waive any legal rights or release researcher or funder from negligence
- **Complete but concise**
  - Sufficient information that a reasonable person would want to make a decision
- **Comprehensive**
  - Purpose and procedures of the research study
  - Length of subject's involvement
  - Benefits and risks or discomforts
  - Compensation, if any, for research-related injury
  - Disclosure of alternative treatments if available
  - Confidentiality of records
  - Contact persons
  - Right to refuse or withdraw without loss of benefits

Part of the disclosure is documentation of the information that was shared with the subject's signature denoting agreement to participate. A consent form is a written document that includes the elements of informed consent required by the Common Rule (DHHS, 2017a). In addition, a consent form may include other information required by the institution in which the study is to be conducted or by the agency funding the study. For federally funded clinical trials, a copy of the IRB-approved consent form must be posted on a publicly available website (DHHS, 2017a).

Comprehension

Informed consent implies not only that the researcher has imparted information to the subjects but also that the prospective subjects have comprehended that information. The researcher must take the time to teach the subjects about the study. The amount of information to be taught depends on the subject's knowledge of research and the specific research topic. Researchers need to discuss the benefits and risks of a study in detail, with examples that the potential subjects or participants can understand. Nurses often serve as patient advocates in clinical agencies and need to assess whether patients involved in research understand the purpose and potential risks and benefits of their participation in a study (ANA, 2015; Banner & Zimmer, 2012; Fry et al., 2011).

Competence

Autonomous persons, who are capable of understanding the benefits and risks of a proposed study, are competent to give consent. Persons with diminished autonomy because of legal or mental incompetence or confinement to an institution are not legally competent to consent to participate in research. In the research report, investigators need to indicate the competence of the subjects and the process that was used for obtaining informed consent (Banner & Zimmer, 2012).

Voluntary Agreement

Voluntary agreement means that the prospective subject has decided to take part in a study of his or her own volition, without coercion or any undue influence (DHHS, 2017a). Researchers obtain voluntary agreement after the prospective subject who is competent to make the decision receives the essential information about the study and has demonstrated comprehension of this information. All these elements of informed consent need to be documented in a consent form and discussed in the research report.

Documentation of Informed Consent

The documentation of informed consent depends on the study's level of risk and the requirements of the IRB that approves the study. Most studies require a written consent form that the subject signs. The subject also receives a copy of the consent form. There are three categories of situations in which the process of obtaining and documenting consent are altered.

Studies that involve subjects with diminished autonomy will require a written signed consent form, but an alteration in who signs the form. When potential subjects have some comprehension of the study and agree to participate, they sign the consent form. In addition, the subject's legally authorized representative signs the form. The representative indicates his or her relationship with the subject under the signature. Sometimes nurses are asked to sign a consent form as a witness for a biomedical study. They must know the study purpose and procedures and the subject's comprehension of the study before signing the form. To ensure the consistent implementation of the consent process, nurses and others involved in the consent process are educated about the study and consent process.

For studies in which potential subjects may not be able to read and comprehend the consent form, the IRB may approve an oral presentation of the study or a reading of the study summary. A witness observes the consent process and ensures that the presentation includes the required content of the study summary approved by the IRB. The subject signs a short statement that she or he was provided the summary of the study information and agrees to participate. The researcher and the witness sign the subject's signed short form and the written summary of the study that was orally presented. The subject is given a copy of the short form and the written summary.

In some minimal risk studies, the requirement for written consent is waived. Studies in which a signed consent can be waived usually involve procedures that do not normally require a signature outside of the research context. An example is answering questions about your family structure or relationships with friends. An IRB may approve a waiver when the signed document would be the only connection between the person and the study in situations in which confidentiality is especially a concern. For example, a waiver might be approved with women living with HIV infection who are subjects in a study about disclosing HIV status to friends and family members. Signed consent may also be waived if the potential subjects are members of a culture or community in which signing documents is not the norm (DHHS, 2017a). The researcher would work with the members of the group to identify an alternative mechanism to document the consent, such as using a thumbprint instead of a signature or stating aloud one's agreement to participate.

Studies in which the researcher or data collector interacts with the subjects require obtaining informed consent. The consent process must meet the federal regulations for the conduct of ethical research with human subjects. Research reports often discuss the consent process and identify some of the essential consent information that was provided to the potential subjects. Some mention of the consent process for that study is required, but the depth of the discussion will vary according to the research purpose and types of participants or subjects included in the study. The consent process is usually presented in the methods section under a discussion of study procedures or data collection process. The following critical appraisal guidelines will assist you in examining the consent process of a published study or for a study to be conducted in your clinical agency.

CRITICAL APPRAISAL GUIDELINES

Informed Consent Process

These questions ensure that the subject's right to self-determination is protected. Consider the following questions when critically appraising the consent process of a study:

1. How was informed consent obtained from the subjects or participants?
2. Did the subjects have diminished autonomy because of legal or mental incompetence or confinement to an institution? If the subjects were not competent to give consent, did their legally authorized representatives give consent?
3. Were children included as subjects in the study? Was assent obtained? Did the parents or guardians give permission or consent for the child to participate?
4. Were the subjects vulnerable to undue influence or coercion? If so, what precautions were taken to avoid potential subjects feeling pressured to participate?
5. Was the essential information for consent provided and comprehended by the subjects? Were measures taken to ensure that low-literacy subjects and subjects with diminished autonomy understood the study requirements?
6. Did it seem that the subjects participated voluntarily in the study?

As described previously, Williams et al. (2017) conducted a study of life events, stress, and bullying in ninth graders, with the purpose of examining the contribution of these variables to depression. Because the subjects were children, parental permission and student assent were appropriately obtained, as described in Research Example 4.2. Typically, in a research report, there is minimal discussion about the informed consent process.

RESEARCH EXAMPLE 4.2

Informed Consent

Research Study Excerpt

Ninth graders are often viewed as the lowest on the totem pole in high school. This population may often feel powerless to defend themselves against targeted, aggressive, and hurtful behaviors from older, more physically and socially powerful upper classmen (Fredstrom, Adams, & Gilman, 2011)... The primary investigator explained the study to all 9th graders and then provided packets with a letter to parents, a refusal form, and consent form to sign and return. Adolescents who were eligible to participate signed an assent form before the study began... At the completion of the study, each participant was provided with a $5.00 gift card to a local food establishment and information about mental health counselors who are available at low or no cost. (Williams et al., 2017, pp. 24–25)

Continued

RESEARCH EXAMPLE 4.2—cont'd

Critical Appraisal

The researchers noted that the ninth grade was a difficult transition period because, in the high school system, they are perceived to have low status (Williams et al., 2017). The researcher explained the study to the eligible students and sent packets with a letter, refusal form, and consent form home with the students for their parents to review. Only when parents signed and returned the consent forms were students allowed to participate in the study. When students met the other inclusion criteria, the students were given assent forms to sign. The potential subjects were recognized as having diminished autonomy by virtue of biological age and the legal responsibility of the parents for their children's welfare. Appropriate precautions were taken by obtaining parent consent and student assent. The $5 gift card was reasonable for the amount of time and effort the student volunteered, so no concerns about coercion were raised.

Concerns about the effect of low literacy on students being able to understand the study were decreased by excluding students who were non-English speakers and who were unable to complete the instruments. Based on the information provided in the report, the students participated voluntarily. The components of informed consent—in this case parental permission and student assent—were ethically obtained.

Almost 40% of the students reported depressive symptoms to the extent that they were referred to the school nurse for further evaluation. Cortisol rhythms for the study were normal for over 90% of the students. Overall, self-reported bullying was lower than national rates, but students who described their gender identity as homosexual, bisexual, or unsure were found to have experienced more bullying. Williams et al. (2017) found that depression was significantly correlated with stressful life events, life changes, perceived stress, and bullying, but not with cortisol rhythms. When the combined effects of the variables on depression were examined, perceived stress, bullying, and gender identity explained 59% of the variance in depression. Williams et al. (2017) identified the limitations as being cross-sectional research, limited data points for cortisol levels, and the possibility that a recent event (death of a student in one school the previous week) influenced the findings related to depression (see Chapter 8)The implications for practice are that nurses should have heightened awareness of adolescents at high risk for depression because of gender identity, life changes, bullying, and stress. To ensure identification of depression, nurses may want to use an assessment tool of depression in their practice with adolescents.

UNDERSTANDING INSTITUTIONAL REVIEW

An institutional review board (IRB) is a committee that reviews research to ensure that the investigator is conducting the research ethically. IRBs have the authority to approve, require modifications, and disapprove studies it reviews. If unforeseen problems occur during a study, the IRB is notified and the study stopped until the issue is resolved and the IRB approves the continuation of the study. Universities, hospitals, corporations, and other healthcare organizations have IRBs to promote the conduct of ethical research and protect the rights of prospective subjects at their institutions (Grady, 2015; Ness & Royce, 2017; Resnik, 2015). Federal regulations provide details about the composition and functions of IRBs (DHHS, 2017a).

Institutional Review Board Composition and Function

Each IRB has at least five members of varying backgrounds—cultural, economic, educational, gender, racial—to promote complete, scholarly, and fair review of research commonly conducted in an institution (DHHS, 2017a). At least one member has scientific expertise, and at least one member is a community member without scientific training. The same member or another member is not affiliated with the institution in any way. The members are sensitive to the attitudes of the community it serves and are educated about the federal regulations, institutional policies, and standards of professional conduct by which studies are to be evaluated. If an institution regularly reviews studies with subjects who may be vulnerable to coercion or undue influence, one or more members of the IRB should have experience working with persons who are similar to potential subjects.

IRB members must not have a conflicting interest related to a study conducted in an institution. For example, if a member of the IRB proposes a study to be conducted in the institution, the member could not be involved in the deliberations and decision about the study other than to provide information (DHHS, 2017a).

To be recognized as an IRB for an institution seeking federal funding, the IRB must register with the Office of Human Research Protection (OHRP; DHHS, n.d.) and obtain a federal-wide assurance (FWA; Grady, 2015). An FWA is documentation of the IRB's adoption of an ethical standard, such as the Belmont Report (National Commission for the Protection of Human Subjects of Biomedical and Behavioral Research, 1979), and agreement (assurance) to comply with the Common Rule. To receive an FWA, an IRB must have written policies for membership and processes and maintain records of all studies reviewed and the subsequent decisions (DHHS, 2017a).

Exempt and Expedited Levels of Reviews Conducted by Institutional Review Boards

The functions and operations of an IRB involve the review of research to determine the appropriate level of review. The IRB chairperson and/or committee, not the researcher, decide the level of the review required for each study (DHHS, 2017a). The revised Common Rule has broadened the types of study that are **exempt from review**. Studies that are exempt from review pose no apparent risks to the research subjects. Box 4.5 contains a list of the types of studies that are exempt from review. Once a study is deemed to be exempt, the IRB does not require a continuing review of the study as is required for other levels of review (DHHS, 2017a). Studies conducted by nurses frequently are evaluated as being exempt from review.

Studies may meet the criteria to receive an expedited review if they carry some risks, but the risks are minimal. The IRB chairperson or one or more experienced IRB members conducts the **expedited review**. The types of studies eligible for expedited review did not change with the revision of the Common Rule. Box 4.6 lists the types of studies that may qualify for expedited review

BOX 4.5 CHARACTERISTICS OF STUDIES EXEMPT FROM REVIEW BY INSTITUTIONAL REVIEW BOARD, WITH EXAMPLES

- Will be conducted in established education settings
  - Correlational study of the relationship between the effectiveness of an innovative teaching strategy with class characteristics
- Will use education tests, surveys, interviews, or observation of public behavior with subject not identified and minimal risks with the data not linked to the subject
  - Descriptive study with anonymous online data collection using a social support scale and demographic questionnaire
- Will use a benign behavioral intervention[a] and data that were not linked to subjects
  - Quasi-experimental study comparing knowledge of diabetes gained through playing an online game or through an oral presentation
- Will use data that were publicly available, de-identified, or collected to evaluate government projects or public services
  - Exploratory-descriptive qualitative study of program participants' written evaluation of the services of a federally supported clinic

[a]The Common Rule describes "benign behavioral interventions" as short noninvasive actions that are not expected to have a long-term adverse impact or be embarrassing or offensive (DHHS, 2017a).

US Department of Health and Human Services (DHHS). (2017a). Final revisions to the Common Rule: Protection of human subjects. Code of Federal Regulations, Title 45, Part 46. Retrieved March 11, 2017, from https://www.hhs.gov/ohrp/regulations-and-policy/regulations/finalized-revisions-common-rule/index.html.

BOX 4.6 CHARACTERISTICS OF STUDIES ELIGIBLE FOR EXPEDITED REVIEW BY INSTITUTIONAL REVIEW BOARD, WITH EXAMPLES

Expedited review is reserved for studies with minimal risks; data are collected through one of the following means:

- Small amounts of blood collected by venipuncture or finger stick
  - Quasi-experimental study comparing fast blood sugar readings once a week for persons with diabetes who are receiving weekly phone calls about diet and exercise with those of persons with diabetes receiving usual care
- Biological specimens collected by noninvasive means
  - Descriptive comparative study of blood vessel structures of placentas obtained at delivery from women who had pregnancy-induced hypertension to those of women who were normotensive through pregnancy
- Noninvasive readings or images collected by usual diagnostic procedures
  - Descriptive comparison study of stages of lung cancer based on magnetic resonance imaging scans with traditional X-rays of stage III lung tumors
- Voice, video, or digital recordings of interviews and focus groups
  - Grounded theory study of the experience of mothering adopted children with data collected by interview
- Medical records, when subjects can potentially be identified (if data are de-identified, study may be exempt)
  - Correlational study of nutritional status of patients with community-acquired pressure ulcer to that of patients with hospital-acquired pressure ulcers
- Questionnaires or surveys of cultural beliefs, communication, perception, and social behavior
  - Predictive correlational study of cultural beliefs and use of emergency room by underinsured and uninsured persons

(DHHS, 2017a). Under expedited review procedures, the reviewers may exercise all the authority of the IRB, except disapproval of the research. A research activity may be disapproved only after a complete review by the IRB (DHHS, 2017a). Descriptive studies, in which subjects are asked to respond to questionnaires, usually need only expedited review. Studies approved by expedited review do not require annual review.

Full Reviews Conducted by Institutional Review Boards

A study that carries greater than minimal risks must receive a **full review** by an IRB during a convened meeting. To obtain IRB approval, researchers must describe in their IRB application how they will minimize risks to the subjects, ensure that selection of subjects is equitable, protect the confidentiality and privacy of subjects, and make accommodations for potential subjects who are vulnerable to coercion or undue influence (Grady, 2015; DHHS, 2017a). Parents of infants in neonatal intensive care units (NICUs) are examples of persons who might be susceptible to undue influence because of the complexity of treatment decisions and their own stress (Janvier & Farlow, 2015). Procedures for obtaining informed consent must be clearly described, including appropriate documentation of the consent.

Another researcher responsibility is to have a plan to monitor the results during the study for safety concerns or results that might influence a subject's decision about continued participation in the study (DHHS, 2017a). For example, in a study comparing two medications, the researcher identifies that one medication is causing dramatic improvements in the health of the subjects receiving it. Subjects who are in the other group would need to be notified. They may choose to withdraw from the study, or the researcher may stop the study and offer the effective medications to all subjects.

Whether a study is ethical and approved by an IRB depends a great deal on the balance between the risks and benefits of the study. This means that the IRB evaluates whether the risks to subjects are reasonable in relation to anticipated benefits (DHHS, 2017a). To determine this balance, or **benefit-risk ratio,** the benefits and risks associated with the study's sampling method, consent process, procedures, and potential outcomes of the study are assessed. When there are risks, such as potential emotional or psychological stress, the researcher may have a counselor who has agreed to be available to subjects.

Whether the research is therapeutic or nontherapeutic affects the potential benefits for subjects. In therapeutic research, subjects might benefit from the study procedures in areas such as skin care, range of motion, touch, and other nursing or medical interventions. The benefits might include improved physical condition, which could facilitate emotional and social benefits. Nontherapeutic nursing research does not benefit subjects directly but is important because it generates and refines nursing knowledge for future patients, the nursing profession, and society. If the risks outweigh the benefits, the study probably is unethical and should not be conducted. If the benefits outweigh the risks, the study probably is ethical and has the potential to add to knowledge related to the health of individuals and populations.

Most published studies indicate that IRB approval was obtained, but do not indicate whether the study was exempt from review or received an expedited or full review. A research report needs to identify the IRBs that reviewed and approved a study for implementation clearly. Studies are conducted frequently in more than one clinical facility or are joint projects between universities. Federally funded studies involving multiple institutions are considered cooperative research, and all the institutions are required to accept the approval of one IRB designated by the funding agencies (DHHS, 2017a). In other studies involving multiple institutions, the IRBs may conduct a joint review or accept the review of another institution. The revised Common Rule recommends avoiding duplication of effort in the review of studies (DHHS, 2017a).

CRITICAL APPRAISAL GUIDELINES

Overall Ethical Aspects of a Study

The following guidelines can be used to critically appraise the ethical aspects of a study. When conducting a study, researchers must meet the DHHS (2017a) regulations and applicable state and tribal laws for the conduct of ethical research with human subjects. These critical appraisal guidelines build on the previous guidelines and are intended to help you summarize or draw conclusions about the ethical conduct of the study. Consider the following questions when critically appraising the ethical aspects of a study:

1. Was the study approved by an IRB(s)? Based on your evaluation, which level of review (exempt, expedited, or full) did the study warrant?
2. What measures did the researchers take to minimize the risks and ensure the benefits? Apply the benefit-risk ratio to the study. Were the measures sufficient?
3. Using the previous guidelines about consent, was informed consent ethically obtained from the subjects?
4. Using the previous guidelines about protecting subjects' rights, were the rights of the subjects protected during the study?
5. Summarize your conclusions about the ethical aspects of the study.

The previously described study (Williams et al., 2017) was appropriately reviewed and approved by an IRB and school administrators. For comparison, a second example is provided in Research Example 4.3 of an ethnographic study in an NICU about nurses' beliefs about infant feeding and how the babies were actually fed (Cricco-Lizza, 2016). Ethnographic studies can pose some unique challenges due to observing people in the environment who may not directly participate in the study and have not given consent. Also, the researcher frequently participates in activities of the culture being studied. Over the 14 months of the study, Cricco-Lizza (2016) participated in the daily life of the unit through 128 periods of observations, informally interviewed 114 general informants multiple times, and conducted formal interviews with 18 key informants.

RESEARCH EXAMPLE 4.3

Determining the Ethics of a Study

Research Study Excerpt

This qualitative design used interviewing and participant observation and allowed for personal interactions embedded within the NICU culture... general informants were selected to provide a broad overview of beliefs and practices in the unit. From this group, key informants were followed more extensively to obtain an in-depth view... These informants were observed and formally or informally interviewed to obtain rich details about infant feeding in the NICU. Participant observation facilitated the gathering of information about their actual infant feeding practices while informal and formal interviews allowed for exploration of their specific beliefs... The nursing and medical directors granted permission for data collection in this NICU, and the nurses were informed about the study through the intranet, staff meetings, and face-to-face interactions in the NICU. University- and hospital-based human subjects committees allowed ethical approval for this investigation with the stipulation that nurses provide written informed-consent for the formal tape-recorded interviews... prolonged contact facilitated a deeper exploration of infant feeding beliefs and practices in this NICU. The interviews were labeled with pseudonyms, and the interviews were transcribed verbatim. These transcripts included the words and behaviors of the nurses during the interviews. They were checked line-by-line for accuracy and compared directly against the recordings. (Cricco-Lizza, 2016, pp. e92–e93)

Critical Appraisal

One of the strengths of the study from an ethical standpoint was that the study was approved by the IRBs of the researcher's university and the hospital where the study occurred. Because of the challenges of informed consent and participant observation, the study warranted full review during a meeting of the IRBs. The researcher minimized the risks by obtaining written consent for formal interviews, marking study records with pseudonyms, and informing the nurses and staff on the unit that she was conducting a study and collecting data about what she observed. Cricco-Lizza (2016) enhanced the benefits of the study by using rigorous methods to ensure the credibility of the study findings and protecting the rights of the subjects (nurses in the NICU). The benefits of the study outweighed the risks because ethical procedures used during the study protected the confidentiality of the nurses as much as possible. The study was conducted in an ethical manner.

CURRENT ISSUES IN RESEARCH ETHICS

The constant changes in health care and technology create new challenges in research ethics. In this section, three areas that continue to evolve are issues related to genomics research, using animals in studies, and research misconduct.

Genomics Research

Genomic research is a promising area of science related to human disease and healing. The unique identifiers in each person's genetic code make protecting subjects' rights of self-determination and informed consent uniquely challenging. The Human Genome Project funded by the National Institutes of Health (NIH) recognized from the onset the ethical and legal dilemmas of genomic research. As a result, program funding has included funding specifically for the study of these issues (McEwen, Boyer, & Sun, 2013). "No other area of biomedical research has sustained such a high commitment, backed by dollars, to the examination of ethical issues" (McEwen et al., 2013, p. 375). Despite this investment, issues remain that are related to consent and the future use of genetic data.

Several highly publicized cases have increased awareness and fear among the public. Henrietta Lacks, an African American woman, only 31 years of age, was diagnosed with cervical cancer. She was admitted to John Hopkins University Hospital in 1951 for the usual treatment (Jones, 1997). The specimens collected were taken to the laboratory of a scientist named Dr. Gey. Dr. Gey was trying to identify and reproduce a cell line for research purposes, and generously provided the cell line to other researchers free of charge. These researchers, building on Dr. Gey's work, developed a cell line from those especially hardy tumor cells—a cell line that was successfully used in research (Bledsoe & Grizzle, 2013; Skloot, 2010). Highly effective treatments, such as the polio vaccine and in vitro fertilization, were developed using the cell line. The treatments were extremely profitable for the researchers and the institutions with which they were associated, and resulted in literally billions of dollars being made by selling the cell line to other researchers (McEwen et al., 2013). Mrs. Lacks died never knowing that her tumor cells were used for research, and her family only learned of her contribution to science in 2010. Her family members have not pursued legal retribution, but have chosen to focus on educating the public and scientists to prevent a recurrence.

Unfortunately, unethical studies and unethical research practices continue to occur. Another example of unethical research occurred in the 1990s. At that time, researchers began collecting blood specimens of members of an isolated Native American Indian tribe, the Havasupai, who lived in the Grand Canyon (Caplan & Moreno, 2011). Diabetes mellitus was a devastating disease among their tribe, and the researchers proposed a study to identify genetic clues of disease susceptibility. However, the researchers used the blood specimens to study other topics, such as schizophrenia and tribal origin (McEwen et al., 2013). The tribe sued Arizona State University, the employer of the original researcher, and was awarded a settlement in 2010. Part of the settlement was the release of the remaining blood samples to the tribe to be disposed of in a culturally appropriate way.

A related case occurred with the people of the First Nations in Canada. Researchers collected genetic materials to study arthritis in 2006, and the subjects later asked for the specimens to be returned, based on cultural beliefs (Brief & Illes, 2010).

Among the unresolved issues in genomics research are de-identification of data, subjects withdrawing from a study, additional studies being conducted with specimens already collected, return of information to the research subject, if beneficial to the subject, and ownership of specimens. There is concern that by its very nature, genomic data cannot be completely de-identified (Terry, 2015). Genetic data, even when identifying information has been removed as required (Gray et al., 2017), have the potential of being combined with data from genetic genealogy databases and other publicly available demographic data to re-identify a subject (McEwen et al., 2013).

Broad consent in the revised Common Rule was developed to address some of these concerns (DHHS, 2017a). When individuals allow their biospecimens to be retained for future studies, the broad consent document will include information about whether the researchers will contact the individuals if the research reveals a health problem. The implementation of broad consent will likely increase the capability of research institutes and universities to conduct genomic research. Critical appraisal of genomic research based on a research report includes understanding the decisions made by the researchers, the type of consent that was obtained, and discussion of the issues surrounding human protection from harm.

Using Animals in Research

Potential subjects for research include humans and their genes, as well as plants, laboratory-grown organisms, and computer modeling using existing data sets. If possible, most researchers prefer to use nonanimal subjects because nonanimal subjects are generally less expensive However, for decades animals have been used in the conduct of biomedical and biobehavioral research and have significantly contributed to our understanding of disease processes. Because animals are deemed valuable subjects for selected research projects, the question concerning their humane treatment must be addressed.

Studies have indicated that animals experience a wider variety of harm, including fear and pain, than was previously thought (Ferdowsian, 2011). As a result, some animal rights groups have become empowered to be stronger advocates in protecting animal research subjects. Many scientists, especially physicians, believe that extremists in the animal rights' movement could threaten the future of healthcare research. The goal of these groups is to raise the consciousness of researchers and society to ensure that animals are used wisely and treated humanely in the conduct of research. In response, ethicists have expanded the application of ethical principles to the use of animals in studies (Beauchamp, Ferdowsian, & Gluck, 2014).

Because more nurses are conducting research with animals, the ethics of these studies need to be critically appraised. An important question to address is to determine what mechanisms ensured that the animals were treated humanely in the conduct of the study. The Office of Laboratory Animal Welfare (OLAW), part of the NIH, serves as a federal compliance body for this type of research (DHHS, 2017c). OLAW collaborates with institutions that have been awarded federal funding for research involving laboratory animals. Receiving the funding is contingent on the institution obtaining an assurance, which requires that an institution's policies for laboratory animal welfare meets or exceeds the Public Health Services (PHS) policy (DHHS, 2015).

Institutions' assurance statements about compliance with PHS policy related to the use of laboratory animals have promoted the humane care and treatment of animals in research. In addition, almost 1000 institutions have voluntarily sought and gained accreditation from the American Association for Accreditation of Laboratory Animal Care International (AAALAC). The association was developed to ensure the humane treatment of animals in research (AAALAC, 2017). In conducting research, each investigator must carefully select the type of participant needed; if animals are used in a study, they require humane treatment. In critically appraising studies, you need to ensure that animals were the appropriate subjects for a study and that they were treated humanely during the conduct of the study.

Research Misconduct

The goal of research is to generate sound scientific knowledge, which is possible only through the honest conduct, reporting, and publication of studies. However, since the 1980s, a number of fraudulent studies have been conducted and published in prestigious scientific journals. In response, the Office of Research Integrity (ORI) was created within the federal government.

The ORI, a part of the DHHS, is responsible for defining important terms used in the identification and management of research misconduct. **Research misconduct** is defined as "the fabrication, falsification, or plagiarism in processing, performing, or reviewing research, or in reporting research results. It does not include honest error or differences in opinion" (ORI, 2016b). Research misconduct is an intentional act that involves a significant departure from the acceptable practice of the scientific community for maintaining the integrity of the research record. Before action is taken, an allegation must be confirmed by a preponderance of evidence. **Fabrication in** research is the making up of results and recording or reporting them. Falsification of research is manipulating research materials, equipment, or processes or changing or omitting data or results so that the research is not accurately represented in the research record. Plagiarism is the appropriation of another person's ideas, processes, results, or words without giving appropriate credit, including those obtained through confidential review of others' research proposals and manuscripts. More information on preventing and addressing research misconduct can be found on the ORI website (2017; https://ori.hhs.gov/).

An example of research misconduct is the work of Meredyth M. Forbes, a doctoral student who was involved in studies to understand cellular reproduction that were funded through five grants from the NIH. She admitted to falsifying or fabricating data that were included in at least six publications and eight conference presentations (ORI, 2016a). She agreed never to be involved in federal projects in the future. In an effort to salvage the value of the research, her coinvestigators have been repeating the experiments to obtain accurate data, produce reliable results, and correct the peer-reviewed articles that were published.

The seven cases of research misconduct reported by ORI in 2016 involved cellular studies conducted in laboratories, studies that rarely include nurse researchers. However, research misconduct does occur in the nursing profession (Fierz et al., 2014; Ward-Smith, 2016). Habermann, Broome, Pryor, and Ziner (2010) conducted a study of research coordinators' experiences with scientific misconduct and research integrity and found that research coordinators often learned of the misconduct firsthand, and the principal investigator was usually identified as the responsible party. They identified five major categories of misconduct: "protocol violations, consent violations, fabrication, falsification, and financial conflict of interest" (Habermann et al., 2010, p. 51). They indicated that the definition of research misconduct might need to be expanded beyond fabrication, falsification, and plagiarism.

Research misconduct has resulted in papers in nursing journals being retracted. One example is a paper published by Lewis (2013), on intraprofessional learning, that was retracted. The data reported the previous year by Lewis had been used without the approval or acknowledgment of the research team. Keith (2015) reported in *Retraction Watch* that three papers had been retracted that were published in nursing journals and authored by an international researcher. In each case, the researcher had published two papers reporting the same study, without acknowledgment that the study had already been reported. The ORI reported that another nurse, Scott Weber, was found guilty of research misconduct. He was found to have plagiarized significant portions of published articles, including using previous studies' data in graphs in his publications (DHHS, 2011). He also changed the years of some cited articles in his reference lists to avoid detection of plagiarism. Fortunately, these nurses represent a very small percentage of nurse researchers and authors. Most nurse researchers have a strong commitment to maintaining the integrity of the evidence that they produce.

KEY POINTS

- Four experimental projects have been highly publicized for their unethical treatment of human subjects: the Nazi medical experiments, the Tuskegee Syphilis Study, the Willowbrook Study, and the Jewish Chronic Disease Hospital Study.
- Two historical documents, the Nuremberg Code and the Declaration of Helsinki, have had a strong impact on the conduct of research.
- The principles of respect for persons, beneficence, and justice are the standards for protection of human rights.

- The human rights that require protection in research are the right to: (1) self-determination; (2) privacy; (3) anonymity and confidentiality; (4) fair selection and treatment; and (5) protection from discomfort and harm.
- DHHS (2017a) regulations have been revised with the purpose of continuing to promote ethical conduct in research, avoiding duplication of effort across IRBs, and ensuring the understandability of informed consent documents.
- Informed consent involves the disclosure of essential information about the study, comprehension of the information by a competent subject, and voluntary agreement to participate.
- An IRB consists of a committee of peers who examine studies for ethical concerns with three levels of review: exempt, expedited, and complete.
- The extent of any risk for harm and discomfort as well as the vulnerability of the proposed sample will determine the level of IRB review that is needed, whether exempt research, expedited review, or full board review.
- Genomic research involves unique ethical challenges because of the potential that the subject can be identified by the data, the ability to store biospecimens for future studies, and notification of subjects when future studies identify genetic variations linked to latent diseases.
- Animals are important for the conduct of certain studies, and they must be treated humanely during the study.
- Research misconduct is a serious ethical problem that includes plagiarism, falsification and fabrication of data, and duplicate publication.

REFERENCES

American Association for Accreditation of Laboratory Animal Care International (AAALAC International). (2017). *About AAALAC*. Retrieved March 18, 2017, from https://aaalac.org/about/index.cfm.

American Nurses Association (ANA). (2015). *Code of ethics for nurses with interpretive statements*. Washington, D.C.: Author.

Antal, H., Bunnell, H., McCahan, S., Pennington, C., Wysocki, T., & Blake, K. (2017). A cognitive approach for design of a multimedia informed consent video and website in pediatric research. *Journal of Biomedical Informatics, 66*, 248–258.

Banner, D., & Zimmer, L. (2012). Informed consent in research: An overview for nurses. *Canadian Journal of Cardiovascular Nursing, 22*(1), 26–30.

Beauchamp, T., Ferdowsian, H., & Gluck, J. (2014). Rethinking the ethics of research involving nonhuman animals: An introduction. *Theoretical Medicine and Bioethics, 35*(2), 91–96.

Beecher, H. K. (1966). Ethics and clinical research. *New England Journal of Medicine, 274*(24), 1354–1360.

Berger, R. L. (1990). Nazi science: The Dachau hypothermia experiments. *New England Journal of Medicine, 322*(20), 1435–1440.

Bledsoe, M., & Grizzle, W. (2013). Use of human specimens in research: The evolving United States regulatory, policy, and scientific landscape. *Diagnostic Histopathology, 15*(9), 322–330.

Bourgeosis, F., & Hwang, T. (2017). The Pediatric Research Equity Act moves into adolescence. *Journal of the American Medication Association, 317*(3), 259–260.

Boynton, M., Portnoy, D., & Johnson, B. (2013). Exploring the ethics and psychological impact of deception in psychological research. *IRB: Ethics & Human Research, 35*(2), 7–13.

Brandt, A. M. (1978). Racism and research: The case of the Tuskegee syphilis study. *Hastings Center Report, 8*(6), 21–29.

Brief, E., & Illes, J. (2010). Tangles of neurogenetics, neuroethics, and culture. *Neuron, 68*(2), 174–177.

Caplan, A., & Moreno, J. (2011). The Havasu 'Baaja tribe and informed consent. *The Lancet, 377*(9766), 621–622.

Cricco-Lizza, R. (2016). Infant feeding beliefs and day-to-day feeding practices of NICU nurses. *Journal of Pediatric Nursing, 31*, e91–e98.

Doody, O., & Noonan, M. (2016). Nursing research ethics, guidance and application in practice. *British Journal of Nursing, 28*(25), 803–807.

Eastwood, G. (2015). Ethical issues in gastroenterology research. *Journal of Gasteroenterology and Hepatology, 30*(S1), 8–11.

Farmer, L., & Lundy, A. (2017). Informed consent: Legal and ethical considerations for advanced practice nurses. *Journal of Nurse Practitioners*, *13*(2), 124–130.

Ferdowsian, H. (2011). Human and animal research guidelines: Aligning ethical constructs with new scientific developments. *Bioethics*, *25*(8), 472–478.

Fierz, K., Gennaro, S., Dierickx, K., Van Achterberg, T., Morin, K., & De Geest, S. (2014). Scientific misconduct: Also an issue for nursing science? *Journal of Nursing Scholarship*, *46*(4), 271–280.

Fredstrom, B. K., Adams, R. E., & Gilman, R. (2011). Electronic and school-based victimization: Unique contexts for adjustment difficulties during adolescence. *Journal of Youth and Adolescence*, *40*(4), 405–415.

Fry, S. T., Veatch, R. M., & Taylor, C. (2011). *Case studies in nursing ethics* (4th ed.). Sudbury, MA: Jones & Bartlett Learning.

Grady, C. (2015). Institutional review boards: Purposes and challenges. *Chest*, *148*(5), 1148–1155.

Gray, J. R., Grove, S. K., & Sutherland, S. (2017). *The practice of nursing research: Appraisal, synthesis, and generation of evidence* (8th ed.). St. Louis, MO: Elsevier Saunders.

Habermann, B., Broome, M., Pryor, E. R., & Ziner, K. W. (2010). Research coordinators' experiences with scientific misconduct and research integrity. *Nursing Research*, *59*(1), 51–57.

Halkoaho, A., Pietila, A.-M., Ebbesen, M., Karki, S., & Kangasniemi, M. (2016). Cultural aspects related to informed consent in health research: A systematic review. *Nursing Ethics*, *23*(6), 698–712.

Health Insurance Portability and Accountability Act of 1996. Pub. L. No. 104.191, 110 Stat. 1936 (2003). Retrieved April 8, 2017, from https://www.gpo.gov/fdsys/pkg/PLAW-104publ191/content-detail.html.

Hershey, N., & Miller, R. D. (1976). *Human experimentation and the law*. Rockville, MD: Aspen.

Janvier, A., & Farlow, B. (2015). The ethics of neonatal research: An ethicist's and a parent's perspective. *Seminars in Fetal & Neonatal Medicine*, *20*(6), 436–441.

Jones, H. W. (1997). Record of the first physician to see Henrietta Lacks at the Johns Hopkins Hospital: History of the HeLa cell line. *American Journal of Obstetrics and Gynecology*, *176*(6), s227–s228.

Keith, R. (2015). Investigation ups nursing researcher's retraction count to 3. In *Retraction Watch*. Retrieved March 18, 2017, from http://retractionwatch.com/2015/09/23/3rd-retraction-for-nursing-researcher-after-investigation-finds-overlap.

Kids v Cancer. (2017). *RACE for Children Act*. Retrieved March 16, 2017, from http://www.kidsvcancer.org/race-for-children-act/.

Levine, R. J. (1986). *Ethics and regulation of clinical research* (2nd ed.). Baltimore, MD: Urban & Schwarzenberg.

Lewis, R. (2013). Retraction notice to interprofessional learning in acute care: Developing a theoretical framework. *Nursing Education Today*, *33*(8), 931.

Marshall, C., & Rossman, G. (2016). *Designing qualitative research* (6th ed.). Thousand Oaks, CA: Sage.

McEwen, J., Boyer, J., & Sun, K. (2013). Evolving approaches to the ethical management of genomic data. *Trends in Genetics*, *29*(6), 375–382.

Menikoff, J., Kaneshiro, J., & Pritchard, I. (2017). The Common Rule updated. *The New England Journal of Medicine*, *376*(7), 613–615.

Milgram, S. (1963). Behavioral study of obedience. *Journal of Abnormal and Social Psychology*, *67*(4), 371–378.

Munhall, P. L. (2012). Ethical considerations in qualitative research. In P. L. Munhall (Ed.), *Nursing research: A qualitative perspective*. (5th ed.)(pp. 491–502). Sudbury, MA: Jones & Bartlett Learning.

National Commission for the Protection of Human Subjects of Biomedical and Behavioral Research. (1979). *Belmont Report: Ethical principles and guidelines for research involving human subjects*. Washington, D.C.: U.S. Government Printing Office. DHEW Publication No. (05) 78-0012. Retrieved February 25, 2017, from https://www.hhs.gov/ohrp/regulations-and-policy/belmont-report/.

National Research Council. (2011). *Guide to the care of and use of laboratory animals*. Washington, D.C.: National Academies Press. Retrieved March 18, 2017, from https://grants.nih.gov/grants/olaw/Guide-for-the-Care-and-Use-of-Laboratory-Animals.pdf.

Ness, E., & Royce, C. (2017). Clinical trials and the role of the oncology clinical trials nurse. *Nursing Clinics of North America*, *52*(2), 133–148.

Office of NIH History, National Institute of Health. (1949). *Trials of war criminals before the Nuremberg Military Tribunals*. Control Council Law No. 10, Vol. 2, pp. 181–182. Washington, D.C.: U.S. Government Printing Office. Retrieved February 25, 2017, from https://history.nih.gov/research/downloads/nuremberg.pdf.

Office of Research Integrity (ORI). (2016a). *Case summary: Forbes, Meredyth M.* Retrieved March 18, 2017, from https://ori.hhs.gov/content/case-summary-forbes-meredyth-m.

Office of Research Integrity (ORI). (2016b). *Frequently asked questions.* Retrieved March 18, 2017, from https://ori.hhs.gov/content/frequently-asked-questions#5.

Office of Research Integrity (ORI). (2017). *Home page.* Retrieved March 18, 2017, from https://ori.hhs.gov/https://ori.hhs.gov.

Oulton, K., Gibson, F., Sell, D., Williams, A., Pratt, L., & Wray, J. (2016). Assent for children's participation in research: Why it matters and making it meaningful. *Child: Care, Health and Development, 42*(4), 588–592.

Pediatric Research Equity Act (PREA) of 2003. Title 21. U.S.C. §§ 355. Retrieved April 8, 2017, from https://www.fda.gov/downloads/Drugs/DevelopmentApprovalProcess/DevelopmentResources/UCM077853.pdf.

Resnik, D. (2015). Some reflections on evaluating institutional review board effectiveness. *Contemporary Clinical Trials, 45*(Part B), 261–264.

Reynolds, P. D. (1979). *Ethical dilemmas and social science research.* San Francisco, CA: Jossey-Bass.

Roberts, L., Jadalla, A., Jones-Oyefeso, V., Winslow, B., & Taylor, E. (2017). Researching in collectivist cultures: Reflections and recommendations. *Journal of Transcultural Nursing, 28*(2), 137–143.

Rothman, D. J. (1982). Were Tuskegee and Willowbrook "studies in nature?". *Hastings Center Report, 12*(2), 5–7.

Skloot, R. (2010). *The immortal life of Henrietta Lacks.* New York, NY: Crown Publishers.

Steinfels, P., & Levine, C. (1976). Biomedical ethics and the shadow of Nazism. *Hastings Center Report, 6*(4), 1–20.

Terry, N. (2015). Developments in genetic and epigenetic data protection in behavioral and mental health spaces. *Behavioral Sciences & Law, 33*(5), 653–661.

Trimble, D., Nava, A., & McFarlane, J. (2013). Intimate partner violence and antiretroviral adherence among women receiving care in an urban Southeastern Texas HIV clinic. *Journal of Nurses in AIDS Care, 24*(4), 331–340.

US Department of Health and Human Services (DHHS) (n.d.) *About the Office of Human Research Protection.* Retrieved March 13, 2017, from https://www.hhs.gov/ohrp/regulations-and-policy/index.html.

US Department of Health and Human services (DHHS). (2011). *Findings of research misconduct: Scott Weber.* Retrieved September 2, 2017, from https://grants.nih.gov/grants/guide/notice-files/NOT-OD-12-002.html.

US Department of Health and Human Services (DHHS), National Institutes of Health. (2015). Public Health Service Policy on the Humane Care and Use of Laboratory Animals. Retrieved March 18, 2017, from https://grants.nih.gov/grants/olaw/references/PHSPolicyLabAnimals.pdf.

US Department of Health and Human Services (DHHS). (2017a). Final revisions to the Common Rule: Protection of human subjects. Code of Federal Regulations, Title 45, Part 46. Retrieved March 11, 2017, from https://www.hhs.gov/ohrp/regulations-and-policy/regulations/finalized-revisions-common-rule/index.html.

US Department of Health and Human Services (DHHS). (2017b). *Guidance regarding methods for de-identification of protected health information in accordance with the Health Insurance Portability and Accountability Act (HIPAA) Privacy Rule.* Retrieved March 5, 2017, from https://www.hhs.gov/hipaa/for-professionals/privacy/special-topics/de-identification.

US Department of Health and Human Services (US DHHS). (2017c). Office of Laboratory Animal Welfare (OLAW). Retrieved September 2, 2017, from https://grants.nih.gov/aboutoer/oer_offices/olaw.htm.

US Food and Drug Administration (FDA). (2015). *FDA fundamentals.* Retrieved March 5, 2017, from https://www.fda.gov/AboutFDA/Transparency/Basics/ucm192695.htm.

Ward-Smith, P. (2016). Evidence-based nursing: When the evidence is fraudulent. *Urologic Nursing, 36*(2), 98–99.

Weijer, C. (2000). The ethical analysis of risk. *Journal of Law, Medicine, & Ethics, 28*(4), 344–361.

Williams, S., Turner-Henson, A., Langhinrichsen-Rohling, J., & Azuero, A. (2017). Depressive symptoms in 9th graders: Stress and physiological contributors. *Applied Nursing Research, 34*(4), 24–28.

World Medical Association (WMA). (2013). World Medical Association Declaration of Helsinki: Ethical principles for medical research involving human subjects. *Journal of the American Medical Association, 310*(20), 2191–2194. Retrieved February 5, 2018, from https://www.wma.net/wp-content/uploads/2016/11/DoH-Oct2013-JAMA.pdf.

Because of funding changes, the Agency for Healthcare Research and Quality (AHRQ) National Guideline Clearinghouse website was scheduled for decommissioning as of July 16, 2018. For more information, go to https://www.ahrq.gov/.

CHAPTER

5

Examining Research Problems, Purposes, and Hypotheses

Susan K. Grove

CHAPTER OVERVIEW

LEARNING OUTCOMES

After completing this chapter, you should be able to:

1. Identify research topics, problems, and purposes in published quantitative and qualitative studies.
2. Critically appraise the research problems and purposes in studies.
3. Critically appraise the feasibility of a study problem and purpose.
4. Differentiate among the types of hypotheses (associative vs. causal, simple vs. complex, nondirectional vs. directional, and statistical vs. research).
5. Critically appraise the quality of objectives, questions, and hypotheses in studies.
6. Differentiate the types of variables included in research reports.
7. Critically appraise the conceptual and operational definitions of variables in studies.

We are constantly asking questions to gain a better understanding of ourselves and the world around us. This human ability to wonder and ask creative questions is the first step in the research process. By asking questions, clinical nurses, researchers, and educators are able to identify significant research topics and problems to direct the generation of research evidence for practice. A **research topic** is a concept or broad issue that is important to nursing, such as acute pain, chronic pain management, coping with illness, and health promotion. Each topic contains numerous research problems that might be investigated through quantitative and qualitative studies. For example, chronic pain management is a research topic that includes research problems such as "What is it like to live with chronic pain?" and "What strategies are useful in coping with chronic pain?" Different types of qualitative studies have been conducted to investigate these problems or

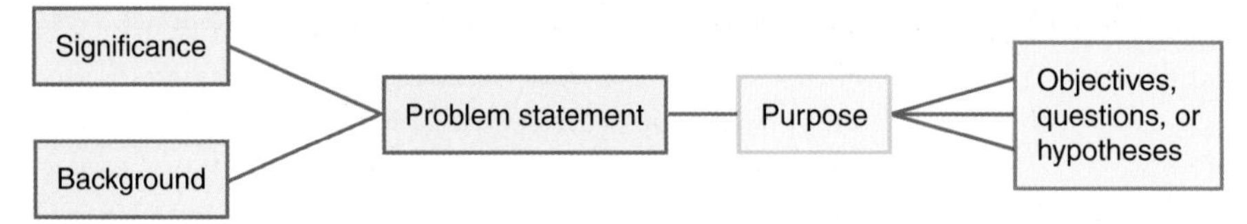

FIG 5.1 Linking research problem, purpose, and objectives, questions, or hypotheses.

areas of concern in nursing (Creswell & Poth, 2018). Quantitative studies have been conducted to address problems such as "What is an accurate and concise way to assess chronic pain?" and "What interventions are effective in managing chronic pain?"

The problem provides the basis for developing the research purpose. The purpose is the goal or focus of a study that guides the development of the objectives, questions, or hypotheses that further focus the intent of the study (Fig. 5.1). Objectives, questions, or hypotheses can be developed to bridge the gap between the more abstractly stated problem and purpose and the detailed design for conducting the study. However, many studies do not include objectives, questions, or hypotheses and are guided by the study problem and purpose. The study purpose, objectives, questions, and hypotheses include the variables, relationships among the variables, and often the population to be studied. In qualitative research, the purpose and sometimes broadly stated research questions or objectives guide the study of selected research concepts.

This chapter includes content that will assist you in identifying problems and purposes in a variety of quantitative and qualitative studies. Objectives, questions, and hypotheses are discussed, and the different types of study variables are introduced. Also presented are guidelines that will assist you in critically appraising the problems, purposes, objectives, questions, hypotheses, and variables or concepts in published quantitative and qualitative studies.

WHAT ARE RESEARCH PROBLEMS AND PURPOSES?

A **research problem** is an area of concern in which there is a gap in the knowledge needed for nursing practice. Research is required to generate essential knowledge to address the practice concern, with the ultimate goal of providing evidence-based nursing care (Brown, 2018; Melnyk & Fineout-Overholt, 2015). The research problem in a study (1) indicates the significance of the problem; (2) provides a background for the problem; and (3) includes a problem statement (Box 5.1). The **significance of a research problem** indicates the importance of the problem to nursing and health care and to the health of individuals, families, and communities. The **background for a problem** briefly identifies what we know about the problem area, and the **problem statement** identifies the specific gap in the knowledge needed for practice. Not all published studies include a clearly expressed problem, but the problem usually can be identified in the first page of the report.

The **research purpose** is a clear concise statement of the specific goal or focus of a study. In quantitative studies, the goal of a study might be to identify and describe variables, examine relationships

BOX 5.1 ELEMENTS OF THE RESEARCH PROBLEM

- Significance: Importance of the problem to nursing and health care
- Background: Key knowledge that is known from previous research
- Problem statement: Identified gap in the knowledge needed for practice

in a situation, determine the effectiveness of an intervention, or determine outcomes of health care (Shadish, Cook, & Campbell, 2002). In qualitative studies, the purpose might be to describe perceptions of a phenomenon and give it meaning, develop a theory of a health situation or issue, explore relevant concepts and concerns in nursing, or describe aspects of a culture (Creswell & Poth, 2018). The purpose includes the variables or concepts, the population, and sometimes the setting for the study. A clearly stated research purpose can capture the essence of a study in a single sentence and is essential for directing the remaining steps of the research process. In a research report, the purpose is usually identified and often follows the problem statement (see Fig. 5.1). The guidelines for critically appraising the problems and purposes in studies are presented as follows.

CRITICAL APPRAISAL GUIDELINES

Problems and Purposes in Studies

1. Is the problem clearly and concisely expressed early in the study?
2. Does the problem include the significance, background, and problem statement (see Box 5.1)?
3. Does the purpose clearly express the goal or focus of the study?
4. Is the purpose focused on the study problem statement?
5. Are the study variables and population identified in the purpose?

The research problem and purpose from the study by Ruiz-González and colleagues (2016, p. 13) about the "long-term effects of an intensive-practical diabetes educational program on HbA1c and self-care" are presented as Research Example 5.1. This example is critically appraised using the identified guidelines.

RESEARCH EXAMPLE 5.1

Problem and Purpose of a Quantitative Study

Research Study Excerpt

Problem Significance

Diabetes mellitus is a disease that affects 246 million people world-wide (Steinsbekk, Rygg, Lisulo, Rise, & Fretheim, 2012) and has a high prevalence in the Spanish population... According to the World Health Organization, adequate control of the disease unequivocally requires educating patients and developing their skills to manage their treatment and prevent complications. (Ruiz-González et al., 2016, p. 13)

Problem Background

Education is achieved through diabetes education programs (DEPs)... DEPs are available in various formats and types... and have been widely proven to be useful in improving biological, psychosocial, and behavioral parameters (Steinsbekk et al., 2012). Recent meta-analyses of controlled studies (Hopkins et al., 2012...) have shown improvements ranging from .52% to .81% in levels of hemoglobin (HbA1c)... and also shown considerable improvement in other areas such as self-efficacy and knowledge. (Ruiz-González et al., 2016, p. 13)

Problem Statement

Despite there are many important variables in education and it is important to consider patient's profile..., few studies have included them in the same DEP or have assessed their long-term effects. In addition, the effectiveness of DEPs should be determined by their influence on both biomedical and psychosocial variables. (Ruiz-González et al., 2016, p. 14)

Continued

RESEARCH EXAMPLE 5.1—cont'd

Research Purpose

The purpose of this study was to implement an intensive and practical DEP and evaluate its long-term effects and its impact on psychosocial variables. (Ruiz-González et al., 2016, p.13)

Critical Appraisal

Research Problem

Ruiz-González et al. (2016) presented a clear concise research problem with the relevant areas of (1) significance, (2) background, and (3) problem statement. Diabetes is a significant, complex, chronic illness that requires extensive knowledge to manage effectively. A clear background of the problem was provided by citing findings from two meta-analyses (Hopkins et al., 2012; Steinsbekk et al., 2012) that summarized studies focused on the effectiveness of DEPs on the management of type 1 and type 2 diabetes. The discussion of the problem concluded with a concise problem statement that indicated the gap in the knowledge needed for practice and provided a basis for the study purpose.

Research Purpose

The research purpose frequently is reflected in the title of the study, stated in the abstract, and restated after the literature review. Ruiz-González and associates (2016) included the purpose of their study in all three places. However, the statements of the purpose in the article were varied, which can be confusing to readers. The researchers clearly identified the DEP intervention (independent variable) that was implemented to determine its long-term effects on psychosocial variables (dependent variables). The purpose would have been more complete if it had included the biomedical dependent variables and the population studied, which was adults with type 1 diabetes.

Ruiz-González and colleagues (2016) found that the DEP intervention was effective in improving biomedical and psychological variables, but more psychological strategies are needed in this intervention to motivate adults to make real lifestyle changes. This type of study supports the Quality and Safety Education for Nurses (QSEN, 2017; Sherwood & Barnsteiner, 2017) pre-licensure competency to ensure safe, quality, and cost-effective research-based health care that actively involves patients and families in their care process.

IDENTIFYING THE PROBLEM AND PURPOSE IN QUANTITATIVE AND QUALITATIVE STUDIES

Quantitative and qualitative research approaches enable nurses to investigate a variety of research problems and purposes. Examples of research problems and purposes for different types of quantitative and qualitative studies are presented in this section.

Problems and Purposes in Types of Quantitative Studies

Example research problems and purposes for the different types of quantitative research—descriptive, correlational, quasi-experimental, and experimental—are presented in Table 5.1. If little is known about a topic, researchers usually start with descriptive and correlational studies and progress to quasi-experimental and experimental studies as knowledge expands in an area. An examination of the problems and purposes in Table 5.1 will reveal the differences and similarities among the types of quantitative research. The research purpose usually reflects the type of study that was conducted (Gray, Grove, & Sutherland, 2017). The purpose of descriptive research is to identify and describe concepts or variables, identify possible relationships among variables, and delineate differences between or among existing groups, such as males and females or different ethnic groups.

TABLE 5.1 QUANTITATIVE RESEARCH TOPICS, PROBLEMS, AND PURPOSES

TYPE OF RESEARCH	RESEARCH PROBLEM AND PURPOSE
Descriptive research	*Title of study:* "Hand hygiene opportunities in pediatric extended care facilities [ECF]." (Buet et al., 2013, p. 72)
	Problem: "The population in pediatric ECFs is increasingly complex, and such children are at high risk of healthcare-associated infections (HAIs), which are associated with increased morbidity, mortality, resources use, and cost (Burns et al., 2010) [problem significance]... The Centers for Disease Control and Prevention (CDC)... and the World Health Organization (WHO, 2009) have published evidence-based guidelines confirming the causal relationship between poor infection control practices, particularly hand hygiene (HH), and increased risk of HAIs [problem background]. However, most of the HH research has been focused in adult long term care facilities and acute care settings and findings from such studies are unlikely to be applicable to HH in pediatric ECFs given the different care patterns, including the relative distribution of different devices" [problem statement] (Buet et al., 2013, pp. 72–73).
	Purpose: "The purpose of this observational study was to assess the frequency and type of HH opportunities initiated by clinical (e.g., physicians and nurses) and non-clinical (e.g., parents and teachers) care givers, as well as evaluate HH adherence using the WHO's '5 Moments for HH' observation tool" (Buet et al., 2013, p. 73).
Correlational research	*Title of study:* "Emergency department [ED] weekend presentation and mortality in patients with acute myocardial infraction [AMI]" (de Cordova et al., 2017, p. 20).
	Problem: "Each year in EDs across the United States, 8 million people are evaluated for symptoms that are consistent with AMI, and approximately 400,000 people die [problem significance]... Patients who present to the ED with an AMI require immediate interventions and treatments to increase their chances of survival... The recommended guidelines, according to the American Heart Association and the American College of Cardiology for the management of a patient with AMI includes diagnostic 12-lead electrocardiogram and biochemical markers, administration of aspirin, thrombolytic therapy within 30 minutes of arrival, and/or percutaneous coronary interventions (PCIs) within 90 minutes of arrival [problem background]... Few research teams have specifically examined patient mortality for the patient with AMI in the ED" and for those presenting to the ED on weekends and holidays [problem statement] (de Cordova et al., 2017, pp. 20–21).
	Purpose: "... the purpose of this study was to determine if a weekend and holiday presentation is associated with an increase in mortality among patients with AMI presenting to the ED in New Jersey" (de Cordova et al., 2017, p. 21).
Quasi-experimental research	*Title of study:* "Methods and design of a 10-week multi-component family meals intervention: A two group quasi-experimental effectiveness trial" (Rogers et al., 2017, p. 1).
	Problem: There is an "ongoing childhood obesity public health crisis [problem significance]... American Academy of Pediatrics recommends participation in family meals as a childhood obesity prevention strategy due to the literature demonstrating a protective effect on participation in healthy mealtime routines on child and weight [problem background].... In addition, the majority of current research fails to examine the child health impact of family meals beyond BMI [body mass index]... Future research, specifically intervention work, would also benefit from expansion of the target age range to include younger children (4-7 year olds), who are laying the foundation of their eating patterns and are capable of participating in family meal preparations" [problem statement] (Rogers et al., 2017, pp. 1–2).

Continued

TABLE 5.1 QUANTITATIVE RESEARCH TOPICS, PROBLEMS, AND PURPOSES—cont'd

TYPE OF RESEARCH	RESEARCH PROBLEM AND PURPOSE
	Purpose: The purpose of this study was to determine the effectiveness "of a 10-week multi-component family meals intervention aimed at eliciting positive changes in child diet and weight status" (Rogers et al., 2017, p. 1).
Experimental research	*Title of study:* "Effects of oral care with glutamine in preventing ventilator-associated pneumonia in neurosurgical intensive care unit patients" (Kaya et al., 2017, p. 10).
	Problem: "Ventilator-associated pneumonia (VAP) is one of the most frequent nosocomial infections in intensive care unit patients [problem significance].... One of the measures to prevent the development of VAP is applying good oral care... In recent studies, glutamine was reported to be an essential amino acid that is critical for the regulation of protein synthesis, respiratory fueling, and nitrogen shuttling [problem background].... Different products and protocols in oral care has been the subject for research. However, the number of studies about glutamine is limited" [problem statement] (Kaya et al., 2017, pp 10–11).
	Purpose: The purpose of this study was "to determine the effects of oral care with glutamine in preventing ventilator-associated pneumonia in patients admitted to neurosurgical intensive care unit" (Kaya et al., 2017, p. 10).

Buet and colleagues (2013) conducted a descriptive study to identify the HH opportunities and adherence among clinical and nonclinical caregivers in extended pediatric care facilities. These researchers followed the World Health Organization (WHO) "5 Moments for Hand Hygiene" (WHO, 2009): before touching a patient, before clean or aseptic procedures, after body fluid exposure or risk, after touching a patient, and after touching patient surroundings. Researchers found that HH opportunities were numerous for clinical and nonclinical caregivers, but adherence to HH was low, especially for nonclinical individuals. HH evidence-based guidelines must be followed to prevent healthcare-associated infections.

The purpose of correlational research is to examine the type (positive or negative) and strength of relationships or associations among variables. Positive relationships (designated by a plus [+] sign) indicate that variables change in the same direction; they either increase or decrease together. For example, the more cigarettes an adult smokes each day, the greater his or her risk of lung cancer. Negative relationships (designated by a minus [−] sign) indicate that variables change in the opposite direction; as one variable increases, the other variable decreases. For example, the more minutes that a middle-aged adult exercises each week, the lower the BMI. The strength of relationships varies from −1 to 0 to +1, with −1 indicating a perfect negative relationship, 0 indicating no relationship, and +1 indicating a perfect positive relationship between variables (Grove & Cipher, 2017). Types of relationships are discussed in more detail in the section on hypotheses.

de Cordova, Johansen, Martinez, and Cimiotti (2017, p. 20) conducted a correlational study to determine if "weekend and holiday presentation was associated with increased mortality in EDs [emergency departments] among patients with AMI [acute myocardial infarction]." The researchers clearly identified the problem and purpose for this study (see Table 5.1). de Cordova and colleagues found that weekend and holiday presentations to the ED for AMI were associated with increased mortality, and further research is needed regarding ED resources during the week, weekend, and holidays to promote quality care.

Quasi-experimental studies are conducted to determine the effect of a treatment or independent variable on designated dependent or outcome variables (Shadish et al., 2002). Rogers and colleagues (2017) developed a quasi-experimental study to examine the effectiveness of a multicomponent family meals intervention called Simple Suppers on elementary school children's (age, 4–10 years) diet and weight status. The research problem and purpose for this study are presented in Table 5.1. The researchers might have provided more detail on the problem significance and background in the article. However, they presented the intervention Simple Suppers and the outcomes to be measured in detail. Rogers et al. (2017) recommended further research to determine the effectiveness of this Simple Supper intervention developed for underserved families with elementary school-age children.

Experimental studies are conducted in highly controlled settings using a structured design to determine the effect of one or more independent variables on one or more dependent variables (Gray et al., 2017). Kaya and colleagues (2017, p. 11) conducted a "randomized, controlled, experimental study to determine the effects of oral care with glutamine in preventing ventilator-associated pneumonia in patients admitted to neurosurgical intensive care unit [ICU] in New Jersey." They found that providing oral care with glutamine had no significant effect on the incidence of VAP in the neurosurgical ICU patients. Kaya et al. (2017) recommended additional research with a larger sample size over a longer time period.

Problems and Purposes in Types of Qualitative Studies

The problems formulated for qualitative research identify areas of concern that require investigation to gain new insights, expand understanding, and improve comprehension of the whole. The purpose of a qualitative study indicates the focus of the study, which may be a concept such as pain, an event such as loss of a child, or a facet of a culture such as the healing practices of a specific Native American tribe. In addition, the purpose often indicates the qualitative approach used to conduct the study (Creswell, 2014; Creswell & Poth, 2018; Munhall, 2012). Table 5.2 includes examples

TABLE 5.2 QUALITATIVE RESEARCH TOPICS, PROBLEMS, AND PURPOSES

TYPE OF RESEARCH	RESEARCH PROBLEM AND PURPOSE
Phenomenological research	*Title of study:* "Severe childhood autism: The family lived experience" (Gorlin et al., 2016, p. 580).
	Problem: "Autism is the most prevalent developmental disability in the United States, affecting approximately 1 in 68 children (Center for Disease Control [CDC], 2014). Approximately one-third of the children with autism are considered to have 'severe autism' with significant functional challenges [problem significance]... There has been an effort to clarify autism severity based on a more holistic approach that focuses on the child's daily needs within the context of the family instead of solely on symptoms [problem background]... In many of these studies, however, the severity of the child with autism is not identified... Additionally many of the phenomenological studies rely on the response of one family member, usually the mother to portray the family experience... Extended family members or others considered as family have not been included in the studies reviewed" [problem statement] (Gorlin et al., 2016, pp. 580–582).
	Purpose: "The aim or purpose of this research was to interpret the meaning of the lived experience of families who live with a child who has severe autism" (Gorlin et al., 2016, p. 582).
Grounded theory research	*Title of study:* "A grounded theory study of how nurses integrate pregnancy and full-time employment: Becoming someone different" (Quinn, 2016, p. 170).

Continued

TABLE 5.2 QUALITATIVE RESEARCH TOPICS, PROBLEMS, AND PURPOSES—cont'd

TYPE OF RESEARCH	RESEARCH PROBLEM AND PURPOSE
	Problem: "According to the U.S. Department of Labor (2010), there are approximately 1.7 million nurses in the United State, 40% of whom are women within the childbearing ages of 20-45 years, and more than 65% are employed full-time [problem significance]... Research from 1990 to 2000 reported mostly unfavorable findings related to attitudes surrounding pregnant employees in the workplace... Some employers conversely, embrace their pregnant employees and view them as valuable members of their work teams [problem background]... Nursing, as an international industry, has not explored how its female workforce (i.e., nurses) integrates pregnancy and employment" [problem statement] (Quinn, 2016, pp. 170–171).
	Purpose: "The purpose of this research was to explore how primiparous U.S. nurses integrated pregnancy and full-time employment" (Quinn, 2016, p. 170).
Exploratory-descriptive qualitative research	*Title of study:* "Women's perceptions of biases and barriers in their myocardial infarction triage experience" (Arslanian-Engoren & Scott, 2016, p. 166).
	Problem: "Every 10 minutes a woman dies from a myocardial infarction (MI). Yet, symptoms of impending MI in women are less likely to be recognized than in men [problem significance].... Investigators have examined the cardiac triage decisions of ED nurses, who are often the first healthcare provider to evaluate and triage women for MI and initiate guideline recommendations. Results indicated that nurses do not always recognize women's cardiac symptoms and their practice does not consistently adhere to MI evidence-based guidelines [problem background]... Less is known about the personal experiences of women within the ED healthcare system that may affect the accuracy or timeliness of nurses' cardiac triage decisions" [problem statement] (Arslanian-Engoren & Scott, 2016, pp. 166–167).
	Purpose: "Therefore, the purpose of this study was to examine the cardiac triage experiences of women who presented to the ED with an acute MI" (Arslanian-Engoren & Scott, 2016, p. 167).
Ethnographic research	*Title of study:* "Perceptions and experiences of using a nipple shield among parents and staff: An ethnographic study in neonatal units" (Flacking & Dykes, 2017, p. 1).
	Problem: "Breast milk mediates unequalled beneficial effects regarding nutritional, immunological, and cognitive outcomes in preterm infants (<37 gestational weeks, gw), therefore international recommendations state that infants should be exclusively breastfed for the first 6 months of life [problem significance]... Although research shows that preterm infants display rooting, efficient areolar grasp, and repeated short sucking bursts from 29 weeks, and occasional long sucking bursts and repeated swallowing from 31 weeks, the transition from tube feeding to exclusive breastfeeding at the breast takes time [problem background]... However, the use of nipple shields is very controversial and study results are contradictory. Furthermore, no study has previously explored the parents' and staffs' perspective and experiences of using a nipple shield in neonatal units" [problem statement] (Flacking & Dykes, 2017, pp. 1–2).
	Purpose: The purpose of this ethnographic study " is to explore perceptions and experiences of using a nipple shield among parents and staff in neonatal units" (Flacking & Dykes, 2017, p. 2).

ED, Emergency department; *gw*, gestational weeks.

of research problems and purposes for the types of qualitative research—phenomenological, grounded theory, exploratory-descriptive, and ethnographic—commonly found in the nursing literature and included in this text.

Phenomenological research is conducted to promote a deeper understanding of complex human experiences as they have been lived by the study participants (Creswell & Poth, 2018). Gorlin, McAlpine, Garwick, and Wieling (2016) conducted a phenomenological study to examine the experiences of families living with a child with severe autism. The research problem and purpose for this study were clearly developed in the article and are presented in Table 5.2. Gorlin and colleagues' (2016, p. 596) study findings "illuminated the extensive hardships and challenges of families who have a child with severe autism; identified needed resources; and illuminated how families formed hybrid families for additional support."

In grounded theory research, the problem identifies the area of concern, and the purpose indicates the focus of the theory to be developed to account for a pattern of behavior of those involved in the study (Charmaz, 2014). For example, Quinn (2016, p. 170) conducted "a grounded theory study of how nurses integrate pregnancy and full-time employment." The problem and purpose were clearly stated in this study and are presented in Table 5.2. Quinn (2016, p. 173) found that "Becoming someone different emerged as the basic social process of how RNs (registered nurses) integrate full-time employment and pregnancy. Four categories—looking different, feeling different; expectations while expecting; connecting differently; and transitioning labor—were identified from the data analysis."

Exploratory-descriptive qualitative research is being conducted by several researchers to describe unique concepts, issues, health problems, or situations that lack clear description or definition. Kim, Sefcik, and Bradway (2017) conducted a systematic review to describe the characteristics of exploratory-descriptive qualitative studies, which often provide the basis for future qualitative and quantitative research. Arslanian-Engoren and Scott (2016) conducted an exploratory-descriptive qualitative study of "women's perceptions of biases and barriers in their myocardial infarction (MI) triage experience." The research problem and purpose for this study were clearly presented in the research report (see Table 5.2). These researchers found that women with an MI perceived multiple barriers to their prompt diagnosis and treatment in an ED. Thus Arslanian-Engoren and Scott (2016, p. 171) recommended research to "evaluate interventions to improve the care delivery processes, reduce barriers, and facilitate the prompt and accurate treatment of women for acute MI."

In ethnographic research, the problem and purpose identify the culture and specific attributes of the culture that are to be examined, described, analyzed, and interpreted to reveal the social actions, beliefs, values, and norms of the culture (Creswell & Poth, 2018). Flacking and Dykes (2017, p. 1) conducted an ethnographic study of the "perceptions and experiences of using a nipple shield among parents and staff… in neonatal units." Table 5.2 includes the concisely developed research problem and purpose for this ethnographic study. The researchers concluded that using a nipple shield had both positive and negative aspects. The nipple shield facilitated the premature neonate's attachment to the breast and the quality of nutritional intake but was a barrier to the relationship between mother and infant during breastfeeding. The nipple shield is often viewed as a short-term solution, and nurses must take into consideration the particular needs of the mother and baby.

DETERMINING THE SIGNIFICANCE OF A STUDY PROBLEM AND PURPOSE

A research problem and purpose is significant when it has the potential to generate or refine relevant knowledge that directly or indirectly affects nursing practice (Gray et al., 2017). When critically appraising the significance of the problem and purpose in a published study, you need to determine whether the researchers made a clear link of how the findings (1) might be applied in nursing practice, (2) expanded on previous research, (3) improved understanding of a problem by developing theory, and/or (4) added knowledge to current nursing research priorities.

Application to Nursing Practice

Practice-focused studies are significant because they address clinical concerns and generate findings for application to nursing practice. In addition, studies with significant research problems promote healthy patient and family outcomes, decrease morbidity and mortality, and reduce the costs of care. The ultimate goal is providing evidence-based practice (EBP), in which nursing care is based on the most current research (Melnyk, Gallagher-Ford, Fineout-Overholt, 2017).

Several studies have focused on the effects of nursing interventions or on ways to improve these interventions. For example, in the Ruiz-González et al. (2016) study that was introduced earlier, a DEP was implemented to improve biomedical (e.g., HbA1c) and psychosocial (e.g., self-care) variables in adults with type 1 diabetes. Rogers et al. (2017) developed a multicomponent family meal intervention to improve children's diets and weight status, with the goal of reducing childhood obesity. Intervention-focused studies have the potential to generate significant, practical, and credible knowledge that can be applied to patient care to promote quality and safe patient- and family-centered care (Brown, 2018; Sherwood & Barnsteiner, 2017).

Expands Previous Research

For knowledge to advance, researchers design their studies based on the findings of previous research. In a research article, the introduction and literature review sections include relevant studies that provide a basis for the current study. Often, a summary of the current literature indicates what is known and not known in the problem area being studied (see Chapter 6). The gaps in the current knowledge base (problem statement) provide support for the study's purpose (see Fig. 5.1). Ruiz-González et al. (2016) based their study on findings indicating that DEPs were effective in helping patients manage their type 1 diabetes. Then, they focused their study on what was not known regarding the long-term effects of DEPs on both biomedical and psychosocial outcomes of adults with type 1 diabetes.

Most study problems and purposes are based on previous research, as indicated by the research sources in the study's reference list. Studies from research and clinical practice journals are cited, indicating the findings on which the current study was based. You can review the reference list from the Ruiz-González et al. (2016) study to identify the types of studies and journals cited in this article.

Promotes Theory Testing or Development

Another way that knowledge grows is when researchers design studies to refine or expand theoretical understanding of a clinical problem. Significant problems and purposes in quantitative studies are supported by theory, and often the focus of these studies is theory testing (Chinn & Kramer, 2015). The focus of a qualitative study may be to develop a theory (Creswell & Poth, 2018). For example, Quinn (2016) conducted a grounded theory study to develop a theory that described how US nurses integrated pregnancy and full-time employment. A detailed discussion of the different types of theories tested and/or developed through research is presented in Chapter 7.

Addresses Nursing Research Priorities

There are literally thousands of topics that a nurse researcher could study. To have the most benefit, researchers need to study problems that are the most important to nursing. Over the last 50 years, expert researchers, professional organizations, and funding agencies have identified research priorities to encourage studies in the areas important for nursing. Many professional nursing organizations use their websites to communicate current research priorities. For example, the current research priorities of the American Association of Critical Care Nurses (AACN, 2017) are identified on their website (https://www.aacn.org/nursing-excellence/grants/research-priority-areas) as: "(1) effective and appropriate use of technology to achieve optimal patient assessment, management, and/or outcomes; (2) creation of a healing, humane environment; (3) processes and systems that foster the optimal contribution of critical care nurses; (4) effective approaches to symptom management; and (5) prevention and management of complications" (AACN, 2017).

You can access the AACN (2017) research priorities without being a member of the organization, but some organizations, such as the Oncology Nursing Society and Society of Pediatric Nurses require you to sign into their website to access research priorities and activities.

The National Institute of Nursing Research (NINR) is the key agency for promoting nursing research in the United States. The NINR (2017) funds clinical and basic research and supports research training to promote the development of a scientific basis for clinical practice. A major initiative of the NINR is the development of a national nursing research agenda that involves identifying nursing research priorities, outlining a plan for implementing priority studies, and providing funds to support these priority projects.

The focus of the NINR's (2016) Strategic Plan was "advancing science and improving lives." The research agenda "focuses on areas of science in which the health needs are greatest, and in which NINR-supported research can have the largest impact." The research priorities for the NINR include four areas of scientific focus:

- Symptom science: promoting personalized health strategies
- Wellness: promoting health and preventing illness
- Self-management: improving quality of life for individuals with chronic conditions
- End-of-life and palliative care: the science of compassion

"Two other areas, promoting innovation and developing the nurse scientists of the 21st century, are emphasized in all areas of NINR's research programs. The plan is intended to be a living document, one which can be adapted as new opportunities and challenges arise" (NINR, 2016; https://www.ninr.nih.gov/sites/www.ninr.nih.gov/files/NINR_StratPlan2016_reduced.pdf.)

Another federal agency with emphasis on facilitating healthcare research is the Agency for Healthcare Research and Quality (AHRQ). "The AHRQ mission is to produce evidence to make health care safer, higher quality, more accessible, equitable, and affordable, and to work within the U.S. Department of Health and Human Services and with other partners to make sure that the evidence is understood and used" (AHRQ, 2016; https://www.ahrq.gov/cpi/about/ mission/index.html). The research priorities and funded projects are presented on the AHRQ (2017) website (http://www.ahrq.gov/legacy/fund/ragendix.htm).

Some of the research priorities identified by the AHRQ include the following:

- Optimizing care to people with multiple chronic conditions
- Quality care for low-income and racial and ethnic minority patients
- Research focused on translation, implementation, and diffusion of research into practice and policy
- Research to promote career development

The *Healthy People 2020* website identifies and prioritizes the health topics and objectives of all age groups over the next decade (US Department of Health and Human Services [DHHS], 2017). These health topics and objectives direct future research in the areas of health promotion, illness prevention, illness management, and rehabilitation and can be accessed online at https://www.healthypeople.gov/2020/topics-objectives. Work is currently in progress for developing the topics and objectives for *Healthy People 2030*.

The WHO (2017) stresses the importance of research in building a healthier future for people all over the world. The WHO (2017) has offices in more than 190 countries and encourages the identification of priorities for a common nursing research agenda among these countries. A quality healthcare delivery system and improved patient and family health have become global goals. By 2020, the world's population is expected to increase by 94%, with the older adult population increasing by almost 240%. Seven of every 10 deaths are expected to be caused by noncommunicable diseases, such as chronic conditions (e.g., heart disease, cancer, depression) and injuries (unintentional and intentional). The priority areas for research identified by WHO are to:

> *(1) improve the health of the world's most marginalized populations; (2) study new diseases that threaten public health around the world; (3) conduct comparative analyses of supply and demand of the health workforce of different countries; (4) analyze the feasibility, effectiveness, and quality of education and practice of nurses; (5) conduct research on healthcare delivery modes; and (6) examine the outcomes for healthcare agencies, providers, and patients around the world.*
>
> ***WHO, 2017; http://www.who.int/entity/en***

In summary, expert nurse researchers, professional nursing organizations, and national and international agencies and organizations have identified research priorities to direct the future conduct of healthcare research to improve the outcomes for patients and families, nurses, and healthcare systems. When conducting a critical appraisal of a study, you need to examine the study's contribution to nursing practice and determine whether the study's problem and purpose are based on previous research, theory, and current research priorities.

EXAMINING THE FEASIBILITY OF A STUDY PROBLEM AND PURPOSE

A critical appraisal of research begins by determining the feasibility of the problem and purpose of the study. The **feasibility of a study** is determined by examining the researchers' expertise; money commitment; availability of subjects, facilities, and equipment; and the study's ethical considerations (Gray et al., 2017; Rogers, 1987). The feasibility of Ruiz-González and colleagues' (2016) study of the long-term effects of a DEP on biological and psychosocial variables in adults with type 1 diabetes was critically appraised and presented as an example. You can review this study's problem and purpose at the beginning of this chapter and locate this study through your library. The critical appraisal involves addressing the following questions about a study's feasibility.

? CRITICAL APPRAISAL GUIDELINES

Examining the Feasibility of a Study's Problem and Purpose

1. Did the researchers have the research, clinical, and educational expertise to conduct the study?
2. Was the study funded by local or national organizations or agencies? Did clinical agencies provide support for the study?
3. Did the researchers have adequate subjects, settings, and equipment to conduct their study?
4. Was the purpose of the study ethical?

Researcher Expertise

The research problem and purpose studied need to be within the area of expertise of the researchers. Research reports usually identify the education of the researchers and their current positions, which indicate their expertise to conduct a study. Doctor of philosophy (PhD) and postdoctorate degrees indicate very strong educational preparation for conducting research. Also, examine the reference list to determine whether the researchers have conducted additional studies in this area. If you need more information, you can search the Internet for the researchers' accomplishments and involvement in research.

Ruiz-González (principal author), Guardia-Archilla, Rodríguez-Morales, Molina, and Casares were all master's-prepared and working in the areas of endocrinology and nutrition at two different university hospitals. University hospitals usually have a strong focus on research and conduct a variety of studies. Fernández-Alcántara was also master's-prepared and working in the university-based Mind, Brain, and Behavior Research Center. Santos-Roig was PhD-prepared and working in a university school of psychology. The reference list included no previous publications by these authors. Ruiz-González and colleagues (2016) demonstrated extremely strong clinical expertise in the areas of diabetes, endocrinology, nutrition, and psychology. Two authors were university-based and affiliated with research centers. The research and educational expertise of these authors was somewhat limited, with most being master's-prepared and none having previous publications in this area.

Money Commitment

The problem and purpose studied are influenced by the amount of money available to the researchers. The cost of a research project can range from a few dollars for a student's small study to hundreds of thousands and even millions of dollars for complex projects. Critically appraising the feasibility of a study involves examining the financial resources available to the researchers in conducting their study. Sources of funding for a study usually are identified in the article.

Studies might be funded by grants from national institutions (e.g., NINR, 2017; AHRQ, 2017), professional organizations, or private foundations. The researchers may have received financial assistance from companies that provided necessary equipment or support from the agencies where they conducted the study. Receiving funding for a study indicates that it was reviewed by peers who chose to support the research financially. The study by Ruiz-González et al. (2016, p. 13) was "funded by the Regional Ministry of Health of Andalusia, Spain." These researchers were also supported in implementing the DEP intervention and collecting essential study data at the day clinic where the study was conducted. Ruiz-González et al. (2016) clearly identified the regional funding for their study and clinical agency support.

Availability of Subjects, Facilities, and Equipment

Researchers need to have adequate sample size, facilities, and equipment to implement their study. Most published studies indicate the sample size and setting(s) in the methods section of the research report. Often, nursing studies are conducted in natural or partially controlled settings, such as a home, school, hospital unit, or clinic. Many of these facilities are fairly easy to access, and the hospitals and clinics often provide access to adequate numbers of patients. Ruiz-González and colleagues' (2016) study included an initial sample of 115 patients with type 1 diabetes who attended a diabetic outpatient clinic. However, the final sample included only 40 participants after this year-long study. Adequate subjects were available through the diabetic clinic, but the 34.7% retention rate ($[40 \div 115] \times 100\% = 0.347 \times 100\% = 34.7\%$) could have affected the study results.

A review of the methods section of the research article will determine if adequate and accurate equipment was available. Nursing studies frequently require a limited amount of equipment, such as a tape or video recorder for interviews; physiological measures, such as laboratory values, vital signs, or BMI; and Internet-based or hard copy scales. Ruiz-González et al. (2016) assessed all participants' biomedical variables (HbA1c, lipid levels, BMI) and psychosocial variables (knowledge of diabetes, self-reported self-care behaviors, perceived barriers, self-efficacy) before and after implementing the DEP in the clinic. Thus the subjects, equipment, and facility were adequate to conduct this study.

Ethical Considerations

The purpose selected for investigation must be ethical, which means that the subjects' rights and the rights of others in the setting are protected (Gray et al., 2017). An ethical study confers more benefits than risks in its conduct and will generate useful knowledge for practice. Chapter 4 provides a detailed discussion of ethics in quantitative and qualitative research. Ruiz-González and colleagues (2016, p. 15) provided a clear discussion of the ethical aspects of their study in the following: "Patients were informed of the objectives of the study and gave written informed consent prior to test administration. The study was approved by the Ethics Committee of San Cecilio University Hospital."

EXAMINING RESEARCH OBJECTIVES, QUESTIONS, AND HYPOTHESES IN RESEARCH REPORTS

Research objectives, questions, and hypotheses evolve from the problem, purpose, literature review, and sometimes the study framework to direct the remaining steps of the research process (see Fig. 5.1). Many researchers only identify a problem and purpose to guide their quantitative or qualitative studies. However, some studies include specific objectives, questions, or hypotheses to guide the methodology, organize the results, and clarify the findings. In a published study, the objectives, questions, or hypotheses usually are presented after the literature review section, right before the methods section. The content in this section will assist you in identifying and critically appraising the objectives, questions, and hypotheses in studies.

Research Objectives

A **research objective** is a clear, concise, declarative statement expressed in the present tense to identify the goals of the study. The objectives are sometimes referred to as aims and are generally presented in descriptive and correlational quantitative studies. For clarity, an objective usually focuses on one or two variables and indicates whether they are to be identified or described. Sometimes the focus of objectives is to identify relationships among variables or determine differences between two or more existing groups, such as females and males, for selected variables.

Qualitative research is most appropriate when the focus of the study is to obtain a personal perspective of a situation, experience, or event (Creswell & Poth, 2018; Henson & Jeffrey, 2016). The research objectives or aims formulated for quantitative and qualitative studies have some similarities because they focus on exploration, description, and determination of relationships. However, the objectives directing qualitative studies are commonly broader in focus and include concepts that are more complex and abstract than those of quantitative studies. The aims in qualitative studies focus on participants' experiences of certain events and health conditions, theory development, understanding of cultures of groups and institutions, and description of challenges, reasons for behaviors, and perceptions of specific care or interventions in nursing practice (Creswell & Poth, 2018; Kim et al., 2017).

Guillaume, Crawford, and Quigley (2016, p. 65) included aims to direct their study of the "characteristics of the middle-age adult inpatient fall." These researchers demonstrated the logical flow from research problem and purpose to research aims (see Fig. 5.1) in reporting their quantitative descriptive study, presented in Research Example 5.2. The questions in the following box were used to conduct a critical appraisal of this study.

CRITICAL APPRAISAL GUIDELINES

Research Objectives and Questions

1. Are the objectives (aims) or questions clearly and concisely expressed in the study?
2. Are the study objectives or questions based on the study purpose?
3. Do the objectives or questions appear to direct the study methodology, organize the study results, and facilitate the interpretations of findings?

RESEARCH EXAMPLE 5.2

Problem, Purpose, and Aims or Objectives

Research Study Excerpt

Research Problem

Falls with injuries remains one of the most reportable, serious, and costly type of adverse events that occur in United States (U.S.) hospitals, resulting in detrimental morbidity and mortality outcomes... In acute care hospitals, an estimated 1,000 falls occur per hospital each year regardless of size, with over one million inpatient falls reported annually at the national level [problem significance].... The recent fall study by Williams et al. (2014) also identified that middle-aged inpatients 51–60 years old (n = 5,561) had the highest reported fall rates, followed by patients age 61–70 years (n = 4,699) [problem background].... While predictors of falls and injuries have been studied across all adult inpatients..., research has not specifically addressed the fall risk characteristics in the middle-age [problem statement]. (Guillaume et al., 2016, pp. 65–66)

Research Purpose

The purpose of this study was to describe the characteristics of middle-age adult inpatients' [ages 45–64] that fall, along with their fall and fall injury risk factors. (Guillaume et al., 2016, p. 66)

Research Aims

The aims were to (a) describe falls and fall injury risk factors; (b) describe unit-specific data, fall numbers with type of falls, injuries from falls, and prevention strategies; and (c) compare the incidence of fall and fall injury rates of the middle-age (45–64) patients with the hospital adult age groups (21–44 and 65–90). (Guillaume et al., 2016, p. 66)

Critical Appraisal

Guillaume and colleagues (2016) identified a significant problem regarding inpatient falls for middle-aged adults that had not been adequately studied. The problem statement clearly indicated what was not known and provided a basis for the purpose and aims of this study. The purpose clearly indicated that the focus of the study was to describe the characteristics of middle-age adult inpatient falls. The study aims built on the problem and purpose and provided more clarity regarding the specific goals of the study. These aims were very useful in organizing the study results and interpreting the findings. The specific variables described and compared related to falls were identified in the study aims. The first two aims were focused on description and the last on comparing fall and fall injury rates of middle-age adults with two other hospital adult age groups.

Research Questions

A research question is a clear, concise, interrogative statement that is worded in the present tense, includes one or more variables, and is expressed to guide the implementation of studies. The foci of research questions in quantitative studies are description of variable(s), examination of relationships among variables, use of independent variables to predict a dependent variable, and determination of differences between two or more groups regarding selected variable(s). These research questions are usually narrowly focused and inclusive of the study variables and population. It is really a matter of choice whether researchers identify objectives or questions in their study but, more often, questions are stated to guide descriptive and correlational quantitative studies. Hypotheses should be developed to direct quasi-experimental and experimental quantitative studies (Shadish et al., 2002).

Hernandez, Morgan, and Parshall (2016, p. 481) conducted a descriptive correlational study to examine the "resilience, stress, stigma, and barriers to mental healthcare in U.S. Air Force [USAF] nursing personnel." These researchers identified a purpose and research questions to direct the implementation of their study, presented in Research Example 5.3. The critical appraisal guidelines for examining research objectives or questions in a study, presented earlier, were applied to this example.

RESEARCH EXAMPLE 5.3

Purpose and Research Questions From a Quantitative Study

Research Study Excerpt

Research Purpose

This study assessed the extent to which stigma and barriers to accessing MH [mental health] services as perceived by USAF nursing personnel are associated with resilience, stress, previous deployment, or demographic characteristics. (Hernandez et al., 2016, p. 481)

Research Questions

1. *What are USAF nursing personnel's levels of stigma and barriers to accessing MH services, stress, and resilience?*
2. *What are the magnitude and direction of associations among stigma and barriers to accessing MH services, stress, and resilience in USAF nursing personnel?*
3. *Are the demographic characteristics, military grade, past deployment, and access to MH services related to stigma and barriers to accessing MH services, stress, and resilience among USAF nursing personnel?* (Hernandez et al., 2016, p. 482)

Critical Appraisal

Hernandez and colleagues (2016) clearly stated their study purpose, and the research questions evolved from the purpose and clarified the goals of their study. Question 1 focused on a description of nursing personnel's levels of stigma and barriers to accessing MH services. Questions 2 and 3 focused on examining relationships or associations among the study variables. These questions were addressed by the study methodology, results, and findings. Hernandez et al. (2016, p. 481) found that a large percentage of the USAF nursing personnel had "concerns that accessing MH services may adversely affect their careers and how they are viewed by unit leaders and peers. In addition, higher levels of concern about stigma were associated with higher levels of stress and lower levels of resilience."

The research questions directing qualitative studies are often limited in number, broadly focused, and inclusive of variables or concepts that are more complex and abstract than those of quantitative studies. Marshall and Rossman (2016) indicated that the questions developed to direct qualitative research might be theoretical, which can be studied with different populations or in a variety of sites, or the questions could be focused on a particular population or setting. The study questions formulated are very important for the selection of the qualitative research method used to conduct the study (Creswell & Poth, 2018).

Roll and Bowers (2017) conducted a qualitative study to describe how healthy aging is promoted for individuals with developmental disabilities. These investigators developed research questions to guide their study. The purpose and questions from this study are presented in Research Example 5.4.

RESEARCH EXAMPLE 5.4

Purpose and Research Questions From a Qualitative Study

Research Study Excerpt

Research Purpose

This qualitative study "sought to describe and analyze one innovative community nursing outreach program that emerged in 2009 in response to the observed health disparities and unmet health needs of people with I/DD [intellectual and developmental disabilities]" (Roll & Bowers, 2017, p. 236).

Research Questions

1. *Why did this community outreach nursing program (CONP) for people with I/DD emerge?*
2. *What is the daily work of the community outreach nurses in this program with the goal of promoting healthy aging of individuals with I/DD in the community?* (Roll & Bowers, 2017, p. 237)

Critical Appraisal

Roll and Bowers (2017) clearly identified their study purpose and the research questions clarified the goals of the study. Question 1 focused on identifying and describing why the CONP for people with I/DD emerged, and question 2 focused on a description of the daily work of nurses in the CONP. These questions were the focus of data collection and analysis and provided organization to the discussion of findings. Roll and Bowers (2017, p. 234) found that the CONP was implemented to improve communication between primary care providers and individuals with I/DD. The nurses' daily work included "health education, advocacy for the safe return home,... and enabling social participation" of individuals with I/DD.

Hypotheses

A hypothesis is a formal statement of the expected relationship(s) between two or more variables in a specified population. The hypothesis translates the research problem and purpose into a clear explanation or prediction of the expected results or outcomes of selected quantitative studies. A clearly stated study hypothesis includes the independent variables to be manipulated or measured, indicates the proposed outcomes or dependent variables to be measured, and identifies the population to be studied. Different types of variables are discussed in more detail at the end of this chapter. Hypotheses also influence the study design, sampling method, data collection and analysis process, and interpretation of findings (Fawcett & Garity, 2009; Grove & Cipher, 2017). Quasi-experimental and experimental quantitative studies are conducted to test the effectiveness of a treatment or intervention; these types of studies should include hypotheses to predict the study outcomes. Predictive correlational studies that measure independent variables to predict a dependent variable often include hypotheses (Gray et al., 2017). In this section, types of hypotheses are described, and the elements of a testable hypothesis are discussed, so that you can critically appraise hypotheses in published studies.

Types of Hypotheses

Different types of relationships and numbers of variables are identified in hypotheses. A study might have one, four, or more hypotheses, depending on its complexity. The type of hypothesis developed is based on the purpose of the study. Hypotheses can be described using four categories that are identified in Box 5.2 and described in this section.

Associative versus causal hypotheses. The relationships identified in hypotheses are associative or causal. An associative hypothesis proposes relationships among variables that occur or exist together in the real world so that when one variable changes, the other changes (Gray et al., 2017).

BOX 5.2 TYPES OF HYPOTHESES

- Associative versus causal hypotheses
- Simple versus complex hypotheses
- Nondirectional versus directional hypotheses
- Statistical versus research hypotheses

Associative hypotheses identify relationships among variables in a study but do not indicate that one variable *causes* an *effect* on another variable. McKee, Long, Southward, Walker, and McCown (2016) conducted a predictive correlation study to determine the factors that were predictive of childhood obesity. They "hypothesized that children of overweight or obese parents are more likely to be obese" (McKee et al., 2016, p. 197). This associative hypothesis predicts two positive relationships between overweight parents and obese children and between obese parents and obese children. The relationships in this hypothesis are diagrammed as follows:

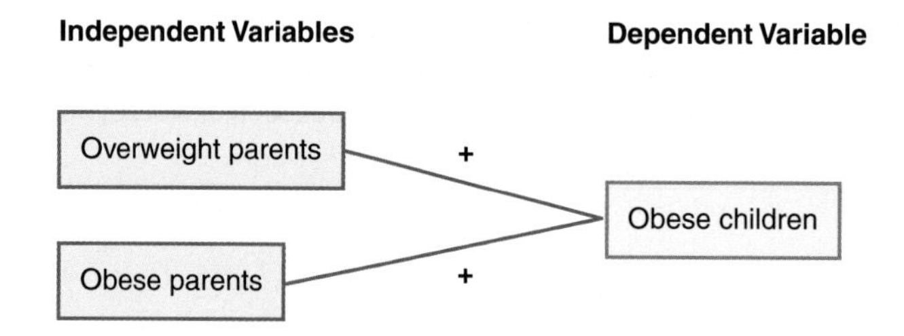

The lines that connect the three variables are straight, without arrows, which indicate linear relationships or associations. McKee et al. (2016, p. 200) found "that the second greatest predictor of childhood obesity was having at least one obese parent, and the third greatest predictor was having at least one overweight parent."

A **causal hypothesis** proposes a cause and effect interaction between two or more variables, referred to as independent and dependent variables. The independent variable (treatment or intervention) is manipulated by the researcher to cause an effect on the dependent or outcome variable. The researcher then measures the dependent variable to examine the effect created by the independent variable (Waltz, Strickland, & Lenz, 2017). A format for stating a causal hypothesis is the following.

Study participants in the experimental group, who are exposed to the independent variable (intervention), demonstrate greater change, as measured by the dependent variable, than those in the comparison group who received standard care.

The study by Ruiz-González et al. (2016), presented earlier, was conducted to examine the long-term effects of a DEP (independent variable) on biomedical and psychosocial measures (dependent variables). This study included the following causal hypothesis: "after the DEP, patients will have lower levels of A1c hemoglobin, greater theoretical and practical knowledge about diabetes, fewer barriers [to self-care], higher frequency of self-care, and greater self-efficacy." This hypothesis included seven variables—one independent variable (DEP) that was implemented to create an effect on the six dependent variables (HbA1c, theoretical and practical knowledge about diabetes, barriers to self-care, self-care, and self-efficacy). This causal hypothesis might be diagrammed as follows, with an arrow (→) to indicate cause and effect versus associative relationships:

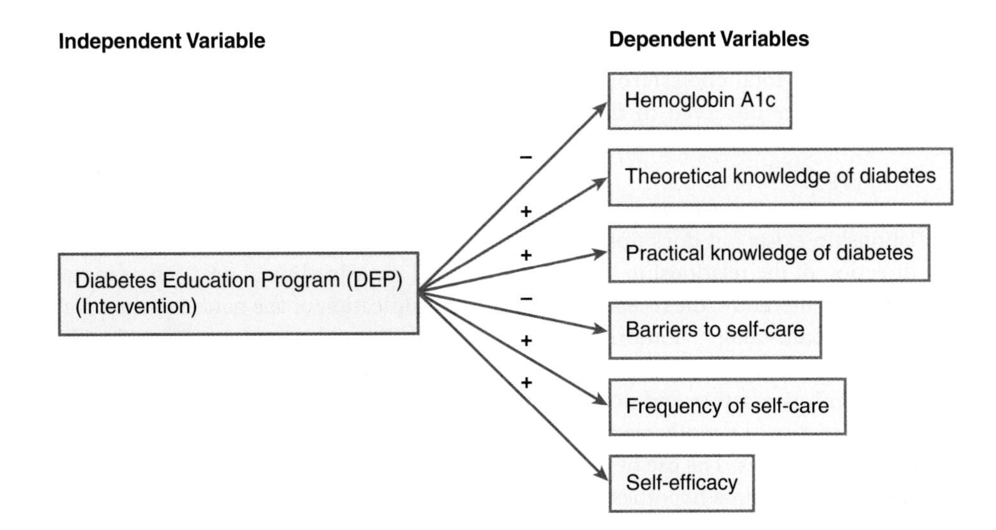

This causal hypothesis identifies two negative and four positive relationships. The DEP was expected to decrease HbA1c and barriers to self-care and to increase knowledge of diabetes, frequency of self-care, and self-efficacy. The study by Ruiz-González et al. (2016, p. 13) supported this hypothesis because "significant changes were maintained at one-year follow-up in hemoglobin A1c, barriers to self-care, frequency of self-care, knowledge about the disease, and perceived self-efficacy."

Simple versus complex hypotheses. Hypotheses are either simple or complex (see Box 5.2). A **simple hypothesis** states the relationship (associative or causal) between two variables. McKee and colleagues (2016, p. 197) stated a simple associate hypothesis in their study of predictors of childhood obesity. They hypothesized that children whose weight status is "misperceived by their parents are more likely to be obese." This hypothesis might be diagrammed as follows:

Parents' misperception of child's weight —+— child more likely to be obese.

The study by McKee et al. (2016) supported this hypothesis because 86.2% of the parents misperceived their child's weight as healthy when the child was actually overweight or obese. These researchers found that the parents' misperception of their child's weight status was the strongest predictor of childhood obesity.

A **complex hypothesis** states the relationships (associative or causal) among three or more variables. The study by Ruiz-González and colleagues (2016) included the following complex causal hypothesis: "the DEP patients will show improvements in biomedical measures, particularly in cardiovascular risk factors such as cholesterol (total and LDL [low density lipoprotein]) and body mass index [BMI]" (Ruiz-González et al., 2016, p. 14). This hypothesis might be diagrammed as follows:

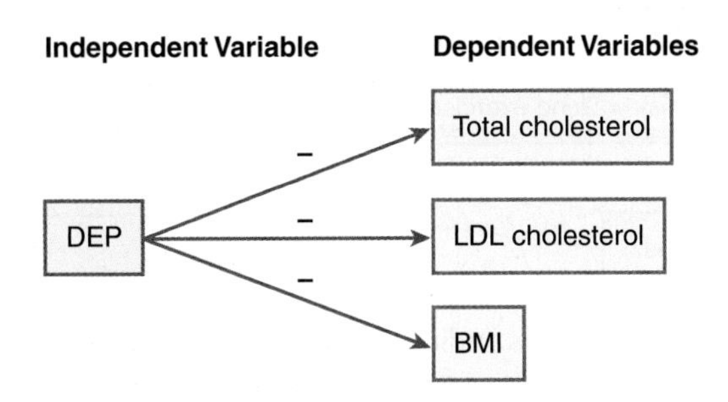

The researchers examined the effect of DEP (an independent variable) on the dependent variables of total cholesterol, LDL, and BMI. This hypothesis was not supported because no changes were observed in the BMI or the total and LDL cholesterol values. Thus the Ruiz-González et al. (2016) study had mixed results, with one hypothesis supported and the other not supported.

Nondirectional versus directional hypotheses. A nondirectional hypothesis states that a relationship exists but does not predict the nature (positive or negative) of the relationship. If the direction of the relationship being studied is not clear in clinical practice or in the theoretical or empirical literature, the researcher has no clear indication of the nature of the relationship. Under these circumstances, nondirectional hypotheses are developed, such as "hours playing video games is related to body mass index in school-age children." This is an example of a simple (two variables), associative, and nondirectional hypothesis.

A directional hypothesis states the nature (positive or negative) of the interaction between two or more variables. The use of terms such as *positive, negative, less, more, increase, decrease, greater, higher*, or *lower* in a hypothesis indicates the direction of the relationship. Directional hypotheses are developed from theoretical statements (propositions), findings of previous studies, and clinical experience. As the knowledge on which a study is based increases, researchers are able to make a prediction about the direction of a relationship between the variables being studied. For example, McKee and colleagues (2016, p. 197) stated a directional hypothesis: "parents will be *more* likely to misperceive the weight status of younger children." The italicized word indicates the nature of the relationship in this simple, associative, directional hypothesis. This hypothesis includes a negative relationship that might be diagrammed as follows:

Parents more likely to misperceive weight status ——(−)—— for younger children

The study by McKee et al. (2016) supported this hypothesis because the parents significantly misperceived the weight status of their younger children as being healthy when they were actually overweight or obese.

A causal hypothesis predicts the effect of an independent variable on a dependent variable, specifying the direction of the relationship. The independent variable increases or decreases each dependent variable; thus all causal hypotheses are directional. Huang, Chang, and Lai (2016) conducted a quasi-experimental study to determine the effects of music and exercise on insomnia in older adults. One of the hypotheses examined in this study was that "Participants who perform brisk walking exercise combined with music in the evening for two nights exhibit higher sleep quality scores than no-exercise baseline scores" (Huang et al., 2016, p.105). The hypothesis might be diagrammed as follows:

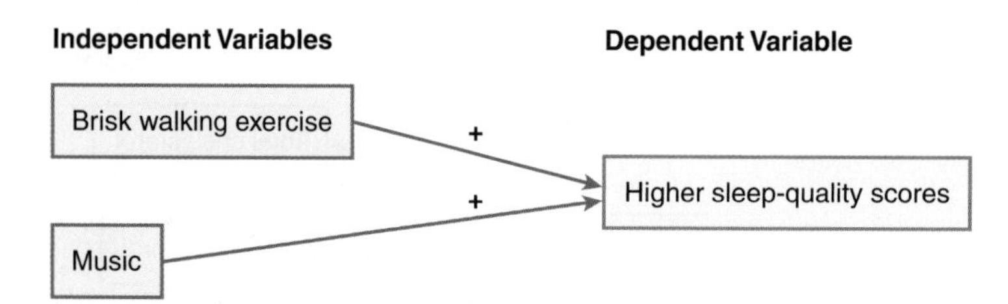

This causal hypothesis (as indicated by the *arrows*) is complex (three variables), directional (higher sleep scores), and positive (exercise and music increase sleep scores). The results of this

study were statistically significant, supporting this hypothesis that exercise and music interventions did improve the quality of aging adults' sleep scores.

Statistical versus research hypotheses. Hypotheses are either research or statistical (see Box 5.2). The statistical hypothesis, also referred to as a null hypothesis (H_0), is used for statistical testing and for interpreting statistical outcomes. Even if the null hypothesis is not stated, it is implied because it is the converse of the research hypothesis (Grove & Cipher, 2017). Some researchers state the null hypothesis because it is more easily interpreted on the basis of the results of statistical analyses. The null hypothesis is also used when the researchers believes that there is no relationship between two variables and when theoretical or empirical information is inadequate to state a research hypothesis. Null hypotheses can be simple or complex and associative or causal but are always nondirectional because the null hypothesis states there is no relationship between variables or differences between groups. Huang and colleagues (2016, p. 105) stated the following null hypothesis in their study: "Subjective sleep quality scores do not differ between listening to soothing music and performing brisk walking exercise combined with music." The null hypothesis was supported because the "results revealed that both the soothing music and brisk walking exercise combined with music exhibited the same effects on subjective sleep quality" (Huang et al., 2016, p. 107).

A research hypothesis is the alternative hypothesis (H_1 or H_A) to the null or statistical hypothesis and states that a relationship exists between two or more variables. All the hypotheses stated earlier in this chapter have been research hypotheses. Research hypotheses can be simple or complex, nondirectional or directional, and associative or causal.

CRITICAL APPRAISAL GUIDELINES

Hypotheses in Studies

1. Are the hypotheses formally stated in the study? If the study is quasi-experimental or experimental, hypotheses are needed to direct the study.
2. Do the hypotheses clearly identify the relationships among the variables of the study?
3. Are the hypotheses associative or causal, simple or complex, directional or nondirectional, and research or null (statistical; see Box 5.2)?
4. If hypotheses are included in a study, are they used to organize research results and interpret study findings?

The study by Ruiz-González and colleagues' (2016), introduced earlier, focused on the effects of a DEP on biomedical and psychosocial variables in adults with type 1 diabetes. These researchers developed causal hypotheses to direct the conduct of their study, presented in Research Example 5.5.

RESEARCH EXAMPLE 5.5

Hypothesis

Research Study Excerpt

The following hypotheses were developed: (1) after the DEP patients will have lower levels of HbA1c, greater theoretical and practical knowledge about diabetes, fewer barriers, higher frequency of self-care, and greater self-efficacy; (2) these changes will remain stable at six-month and one-year follow-up; (3) after the DEP patients will show improvements in biomedical measures, particularly in cardiovascular risk factors, such as cholesterol (total and LDL) and body mass index. (Ruiz-González et al., 2016, p. 14)

Continued

RESEARCH EXAMPLE 5-5—cont'd

Critical Appraisal

Ruiz-González and colleagues (2016) stated causal hypotheses, which are appropriate for quasi-experimental research that examines the effects of an intervention on selected dependent variables. The study included three complex, causal, and directional research hypotheses. Hypotheses 1 and 3 were clearly stated and identified the DEP intervention and the specific psychosocial variables (knowledge of diabetes, barriers, self-care, and self-efficacy) and biomedical variables (HbA1c, total cholesterol, LDL, and BMI) that were measured. These two hypotheses were diagrammed earlier in this section and clarify the relationships between the independent and dependent variables. Hypothesis 2 focused on the prediction of the relationships among the variables over time (6 months and a year). The results section of the article was focused on the study variables and did not clearly address whether the hypotheses were supported or not.

Testable Hypothesis

The value of a hypothesis ultimately is derived from whether it is testable in the real world. A **testable hypothesis** is one that clearly predicts the relationships among variables and contains variables that are measurable or able to be manipulated in a study. The independent variable must be clearly defined, often by a protocol, so that it can be implemented precisely and consistently as an intervention in a study. The dependent variable must be clearly defined to indicate how it will be precisely and accurately measured (see the next section on defining study variables).

A testable hypothesis also needs to predict a relationship that can be "supported" or "not supported," as indicated by the data collected and analyzed. If the hypothesis states an associative relationship, correlational analyses are conducted on the data to determine the existence, type, and strength of the relationship between the variables studied. The hypothesis that states a causal link between the independent and dependent variables is evaluated using statistical analyses, such as the *t*-test or analysis of variance (ANOVA), that examine differences between the means of the dependent variables for the experimental and comparison or control groups (Grove & Cipher, 2017; see Chapter 11). It is the statistical or null hypothesis (stated or implied) that is tested to determine whether the independent variable produced a significant effect on the dependent variable.

Hypotheses are clearer without specifying the presence or absence of a significant difference because determination of the level of significance is only a statistical technique applied to sample data. In addition, hypotheses should not identify methodological points, such as techniques of sampling, measurement, and data analysis (Grove & Cipher, 2017). Therefore such phrases as *measured by*, *in a random sample of*, and *using ANOVA* are inappropriate because they limit the hypothesis to the measurement methods, sample, or analysis techniques identified for one study. In addition, hypotheses need to reflect the variables and population outlined in the research purpose.

In summary, the research objectives, questions, and hypotheses must be clearly focused and concisely expressed in studies. Both objectives and questions are used in qualitative studies and descriptive and correlational quantitative studies, but questions are more common. Some correlational studies focus on predicting relationships and may include hypotheses. Quasi-experimental and experimental studies should be directed by hypotheses.

UNDERSTANDING STUDY VARIABLES AND RESEARCH CONCEPTS

The research purpose and objectives, questions, and hypotheses include the variables or concepts to be examined in a study. **Variables** are qualities, properties, or characteristics of persons, things, or situations that change or vary. Variables should be concisely defined to promote their measurement or manipulation in quantitative or outcomes studies (Chinn & Kramer, 2015; Waltz et al., 2017). Research concepts are usually studied in qualitative research, are at higher levels of abstraction than variables, and are not manipulated in studies (Creswell & Poth, 2018). In this section, different types of variables are described, and conceptual and operational definitions of variables are discussed. The research concepts investigated in qualitative research are also discussed.

Types of Variables in Quantitative Research

Variables are classified into a variety of types to explain their use in research. Some variables are manipulated; others are controlled. Some variables are identified but not measured; others are measured with refined measurement devices. The types of variables presented in this section include research, independent, dependent, and extraneous variables (Gray et al., 2017; Waltz et al., 2017).

Research Variables

Descriptive and correlational quantitative studies involve the investigation of research variables. **Research variables** are the qualities, properties, or characteristics identified in the research purpose and objectives or questions that are measured in a study. Research variables are included in a study when the intent is to observe or measure variables as they exist in a natural setting, without the implementation of a treatment. Thus no independent variables are manipulated, and no cause and effect relationships are examined. Buet and associates (2013) described the research variables of HH opportunities and HH adherence for clinical caregivers (e.g., nurses, physicians) and non-clinical caregivers (e.g., parents, teachers) in pediatric extended-care facilities (see Table 5.1 for the study problem and purpose).

Independent and Dependent Variables

The relationship between independent and dependent variables is the basis for formulating hypotheses for correlational, quasi-experimental, and experimental studies. In predictive correlational studies, the variables measured to predict a single dependent variable are called *independent variables* (Grove & Cipher, 2017). For example, McKee and colleagues (2016) conducted a predictive correlational study to determine if the independent variables of parents' misperceptions of their child's weight status (healthy, overweight, obese), parents' weight status as either overweight or obese, and the age of child were used to predict the likelihood of childhood obesity (dependent variable). The hypotheses from this study were presented earlier and were supported by the study results.

The term **independent variable** is more frequently used to identify an intervention that is manipulated or varied by the researcher to create an effect on the dependent variable. The independent variable is also called an intervention, treatment, or experimental variable. A **dependent variable** is the outcome that the researcher wants to predict or explain. Changes in the dependent variable are presumed to be caused by the independent variable. Strohfus and colleagues (2017) conducted a study to examine the effects of peer-to-peer immunization education and training on health personnel's knowledge and the immunization rates in their medical offices. These researchers stated the following null hypothesis: "there would be no significant increase and retention of knowledge, and no increased immunization rates after the education was provided" (p. 132). The independent variable was the immunization education and training that was implemented to determine its effects on 113 health personnel's knowledge and the immunization rates in 28 medical offices. Strohfus et al. (2017, p. 133) found that "overall knowledge increased by 7.8% (n = 113) 12-months post education," and the immunization rates increased significantly in the medical offices.

Extraneous Variables

Extraneous variables exist in all studies and can affect the measurement of study variables and the relationships among these variables. Extraneous variables are of primary concern in quantitative studies examining the effects of interventions because they can interfere with obtaining a clear understanding of the relational or causal dynamics within these studies. These variables are classified as recognized or unrecognized and controlled or uncontrolled. Some extraneous variables are not recognized until the study is in progress or has been completed, but their presence influences the study outcome.

Researchers attempt to recognize and control as many extraneous variables as possible in quasi-experimental and experimental studies, and specific designs, intervention protocols, and sample criteria have been developed to control the influence of extraneous variables that might influence the outcomes of these studies. Ruiz-González et al. (2016, p. 14) selected a quasi-experimental design "where every single participant is subjected to every single treatment (including control)… The fact that subjects act as their own control provides a way of reducing the amount of error arising from natural variance between individuals." The sample exclusion criteria ensured that individuals with physical and psychological impairments were not included in the study, reducing additional potential for error. The scales used to measure knowledge of diabetes, self-care behaviors, barriers, and self-efficacy were presented in detail. However, the intervention (DEP) lacked detail in the article; having a protocol that was evidence-based for the intervention would have reduced the potential for error. The processes for measuring the biomedical variables (total cholesterol, LDL, and BMI) lacked description.

The extraneous variables that are not recognized until the study is in process, or are recognized before the study is initiated but cannot be controlled, are referred to as confounding variables. Sometimes, extraneous variables can be measured during the study and controlled statistically during analysis. However, extraneous variables that cannot be controlled or measured are a design weakness and can hinder the interpretation of findings (see Chapter 8). As control in correlational, quasi-experimental, and experimental studies decreases, the potential influence of confounding variables increases.

Environmental variables are a type of extraneous variable that compose the setting in which the study is conducted. Examples of these variables include climate, family, healthcare system, and governmental organizations. If a researcher is studying people in an uncontrolled or natural setting, it is impossible and undesirable to control all the extraneous variables. In qualitative and some quantitative studies (descriptive and correlational), little or no attempt is made to control extraneous variables. The intent is to study participants in their natural environment, without controlling or altering that setting or situation (Creswell, 2014; Creswell & Poth, 2018). The environmental variables in quasi-experimental and experimental research can be controlled by using a laboratory setting or a specially constructed research unit in a hospital.

Environmental control is an extremely important part of conducting an experimental study. For example, Kaya and colleagues (2017) conducted an experimental study in a neurosurgical ICU, which is a highly controlled clinical setting (see Table 5.1). The controlled setting, structured intervention of oral care with glutamine, and detailed measurement of VAP decreased the potential impact of extraneous variables on the study outcomes.

Conceptual and Operational Definitions of Variables in Quantitative Research

A variable is described in a study by the development of conceptual and operational definitions. A conceptual definition provides the theoretical meaning of a variable (Chinn & Kramer, 2015) and is often derived from a theorist's definition of a related concept. In a published study, the framework

TABLE 5.3 LINKING CONCEPTS TO VARIABLES AND IDENTIFYING TYPES OF VARIABLES

CONCEPT	VARIABLE	TYPE OF VARIABLE
Diabetes education	Diabetes education program	Independent
Psychosocial measures	Theoretical knowledge diabetes	Dependent
	Practical knowledge diabetes	Dependent
	Barriers	Dependent
	Self-care	Dependent
	Self-efficacy	Dependent
Biomedical measures	Hemoglobin A1c	Dependent
	Total cholesterol	Dependent
	Low density lipoprotein	Dependent
	Body mass index	Dependent

Data from Ruiz-González, I., Fernández-Alcántara, M., Guardia-Archilla, T., Rodríquez-Morales, S., Molina, A., Casares, D. et al. (2016). Long-term effects of an intensive-practical diabetes education program on HbA1c and self-care. *Applied Nursing Research, 31*(1), 13-18.

includes concepts and their definitions, and the variables are selected to represent these concepts (see Chapter 7 for more details). The variables are conceptually defined, indicating the link with the concepts in the framework. An **operational definition** is derived from a set of procedures or progressive acts that a researcher performs to receive sensory impressions (e.g., sound, visual, tactile impressions) that indicate the existence or degree of existence of a variable (Waltz et al., 2017). Operational definitions need to be independent of time and setting so that variables can be investigated at different times and in different settings using the same operational definitions. An operational definition is developed so that a variable can be measured or manipulated in a concrete situation; the knowledge gained from studying the variable will increase the understanding of the theoretical concepts that this variable represents.

Table 5.3 includes the concepts and variables from the study by Ruiz-González et al. (2016) of the effects of the DEP on the management of type 1 diabetes. Reading across the table, you see the link of each concept to the variable(s), and the type of variable is identified. The conceptual and operational definitions for the independent variable DEP and one of the dependent variables, HbA1c, are presented in Research Example 5.6. The guidelines identified in the following box were used to critically appraise the variables and their definitions in this study.

CRITICAL APPRAISAL GUIDELINES

Study Variables

1. Are the variables clearly identified in the study purpose and/or research objectives, questions, or hypotheses?
2. What types of variables are examined in the study? Are independent and dependent variables or research variables examined in the study?
3. If a quasi-experimental or experimental study is conducted, are the extraneous variables identified and controlled?
4. Are the variables conceptually defined?
5. Are the variables clearly operationally defined?

RESEARCH EXAMPLE 5.6

Conceptual and Operational Definitions of Variables

Independent Variable: Diabetes Education Program (DEP)

Conceptual Definition

The DEP was based on the study framework concept of therapeutic education implemented to "help patients develop skills to conduct behaviors leading to better health-related parameters and quality of life" (Ruiz-González et al., 2016, p. 13). The DEP included evidence-based coaching strategies designed to improve intermediate and long-term outcomes for individuals with type 1 diabetes (Steinsbekk et al., 2012).

Operational Definition

The DEP "sessions included a theoretical part, devoted to teaching the topics that are considered essential in the education of patients with diabetes (illness, diet, exercise, insulin and hypoglycemia, self-analysis, self-management, macro and microvascular complications). Also the sessions include a practical part, in which patients put their skills into practice (e.g., self-monitoring and self-care, insulin injections, carbohydrate counting)" (Ruiz-González et al., 2016, p. 15).

Dependent Variable: Hemoglobin (HbA1c)

Conceptual Definition

HbA1c is a biomedical measure of an individual's success in managing their type 1 diabetes (Ruiz-González et al., 2016).

Operational Definition

HbA1c is a laboratory value that reflects the average blood sugar reading for a patient over 90 days.

Critical Appraisal

These independent and dependent variables were clearly identified in the research purpose and hypotheses stated earlier. The conceptual definitions for the DEP and HbA1c were based on the study concepts (see Table 5.3). The operational definitions for the variables were found in the methods section of the research report. The conceptual definitions for DEP and HbA1c were strong, but the operational definitions might have included more detail to direct the implementation of the DEP intervention and the measurement process for HgA1c in the study.

Research Concepts Investigated in Qualitative Research

The variables in quasi-experimental and experimental research are narrow and specific in focus and can be quantified (converted to numbers) or manipulated using specified steps that are often developed into a protocol. In addition, the variables are objectively defined to decrease researcher bias, as indicated in the previous section. Qualitative research is more abstract, subjective, and holistic than quantitative research and involves the investigation of research concepts versus research variables. Research concepts include the ideas, experiences, situations, events, or cultures that are investigated in qualitative research. For example, Gorlin and colleagues (2016) conducted a qualitative study to explore the phenomenon of living with severe childhood autism. The problem and purpose for this phenomenological study are presented in Table 5.2, and the following research question directed the study: "What is the lived experience of the family living with a child who has severe autism?" (Gorlin et al., 2016, p. 582). The research concept explored was "experiences of living with severe autism" as perceived by the family. In many qualitative studies, the focus of the study is to define or describe the concept(s) being studied (Creswell & Poth, 2018). In this study, the concept of living with severe autism illuminated the extensive hardships and challenges for families and identified their needed resources (Gorlin et al., 2016). More details on the research concepts studied in qualitative research can be found in Chapter 3.

Demographic Variables

Demographic variables are attributes of subjects that are collected to describe the sample. The demographic variables are identified by the researcher when a proposal is developed for conducting a study. Some common demographic variables are age, education, gender, ethnic origin (race), marital status, income, job classification, and medical diagnosis. Once data are collected from the study participants on these demographic variables and analyzed, the results are called demographic or sample characteristics used to describe the sample (see Chapter 9). A study's demographic characteristics can be presented in table format and/or narrative. Gorlin and colleagues (2016) identified the types of family members included in the study in the narrative of their article and presented the demographic characteristics in a table, as seen in Research Example 5.7.

RESEARCH EXAMPLE 5.7

Demographic Characteristics

Research Study Excerpt

Almost half of the mothers (5 out of 11) identified members outside the immediate family and home—such as grandparents, an aunt, or a friend—as part of their family. Participants included: 11 mothers, 4 fathers, 4 grandmothers, 1 aunt, 1 sibling, and 1 friend... Demographics of the 22 individual family participants are described in [Table 4]. (Gorlin et al., 2016, p. 584)

TABLE 4 Demographic Characteristics of Individual Family Participants ($N = 22$)

Variable	Frequency	%
Relationship to Child[a]		
• Mother	11	50
• Father	4	18
• Grandmother	4	18
• Aunt	1	4
• Friend	1	4
• Sibling	1	4
Gender		
• Male	4	18
• Female	18	82
Age Range		
• 20–30	2	9
• 31–40	7	32
• 41–50	7	32
• 51–60	2	9
• 61–75	4	18
Race		
• White European American	15	68
• African American	3	14
• Southeast Asian	1	4
• Multiracial	3	14

Continued

RESEARCH EXAMPLE 5.7—cont'd

TABLE 4 Demographic characteristics of individual family participants (*N* = 22)—cont'd

Variable	Frequency	%
Religion		
• Practicing Christian	12	54
• Nonpracticing Christian	5	23
• No affiliation	3	14
• Agnostic	2	9
Highest Level of Education		
• High school degree	3	14
• 1–2 years of college	8	36
• 4-year college	7	32
• Graduate degree	4	18

[a]Percentage may not equal 100 due to rounding to nearest integer.

Adapted from Gorlin, J. B., McAlpine, C. P., Garwick, A., & Wieling, E. (2016). Severe childhood autism: The family lived experience. *Journal of Pediatric Nursing, 31*(6), 586.

Critical Appraisal

The demographic variables identified in Table 4 included relationship to the child, gender, age range, race, religion, and highest level of education. Data on many of these demographic variables are commonly collected and analyzed to describe study samples. The Gorlin et al. (2016) sample characteristics can be used to compare this sample with the samples from other studies. The researchers clearly identified the 22 study participants and provided a quality description of their demographic characteristics in Table 4.

KEY POINTS

- The research problem is an area of concern in which there is a gap in the knowledge base needed for nursing practice. The problem includes significance, background, and problem statement.
- The research purpose is a concise clear statement of the specific goal or focus of the study.
- A significant problem and purpose identify findings for nursing practice, expand previous research, promote theory development, and/or address current research priorities in nursing.
- Study feasibility is evaluated by examining the researchers' expertise, costs and funding, availability of subjects, facilities, and equipment, and the study's ethical considerations.
- Research objectives, questions, or hypotheses are formulated to bridge the gap between the more abstractly stated research problem and purpose and the detailed quantitative design, results, and interpretation of findings.
- A qualitative study often includes the problem, purpose, and research questions or aims to direct the study.
- A hypothesis is the formal statement of the expected relationship(s) between two or more variables in a specified population in a quantitative study.
- Quasi-experimental and experimental studies should include hypotheses that predicted the potential outcomes for the study.
- Hypotheses can be described using four categories: (1) associative versus causal; (2) simple versus complex; (3) nondirectional versus directional; and (4) statistical versus research.
- Variables are qualities, properties, or characteristics of persons, things, or situations that change or vary.

- Research variables are the qualities, properties, or characteristics that are observed or measured in descriptive and correlational studies.
- An independent variable is an intervention or treatment that is manipulated or varied by the researcher to create an effect on the dependent variable.
- A dependent variable is the outcome that the researcher wants to predict or explain.
- In predictive correlational studies, independent variables are measured to predict a dependent variable.
- A variable is described in a study by developing conceptual and operational definitions.
- A conceptual definition provides the theoretical meaning of a variable and is derived from a theorist's definition of a related concept.
- Operational definitions indicate how a treatment or independent variable will be implemented and how the dependent or outcome variable will be measured.
- Research concepts include the ideas, experiences, situations, events, or behaviors that are investigated in qualitative research.
- Research concepts are defined and described during the conduct of qualitative studies.
- Demographic variables are collected and analyzed to determine demographic or sample characteristics for describing the study subjects or participants.

REFERENCES

Agency for Healthcare Research and Quality (AHRQ). (2016). *About AHRQ: Mission and budget*. Retrieved January 9, 2017, from https://www.ahrq.gov/cpi/about/mission/index.html.

Agency for Healthcare Research and Quality (AHRQ). (2017). *AHRQ research funding priorities and special emphases notices*. Retrieved November 27, 2017, from https://www.ahrq.gov/funding/priorities-contacts/special-emphasis-notices/index.html.

American Association of Critical Care Nurses (AACN). (2017). *AACN's research priority areas*. Retrieved February 12, 2017, from https://www.aacn.org/nursing-excellence/grants/research-priority-areas.

Arslanian-Engoren, C., & Scott, L. D. (2016). Women's perceptions of biases and barriers in their myocardial infarction triage experience. *Heart & Lung, 45*(3), 166–172.

Brown, S. J. (2018). *Evidence-based nursing: The research-practice connection* (4th ed.). Sudbury, MA: Jones & Bartlett.

Buet, A., Cohen, B., Marine, M., Scully, F., Alper, P., Simpser, E., et al. (2013). Hand hygiene opportunities in pediatric extended care facilities. *Journal of Pediatric Nursing, 28*(1), 72–76.

Burns, K. H., Casey, P. H., Lyle, R. E., Bird, T. M., Fussell, J. J., & Robbins, J. M. (2010). Increasing prevalence of medically complex children in U.S. hospitals. *Pediatrics, 126*(4), 638–646.

Centers for Disease Control and Prevention (CDC). (2014). *Prevalence of autism spectrum disorder among children aged 8 years—Autism and developmental disabilities monitoring network, 11 sites, United States, 2010. Morbidity and Mortality Weekly Reports (MMWR)*. Retrieved February 11, 2017, from https://www.cdc.gov/mmwr/pdf/ss/ss6302.pdf.

Charmaz, K. (2014). *Constructing grounded theory* (2nd ed.). Los Angeles, CA: Sage.

Chinn, P. L., & Kramer, M. K. (2015). *Knowledge development in nursing: Theory and process* (9th ed.). St. Louis, MO: Elsevier Mosby.

Creswell, J. W. (2014). *Research design: Qualitative, quantitative, and mixed methods approaches* (4th ed.). Thousand Oaks, CA: Sage.

Creswell, J. W., & Poth, C. N. (2018). *Qualitative inquiry & research design: Choosing among five approaches* (4th ed.). Thousand Oaks, CA: Sage.

de Cordova, P. B., Johansen, M. L., Martinez, M. E., & Cimiotti, J. P. (2017). Emergency department weekend presentation and mortality in patients with acute myocardial infarction. *Nursing Research, 66*(1), 20–27.

Fawcett, J., & Garity, J. (2009). *Evaluating research for evidence-based nursing practice*. Philadelphia, PA: F. A. Davis.

Flacking, R., & Dykes, F. (2017). Perceptions and experiences of using a nipple shield among parents and staff: An ethnographic study in neonatal units. *BMC Pregnancy and Childbirth, 17*(1), 1–8.

Gorlin, J. B., McAlpine, C. P., Garwick, A., & Wieling, E. (2016). Severe childhood autism: The family lived experience. *Journal of Pediatric Nursing, 31*(6), 580–597.

Gray, J. R., Grove, S. K., & Sutherland, S. (2017). *The practice of nursing research: Appraisal, synthesis, and generation of evidence* (8th ed.). St. Louis, MO: Elsevier Saunders.

Grove, S. K., & Cipher, D. J. (2017). *Statistics for nursing research: A workbook for evidence-based practice* (2nd ed.). St. Louis, MO: Elsevier.

Guillaume, D., Crawford, S., & Quigley, P. (2016). Characteristics of the middle-age adult inpatient fall. *Applied Nursing Research, 31*(1), 65–71.

Henson, A., & Jeffrey, C. (2016). Turning a clinical question into nursing research: The benefits of a pilot study. *Renal Society of Australasia Journal, 12*(3), 99–105.

Hernandez, S. H., Morgan, B. J., & Parshall, M. B. (2016). Resilience, stress, stigma, and barriers to mental healthcare in U.S. Air Force nursing personnel. *Nursing Research, 65*(6), 481–486.

Hopkins, D., Lawrence, I., Mansell, P., Thompson, G., Amiel, S., Campbell, M., et al. (2012). Improved biomedical and psychological outcomes 1 year after structured education in flexible insulin therapy for people with type 1 diabetes: The UK DAFNE experience. *Diabetes Care, 35*(8), 1638–1642.

Huang, C., Chang, E., & Lai, H. (2016). Comparing the effects of music and exercise with music for older adults with insomnia. *Applied Nursing Research, 32*(1), 104–110.

Kaya, H., Turan, Y., Tunali, Y., Aydin, G., Yüce, N., Gürbüz, S., & Tosun, K. (2017). Effects of oral care with glutamine in preventing ventilator-associated pneumonia in neurosurgical intensive care unit patients. *Applied Nursing Research, 33*(1), 10–14.

Kim, H., Sefcik, J. S., & Bradway, C. (2017). Characteristics of qualitative descriptive studies; A systematic review. *Research in Nursing & Health, 40*(1), 23–42.

Marshall, C., & Rossman, G. B. (2016). *Designing qualitative research* (6th ed.). Los Angeles, CA: Sage.

McKee, C., Long, L., Southward, L. H., Walker, B., & McCown, J. (2016). The role of parental misperception of child's body weight in childhood obesity. *Journal of Pediatric Nursing, 31*(2), 196–203.

Melnyk, B. M., & Fineout-Overholt, E. (2015). *Evidence-based practice in nursing & healthcare: A guide to best practice* (3rd ed.). Philadelphia, PA: Wolters Kluwer.

Melnyk, B. M., Gallagher-Ford, L., & Fineout-Overholt, E. (2017). *Implementing evidence-based practice competencies in health care*. Indianapolis, IN: Sigma Theta Tau International.

Munhall, P. L. (2012). *Nursing research: A qualitative perspective* (5th ed.). Sudbury, MA: Jones & Bartlett Learning.

National Institute of Nursing Research (NINR). (2016). *The NINR Strategic Plan: Advancing science, improving lives*. Retrieved February 20, 2017, from https://www.ninr.nih.gov/sites/www.ninr.nih.gov/files/NINR_StratPlan2016_reduced.pdf.

National Institute of Nursing Research (NINR). (2017). *About NINR*. Retrieved November 27, 2017, from https://www.ninr.nih.gov/aboutninr.

Quality and Safety Education for Nurses (QSEN). (2017). *QSEN competencies: Pre-licensure knowledge, skills, and attitudes (KSAs)*. Retrieved November 27, 2017, from http://qsen.org/competencies/pre-licensure-ksas/.

Quinn, P. (2016). A grounded theory study of how nurses integrate pregnancy and full-time employment. *Nursing Research, 65*(3), 170–178.

Rogers, B. (1987). Research corner: Is the research project feasible? *American Association of Occupational Health Nurses Journal, 35*(7), 327–328.

Rogers, C., Anderson, S. E., Dollahite, J. S., Hill, T. F., Holloman, C., Miller, C. K., et al. (2017). Methods and design of a 10-week multi-component family meals intervention: A two group quasi-experimental effectiveness trial. *BMC Public Health, 17*(1), 1–15.

Roll, A. E., & Bowers, B. J. (2017). Promoting healthy aging of individuals with developmental disabilities: A qualitative case study. *Western Journal of Nursing Research, 39*(2), 234–251.

Ruiz-González, I., Fernández-Alcántara, M., Guardia-Archilla, T., Rodríquez-Morales, S., Molina, A., Casares, D., et al. (2016). Long-term effects of an intensive-practical diabetes education program on HbA1c and self-care. *Applied Nursing Research, 31*(1), 13–18.

Shadish, W. R., Cook, T. D., & Campbell, D. T. (2002). *Experimental and quasi-experimental designs for generalized causal inference*. Chicago, IL: Rand McNally.

Sherwood, G., & Barnsteiner, J. (2017). *Quality and safety in nursing: A competency approach to improving outcomes* (2nd ed.). Ames, IA: Wiley-Blackwell.

Steinsbekk, A., Rygg, L. O., Lisulo, M., Rise, M. B., & Fretheim, A. (2012). Group based diabetes self-management education compared to routine treatment for people with type 2 diabetes mellitus: A systematic review with meta-analysis. *BMC Health Services Research, 12*, 213. Retrieved January 30, 2018 from http://www.biomedcentral.com/1472-6963/12/213.

Strohfus, P. K., Kim, S. C., Palma, S., Duke, R. A., Remington, R., & Roberts, C. (2017). Immunizations challenge healthcare personnel and affects immunization rates. *Applied Nursing Research, 33*(1), 131–137.

US Department of Health and Human Services (U.S. DHHS). (2017). *Healthy People: 2020 Topics and objectives*. Retrieved January 25, 2017 from https://www.healthypeople.gov/2020/topics-objectives.

US Department of Labor. (2010). *Quick stats of women workers 2010*. Retrieved February 12, 2017 from https://www.dol.gov/wb/factsheets/qs-womenwork2010.htm.

Waltz, C. F., Strickland, O. L., & Lenz, E. R. (2017). *Measurement in nursing and health research* (5th ed.). New York, NY: Springer Publishing Company.

Williams, T., Szekendi, M., & Thomas, S. (2014). An analysis of patient falls and fall prevention programs across academic medical centers. *Journal of Nursing Care Quality, 29*(1), 19–29.

World Health Organization (WHO). (2009). *Guidelines for hand hygiene in health care*. Retrieved February 20, 2017 from http://who.int/gpsc/5may/tools/9789241597906/en.

World Health Organization (WHO). (2017). *About WHO*. Retrieved January 25, 2017 from http://www.who.int/about/en/.

Because of funding changes, the Agency for Healthcare Research and Quality (AHRQ) National Guideline Clearinghouse website was scheduled for decommissioning as of July 16, 2018. For more information, go to https://www.ahrq.gov/.

CHAPTER

6

Understanding and Critically Appraising the Literature Review

Christy J. Bomer-Norton

CHAPTER OVERVIEW

LEARNING OUTCOMES

After completing this chapter, you should be able to:

1. Discuss the purposes of the literature review in quantitative and qualitative research.
2. Critically appraise the literature review section of a published study for current quality sources, relevant content, and synthesis of relevant content.
3. Conduct a computerized search of the literature.
4. Write a literature review from a synthesis of critically appraised literature to promote the use of evidence-based knowledge in nursing practice.

A high-quality review of literature contains the current theoretical and scientific knowledge about a specific topic. The review identifies what is known and unknown about that topic. Nurses in clinical practice review the literature to synthesize the available evidence to find a solution to a problem in practice, or because they want to remain current in their practice. As students and nurses read studies, they must critically appraise the literature review, as well as the other components of the study. Critically appraising a review of the literature begins with understanding the purpose of the literature review in quantitative and qualitative studies and the relative quality of the different types of references that are cited. The critical appraisal guidelines for literature reviews listed in this chapter can be applied to both quantitative and qualitative studies. In addition, example critical appraisals of the literature reviews in both quantitative and qualitative studies are provided.

A **review of literature** is the process of finding relevant research reports and theoretical sources, critically appraising these sources, synthesizing the results, and developing an accurate and complete reference list. As a foundation for this process, this chapter includes information on how to find references, select those that are relevant, organize what you find, and write a logical summary of the findings.

You may be required to review the literature as part of a course assignment or project in the clinical setting, especially projects in Magnet hospitals. Nurses in Magnet hospitals must implement evidence-based practice (EBP), identify problems, and assist with data collection for studies (American Nurses Credentialing Center [ANCC], 2017). Reviewing the literature is a first step in implementing EBP and identifying research problems.

PURPOSE OF THE LITERATURE REVIEW

Literature reviews in published research reports provide the background for the problem studied. Such reviews include: (1) describing the current knowledge of a practice problem; (2) identifying the gaps in this knowledge base; and (3) explaining how the study being reported has contributed to building knowledge in this area. The scope of a literature review must be broad enough to allow the reader to become familiar with the research problem and narrow enough to include only the most relevant sources.

Purpose of the Literature Review in Quantitative Research

The review of literature in quantitative research is conducted to direct the planning and execution of a study. The major literature review is performed at the beginning of the research process (before the study is conducted). A limited review is conducted after the study is completed to identify studies published since the original literature review, especially if it has been 1 year or longer since the study began. Additional articles may be retrieved to find information relevant to interpreting the findings. The results of both reviews are included in the research report. The purpose of the literature review is similar for the different types of quantitative studies—descriptive, correlational, quasi-experimental, and experimental.

Quantitative research reports may include citations to relevant sources in all sections of the report. The researchers include sources in the introduction section to summarize the background and significance of the research problem. Citations about the number of patients affected; cost of treatment; and consequences in terms of human suffering, physical health, disability, and mortality may be included. The review of literature section may not be labeled but may be integrated into the introduction. The review includes theoretical and research references that document current knowledge about the problem studied.

A quantitative researcher develops the framework section of a proposal or article from the theoretical literature and sometimes from research reports, depending on the focus of the study. Similar to the review of literature, the research framework may not be labeled but may be integrated into the introduction, review, or background of a study. A chosen theoretical framework is an organizational tool that places a study within a larger body of knowledge. A study is like a puzzle piece that has a place and context within the larger puzzle (the framework). Theoretical frameworks are described in detail in Chapter 7.

The methods section of the research report describes the design, the sample and the process for obtaining the sample, measurement methods, treatment, data collection process, and a list of the statistical analyses conducted. References may be cited in various parts of the methods section as support for the appropriateness of the methods used in the study. The results section includes the results of the statistical analyses, but also includes sources to validate the analytical techniques that were used to address the research questions or hypotheses (Grove & Cipher, 2017). Sources might also be included to compare the analysis of the data in the present study with the results of previous studies. The discussion section of the research report provides a comparison of the findings with other studies' findings, if not already included in the results section. The discussion section also incorporates conclusions that are a synthesis of the findings from previous research and those from the present study.

Purpose of the Literature Review in Qualitative Research

In qualitative research reports, the introduction will be similar to the same section in the quantitative study report because the researchers document the background and significance of the research problem. Researchers often include citations to support the need to study the selected topic (Creswell & Poth, 2018). However, additional review of the literature may not be cited for two reasons. One reason is that qualitative studies are often conducted on topics about which we know very little, so little literature is available to review. The other reason is that some qualitative researchers deliberately do not review the literature deeply before conducting the study; because they do not want their expectations about the topic to bias their data collection, data analysis, and findings (Munhall, 2012). This is consistent with the expectation that qualitative researchers remain open to the perspectives of the participants. In the methods, results, and discussion sections, qualitative researchers will incorporate literature to support the use of specific methods and place the findings in the context of what is already known.

The purpose, extent, and timing of the literature review vary across the different qualitative approaches (Gray, Grove, & Sutherland, 2017). Phenomenologists are among those who are likely to delay literature review until after data collection and initial analysis have been completed (Munhall, 2012). These researchers will review the literature in the later stages of the analysis and as they interpret the findings in the larger context of theoretical and empirical knowledge. Grounded theory researchers include a minimal review of relevant studies at the beginning of the research process. This review is merely a means of making the researcher aware of what studies have been conducted and that a research problem exists (Corbin & Strauss, 2008), but the information from these studies is not used to direct data collection or theory development for the current study (Walls, Pahoo, & Fleming, 2010). The researcher uses the literature primarily to explain, support, and extend the theory generated in the study (Charmaz, 2014).

The review of literature in ethnographic research is similar to that in quantitative research. In early ethnographies of unexplored groups of people in distant locations, culture-specific literature was not available to review before data collection. Theoretical and philosophical literature, however, was available and continues to be used to provide a framework or perspective through which researchers approach data collection. The research problem for an ethnography study is based on a review of the literature that identifies how little is known about the culture of interest (Creswell & Poth, 2018). The review also informs the research process by providing a general understanding of the cultural characteristics to be examined. For example, the literature review for an ethnography of nursing in Uganda would reveal that the healthcare system has referral hospitals, district hospitals, and health centers. With this information, the researcher might decide to develop a data collection plan to observe nurses in each setting, or the researcher might decide to narrow the ethnography to health centers. Another example would be the ethnographer studying health behaviors of Burmese refugees in a specific neighborhood. From the literature, the researcher has learned that older community members are highly respected and, as a result, the researcher would seek support of older refugees to facilitate access to others in the community. Ethnographers return to the literature during analysis and interpretation of the data to expand the readers' understanding of the culture.

Researchers using the exploratory-descriptive qualitative approach may be conducting the study because they have reviewed the literature and found that little knowledge is available. Exploratory-descriptive qualitative researchers want to understand a situation or practice problem better so that solutions can be identified (Gray et al., 2017). Chapter 3 contains additional information about literature reviews in qualitative studies.

SOURCES INCLUDED IN A LITERATURE REVIEW

The **literature** is all written sources relevant to the topic that you have selected, including articles published in periodicals or journals, Internet publications, monographs, encyclopedias, conference papers, theses, dissertations, textbooks, and other books. Websites and reports developed by relevant and reliable government agencies, intergovernmental organizations, and professional organizations may also be included. Each source reviewed by the author and used to write the review is cited. A **citation** is the act of quoting a source, paraphrasing content from a source, using it as an example, or presenting it as support for a position taken. Each citation should have a corresponding reference in the reference list. The **reference** is documentation of the origin of the cited quote or paraphrased idea and provides enough information for the reader to locate the original material. This information is typically the original author's name, year, and title of publication and, when necessary, periodical or monograph title, volume, pages, and other location information as required by standard style writing manuals. The style developed by the American Psychological Association (APA, 2010) is commonly used in nursing education programs and journals. More information about APA style is provided later in this chapter.

Types of Publications

An **article** is a paper about a specific topic and may be published together with other articles on similar themes in journals (periodicals), encyclopedias, or edited books. As part of an edited book, articles may be called chapters. A **periodical** such as a journal is published over time and is numbered sequentially for the years published. This sequential numbering is seen in the year, volume, issue, and page numbering of a journal. A **monograph,** such as a book on a specific subject, a record of conference proceedings, or a pamphlet, is usually a one-time publication. Periodicals and monographs are available in a variety of media, including online and in print. An **encyclopedia** is an authoritative compilation of information on alphabetized topics that may provide background information and lead to other sources, but is rarely cited in academic papers and publications. Some online encyclopedias are electronic publications that have undergone the same level of review as published encyclopedias. Other online encyclopedias, such as Wikipedia, are in an open, editable format and, as a result, the credibility of the information is variable. Using Wikipedia as a professional source is controversial (Luyt, Ally, Low, & Ismail, 2010; Younger, 2010). When you are writing a review of the literature, Wikipedia may provide ideas for other sources that you may want to find, but check with your faculty about whether Wikipedia or any other encyclopedia may be cited for course assignments.

Major professional organizations may publish papers selected by a review process that were presented at their conference, called **conference proceedings**. These publications may be in print or online. Conference proceedings may include the findings of pilot studies and preliminary findings of ongoing studies. A **thesis** is a report of a research project completed by a postgraduate student as part of the requirements for a master's degree. A **dissertation** is a report of an extensive, sometimes original, research project that is completed as the final requirement for a doctoral degree. Theses and dissertations can be cited in a literature review. In some cases, an article may be published based on the student's thesis or dissertation.

Academic journals are periodicals that include research reports and nonresearch articles related to a specific academic discipline and/or research methodology. **Clinical journals** are periodicals that include research reports and nonresearch articles about practice problems and professional issues in a specific discipline. Table 6.1 includes examples of academic and clinical nursing journals that publish a substantial amount of nursing research.

TABLE 6.1 SOME NURSING JOURNALS THAT PUBLISH A SUBSTANTIAL AMOUNT OF RESEARCH

NUMBERS OF RESEARCH ARTICLES	ACADEMIC JOURNALS	CLINICAL JOURNALS
20 to 40 articles annually	*Clinical Nursing Research* *Journal of Research in Nursing* *Research in Nursing & Health*	*American Journal of Maternal Child Nursing*
40 to 60 articles annually	*Nursing Research* *Western Journal of Nursing Research* *Journal of Nursing Scholarship*	*Heart & Lung* *The Journal of Acute and Critical Care* *Journal of Psychiatric and Mental Health Nursing* *Archives of Psychiatric Nursing*
More than 60 articles annually	*International Journal of Nursing Studies* *Applied Nursing Research*	*Journal of Pediatric Nursing*

Adapted from Gray, J. R., Grove, S. K., & Sutherland, S. (2017). *The practice of nursing research: Appraisal, synthesis, and generation of evidence* (8th ed.). St. Louis, MO: Elsevier Saunders, p. 81.

You are familiar with **textbooks** as a source of information for academic courses. Other books on theories, methods, and events may also be cited in a literature review. To evaluate the quality of a book, consider the qualifications of the author related to the topic, and review the evidence that the author provides to support the book's premises and conclusions. With textbooks and other books, chapters in an edited book might have been written by different people, which are cited differently than the book as a whole (addressed later in this chapter). This is important to note when checking citations and writing your own literature reviews.

Electronic access to articles and books has increased dramatically, making many types of published literature more widely available. In addition, **websites** are an easily accessible source of information. However, not all websites are valid and appropriate for citation in a literature review. Websites may contain information that is not scientifically sound or is biased by commercial interest. For example, the website of a pharmaceutical company that sells diuretic medications may not be an appropriate source for hypertension treatment statistics. In contrast, websites prepared and sponsored by government agencies such as the Centers for Disease Control and Prevention, intergovernmental organizations such as the World Health Organization, and professional organizations such as the American Nurses Association are considered appropriate references to cite.

Content of Publications

References cited in literature reviews contain two main types of content, theoretical and empirical. **Theoretical literature** includes concept analyses, models, theories, and conceptual frameworks that support a selected research problem and purpose. Theoretical sources can be found in books, periodicals, and monographs. Nursing theorists have written books to describe the development and content of their theories. Other books contain summaries of several theories. In a published study, theoretical and conceptual sources are described and summarized to reflect the current understanding of the research problem and provide a basis for the research framework.

Empirical literature in a literature review section of an article refers to knowledge derived from research. In other words, the knowledge is based on data from research (data-based). **Data-based literature** consists of reports of research and published studies found in journals, on the Internet, or in books; and unpublished studies, such as master's theses and doctoral dissertations.

Quality of Sources

Most references cited in quality literature reviews are primary sources that are peer-reviewed. A **primary source** is written by the person who originated or is responsible for generating the ideas published. A research report written by the researchers who conducted the study is a primary source. A theorist's development of a theory or other conceptual content is a primary source. A **secondary source** summarizes or quotes content from primary sources. Authors of secondary sources paraphrase the works of researchers and theorists and present their interpretation of what was written by the primary author. As a result, information in secondary sources may be misinterpretations of the primary authors' thoughts. Secondary sources are used only if primary sources cannot be located, or the secondary source provides creative ideas or a unique organization of information not found in a primary source. **Peer-reviewed** means that the author of the research report, clinical description, or theoretical explanation submitted a manuscript to a publication editor, who identified scholars familiar with the topic to review the manuscript. These scholars provide input to the editor about whether the manuscript in its current form is accurate, meets standards for quality, and is appropriate for the journal. A peer-reviewed paper has undergone significant scrutiny and its content is considered trustworthy.

Quality literature reviews include relevant and current sources. **Relevant studies** are those with a direct bearing on the problem of concern. **Current sources** are those published within 5 years before publication of the manuscript. Sources cited should be comprehensive as well as current. Some problems have been studied for decades, and the literature review often includes seminal and landmark studies that were conducted years ago. **Seminal studies** are the first studies on a particular topic that signaled the beginning of a new way of thinking on the topic and sometimes are referred to as classic studies. **Landmark studies** are significant research projects that have generated knowledge that influences a discipline and sometimes society as a whole. Such studies frequently are replicated or serve as the basis for the generation of additional studies. Some authors may describe a landmark study as being a groundbreaking study. Thus citing a few older studies significant to the development of knowledge on the topic being reviewed is appropriate. Most publications cited, however, should be current. **Replication studies** are reproductions or repetitions of a study that researchers conducted to determine whether the findings of the original study could be found consistently in different settings and with different study participants. Replication studies are important to build the evidence for practice. A replication study that supports the findings of the original study increases the credibility of the findings and strengthens the evidence for practice. A replication that does not support the original study findings raises questions about the credibility of the findings.

Syntheses of research studies, another type of data-based literature, may be cited in literature reviews. A research synthesis may be a systematic review of the literature, meta-analysis of quantitative studies, meta-synthesis of qualitative studies, or a mixed-methods systematic review. These publications are valued for their rigor and contributions to EBP (see Chapters 1 and 13).

CRITICALLY APPRAISING LITERATURE REVIEWS

Appraising the literature review of a published study involves examining the quality of the content and sources presented. A correctly prepared literature review includes what is known and not known about the study problem and identifies the focus of the present study. As a result, the review provides a basis for the study purpose and may be organized according to the variables (quantitative) or concepts (qualitative) in the purpose statement. The sources cited must be relevant and current for the problem and purpose of the study. The reviewer must locate and review the sources or respective abstracts to determine whether these sources are relevant. To judge whether all the relevant sources are cited, the reviewer must search the literature to determine the relevant sources. This is very time-consuming and usually is not done for appraising an article. However, you can review the reference list and determine the focus of the sources, the number of data-based and theoretical sources cited, and where and when the sources were published. Sources should be current, up to the date when the paper was accepted for publication. Most articles indicate when they were accepted for publication on the first page of the study.

Although the purpose of the literature review for a quantitative study is different from the purpose of the literature review for a qualitative study, the guidelines for critically appraising the literature review of quantitative and qualitative studies are the same. However, because the purposes of literature reviews are different, the type of sources and the extent of the literature cited may vary.

CRITICAL APPRAISAL GUIDELINES

Literature Reviews

1. Quality sources
   - Are most references from peer-reviewed sources (Aveyard, 2014)?
   - Are most references primary sources?
   - Do the authors justify citing references that are not peer-reviewed, primary sources?
2. Current sources
   - Are the references current (number and percentage of sources published in the last 10 years and in the last 5 years)?
   - Are references older than 10 years landmark, seminal, or replication studies?
   - Are references older than 10 years cited to support measurement methods or theoretical content?
3. Relevant content
   - Is the content directly related to the study concepts or variables?
   - Are the types of sources and disciplines of the source authors appropriate for the study concepts or variables?
4. Synthesis of relevant content
   - Are the studies critically appraised and synthesized (Aveyard, 2014; Fawcett & Garity, 2009; Gray et al., 2017; Hart, 2009; Machi & McEvoy, 2016)?
   - Is a clear concise summary presented of the current empirical and theoretical knowledge in the area of the study, including identifying what is known and not known (Machi & McEvoy, 2016; O'Mathuna & Fineout-Overholt, 2015)?
   - Does the study address a gap in the literature identified in the literature review?

Critical Appraisal of a Literature Review in a Quantitative Study

Moscou-Jackson, Allen, Kozachik, et al. (2016, p. 38) conducted a cross-sectional analysis of a prospective cohort study (see Chapter 8 for designs) "to (1) describe the prevalence of insomnia symptoms and (2) identify biopsychosocial predictors in community-dwelling adults with SCD [sickle cell disease]." The section entitled "Background" is critically appraised as an example of a literature review in a quantitative study. In addition to the references included in the review of the literature, these authors cited references throughout the research report. All the cited references are considered in the critical appraisal, except the unpublished scale by Sanders-Phillips and Harrell (n.d.). Because the source was undated, its currency could not be assessed.

The citations for the (Moscou-Jackson, Allen, Kozachik, et al., 2016) quantitative study and the background literature section are presented in Research Example 6.1.

RESEARCH EXAMPLE 6.1

Literature Review: Quantitative

Research Study Excerpt

Background: *An estimated 90,000 to 100,000 people in the United States are reported to have sickle cell disease (SCD), a serious genetic disorder resulting from an abnormal hemoglobin gene, HbS (National Heart Lung and Blood Institute, 2015)...*

Two known predictors of sleep disturbances in patients with SCD include depression (Palermo & Kiska, 2005; Wallen et al., 2014) and pain (Valrie et al., 2007; Wallen et al., 2014)... In addition, disease severity and disease activity are consistently identified across studies as risk factors for sleep problems among chronic disease populations (Chandrasekhara, Jayachandran, Rajasekhar, Thomas, & Narisimulu, 2009; Frech et al., 2011; [Martínez-Lapiscina, Erro, Ayuso, & Jericó], 2012).

While a few studies have investigated sleep disturbances in adults with SCD (Sogutlu et al., 2011; Wallen et al., 2014), no studies to date have systematically investigated insomnia symptoms in this population. (Moscou-Jackson, Allen, Kozachik, et al., 2016)

Critical Appraisal

1. Quality Sources

Quality sources were chosen by Moscou-Jackson, Allen, Kozachik, et al. (2016) for their literature review. They cited 46 references in their research report, the majority of which were original research and primary sources. In the references, 39 (85%) were from academic or clinical journals, all of which were peer reviewed. References not from journals were obtained from credible sources, such as a federal agency, the National Institutes of Health, Heart, the Lung and Blood Institute, or the American Psychiatric Association. The accuracy of cited references is very important; a few citation errors were noted in the text and in the reference list of Moscou-Jackson, Allen, Kozachik, et al. (2016). Corrections are noted in brackets.

2. Current Sources

As noted, the unpublished scale by Sanders-Phillips and Harrell (n.d.) was undated; therefore it could not be assessed for currency. The other 45 cited references were appraised for currency. One reference, Moscou-Jackson, Allen, Smith, and Haywood (2016) with the date labeled at "in press" in the reference list was not published at the time of the Moscou-Jackson, Allen, Kozachik, et al. (2016) article, but the publication date of 2016 was verified and the reference is included in the appraisal. Of the references, 34 (76%) were published in the past 10 years (in or since 2006) and 21 (47%) were published in the past 5 years (in or since 2011). Measurement tool references were among the 11 references older than 10 years that Moscou-Jackson, Allen, Kozachik, et al. (2016) cited and were appropriate for inclusion.

3. Relevant Content

Moscou-Jackson, Allen, Kozachik, et al. (2016) included references directly related to the study variables, including SCD, sleep, pain, and depression. References to support the reliability, validity, and scoring of the instruments used to measure insomnia, pain, depression, and life stress were included. The journals cited were from a broad array of disciplines appropriate for the research topic including nursing, medicine, public health, behavioral science, and interdisciplinary sources. The Theory of Unpleasant Symptoms developed by Lenz, Pugh, Milligan, Gift, & Suppe (1997) was used as the framework for the study and was the only theoretical source cited.

4. Synthesis of Relevant Content

In their review, Moscou-Jackson, Allen, Kozachik, et al. (2016) focused their discussion on the relevance of the references to the study variables rather than on the strengths of those references. The review could have been strengthened by critical appraisal of the studies included in the review. The review provided a logical argument supporting the study methodology and the purpose of the study. The logical argument, along with the quality and relevance of the sources, are strengths of the review.

Continued

RESEARCH EXAMPLE 6.1—cont'd

The first paragraph of the review provided a brief background on the physiology of SCD and the numbers of individuals affected by SCD in the United States. This information provided context for the entire review. Literature reviews often start with the background and significance of the problem to highlight the negative impact of the specific problem and the potential value of the research. In the second paragraph of the review, Moscou-Jackson, Allen, Kozachik, et al. (2016) provided evidence of sleep issues among those with SCD.

Moscou-Jackson, Allen, Kozachik, et al. (2016) synthesized information on the identified predictors of sleep issues among those with SCD and provided two references for each of the predictors. They also synthesized information and noted that "disease severity and disease activity are consistently identified across studies as risk factors for sleep problems among chronic disease populations" (Moscou-Jackson, Allen, Kozachik, et al., 2016, p. 39). Researchers often synthesize information on what is known in a similar population to justify the use of a variable in their current study when information on that variable is unavailable in their population of patients with SCD.

The researchers provided a clear synthesis of the information known and unknown about SCD and sleep issues. Moscou-Jackson, Allen, Kozachik, et al. (2016, p. 39) clearly identified a gap in the literature: "While a few studies have investigated sleep disturbances in adults with SCD (Sogutlu et al., 2011; Wallen et al., 2014), no studies to date have systematically investigated insomnia symptoms in this population." The purpose of the study was to address this gap in the literature. Often, in a review of literature, as seen in the article by Moscou-Jackson, Allen, Kozachik, et al. (2016), the gap in literature is presented just before the purpose of the study as justification for the current study.

Moscou-Jackson, Allen, Kozachik, et al. (2016, p. 38) found "a slight majority (55%) of the sample reported clinically significant insomnia symptomatology... While insomnia symptoms were associated with a number of biopsychosocial characteristics, depressive symptoms and acute pain were the only independent predictors." These researchers recommended that adults affected by SCD be assessed for insomnia and treated as needed. Recognition and referral for pain and depression should also be a focus of care.

Critical Appraisal of a Literature Review in a Qualitative Study

The grounded theory study conducted by Koehn, Ebright, and Draucker (2016) is presented as an example of critical appraisal of a qualitative study literature review. The research report of their study of "licensed nurses' decision-making with regard to reporting medical errors" (p. 566) does not have a section titled "Literature Review." Koehn et al. (2016) cited references primarily in the introduction, as well as the discussion and recommendations sections. The "Introduction" section and references are used as an example for a critical appraisal of a literature review in a qualitative study (pp. 566–567). The key literature review content for the Koehn et al. (2016) study is presented in Research Example 6.2.

RESEARCH EXAMPLE 6.2

Literature Review: Qualitative

Research Study Excerpt

A 2000 Institute of Medicine (IOM) report To Err Is Human *provided estimates of the number of medical errors that occur nationwide and concluded that 44,000 to 98,000 patients die annually as a result of preventable medical errors (Kohn, Corrigan, & Donaldson, 2000)... Accurate counts of deaths or injuries attributed to medical errors are hard to obtain due to variations in legal, cultural, and administrative approaches to reporting errors (Anderson, Kodate, Walters, & Dodds, 2013; Loeb & O'Leary, 2004)... In many institutions, the work-place culture regarding error reporting remains one of blame, and nurses are often concerned about personal repercussions associated with reporting errors (Blair, Kable, Courtney-Pratt, & Doran, [2016]; Castel, Ginsburg, Zaheer, & Tamin, 2015; Cook et al., 2004; Espin et al., 2006; Jeffe et al., 2004; Stratton, Blegen, Pepper, & Vaughn, 2004; Taylor et al., 2004; Uribe et al., 2002)... A better understanding of nurses' decision-making regarding error reporting and workplace factors that influence their decisions can inform the frequency and accuracy of error reporting by nurses.* (Koehn et al., 2016, p. 566)

Critical Appraisal

1. Quality Sources

Koehn and associates (2016) chose quality sources for their literature review. They cited 67 references in their research report, most of them primary sources of original research. A total of 53 (79%) of references were from academic or clinical journals, all of which were peer reviewed. For example, the following reference was among those cited by Koehn and colleagues (2016):

Prang, I., and Jelsness-Jørgensen, L. (2014). Should I report? A qualitative study of barriers to incident reporting among nurses working in nursing homes. *Geriatric Nursing, 35*(6), 441–447.

Prang and Jelsness-Jørgensen (2014) conducted this qualitative study; therefore the reference is a primary source. The clinical journal *Geriatric Nursing* was confirmed to be a peer-reviewed journal by accessing the journal's website at https://www.journals.elsevier.com/geriatric-nursing (Geriatric Nursing, 2017).

2. Current Sources

Koehn and associates (2016) cited 67 references. Of these sources, 52 (78%) were published 10 years before this study (in or since 2006), and 32 (48%) were published 5 years before this study (in or since 2011). Because qualitative researchers often study topics that have limited research, it is not uncommon for the literature cited to be older references. The oldest reference, Glaser and Strauss (1967), is a classic theoretical source cited in the methods section.

3. Relevant Content

Koehn and colleagues (2016) selected references directly related to the study concepts, including medical errors, medication errors, safety, interruptions, and reporting. The authors and journals cited were mainly from the disciplines of nursing and medicine.

4. Synthesis of Relevant Content

Koehn et al. (2016) provided a robust review of literature, especially for a qualitative study. They did not critically appraise the strengths and weaknesses of the cited studies, which is a weakness of this review.

The first paragraph provided background and significance of the problem, including estimates of the numbers of medical errors and resultant deaths. In subsequent paragraphs, Koehn et al. (2016) continued to describe issues related to medical errors and provided justification for the study. They synthesized challenges in measuring the rates and outcomes of medical errors precisely. Improvements in the number of medical errors have not been seen, despite the interventions developed to reduce errors. Multiple sources have indicated that error reporting still results in blame for nurses who fear for their future when reporting errors.

In the last paragraph, Koehn and colleagues (2016, p. 567) stated the gap in the literature somewhat implicitly; "A better understanding of nurses' decision-making regarding error reporting and workplace factors that influence their decisions can inform the frequency and accuracy of error reporting by nurses." The purpose of their study addressed this gap and was provided directly after it.

Koehn and colleagues' (2016) study resulted in a theory that described the process before, during, and after an error occurred. "The model included five stages: Being Off Kilter, Living the Error, Reporting or Telling About the Error, Living the Aftermath, and Lurking in Your Mind" (p. 566). They recommended "initiatives to improve error reporting and to support nurses who have made errors" (Koehn et al., 2016, p. 566).

REVIEWING THE LITERATURE

Reviewing the literature is a frequent expectation in nursing education programs. Students may be overwhelmed and intimidated by this expectation, concerns that can be overcome with information and a checklist of steps to follow in the process. The steps of the literature review (Box 6.1) are discussed; these provide an outline for the rest of the chapter. In addition, this section will include common student questions, with answers.

Preparing to Review the Literature

Preparation before a complex task can give structure to the process and increase the efficiency and effectiveness of these efforts. This section provides information about the purpose of a literature review and selecting the databases to be searched (see Box 6.1).

Clarify the Purpose of the Literature Review

Your approach to reviewing the literature will vary, according to the purpose of the review. Reviewing the literature for a course assignment requires a clear understanding of the assignment. These reviews will vary depending on the level of educational program, purpose of the assignment, and expectations of the instructor. Note the acceptable length of the written review of the literature to be submitted. Usually, the focus of course assignment literature reviews will be a summary of information on the selected topic and the implications of the information for clinical practice.

Students repeatedly ask, "How many articles should I have? How far back in years should I go to find relevant information?" The answer to both those questions is an emphatic "It depends." Faculty for undergraduate courses may provide you with guidelines about the number and types of articles you are required to include in an assignment or project. Graduate students are expected to conduct a more extensive review for course papers and research proposals for theses or dissertations. How far back in the literature you need to search depends on the topic. You need to locate

BOX 6.1 STEPS OF THE LITERATURE REVIEW

A. Preparing to review the literature
   1. Clarify the purpose of the literature review.
   2. Select electronic databases and search terms.

B. Conducting the search
   3. Search the selected databases.
   4. Use a table to document the results of your search.
   5. Refine your search.
   6. Review the abstracts to identify relevant studies.
   7. Obtain full-text copies of relevant articles.
   8. Ensure that information needed to cite the source is recorded.

C. Processing the literature
   9. Read the articles.
   10. Appraise, analyze, and synthesize the literature.

D. Writing the review of the literature
   11. Develop an outline to organize information from the review.
   12. Write each section of the review.
   13. Create the reference list.
   14. Check the review and the reference list.

the seminal and landmark studies and other relevant sources in the field of interest. A librarian or course faculty member may be able to assist you in determining the range of years to search for a specific topic.

Another reason you may be conducting a review of the literature is to examine the strength of the evidence and synthesize the evidence related to a practice problem. EBP guidelines are developed through the synthesis of the literature on the clinical problem. The purpose of this type of literature review is to identify all studies that included a particular intervention, critically appraise the quality of each study, synthesize the studies, and draw conclusions about the effectiveness of a particular intervention. When available, replication studies, systematic reviews, meta-analyses, meta-syntheses, and mixed-methods systematic reviews are important publications to include. It is also important to locate and include previous evidence-based papers that examined the evidence of a particular intervention because the conclusions of these authors are highly relevant. Other types of literature syntheses related to promoting evidence-based nursing practice are described in Chapter 13.

Select Electronic Databases and Search Terms

Because electronic access to the literature is so readily available, reviewing the literature can be overwhelming. General search engines such as Google, Google Scholar, or Yahoo will identify scholarly publications, but may include sources that are not reliable. Sources obtained from a general search engine should be assessed for quality, such as evidence of peer review. Additionally, the sources you identify from a general search engine may not be the most current. To find current literature, learn to use computerized **bibliographic databases,** such as The Cumulative Index to Nursing and Allied Health Literature (CINAHL) and Science Direct. These are valuable tools to easily search for relevant empirical or theoretical literature, but different databases contain citations for articles from different disciplines. Table 6.2 includes electronic databases valuable for nursing literature reviews. Depending on the focus of your review, you will be able to select relevant databases to search.

Searching professional electronic databases has many advantages, but one challenge is that you will have to select relevant sources from a much larger number of articles. You can narrow the number of articles and retrieve fewer but relevant articles by using keywords to search. **Keywords** are terms that serve as labels for publications on a topic. For example, a quasi-experimental study focused on providing text message reminders to patients living with heart failure who are taking five or more medications might be found by searching for keywords, such as electronic communication, instant messaging, medication adherence, patient teaching, quasi-experimental designs, and heart failure. When you find one article on your topic, look under the abstract to determine whether the search terms are listed. Using search terms or keywords to search is a skill you can teach yourself, but also remember that a librarian is an information specialist. Consulting a librarian may save you time and make searching more effective.

Conducting the Literature Review

Search the Selected Databases

The actual search of the databases may be the easiest step of the process. One method of decreasing search time is to search multiple databases simultaneously, an approach that is possible when several databases are available within a search engine, such as the Elton B. Stephens Company host (EBSCOhost). To avoid duplicating your work, keep a list of searches that you have completed. This is especially important if you have limited time and will be searching in several short sessions, instead of one long one.

TABLE 6.2 DATABASES FREQUENTLY USED FOR NURSING LITERATURE REVIEWS

NAME OF DATABASE	DATABASE CONTENT
Cumulative Index to Nursing and Allied Health Literature (CINAHL)	Nursing and allied health journals that publish clinical, theoretical, and research articles, including many full-text articles
Google Scholar	Broad-based academic writing, including articles from many disciplines
MEDLINE	Biomedical journals relevant to healthcare professionals deemed reputable by the National Library of Medicine; includes abstracts with links to some full-text sources
PubMed	Free access to MEDLINE available to patients and other consumers
PsycARTICLES	Journals published by the American Psychological Association (APA) and affiliated organizations
Academic Search Complete	Multidisciplinary databases, including articles from many disciplines
Health Source: Nursing/Academic Edition	Journals published for physicians, nurses, and other healthcare professionals, includes many full-text articles and medication education materials for patients
Psychological and Behavioral Sciences Collection	Psychiatry, psychology, and behavioral health journals

Use a Table or Other Method to Document the Results of Your Search

A very simple way to document your search is to use a table. On the table, you will record the search terms, time frame you used, and the results. With most electronic databases, you can sign up for an account and keep your search history online. Reference management software, such as RefWorks (http://www.refworks.com) and EndNotes (http://www.endnote.com), can make tracking the references you have obtained through your searches considerably easier. You can use reference management software to conduct searches and store the information on all search fields for each reference obtained in a search. Within the software, you can store articles in folders with other similar articles. For example, you may have a folder for theory sources, another for methodological sources, and a third for relevant research topics. As you read the articles, you can also insert comments into the reference file about each one. By exporting search results from the bibliographic database to your reference management software, all the needed citation information and abstract are readily available to you electronically when you write the literature review.

Refine Your Search

A search may identify thousands of references, many more than you can read and include in any literature review. Open a few articles that were identified, and see what key terms were used. Reconsider the topic and determine how you can narrow your search. One strategy is to decrease the range of years you are searching. Some electronic databases allow you to limit the search to certain types of articles, such as scholarly, peer-reviewed articles. Combining terms or searching for the terms only in the abstracts will decrease the number of articles identified. For undergraduate course assignments, it may be appropriate to limit the search to only full-text articles. The recommendation would be, however, that graduate students avoid limiting searches to full-text articles because doing so might result in missing sources that are needed. Narrowing a search tightly, you can end up with too few results. When that occurs, you can retry the search with one or more search terms and limitations removed.

Review the Abstracts to Identify Relevant Studies

The abstract provides pertinent information about the article. You can easily determine if the article is a research report, description of a clinical problem, or theoretical article, such as a concept analysis. You will identify the articles that seem to be the most relevant to your topic and the purpose of the review. If looking for evidence on which to base clinical practice, you can identify the research reports and select those conducted in settings similar to yours. If writing a literature review for a course assignment, you will review the abstracts to identify different types of information. For example, you may need information on mortality and morbidity, as well as descriptions of available treatments. Mark the abstracts of the relevant studies or save them in an electronic folder.

Obtain Full-Text Copies of Relevant Articles

Using the abstracts of relevant articles, you will retrieve and save the electronic files of full-text articles on your computer to review more thoroughly. You may want to rename the electronic file using a file name that includes the first author's last name and the year or a file name with a descriptive phrase. For articles not available as full-text online, you can search your library's holdings to determine if the journal is available to you in print form. If your library does not have the journal, you may be able to obtain the article through interlibrary loan. Check with your library's website or a librarian to learn the process for using the interlibrary loan system. If you prefer reading print materials to electronic materials, you may choose to print the articles. It is important to obtain the full-text of the article because the abstract does not include the details needed for a literature review.

Ensure That Information Needed to Cite the Source Is Recorded

As you retrieve and save the articles, note if the article includes all the information needed for the citation. The bibliographic information on a source should be recorded in a systematic manner, according to the format that you will use in the reference list. The purpose for carefully citing sources is that readers can retrieve the reference for themselves, confirm your interpretation of the findings, and gather additional information on the topic. For each reference, you will need the authors' names, year, article title, journal name, journal volume and issue number, and page numbers. If a book chapter has been photocopied or retrieved electronically, ensure that the publisher's name, location, and year of publication are recorded. Notice specifically whether the chapter is in an edited book and if the chapter has an author other than the editor. If you are using electronic personal bibliographic software such as RefWorks, the software records the citation information for you.

Processing the Literature

Processing the literature is among the more difficult phases of the literature review. This section includes reading the articles and appraising, analyzing, and synthesizing the literature.

Read the Articles

As you look at the stack of printed articles or scan the electronic copies of several articles, you may be asking yourself, "Am I expected to read every word of the available sources?" The answer is no. Reading every word of every source would result in you being well read and knowledgeable, but with no time left to prepare the course assignment or paper. With the availability of full-text online articles, you can easily forget the focus of the review. Becoming a skilled reviewer of the literature involves finding a balance and learning to identify the most pertinent and relevant sources. On the other hand, you cannot critically appraise and synthesize what you have not read. Skim over information provided by the author that is not relevant to your task. Learn what is normally included in different sections of an article so you can read the sections pertinent to your task more carefully. Chapter 2 provides ideas on how to read the literature.

Comprehending and critically appraising sources leads to an understanding of the current state of knowledge related to a research problem. Although you may skim or only read selected sections of some references that you find, you will want to read the articles that are most relevant to your topic word for word and probably more than once. **Comprehending a source** begins by reading and focusing on understanding the main points of the article or other sources. Highlight the content that you consider important or make notes in the margins. Record your notes on photocopies or electronic files of articles. The type of information you highlight or note in the margins of a source depends on the type of study or source. With theory articles, you might make note of concepts, definitions, and relationships among the concepts. For a research article, the research problem, purpose, framework, major variables, study design, sample size, measurement methods, data collection, analysis techniques, results, and findings are usually highlighted. You may wish to record quotes (including page numbers) that might be used in a review of a literature section. The decision to paraphrase these quotes can be made later. Also, make notes about what you think about the article, such as how this content fits with other information that you have read.

Appraise, Analyze, and Synthesize the Literature

Analysis is required to determine the value of a reference as you make the decision about what information to include in the review. First, you need to appraise the individual studies critically (see Chapter 12). To critically appraise a study, you need to identify relevant content in the articles and make value judgments about the validity or credibility of the findings. However, the critical appraisal of individual studies is only the first step in developing an adequate review of the literature.

Analysis requires manipulation of what you are finding, literally making it your own (Garrard, 2011). Pinch (1995, 2001) was the first nurse to publish a strategy to synthesize research findings using a literature summary table. Other examples of literature summary tables are provided in Tables 6.3 and 6.4, which show how the column headers might vary, depending on the type of research. Table 6.3 contains key information from the Moscou-Jackson, Allen, Kozachik, et al. (2016) quantitative study as an example. The content in Table 6.4 is from the Koehn et al. (2016) qualitative study. If using reference management software, it may allow you to generate summary tables from information you record about each study.

Another way to manipulate the information you have retrieved and transform it into knowledge is known as *mapping* (Hart, 2009; Machi & McEvoy, 2016). Your nursing faculty may have taught you how to map what you are studying conceptually to make connections between facts and principles (Vacek, 2009). The same strategy can be applied to a literature review to classify the sources by key concepts and arrange them into a graphic or diagrammatic format (Hart, 2009; Machi & McEvoy, 2016). The map may connect studies with similar methodologies or key ideas.

As you continue to analyze the literature you have found, you will make comparisons among the studies. Look for connections, similarities, and themes in the literature. This analysis allows you to appraise the existing body of knowledge critically in relation to the research problem. You may want to record the theories and methods that have been used to study the problem and any flaws with these theories and methods. You will begin to work toward summarizing what you have found by describing what is known and not known about the problem. The information gathered by using

TABLE 6.3 LITERATURE SUMMARY TABLE FOR QUANTITATIVE STUDIES

AUTHOR, YEAR	PURPOSE	FRAMEWORK	SAMPLE	MEASURES	TREATMENT	RESULTS
Moscou-Jackson, Allen, Kozachik, et al. (2016)	"...to (1) describe the prevalence of insomnia symptoms and (2) identify biopsychosocial predictors in community-dwelling adults with SCD [sickle cell disease]." (p 38)	Lenz et al.'s Theory of Unpleasant symptoms	"263 African American adults with SCD" (p. 39)	Demographic data Insomnia Severity index (ISI) 10-item Center for Epidemiologic Studies in Depression (CESD) scale 21-item Urban Life Stress Scale (ULSS) "Do you have daily chronic pain?" Brief Pain Inventory (BPI), SCD genotype (p. 40)	None Nonexperimental	"...a slight majority (55%) of the sample reported clinically significant insomnia symptomatology... While insomnia symptoms were associated with a number of biopsychosocial characteristics, depressive symptoms and acute pain were the only independent predictors (p. 38)"

TABLE 6.4 LITERATURE SUMMARY TABLE FOR QUALITATIVE STUDIES

AUTHOR, YEAR	PURPOSE	QUALITATIVE APPROACH	SAMPLE	DATA COLLECTION	KEY FINDINGS	COMMENTS
Koehn et al. (2016)	"Explored licensed nurses' decision-making with regard to reporting medical errors" (p.566)	Grounded theory	"Thirty nurses from adult intensive care units" (p.566)	Interviews	"The model included five stages: Being Off Kilter, Living the Error, Reporting or Telling About the Error, Living the Aftermath, and Lurking in Your Mind" (p.566)	Support needed for "initiatives to improve error reporting and to support nurses who have made errors" (p.566)

the table formats shown in Tables 6.3 and 6.4 or displayed in a conceptual map can be useful in making these comparisons. Pay special attention to conflicting findings and recommendations for future research because they may provide clues for gaps in knowledge that represent researchable problems.

The synthesis of sources involves thinking deeply about what you have found and identifying the main themes of information that you want to present. Through synthesis, you will cluster and describe connections among what you have found (Hart, 2009). From the clusters of connections, you can begin to draw some conclusions about what is known, and you can make additional connections to the topic being examined. Any written literature review that simply appraises individual studies paragraph by paragraph is inadequate. A literature review that is a series of paragraphs, in which each paragraph is a description of a single study, with no link to other studies being reviewed, does not provide evidence of adequate analysis or synthesis of the literature (Aveyard, 2014).

Note the paragraphs in the Moscou-Jackson, Allen, Kozachik, and colleagues' (2016) review of the literature. They synthesized what is known and unknown by integrating similar findings from sources rather than providing unlinked individual article summaries. The linked information provided justification for the study. They synthesized information from two articles on the significance of studying depression as a predictor in this population. Similarly, two references were cited for pain as a predictor of sleep issues. Their synthesis of potential factors related to sleep among those with SCD drew insight from qualitative research and studies in a similar population of chronic disease, which highlights two important commonly used strategies by researchers when little is known about potential influential factors.

One strategy for synthesizing is to review the tables or conceptual maps that you have developed and make a list of findings that are similar and those that are different. For example, you have read five intervention studies of end-of-life care in children with leukemia. As you review your notes, you notice that four studies were conducted in home settings with samples of children from ages 7 to 10 years and had similar statistically significant results when using a parent-administered intervention. The remaining study, with nonsignificant results, also used a parent-administered intervention, but was set in an inpatient hospice unit and had a sample of younger children. The main ideas that you identify may be that the effectiveness of parent-administered interventions can vary, depending on the setting and age of the child. Another strategy for synthesis is to talk about the articles you have reviewed with another student, nurse, or friend. Verbalizing the characteristics of the studies and explaining them to another person can cause you to think differently about the studies than when you are just reading your notes. Your enhanced thinking may result in the identification of main ideas or conclusions of the review.

Writing the Review of the Literature

Talking about the main ideas of the review can prepare you for the final steps of writing the literature review. Step 11 is organizing your information by developing an outline before writing the major sections of the review (see Box 6.1). The final steps are creating the reference list and checking the review and reference list for correctness.

Develop an Outline to Organize the Information From the Review

Before beginning to write your review, develop an outline based on your synthesis of what you have read, using the sections of the review as major headings in the outline. Depending on the purpose of the written literature review, you will determine what the major sections of the paper will be. Frequently, a comprehensive literature review has four major sections: (1) introduction, (2) discussion of theoretical literature, (3) discussion of empirical literature, and (4) summary.

The introduction and summary are standard sections, but the discussion of sources should be organized by the main ideas that you have identified or the concepts of the theoretical framework that you want to include in the review. Under the major headings of the outline, make notes about which sources you want to mention in the different sections of the paper. The introduction will include the focus or purpose of the review and present the organizational structure of the review. In this section, you should make clear what you will and will not be covering.

The discussion section may be divided into theoretical and empirical subsections or divided by the themes of the review findings. A theoretical literature section might include concept analyses, models, theories, or conceptual frameworks relevant to the topic. The empirical section, if it is a separate section, will include the research findings from the studies reviewed. In addition to the synthesis, you want to incorporate the strengths and weaknesses of the overall body of knowledge, rather than a detailed presentation and critical appraisal of each study. In the summary section of the outline, make notes of your conclusions. A **conclusion** is a statement about the state of knowledge in relation to the topic area, which includes what is known and not known about the area.

Write Each Section of the Review

Start each paragraph with a theme sentence that describes the main idea of the paragraph. Present the relevant studies in each paragraph that support the main idea stated in the theme sentence. End each paragraph with a concluding sentence that transitions to the next claim. Each paragraph can be compared with a train with an engine (theme sentence), freight cars connected to each other (sentences with evidence), and caboose (summary sentence linking to next paragraph).

Avoid using direct quotes from an author. Your analysis and synthesis of the sources will allow you to paraphrase the authors' ideas. **Paraphrasing** involves expressing the ideas clearly and in your own words. The meanings of these sources are then connected to the proposed study. If the written review is not clear or cohesive, you may need to look at your notes and sources again to ensure that you have synthesized the literature adequately. The defects of a study or body of knowledge need to be described, but maintain a respectful tone and avoid being highly critical of theorists' or researchers' work.

As you near the end of the review, write the summary as a concise presentation of the current knowledge base for the research problem. The findings from the studies will have been logically presented in the previous sections so that the reader can see how the body of knowledge in the research area evolved. You will also make conclusions about the gaps in the knowledge base. You need to conclude with the potential contribution of the literature review to the body of nursing knowledge (Aveyard, 2014).

Create the Reference List

Many journals and academic institutions use the format developed by the APA (2010). The sixth edition of the *APA Publication Manual* (2010) provides revised guidelines for citing electronic sources, directly quoting from electronic sources, and creating a reference list. The APA standard for direct quotations from a print source is to cite the author, year, and page of the source on which the quote appears. The reference lists in this text are presented in APA format, with two exceptions. We have not included **digital object identifiers** (DOIs). **DOIs** have become standard for the International Standards Organization (http://www.doi.org), but have not yet received universal support. The use of DOIs seems to be gaining in credibility because the DOI "provides a means of persistent identification for managing information on digital networks" (APA, 2010, p. 188). CrossRef is a registration agency for DOIs so that citations can be linked across databases and disciplines (http://www.crossref.org). Also, when available, we have included the number of the issue in which the article appears. APA requires that you include the issue number only when each issue in a volume (year) begins with page one. When the second issue begins its page numbers based on the last page number of the previous issue, APA does not require the issue number.

The sources included in the list of the references are only those that were cited in the paper. Each citation on an APA-style reference list is formatted as a paragraph with a hanging indent, meaning that the first line is at the left margin and subsequent lines are indented (see citation examples below). If you do not know how to format a paragraph this way, search the Help tool in your word processing program to find the correct command to use. The inclusion of an article published in a print journal in a reference list includes the journal number, volume, issue, and pages. For most journals, the numbering of the volumes of the journal represents all the articles published during a specific year. APA (2010) has requirements for formatting each component of the entry in the reference list for a journal article. Table 6.5 presents the components of common references with the correct formatting.

An entry on a reference list for a book is listed by the author and includes the publisher and its location. The University Press, located in Boulder, Colorado, published a revised edition of Dr. Watson's philosophy of nursing care in 2008. The entry on the reference list would be as follows:

Watson, J. (2008). *Nursing. The philosophy and science of caring* (Revised ed.). Boulder, CO: University Press of Colorado.

Some chapters are compiled by editors, with each chapter having its own author(s). The chapter by Wolf on ethnography is in a qualitative research book edited by Munhall (2012). The chapter title is formatted like an article title, and the page numbers of the chapter are included:

Wolf, M. (2012). Ethnography: The method. In P. L. Munhall (Ed.), *Nursing research: A qualitative perspective* (5th ed.) (p. 285–338). Sudbury, MA: Jones & Bartlett.

When you retrieve an electronic source in ***p**ortable **d**ocument **f**ormat* (pdf), you cite the source in the same way as if you had made a copy of the print version of the article. When you retrieve an electronic source in html (***h**yper**t**ext **m**arkup **l**anguage*) format, you will not have page numbers for the citation. Providing the URL (***u**niform **r**esource **l**ocator*) that you used to retrieve the article is not helpful because it is unique to the path you used to find the article and reflects your search

TABLE 6.5 AMERICAN PSYCHOLOGICAL ASSOCIATION FORMATTING OF CITATIONS

REFERENCE COMPONENT	TYPE OF FONT	CAPITALIZATION	EXAMPLE
Article title	Regular font	• First word of title and subtitle • Proper nouns	Grounded theory methods: Similarities and differences. Nursing students' fears of failing the National Council Licensure Examination (NCLEX)
Journal title	Italicized font	• All key words	*Journal of Clinical Information Systems* *Health Promotion Journal*
Book title	Italicized font	• First word of title and subtitle • Proper nouns	*Qualitative methods: Grounded theory expanded* *Human resources for health in Uganda*

engines and bibliographic databases. The updated APA (2010) standard is to provide the URL for the home page of the journal from which the reader can navigate and find the specific article.

Check the Review and the Reference List

You may complete the first draft of your review of the literature and feel a sense of accomplishment. Before you leave the review behind, a few tasks remain that will ensure the quality of your written review. Begin by rereading the review. It is best to delay this step for a day or at least for a few hours to allow you to take a fresh look at the final written product. One way to identify awkward sentences or disjointed paragraphs is to read the review aloud. Ask a fellow student or trusted colleague to read the review and provide constructive feedback.

A critical final step is to compare the sources cited in the paper with the reference list. Be sure that the authors' names and year of publication match. If you are missing sources on the reference list, add them. If you have sources on the reference list that you did not cite, you must remove them. Downloading citations from a database directly into a reference management system and using the system's manuscript formatting functions reduce some errors but do not eliminate all of them. You want your references to be accurate as a reflection of your attention to detail and quality of your work.

KEY POINTS

- The review of literature in a research report is a summary of current knowledge about a particular practice problem and includes what is known and not known about this problem.
- Reviews of the literature in published studies can be critically appraised for current quality sources, relevant content, and synthesis of relevant content (see the critical appraisal guidelines)
- A review of literature may be necessary to complete an assignment for a course or summarize knowledge for use in practice.
- A checklist for reviewing the literature includes preparing, conducting the search, processing the information, and writing the review.
- Electronic databases allow for the identification of a large number of sources quickly, and the use of keywords can refine the search to the most relevant sources.
- Reference management software should be used to track the references obtained through the searches.
- A literature summary table or conceptual map can be used to help you process the information in numerous studies and identify the main ideas.
- A written review of literature should be grammatically correct, with a logical flow and contain a reference list that is accurate and complete.

REFERENCES

American Nurses Credentialing Center. (2017). *Magnet: Program overview*. Silver Springs, MD: Author. Retrieved March 16, 2017, from http://www.nursecredentialing.org/Magnet/ProgramOverview.

American Psychological Association (APA). (2010). *Publication manual of the American Psychological Association* (6th ed.). Washington, D.C.: Author.

Anderson, J. E., Kodate, N., Walters, R., & Dodds, A. (2013). Can incident reporting improve safety? Healthcare practitioners' views of the effectiveness of incident reporting. *International Journal for Quality in Health Care, 25*(2), 141–150.

Aveyard, H. (2014). *Doing a literature review in health and social care: A practical guide* (3rd ed.). Berkshire, Open University Press.

Blair, W., Kable, A., Courtney-Pratt, H., & Doran, E. (2016). Mixed method integrative review exploring nurses' recognition and response to unsafe practice. *Journal of Advanced Nursing, 72*(3), 488–500.

Castel, E. S., Ginsburg, L. R., Zaheer, S., & Tamim, H. (2015). Understanding nurses' and physicians' fear of repercussions for reporting errors: Clinician characteristics, organization demographics, or leadership factors. *BMC Health Services Research, 15*(1), 326.

Chandrasekhara, P. K. S., Jayachandran, N. V., Rajasekhar, L., Thomas, J., & Narsimulu, G. (2009). The prevalence and associations of sleep disturbances in patients with systemic lupus erythematosus. *Modern Rheumatology, 19*(4), 407–415.

Charmaz, K. (2014). *Constructing grounded theory* (2nd ed.). Los Angeles, CA: Sage.

Cook, A. F., Hoas, H., Guttmannova, K., & Joyner, J. C. (2004). An error by any other name. *American Journal of Nursing, 104*(6), 32–43.

Corbin, J., & Strauss, A. (2008). *Basics of qualitative research* (3rd ed.). Thousand Oaks, CA: Sage.

Creswell, J., & Poth, C. N. (2018). *Qualitative inquiry & research design: Choosing among five approaches* (4th ed.). Thousand Oaks, CA: Sage.

Espin, S., Lingard, L., Baker, G. R., & Regehr, G. (2006). Persistence of unsafe practice in everyday work: An exploration of organizational and psychological factors constraining safety in the operating room. *Quality and Safety in Health Care, 15*(3), 165–170.

Fawcett, J., & Garity, J. (2009). *Evaluating research for evidence-based nursing practice*. Philadelphia, PA: F. A. Davis.

Frech, T., Hays, R. D., Maranian, P., Clements, P. J., Furst, D. E., & Khanna, D. (2011). Prevalence and correlates of sleep disturbance in systemic sclerosis—results from the UCLA Scleroderma Quality of Life Study. *Rheumatology, 50*(7), 1280–1287.

Garrard, J. (2011). *Health sciences literature review made easy: The matrix method* (3rd ed.). Sudbury, MA: Jones & Bartlett.

Geriatric Nursing. (2017). *Elsevier: Geriatric Nursing*. Retrieved May 14, 2017 from, https://www.journals.elsevier.com/geriatric-nursing/.

Glaser, B. G., & Strauss, A. L. (1967). *The discovery of grounded theory: Strategies for qualitative theory*. London: Weidenfeld and Nicolson.

Gray, J. R., Grove, S. K., & Sutherland, S. (2017). *The practice of nursing research: Appraisal, synthesis, and generation of evidence* (8th ed.). St. Louis, MO: Elsevier Saunders.

Grove, S. K., & Cipher, D. J. (2017). *Statistics for nursing research: A workbook for evidence-based practice* (2nd ed.). St. Louis, MO: Elsevier.

Hart, C. (2009). *Doing a literature review: Releasing the social science imagination*. Thousand Oaks, CA: Sage.

Jeffe, D. B., Dunagan, W. C., Garbutt, J., Burroughs, T. E., Gallagher, T. H., Hill, P. R., et al. (2004). Using focus groups to understand physicians' and nurses' perspectives on error reporting in hospitals. *Joint Commission Journal on Quality and Safety, 30*(9), 471–479.

Koehn, A. R., Ebright, P. R., & Draucker, C. B. (2016). Nurses' experiences with errors in nursing. *Nursing Outlook, 64*(6), 566–574.

Kohn, L. T., Corrigan, J., & Donaldson, M. S. (2000). *To err is human: Building a safer health system*. Washington, D.C.: National Academy Press.

Lenz, E. R., Pugh, L. C., Milligan, R. A., Gift, A., & Suppe, F. (1997). The middle-range theory of unpleasant symptoms: An update. *Advances in Nursing Science, 19*(3), 14–27.

Loeb, J. M., & O'Leary, D. S. (2004). The fallacy of the body count: Why the interest in patient safety and why now? In B. J. Youngberg & M. J. Hatlie (Eds.), *The patient safety handbook* (p. 779). Sudbury, MA: Jones & Bartlett Learning.

Luyt, B., Ally, Y., Low, N., & Ismail, N. (2010). Librarian perception of Wikipedia: Threats or opportunities for librarianship? *Libri, 60*(1), 57–64.

Machi, L., & McEvoy, B. (2016). *The literature review: Six steps to success* (3rd ed.). Thousand Oaks, CA: Corwin.

Martínez-Lapiscina, E. H., Erro, M. E., Ayuso, T., & Jericó, I. (2012). Myasthenia gravis: Sleep quality, quality of life, and disease severity. *Muscle & Nerve, 46*(2), 174–180.

Moscou-Jackson, G., Allen, J., Kozachik, S., Smith, M. T., Budhathoki, C., Haywood, C., Jr. (2016). Acute pain and depressive symptoms: Independent predictors of insomnia symptoms among adults with sickle cell disease. *Pain Management Nursing, 17*(1), 38–46.

Moscou-Jackson, G., Allen, J., Smith, M. T., Haywood, C., Jr. (2016). Psychometric validation of the Insomnia Severity Index in adults with sickle cell disease. *Journal of Health Care for the Poor and Underserved, 27*(1), 209–218.

Munhall, P. L. (2012). *Nursing research: A qualitative perspective* (5th ed.). Sudbury, MA: Jones & Bartlett.

National Heart Lung and Blood Institute. (2015). *What is sickle cell disease?* Retrieved June 17, 2015, from http://www.nhlbi.nih.gov/health/health-topics/topics/sca.

O'Mathuna, D. P., & Fineout-Overholt, E. (2015). Critically appraising quantitative evidence for clinical decision making. In B. M. Melnyk & E. Fineout-Overholt (Eds.), *Evidence-based practice in nursing & healthcare: A guide to best practice*. (3rd ed.) (pp. 87–138). Philadelphia, PA: Lippincott Williams & Wilkins.

Palermo, T. M., & Kiska, R. (2005). Subjective sleep disturbances in adolescents with chronic pain: Relationship to daily functioning and quality of life. *Journal of Pain*, *6*(3), 201–207.

Pinch, W. J. (1995). Synthesis: Implementing a complex process. *Nurse Educator*, *20*(1), 34–40.

Pinch, W. J. (2001). Improving patient care through use of research. *Orthopaedic Nursing*, *20*(4), 75–81.

Prang, I. W., & Jelsness-Jørgensen, L. P. (2014). Should I report? A qualitative study of barriers to incident reporting among nurses working in nursing homes. *Geriatric Nursing*, *35*(6), 441–447.

Sogutlu, A., Levenson, J. L., McClish, D. K., Rosef, S. D., & Smith, W. R. (2011). Somatic symptom burden in adults with sickle cell disease predicts pain, depression, anxiety, health care utilization, and quality of life: The PiSCES project. *Psychosomatics*, *52*(3), 272–279.

Stratton, K. M., Blegen, M. A., Pepper, G., & Vaughn, T. (2004). Reporting of medication errors by pediatric nurses. *Journal of Pediatric Nursing*, *19*(6), 385–392.

Taylor, J. A., Brownstein, D., Christakis, D. A., Blackburn, S., Strandjord, T. P., Klein, E. J., & Shafii, J. (2004). Use of incident reports by physicians and nurses to document medical errors in pediatric patients. *Pediatrics*, *114*(3), 729–735.

Uribe, C. L., Schweikhart, S. B., Pathak, D. S., Marsh, G. B., & Fraley, R. R. (2002). Perceived barriers to medical-error reporting: An exploratory investigation. *Journal of Healthcare Management*, *47*(4), 263.

Vacek, J. E. (2009). Using a conceptual approach with a concept map of psychosis as an exemplar to promote critical thinking. *Journal of Nursing Education*, *48*(1), 49–53.

Valrie, C. R., Gil, K. M., Redding-Lallinger, R., & Daeschner, C. (2007). Brief report: Sleep in children with sickle cell disease: An analysis of daily diaries utilizing multilevel models. *Journal of Pediatric Psychology*, *32*(7), 857–861.

Wallen, G. R., Minniti, C. P., Krumlauf, M., Eckes, E., Allen, D., Oguhebe, A., et al. (2014). Sleep disturbance, depression and pain in adults with sickle cell disease. *BMC Psychiatry*, *14*(1), 207.

Walls, P., Pahoo, K., & Fleming, P. (2010). The role and place of knowledge and literature in grounded theory. *Nurse Researcher*, *17*(4), 8–17.

Watson, J. (2008). *Nursing. The philosophy and science of caring* (Revised ed.). Boulder, CO: University Press of Colorado.

Wolf, M. (2012). Ethnography: The method. In P. L. Munhall (Ed.), *Nursing research: A qualitative perspective*. (5th ed.) (pp. 285–338). Sudbury, MA: Jones & Bartlett.

Younger, P. (2010). Using wikis as an online health information resource. *Nursing Standard*, *24*(36), 49–56.

Because of funding changes, the Agency for Healthcare Research and Quality (AHRQ) National Guideline Clearinghouse website was scheduled for decommissioning as of July 16, 2018. For more information, go to https://www.ahrq.gov/.

CHAPTER 7

Understanding Theory and Research Frameworks

Jennifer R. Gray

CHAPTER OVERVIEW

LEARNING OUTCOMES

After completing this chapter, you should be able to:

1. Define theory and the elements of theory (concepts, relational statements, and propositions).
2. Distinguish among the levels of theoretical thinking.
3. Describe the use of middle range theories as frameworks for studies.
4. Describe the purpose of a research framework.
5. Identify research frameworks developed from nursing and other theories.
6. Critically appraise the frameworks in published studies.

Theories are the ideas and knowledge of science. In a psychology course, you may have studied theories of the mind, defense mechanisms, and cognitive development that provide explanations of thinking and behavior. Based on the theoretical views of the mind, different therapies were implemented. In nursing, we also have theories that provide explanations and guide our practice. Our theories explain human responses to illness and other phenomena important to clinical practice. For example, nursing has a theory of comfort that goes beyond the relief of pain to include relaxation and personal growth (Kolcaba, 1994; Krinsky, Murillo, & Johnson, 2014). The theory of comfort is a middle range theory. Middle range theories describe a single phenomenon or process and are less abstract than theories that are more comprehensive. Nurses have also developed a middle range theory to describe the behaviors needed to manage one's weight as well as the cultural, environmental, and psychosocial factors that influence those behaviors (Pickett, Peters, & Jarosz, 2014). Another middle range theory in nursing describes the communication between patients and nurses to manage symptoms (Humphreys et al., 2014). Consistent with the continued focus on quality and safety (Olds & Dolansky, 2017; Sherwood & Barnsteiner, 2017), a theory was developed to describe a culture of safety in a hospital (Groves, 2014; Groves, Meisenbach, & Scott-Cawiezell, 2011). These theories and others that will be described in this chapter provide guidance for nurses conducting research and caring for patients in clinical settings.

When a researcher develops a plan for conducting a quantitative study, the theory on which the study is based is described as the framework for the study. A research framework is a brief explanation of a theory or those portions of a theory that are being used to guide a study or that will be tested in a study. The major ideas of the study, called *concepts,* are included in the framework. The framework, with the concepts and their connections to each other, may be described in words or in a diagram. When the study is conducted, the researcher can then answer the question, "Was this theory correct in its description of reality?" Thus researchers can test the accuracy of theoretical ideas proposed in the theory. In explaining the study findings, the researcher will interpret those findings in relation to the theory (Gray, Grove, & Sutherland, 2017).

Qualitative studies may be based on a theory or may be designed to create a theory. Because the assumptions and underlying philosophy of qualitative research (see Chapter 3) are not the same as quantitative research, the focus of this chapter is on the theories used to guide quantitative studies. To assist you in learning about theories and their use in research, the elements of theory are described, types of theories are identified, and how theories provide frameworks for studies are discussed. You may notice that references in this chapter are older because we cited primary sources for the theories, many of which were developed 10 or more years ago. You are also provided with guidelines for critically appraising research frameworks, and these guidelines are applied to a variety of frameworks from published studies.

UNDERSTANDING THE ELEMENTS OF THEORY

A **theory** is defined as a set of concepts and statements that present a view of a phenomenon. The lower portion of Fig. 7.1 is a diagram of a theory's structure. The core ideas that guide practice and research within a scientific discipline are called *theory.* Note that within the definition of theory are the words *concepts, statements,* and *phenomena.* **Concepts** are terms that abstractly describe and name an object, idea, experience, or phenomenon, thus providing it with a separate identity or meaning (Schaffer, Sandau, & Missal, 2017). Concepts are defined in a particular way to present the ideas relevant to a theory (see Fig. 7.1). The **statements** in a theory describe how the concepts are connected to each other. For example, Toulouse and Kodadek (2016, p. 328) stated that adherence to medications "improves clinical outcomes and reduces the development of complications, patient suffering, and healthcare costs." The concepts are adherence to medications, clinical outcomes, complications, patient suffering, and healthcare costs, and the statement indicates the relationships among them.

A concept, a statement, or a theory may be used to describe a **phenomenon,** the conscious awareness of an experience that comprises the lives of humans (van Manen, 2017). The plural form is **phenomena**. You may understand the phenomenon of anxiety as a result of giving your first injections or the elation of learning you have been accepted into nursing school. As nurses, our patients experience pain, uncertainty, fear, and relief, to name a few of the range of patient experiences related to receiving care. We intervene to relieve the stress and anxiety of patient experiences and move them toward better health.

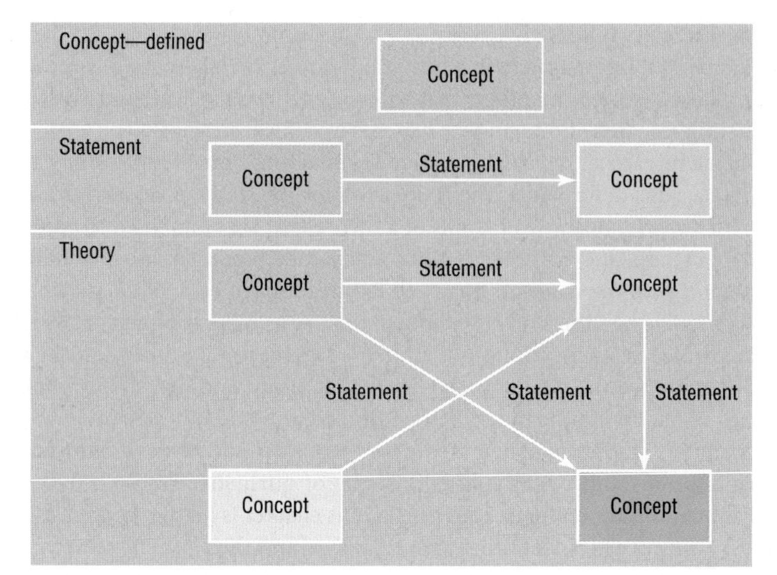

FIG 7.1 Building blocks of theories. (Modified from Gray, J. R., Grove, S. K., & Sutherland, S. [2017]. *Burns and Grove's the practice of nursing research: Appraisal, synthesis, and generation of evidence* [8th ed.]. St. Louis, MO: Elsevier.)

Theory

Theories are abstract, rather than concrete. When you hear the term *social support,* you have an idea about what the phrase means and how you have observed or experienced social support in different situations. The concept of social support is abstract, which means that the concept is the expression of an idea, apart from any specific instance. An **abstract** idea focuses on a general view of a phenomenon. Family social support has been defined by one group of researchers as "an interpersonal process that is centered on the exchange of information… one has the perception or belief of being connected to and feeling loved and esteemed by others" (Gomes et al., 2017, p. 69). **Concrete** refers to realities or actual instances—it focuses on the particular, rather than on the general. For example, in the Gomes et al. (2017) study, social support was facilitated by a telephone intervention to educate and provide emotional support to family caregivers of patients living with diabetes mellitus.

Philosophy

At the abstract level, you may also encounter a philosophy. **Philosophies** are rational intellectual explorations of truths or principles of being, knowledge, or conduct. Philosophies describe viewpoints on what reality is, how knowledge is developed, and which ethical values and principles should guide our practice. Other abstract components of philosophies and theories are **assumptions,** which are statements that are taken for granted or considered true, even though they have not been scientifically tested. For example, a fairly common assumption made by nurses is that "People want to assume control of their own health problems." You may doubt the truth of that assumption, based on your clinical experiences. Nonetheless, theorists begin with some assumptions, explicit or implicit.

Concepts

Nursing's theories describe what is known about person, environment, health, and nursing because these four concepts are the essence of nursing. Person, environment, health, and nursing are known as the metaparadigm concepts of our discipline (Meleis, 2012; Schaffer et al., 2017).

The phenomenon termed *social support* introduced earlier is a concept. A concept is the basic element of a theory. Each concept in a theory needs to be defined by the theorist. The definition of a concept might be detailed and complete, or it might be vague and incomplete and require further development (Chinn & Kramer, 2015). Theories with clearly identified and defined concepts provide a stronger basis for a research framework.

Two terms closely related to concept are *construct* and *variable.* In more abstract theories, concepts have very general meanings that may be a label for a complex idea and are sometimes referred to as constructs. A construct is a broader category or idea that may encompass several concepts. For example, a construct for the concept of social support might be resources. Another concept that is a resource might be household income. At a more concrete level, terms are referred to as variables and are narrow in their definition. Thus a variable is more specific than a concept. The word *variable* implies that the term is defined so that it is measurable and suggests that numerical values of the term are able to vary (are variable) from one instance to another. The levels of abstraction of constructs, concepts, and variables are illustrated with an example in Fig. 7.2. On the *left,* you see a vertical sequence of construct, concept, and variable, with construct being the most abstract and variable being the most concrete. The other two vertical sequences are examples of a construct, concept, and variable.

A variable related to social support might be emotional support. The researchers might define emotional support as a study participant's rating of the extent of emotional encouragement or affirmation that he or she receives during a stressful time. The measurement of the variable is a specific method for assigning numerical values to varying amounts of emotional social support. Study participants could respond to questions on a survey or questionnaire about emotional support, and their individual answers would be reported as scores. For example, the Functional Social Support Questionnaire has a three-item subscale that measures perceived emotional support (Broadhead, Gehlbach, de Gruy, & Kaplan, 1988; Gonzalez-Saenz de Tejada et al., 2016). One of the three items is "People care what happens to me," and the others address whether the respondent feels loved and received praise for doing a good job (Broadhead et al., 1988, p. 722). If researchers used the Functional Social Support Questionnaire in a study, the participant's answers to the three items would be added together as the total score. The total scores on the three questions would be the measurement of the variable of perceived emotional support. (Chapter 10 provides a detailed discussion of measurement methods.)

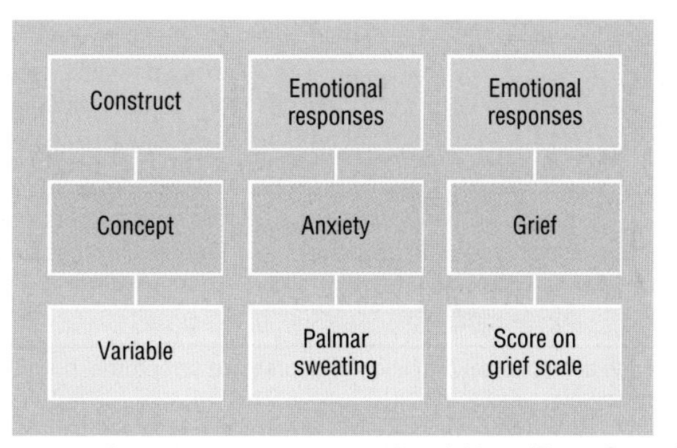

FIG 7.2 Abstract to concrete: Constructs, concepts, and variables. (From Gray, J. R., Grove, S. K., & Sutherland, S. [2017]. *Burns and Grove's the practice of nursing research: Appraisal, synthesis, and generation of evidence* [8th ed.]. St. Louis, MO: Elsevier.)

Defining concepts allows consistency in the way the term is used. Concepts from theories have conceptual definitions that are developed by the theorist and differ from the dictionary definition of a word. A **conceptual definition** is more comprehensive than a denotative (or dictionary) definition and includes associated meanings that the word may have. A conceptual definition is referred to as connotative because the term brings to mind memories, moods, or images, subtly or indirectly. For example, a conceptual definition of home might include feelings of security, love, and comfort, which often are associated with a home, whereas the dictionary definition is narrower and more specific—a home is a dwelling in which a group of people live, who may or may not be related. Some of the words or terms that are used frequently in nursing language have not been clearly defined. Terms used in theory or research need connotative meanings based on professional literature. Connotative definitions are clear statements of the concepts' meaning in the particular theory or study.

The conceptual definition that a researcher identifies or develops for a concept comes from a theory and provides a basis for the operational definition. Remember that in quantitative studies, each variable is ideally associated with a concept, conceptual definition, and operational definition. The operational definition is how the concept can be manipulated, such as an intervention or independent variable, or measured, such as a dependent or outcome variable (see Chapter 5). Conceptual definitions may be explicit or implicit. It is important that you identify the researcher's conceptual definitions of study variables when you critically appraise a study. Coleman (2017) conducted a descriptive correlational study of depression and health-related quality of life of African Americans living with HIV infection ($N = 70$). He identified Wilson and Cleary's (1995) model of health-related quality of life as the study's framework and defined health-related quality of life conceptually and operationally (Table 7.1). Although Coleman (2017) did not conceptually define depressive symptoms, the operational definition of a score of 16 or higher on the Center for Epidemiological Studies Depression scale (see scale in Chapter 10; Radloff, 1977) was explicit.

TABLE 7.1 CONCEPTUAL AND OPERATIONAL DEFINITIONS OF DEPRESSION AND HEALTH-RELATED QUALITY OF LIFE

CONCEPT/VARIABLE	CONCEPTUAL DEFINITION	OPERATIONAL DEFINITION
Health-Related Quality of Life (HRQOL)	"one's ability to function physically and emotionally, and their overall perception of well-being" (Coleman, 2017, p. 139)	Score on the Medical Outcome Study (MOS) 36-Item Short Form Health Survey (SF-36) on a scale of 1–100 (Ware & Sherbourne, 1992) The MOS SF-36 measures "eight health concepts of HRQOL: physical functioning, bodily pain, role limitations, role limitations due to emotional problems, emotional well-being, social functioning, energy/fatigue, and general health" (Coleman, 2017, p. 139).
Depressive Symptoms	Feelings and behaviors associated with negative emotions and sense of hopelessness[a]	Score on the 20-item Center for Epidemiological Studies Depression Scale (Radloff, 1977), a score of 16 or higher indicates depressive symptoms

[a]Coleman (2017) did not state a conceptual definition of depressive symptoms, but the definition in this table was inferred from the study framework.

Based on Coleman, C. (2017). Health-related quality of life and depressive symptoms among seropositive African Americans. *Applied Nursing Research, 33*(1), 138–141.

Statements

A statement clarifies the type of relationship that exists between or among concepts. For example, in the study just mentioned, Coleman (2017) identified several statements among the concepts. One statement was "physical functioning, role limitations, social functioning, general health, and energy fatigue [aspects of HRQOL] were conceptualized to have an impact on depression" (Coleman, 2017, p. 139).

The statements of relationships are what are tested through research. The researcher obtains data for the variables that represent the concepts in the study's framework and analyzes the data for possible significant relationships among the variables using specific statistical tests (Grove & Cipher, 2017). Testing a theory involves determining the truth of each statement in the theory. As more researchers provide evidence about the relationships among concepts, the accuracy or inaccuracy of the statements is determined. Many studies are required to validate all the statements in a theory.

In theories, propositions are a label given to statements describing relationships among concepts. Theories that are more abstract contain relational statements that are called *general propositions* (Gray et al., 2017). Stating a relationship in a more narrow way makes the statement more concrete and testable and results in a specific proposition. Specific propositions in less abstract frameworks (middle range theories) may lead to hypotheses. Hypotheses are developed based on propositions from a grand or middle range theory that comprise the study's framework. Hypotheses, written at a lower level of abstraction, are developed to be tested in a study (see Chapter 5). Statements at varying levels of abstraction that express relationships between or among the same conceptual ideas can be arranged in hierarchical form, from general to specific. Table 7.2 provides examples of relationships between two concepts that are written as general propositions, specific propositions, and hypotheses.

LEVELS OF THEORETICAL THINKING

Theories can be abstract and broad or they can be more concrete and specific. Between abstract and concrete, there are several levels of theoretical thinking. Understanding the degree of abstraction or level of theoretical thinking will help you to critically appraise whether a theory is applicable to the research problem in a study.

TABLE 7.2 **EXAMPLES OF A GENERAL PROPOSITION, SPECIFIC PROPOSITION, AND HYPOTHESIS**

General Proposition	Health-related quality of life is related to depression.
Specific Proposition	Among persons on antiretroviral therapy for HIV infection, domains of health-related quality of life are related to depressive symptoms.
Hypothesis	Among African American persons on antiretroviral therapy for HIV infection, poor physical functioning and increased role limitations are related to increased frequency and severity of depressive symptoms.

Based on Coleman, C. (2017). Health-related quality of life and depressive symptoms among seropositive African Americans. *Applied Nursing Research, 33*(1), 138–141.

Grand Nursing Theories

Early nurse scholars labeled the most abstract theories as **conceptual models** or conceptual frameworks. Today, we refer to the more abstract nursing theories as **grand nursing theories** because they encompass nursing actions and patient responses in multiple settings. For example, Roy (Roy & Andrews, 2008) developed a model in which adaptation was the primary phenomenon of interest to nursing. This model identifies the elements considered essential to adaptation and describes how the elements interact to produce adaptation and thus health. In contrast, Orem (Orem & Taylor, 2011) presents her descriptions of health phenomena in terms of self-care, self-care deficits, and nursing systems. Table 7.3 lists four well-known grand nursing theories, with a brief explanation of their content.

Building a body of knowledge related to a particular grand nursing theory requires an organized program of research and a group of scholars. The Roy Adaptation Model (RAM) has been used as the basis for studies for over 25 years. The Roy Adaptation Association is a group of researchers who "analyze, critique, and synthesize all published studies in English based on the RAM" (Roy, 2011, p. 312). Roy's Adaptation Model continues to be used to guide studies. One example is a pilot study to assess the incidence of acute stress disorder among persons hospitalized following a traumatic injury (Frank, Schroeter, & Shaw, 2017).

The Society of Rogerian Scholars continues to conduct studies and develop knowledge related to Martha Rogers' Science of Unitary Human Beings. The society publishes an online journal called *Visions: The Journal of Rogerian Nursing Science* (http://www.societyofrogerian scholars.org/visions.html). The International Orem Society publishes an issue each year of their online journal, *Self-Care, Dependent-Care, & Nursing*, to disseminate research and clinical applications of Dorothea Orem's theory of self-care. These are examples of researchers who maintain a network to communicate with each other and other nurses about their work with a specific theoretical approach.

TABLE 7.3 SELECTED GRAND NURSING THEORIES

NAME	AUTHOR (YEAR)	BRIEF DESCRIPTION
Adaptation Model	Roy and Andrews (2008)	In response to focal, contextual, and residual stimuli, people adapt by using a variety of processes and systems, some of which are automatic and some of which are learned. The overall goal is to return to homeostasis and promote growth.
Self-Care Deficit Theory of Nursing	Orem (2001) Orem & Taylor (2011)	Individuals' ability to care for themselves is affected by developmental stage, presence of disease, and available resources and may result in a self-care deficit. The goal of nursing is to provide care in proportion to the person's self-care capacity.
Science of Unitary Human Beings	Rogers (1970)	Persons, who are unitary human beings, and the environment around them are energy fields that interact as open systems. The energy fields may produce patterns that can be used for identification.
Theory of Goal Attainment	King (1992)	Within systems, persons are goal-oriented. The nurse and the patient set mutually agreed-upon goals. Through interaction, the nurse educates, supports, and guides the patient toward the goals.

Middle Range and Practice Theories

Middle range theories are less abstract and narrower in scope than grand nursing theories, but are more abstract than theories that apply to only a specific situation (Liehr & Smith, 2017). These types of theories describe experiences such as uncertainty in acute or chronic illness (Mishel, 1988, 1990), self-transcendence over one's life span (Reed, 1991), and unpleasant symptoms (Lenz, Pugh, Milligan, Gift, & Suppe, 1997). Because middle range theories are more closely linked to clinical practice and research than grand nursing theories, nurses providing patient care and nurse researchers find them to be helpful. They may emerge from a grounded theory study, be deduced from a grand nursing theory or may be created through a synthesis of the literature on a particular topic (Liehr & Smith, 2017). Liehr and Smith (2017) identified nine middle range theories about which at least three peer-reviewed articles had been published. Table 7.4 lists these middle range theories. Middle range theories are sometimes called substantive theories because they are closer to the substance of clinical practice. Substantive theories have clearly identified concepts, definitions of concepts, and relational statements. Thus they are more commonly applied as frameworks in nursing studies.

Practice theories are a type of middle range theories that are more specific. They are designed to propose specific approaches to particular nursing practice situations. Some scholars call them *situation-specific theories.* Riegel, Dickson, and Faulkner (2016) published a description of the situation-specific theory of heart failure self-care. Riegel et al. (2016) identified self-care to include taking medications as prescribed, monitoring symptoms, and taking action when a symptom indicates a significant problem. To be able to take these actions, the person with heart failure must undertsand the purpose of each medication, symptoms that indicate worsening heart failure, and when to call the healthcare provider. As seen in this example, applying a middle range theory to a specific situation identifies appropriate nursing actions. For this reason, practice theories are sometimes referred to as prescriptive theories. Evidence-based practice guidelines are a good source for practice and prescriptive theories (see Chapter 13).

TABLE 7.4 MIDDLE RANGE THEORIES FOR NURSING[a]

THEORY	RELEVANT THEORETICAL SOURCES
Caring	Swanson (1991)
Comfort	Kolcaba (1994)
Inner strength	Roux, Dingley, and Bush (2002)
Nursing intellectual capital	Covell (2008)
Self-transcendence	Reed (1991)
Transitions	Meleis (2010)
Uncertainty in illness	Mishel (1988, 1990)
Unpleasant symptoms	Lenz et al. (1997)
Women's anger	Thomas (1991)

[a]Liehr and Smith (2017) identified these nine middle range theories as having ongoing use.

Research Frameworks

A research framework is an abstract and logical structure of meaning, such as a portion of a theory, which guides the development of the study and enables the researcher to link the findings to nursing's body of knowledge (Lor, Backonja, & Lauver, 2017). For clarity, we are using the term *research framework* to refer to the concepts and relationships being addressed in a study. Lor et al. (2017) provided guidance on how theories can be used to guide descriptive and experimental studies. For descriptive studies, researchers can use "concepts from the theory to inform data collection"; researchers conducting experimental studies will find that "concepts from the theory guide overall design" (Lor et al., 2017, p. 4). Perhaps the researcher expects one variable to cause a change in another variable, such as the independent variable of an aerobic exercise program affecting the dependent variable of weight loss. In a well-developed quantitative study, the researcher explains abstractly in the framework why one variable is expected to influence the other. The idea is expressed concretely as a hypothesis to be tested through the study methodology.

Every quantitative study has an implicit or explicit framework. This is true whether the study has a physiological, psychological, social, or cultural focus. A clearly expressed framework is one indication of a well-developed quantitative study. The researcher develops or applies the framework to explain the concepts contributing to or partially causing an outcome. The researcher cites articles and books in support of the explanation.

One strategy for expressing a theory or research framework is a diagram with the concepts and relationships graphically displayed. These diagrams are sometimes called maps or models (Gray et al., 2017). A model includes all the major concepts in a research framework. Arrows between the concepts indicate the proposed linkages between them. Each linkage shown by an arrow is a graphic illustration of a relational statement (proposition) of the theory. Lor et al. (2017) have described how they choose a theory to guide their research and presented a model for the Theory of Care-Seeking Behavior (Fig. 7.3). In the figure, clinical and sociodemographic factors are seen to influence affect, beliefs, norms, and habits. Care-seeking behaviors are affected by clinical and sociodemographic factors and by affect, beliefs, norms, and habit. The relationships between affect, belief, norms, and habits and care-seeking behavior are moderated by external conditions.

Unfortunately, in some quantitative studies, the ideas that compose the framework remain nebulous and are vaguely expressed. Although the researcher believes that the variables being studied

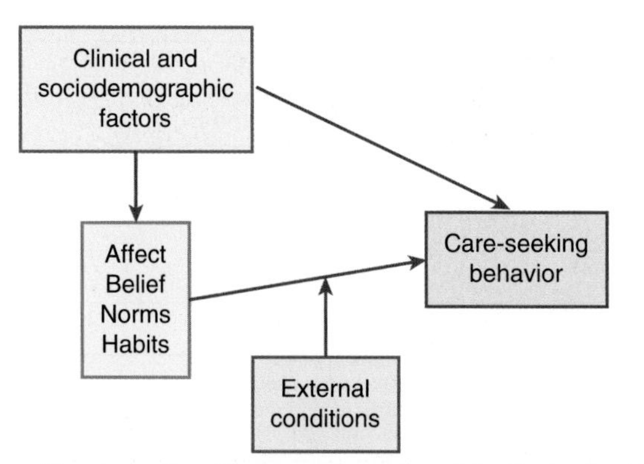

FIG 7.3 Theory of care-seeking behavior. (Redrawn from Lor, M., Backonja, U., & Lauver, D. [2017]. How could nurse researchers apply theory to generate knowledge more efficiently? *Journal of Nursing Scholarship,* 49(5), 580–589.)

are related in some fashion, this notion is expressed only in concrete terms. The researcher may make little attempt to explain why the variables are thought to be related. However, the rudiment of a research framework is the expectation (perhaps not directly expressed) that one or more variables are linked to other variables. Sometimes, basic ideas for the framework are expressed in the introduction or literature review and are described as linkages among variables found in previous studies, but then the researcher stops, without fully developing the ideas as a framework. These are referred to as **implicit frameworks**. In most cases, a careful reader can extract an implicit framework from the text of the research report. When researchers do not clearly describe the framework, you may want to draw a model based on the information provided. Having a model helps you visualize the framework and how the variables in the study are linked. Implicit frameworks provide limited guidance for the development and conduct of a study and limit the contribution of the study findings to nursing knowledge.

Research frameworks can come from grand nursing theories, middle range theories from nursing and other professions, and syntheses of concepts and relationships from more than one theory and syntheses of research findings. In some quantitative studies, the framework that is newly proposed can be called a **tentative theory**. Syntheses of concepts and relationships from more than one theory or syntheses of research findings are also examples of tentative theories that are usually developed for a particular study.

Frameworks for physiological studies are usually derived from physiology, genetics, pathophysiology, and physics. This type of theory is called scientific theory. **Scientific theory** has extensive research evidence to support its claims. Framework concepts are clearly linked to study variables, and valid and reliable methods exist for measuring each concept, related variable, and relational statement in scientific theories. Because the knowledge in these areas has been well tested through research, the theoretical relationships are often referred to as laws and principles. In addition, propositions can be developed and tested using these laws and principles and then applied to nursing problems. However, scientific theories remain open to possible contrary evidence that would require their revision. For example, before this century, scientists believed that they knew the functions and interactions of various genes. The knowledge gained through the Human Genome Project (http://www.genome.gov/10001772) has required that scientists revise some of their theories.

EXAMPLES OF CRITICAL APPRAISAL OF RESEARCH FRAMEWORKS

The quality of a framework in a quantitative study needs to be critically appraised to determine its usefulness for directing the study and interpreting the study findings. The questions that follow have been developed to assist you in evaluating the quality of a study's framework.

CRITICAL APPRAISAL GUIDELINES

Framework of a Study

1. Is a research framework explicitly identified and described in the study? If so, what is the name of the theory and theorist used for the framework?
2. Are the concepts in the framework conceptually defined?
3. Are the operational definitions of the variables consistent with their associated conceptual definitions?
4. Do the researchers clearly identify the relationship statement(s) or proposition(s) from the framework being examined by the study design?
5. Are the study findings linked back to the framework?

Critically appraising a framework of a quantitative study requires that you go beyond the framework itself to examine its linkages to other components of the study, such as the design, measurement of the variables, and implementation of an intervention, if applicable. Begin by identifying the concepts and conceptual definitions from the written text in the introduction, literature review, or discussion of the framework. Then you must judge the adequacy of the linkages of concepts to variables, measurement of research or dependent variables, and implementation of independent variables. You also need to determine if the study findings have been linked back to the research framework. Researchers usually link the findings back to the framework and other literature in the discussion section of the research report. In this section, the critical appraisal guidelines are applied to frameworks that have been derived from a grand nursing theory, middle range theory, tentative theory, and a scientific (physiological) theory.

Framework From a Grand Nursing Theory

One of the challenges with grand nursing theories is their abstractness and difficulty in measuring their concepts. Some researchers have deduced middle range theories from grand nursing theories and used middle range theories to guide their studies. Other researchers have used a grand nursing theory as an overall framework but have not directly linked the variables to the theory constructs.

Behavior modification after an acute myocardial infarction (AMI) is critical to reduce cardiac risk and prevent a reoccurrence. Following an AMI, research findings have been "promising but mixed" related to motivating behavior change to reduce cardiac risks by adapting healthy behaviors. Park, Song, and Jeong (2017) conducted a randomized experimental study to test the effects of a theory-based intervention on outcomes following a first AMI. The intervention was based on a proposition of King's Goal Attainment Theory (King, 1992), one of nursing's grand theories. Park et al. (2017) noted, "the strategies applied to motivate individuals to perform and maintain health behaviors are far from optimal" (Park et al., 2017, p. 9). The researchers made the use of the grand theory explicit in Research Example 7.1.

RESEARCH EXAMPLE 7.1

Grand Nursing Theory as a Framework

Research Study Excerpt

Based on King's framework, goal-oriented strategies can be applied to...ensure effective behavioral modification through the process of interaction, where the patient and the health professional mutually identify the specific cardiovascular risks that the individual has, and agree to pursue the goal of risk management together. Based on the theory of goal attainment, the present study applied a goal-oriented education program to individuals with a first episode of myocardial infarction to evaluate the program effects on cardiovascular risks, health behaviors, and quality of life over 6 months...

The patients who were assigned to the experimental group received the goal-attainment-theory-based education program by a nurse educator from the research team before their discharge to set the mutually agreed goals of risk management and to obtain information on how to modify their health behaviors with the aim of achieving the goals. The patients who were assigned to the control group received the 20-min. formal education on cardiovascular risk management and lifestyle modification by nurse coordinator. This formal education was available as routine care to all patients with AMI admitted to the cardiac units of a university hospital where the study was conducted...

Our findings showed that a nurse-led tailored risk management program with goals being set by each individual has potential for effective cardiovascular risk management through lifestyle modification both initially and over the long term, consequently leading to improvements in the health-related QOL (quality of life)...

Some limitations should be considered when interpreting the findings of this study. First, the participants in both groups received routine lifestyle modification guidance along with aggressive pharmacological treatment after their first episode of AMI. This may have reduced the effect size of the program and, combined with smallness of the sample, would lead to type II error...blinding was not applied during the follow-up assessments due to the features of the education program, leading to the potential bias in assessment. The findings should be considered suggestive, since most of the changes between groups were from self-reported measures... The nurse-led education program with individualized goal-oriented approach can easily be integrated to the current medical treatment system to lead more effective lifestyle modification. (Park et al., 2017, pp. 9, 10–11, 15)

Critical Appraisal

The Theory of Goal Attainment by King (1992) was explicitly identified as the study's framework. The intervention was based on one of King's theoretical propositions that mutually agreed-upon goals developed through interaction will result in behavior change (Park et al., 2017). The researchers, however, did not indicate that the statement was a proposition from the theory. The intervention was conceptually defined based on King's (1992) theory and operationalized using a protocol. There was congruence between the conceptual and operational definitions. Other concepts of the theory were not defined or measured in the study. Park et al. (2017) did not link the study findings back to the framework in the discussion section of their report. The use of the grand theory to guide the intervention was appropriate and added strength to the study but needed to be linked to the dependent variables and the study findings.

Based on a power analysis, 64 participants receiving inpatient cardiac rehabilitation were recruited into the study and randomly assigned to the intervention or usual care group. The research assistants interviewed the participants in the first 2 days after admission to collect data about the outcome variables of quality of life, risk factors, and health behaviors (Park et al., 2017). They also collected demographic and medical information from the medical records. The research assistants were blinded to group assignment.

No significant differences in the outcome variables were found between the intervention and usual care groups at baseline. Participants in both groups reduced their cardiovascular risks in the first 6 months after the AMI, with no significant differences found related to the intervention (Park et al., 2017). However, the intervention had an effect on health behaviors, the mental component of quality of life (QOL), and blood glucose control, with the intervention group reporting higher scores on those measures at 6 months.

The researchers posited the need for future studies of the long-term effects of the theory-based intervention. Mutual goal setting, one of the main concepts of King's theory, warrants study in other populations with the need to make long-term changes in health behaviors.

Framework Based on Middle Range Theory

Many frameworks for nursing studies are based on middle range theories. These studies test the validity of the middle range theory and examine the parameters within which the middle range theory can be applied. Some nursing researchers have used middle range theories developed by non-nurses. Other researchers have used middle range theories that they or other nurses have developed to explain nursing phenomena. In either case, middle range theories should be tested before being applied to nursing practice.

Reinoso (2016) used Mishel's middle range nursing theory, the Theory of Uncertainty for Acute and Chronic Illness (1988), as the framework for a study of psychological stress among persons living with chronic hepatitis C. Reinoso (2016, p. 445) noted that uncertainty about the extent and prognosis of the infection is the "ultimate psychological stressor." The gap in knowledge, which is the statement of the research problem, was not clearly identified but can be inferred from the literature review of studies in which uncertainty was a variable. Reinoso (2016) noted previous studies that had unexpected results related to uncertainty did not include the conditions contributing to uncertainty. Within the description of the middle range theory, the main concept of uncertainty was defined as "the cognitive state the individual creates when he or she is not able to properly structure or categorize an event because of a lack of sufficient cues" (Reinoso, 2016, p. 446). Reinoso linked uncertainty to psychological stress and described the study framework in Research Example 7.2.

RESEARCH EXAMPLE 7.2

Middle Range Theory as a Framework

Research Study Excerpt

Mishel's uncertainty in illness theory provides a substantive theory in which to frame a study on the uncertainties faced by those individuals diagnosed with chronic hepatitis C... The aim of this research study was to examine the correlation, both direction and strength, between uncertainty and the antecedents of Mishel's uncertainty in illness theory. The research question that guided the study was: What is the relationship between the antecedents of Mishel's theory (ie, health care authority figures, years since diagnosis, treatment experience, and social network) and the chronic hepatitis C individual's perception of uncertainty?... A cross-sectional, correlational design was used to assess the direction and strength of relationships among variables.... Uncertainty as the dependent variable was correlated with other variables to evaluate the degree of relationship these variables share... Higher scores measuring health care authority figures were associated with more perceived uncertainty... higher levels of social network were associated with less perceived uncertainty...Years since diagnosis and the treatment experience were unrelated to uncertainty... connecting individuals diagnosed with hepatitis C to resources in the community may further assist in those navigating illness events... those with an expanded social network have less uncertainty and vice versa.... The findings can be utilized to help create interventions catered toward this population to decrease perceived uncertainty and to develop a more cohesive understanding of illness events. (Reinoso, 2016, pp. 445, 446, 450, 451)

Critical Appraisal

The Theory of Uncertainty in Illness (Mishel, 1988) was explicitly identified as the research framework for the study (Reinoso, 2016). A conceptual definition of uncertainty was provided, but no conceptual definitions of the uncertainty antecedents were found in the report. The operational definitions of each variable were explicit. The conceptual and operational definitions of uncertainty were congruent. Relationships between the antecedents of uncertainty and uncertainty itself were identified as the relationships being studied.

Reinoso (2016) linked the findings to the theory and described a possible application to clinical practice. The higher scores related to healthcare authority figures indicated increased distrust or dissatisfaction with the provider, nurses, and other professionals (Reinoso, 2016). When the patient perceived conflicts or discrepancies in the information provided by these persons, uncertainty was higher. Reinoso (2016, p. 451) identified that the negative relationship between social networks and uncertainty had clinical implications by placing responsibility on healthcare providers "to understand the importance social networks play in the interpretation of illness events and connect patients to such networks".

Framework From a Tentative Theory

Findings from completed studies reported in the literature can be a rich source of frameworks when synthesized into a coherent, logical set of relationships. The findings from studies, especially when combined with concepts and relationships from middle range theories or non-nursing theories, can be synthesized into a tentative theory that provides a framework for a particular study.

Duarte and Pinto-Gouveia (2017) conducted a descriptive, correlational cross-sectional study with hospital nurses (n = 298) to test a theoretical model based on research findings related to empathy, empathy-based pathogenic guilt, and professional quality of life. They noted that empathy had been associated with positive outcomes for patients, such as compliance with treatment, and with effective care and less burnout for healthcare professionals. Empathy had also been associated with guilt feelings that may become pathogenic when excessive or misdirected and affect professional quality of life. Professional quality of life was defined as being comprised of burnout and compassion fatigue. These complex relationships were measured and examined using a nonprobability sample (Research Example 7.3).

RESEARCH EXAMPLE 7.3

Tentative Theory as a Framework

Research Study Excerpt

Empathy is at the core of nursing practice... Empathic concern was defined as feelings of care about the welfare of others and becoming upset over their misfortunes. Personal distress was defined as feelings of distress and anxiety when witnessing another's negative state. These two dimensions are considered the affective components of empathy. In contrast to the prosocial effects of perspective taking and empathic concern, personal distress does not appear to have positive effects on personal relations... empathy is closely related to guilt, so that more empathic people are more likely to experience guilt than less empathic people... We particularly focused on survivor guilt and omnipotence guilt, both of which involve an exaggerated sense of responsibility for others... Omnipotent responsibility guilt also arises out of empathy and involves an exaggerated sense of responsibility and concern for the happiness and well-being of others... In certain jobs where one is responsible for others' lives and wellbeing, such as nursing, guilt can be especially acute when things go wrong. However, few studies to date explored the impact of feelings of guilt in nurses' well-being... Self-report questionnaires were used to test the study's aims... test a theoretical model of the relationships between empathy dimensions (empathic concern and perspective taking), empathy-based pathogenic guilt and professional quality of life. We hypothesized that when empathy is associated with pathogenic guilt, i.e. survival and omnipotence guilt, it may contribute for professional ill-being (compassion fatigue and burnout symptoms). Because perspective taking was not significant associated with compassion fatigue we did not test a mediation model. Fig. 1 presents a conceptual diagram of the mediation models. (Duarte & Pinto-Gouveia, 2017, pp. 42–44).

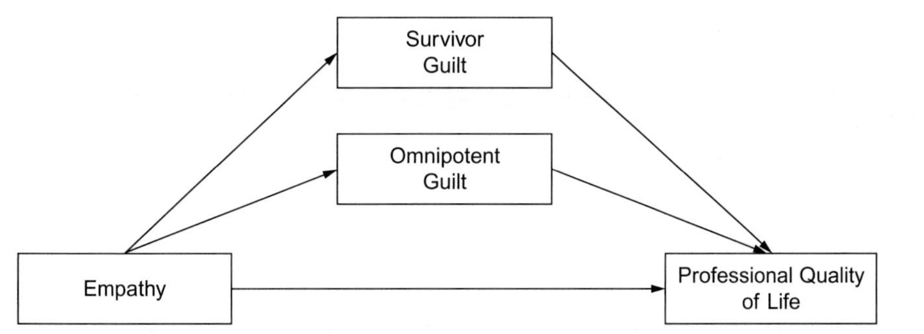

FIG 1 Conceptual diagram of the direct and indirect effects of empathy on professional quality of life. (From Duarte, J., & Pinto-Gouveia, J. [2017]. Empathy and feelings of guilt experienced by nurses: A cross-sectional study of their role in burnout and compassion fatigue symptoms. *Applied Nursing Research, 35*[1], 42–47.)

Continued

RESEARCH EXAMPLE 7.3—cont'd

Critical Appraisal

The tentative research framework was proposed based on prior study findings and conclusions. The concepts were defined and linked to the variables and appropriate instruments for measurement. There was congruence between the inferred conceptual and operational definitions. The statements of the tentative relationships among the concepts were complex, a fact supported by the direct and indirect effects found among the concepts. In the Discussion section, Duarte and Pinto-Gouveia (2017) acknowledged study limitations and identified implications appropriate to their results. Future studies were recommended to "replicate these findings, in larger samples, using experimental and longitudinal designs to test particular hypotheses based on the present findings, and with alternative ways to measure these processes" (Duarte & Pinto-Gouveia, 2017).

Framework for a Physiological Study

Developing a physiological framework to express the logic on which the study is based is clearly helpful to the researcher and readers of the published study. The critical appraisal of a physiological framework is no different from that of other frameworks. However, concepts and conceptual definitions in physiological frameworks may be less abstract than concepts and conceptual definitions in psychosocial studies. Concepts in physiological studies might be such terms as *cardiac output, dyspnea, wound healing, blood pressure, tissue hypoxia, metabolism,* and *functional status.*

Amiri and Turner-Henson (2017) conducted a cross-sectional study with a sample of 88 expectant mothers in their second trimester to determine the effects of formaldehyde (FA) exposure on intrauterine fetal growth. The concepts include intrauterine fetal growth restriction, oxidative stress, and FA exposures. In Research Example 7.4, you will see that a biological model was used as the study framework. In addition, Fig. 7.4 displays the three primary relationships in the model that were the focus of the study. The diagram was simplified to clarify the primary relationships of the model. Amiri and Turner-Henson (2017) did not have explicit conceptual and operational definitions. Table 7.5 provides the conceptual and operational definitions we developed from the article.

RESEARCH EXAMPLE 7.4

Physiological Theory as a Framework

Research Study Excerpt

There is limited empirical evidence about levels of FA exposure in pregnant women and its relationship to fetal growth. We adopted a biological model from Kannan, Misra, Dvonch, and Krishnakumar (2006), who showed the relationship between particulate matter, as an outdoor air pollutant, and pregnancy outcomes, considering the effect of oxidative stress as a biological pathway in this relationship. We examined the relationship between FA exposure and fetal growth in the second trimester and the potential mediating role of oxidative stress in the relationship between FA exposure and fetal growth.... We used a cross-sectional design with participants recruited from urban obstetrics and gynecology clinics (one public, two private) in the Southeast region of the United States... After informed consent was obtained, the first author, as solo data collector, interviewed the participants about demographic characteristics, obstetric history, and residential dwelling characteristics… Participants were instructed to wear the FA badge for 24 hours while they were at home, work, school, and other locations. We asked participants to place the badge on a chair or a stand near their head while they slept and when they showered… These measurements were obtained through review of participants' ultrasonography reports from the electronic health record. Ultrasonographic measurements were reported by certified ultrasonography technicians at each clinic site…

No significant correlations were found between maternal age, education, marital status, yearly family income, and fetal ultrasonographic biometry measurements… There was a significant difference in EFW [estimated fetal weight] percentile medians with the White group having the greatest median… There was no significant relationship between gravida, maternal smoking status, or interval between pregnancies and fetal ultrasonographic biometric measurements… greater FA exposure (>.03 ppm) was found to be significantly associated with BPD [biparietal diameter]… greater FA exposure was associated with short FL [femur length]… the mediating role of oxidative stress in the relationship between FA exposure level and BPD… was not supported in this study. (Amiri & Turner-Henson, 2017, pp. 53–54, 56–58)

Critical Appraisal

Amiri and Turner-Henson (2017) identified the biological model by Kannan et al. (2006) as the research framework, but did not provide explicit conceptual definitions of the study's variables. Conceptual definitions were constructed from the information provided in the introduction and background section of the article (see Table 7.5) and operational definitions were extracted from the study procedures section of the article. The inferred conceptual and operational definitions as abstracted from the study seemed consistent with each other, but explicitly defined concepts would have strengthened the use of the model. Hypothesized relationships among the variables were identified for the descriptive correlational design.

The researchers provided implications for nursing education, practice, and research, but did not discuss the implications for the biological model that was the research framework. In the discussion section, the researchers note that information about the effects of FA exposure on fetal growth has been very limited, making the results of this study significant despite the sample attrition. Other researchers have shown that oxidative stress had a meditating effect on the relationship between FA exposure and biparietal diameter; however, no significant effect was found in this study and the researchers consider several measurement challenges that may have affected the results. The clinical implications are that nurses need to learn more about environmental exposures. Amiri and Turner-Henson (2017, p. 59) state, "Assessment of environmental risks during pregnancy should be a standard part of prenatal care. Nurses should educate women… on risk reduction strategies to avoid toxic exposures."

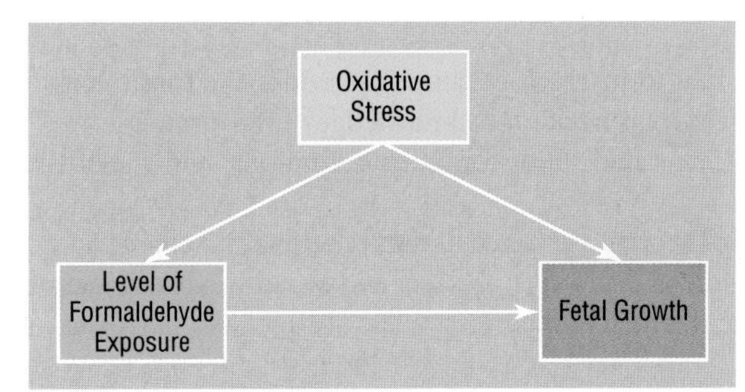

FIG 7.4 Proposed model of the relationships between level of formaldehyde exposure, oxidative stress, and intrauterine fetal growth. (Based on Amiri, A., & Turner-Henson, A. [2017]. The roles of formaldehyde exposure and oxidative stress in fetal growth in the second trimester. *Journal of Gynecological, Obstetrics, and Neonatal Nurses [JOGNN], 46*[1], 51–62.)

TABLE 7.5 CONCEPTUAL AND OPERATIONAL DEFINITIONS OF VARIABLES

VARIABLE	CONCEPTUAL DEFINITION	OPERATIONAL DEFINITION
Intrauterine fetal growth reduction	"any deviation in fetal growth or failure to reach growth potential… associated with greater prenatal mortality and morbidity rates" (Amiri & Turner-Henson, 2017, p. 51).	Biparietal diameter, head circumference, abdominal circumference, femur length, and ratio of abdominal circumference to femur length obtained from the second trimester ultrasonography report in the electronic health record of each participant. The measurements were converted to biometry percentiles based on fetal gender and race.
Formaldehyde (FA) exposure	A hazardous air pollutant that is a known human carcinogen and enhances oxidative stress.	Measured by high-performance liquid chromatography analysis of vapor monitor badge worn by the participants, reported in part per million and compared to environmental standards.
Urine cotinine	A biomarker of tobacco smoke, a source of indoor FA exposure.	Measured using a urinary ELISA assay, with the lowest reliable detection level of 2ng/ml; assay completed by primary investigator.
Oxidative stress	Imbalance of the "production of reactive oxidant molecules goes beyond the capacity of the cell's antioxidant defense mechanism" (p. 53), associated with poor pregnancy outcomes.	Urinary 15-isoprostane F_{21} was measured using urinary isoprostane ELISA kits.
Creatinine	Protein waste products in the urine that are an indicator of renal function and affect the specific gravity of the urine; can be used to standardize other urinary tests.	Level of substance determined by colorimetric analytic method as reported by a national laboratory service.

Based on Amiri, A., & Turner-Henson, A. (2017). The roles of formaldehyde exposure and oxidative stress in fetal growth in the second trimester. *Journal of Gynecological, Obstetrics, and Neonatal Nurses (JOGNN), 46*(1), 51–62.
ELISA, Enzyme-linked immunosorbent assay.

KEY POINTS

- Theory is essential to research because it provides the framework for developing a study and links the study findings back to the knowledge of the discipline.
- A theory is an integrated set of concepts, definitions, and statements that presents a view of a phenomenon.
- The elements of theories are concepts and relational statements.
- Grand nursing theories are very abstract and broadly explain phenomena of interest.
- Middle range and tentative theories are less abstract and narrower in scope than grand nursing theories.
- Every study has a framework, although some frameworks are poorly expressed or are implicit.
- A research framework is an abstract, logical structure of meaning, such as a portion of a theory, which guides the development of the study and enables the researcher to link the findings to nursing's body of knowledge.

- To be used effectively, the research framework must include the concepts and the conceptual and operational definitions. The relational statements or propositions being examined need to be clear and represented by a model or map.
- Frameworks for studies may come from grand nursing theories, middle range theories, research findings, non-nursing theories, tentative theories, and scientific theories.
- Scientific theories are derived from physiology, genetics, pathophysiology, and physics and are supported by extensive evidence.
- Critically appraising a framework requires the identification and evaluation of the concepts, their definitions, and the statements linking the concepts. The study findings should be linked back to the research framework to determine its usefulness in describing reality.

REFERENCES

Amiri, A., & Turner-Henson, A. (2017). The roles of formaldehyde exposure and oxidative stress in fetal growth in the second trimester. *Journal of Gynecological, Obstetrics, and Neonatal Nurses (JOGNN), 46*(1), 51–62.

Broadhead, W. E., Gehlbach, S. H., de Gruy, F., & Kaplan, B. H. (1988). The Duke-UNC Functional Social Support Questionnaire: Measurement of social support in family medicine patients. *Medical Care, 26*(7), 709–723.

Chinn, P. L., & Kramer, M. K. (2015). *Integrated theory and knowledge development in nursing* (9th ed.). St. Louis, MO: Elsevier Mosby.

Coleman, C. (2017). Health-related quality of life and depressive symptoms among seropositive African Americans. *Applied Nursing Research, 33*(1), 138–141.

Covell, C. L. (2008). The middle-range theory of nursing intellectual capital. *Journal of Advanced Nursing, 63*(1), 94–103.

Duarte, J., & Pinto-Gouveia, J. (2017). Empathy and feelings of guilt experienced by nurses: A cross-sectional study of their role in burnout and compassion fatigue symptoms. *Applied Nursing Research, 35*(1), 42–47.

Frank, C., Schroeter, K., & Shaw, C. (2017). Addressing traumatic stress in the acute traumatically injured patient. *Journal of Trauma Nursing, 24*(2), 78–84.

Gomes, L., Coelho, A., dos Santos Gomides, D., Foss-Freitas, M., Foss, M., & Pace, A. (2017). Contribution of family social support to the metabolic control of people with diabetes mellitus: A randomized controlled clinical trial. *Applied Nursing Research, 36*(1), 68–76.

Gonzalez-Saenz de Tejada, M., Bilbao, A., Baré, M., Briones, E., Sarasqueta, C., Quintana, J., & Escobar, A. (2016). Association of social support, functional status, and psychological variables with changes in health-related quality of life outcomes in patients with colorectal cancer. *Psycho-Oncology, 25*(8), 891–897.

Gray, J., Grove, S., & Sutherland, S. (2017). *The practice of nursing research: Appraisal, synthesis, and generation of evidence* (8th ed.). St. Louis, MO: Elsevier Saunders.

Grove, S. K., & Cipher, D. J. (2017). *Statistics for nursing research: A workbook for evidence-based practice* (2nd ed.). St. Louis, MO: Elsevier.

Groves, P. (2014). The relationship between safety culture and patient outcomes: Results from pilot meta-analysis. *Western Journal of Nursing Research, 36*(1), 66–83.

Groves, P., Meisenbach, R., & Scott-Cawiezell, J. (2011). Keeping patients safe in healthcare organizations: A structuration theory of safety culture. *Journal of Advanced Nursing, 67*(8), 1846–1855.

Humphreys, J., Janson, S., Donesky, D., Dracup, K., Lee, K. A., Puntillo, K., et al. (2014). Theory of symptom management. In M. J. Smith & P. R. Liehr (Eds.), *Middle range theory for nursing* (3rd ed., pp. 141–164). New York, NY: Springer Publishing.

Kannan, S., Misra, D., Dvonch, J., & Krishnakumar, A. (2006). Exposures to airborne particulate matter and adverse perinatal outcomes: A biologically plausible mechanistic framework for exploring potential effect modification by nutrition. *Environmental Health Perspectives, 114*(11), 1636–1642.

King, I. (1992). Interpersonal relations: A theoretical framework for application in nursing practice. *Nursing Science Quarterly, 5*(1), 13–18.

Kolcaba, K. (1994). A theory of comfort for nursing. *Journal of Advanced Nursing, 19*(6), 1178–1184.

Krinsky, R., Murillo, I., & Johnson, J. (2014). A practical application of Katharine Kolcaba's comfort theory to cardiac patients. *Applied Nursing Research, 27*(1), 147–150.

Lenz, E. R., Pugh, L. C., Milligan, R., Gift, A., & Suppe, F. (1997). The middle range theory of unpleasant symptoms: An update. *Advances in Nursing Science, 19*(3), 14–27.

Liehr, P., & Smith, M. (2017). Middle range theory: A perspective on development and use. *Advances in Nursing Science, 40*(1), 51–63.

Lor, M., Backonja, U., & Lauver, D. (2017). How could nurse researchers apply theory to generate knowledge more efficiently? *Journal of Nursing Scholarship, 49*(5), 580–589.

Meleis, A. I. (2010). *Transitions theory: Middle range and situation specific theories in nursing research and practice*. New York, NY: Springer Publishing.

Meleis, A. I. (2012). *Theoretical nursing: Development and progress* (5th ed.). Philadelphia, PA: Wolters Kluwer/ Lippincott Williams & Wilkins.

Mishel, M. H. (1988). Uncertainty in illness. *Journal of Nursing Scholarship, 20*(4), 225–232.

Mishel, M. H. (1990). Reconceptualization of the uncertainty in illness theory. *Journal of Nursing Scholarship, 22*(3), 256–262.

Olds, D., & Dolansky, M. (2017). Quality and safety research: Recommendations from the Quality and Safety Education for Nurses (QSEN) Institute. *Applied Nursing Research, 35*, 126–127.

Orem, D. E. (2001). *Nursing: Concepts of practice* (6th ed.). St. Louis, MO: Mosby.

Orem, D. E., & Taylor, S. G. (2011). Reflections on nursing practice science: The nature, the structure, and the foundation of nursing science. *Nursing Science Quarterly, 24*(1), 35–41.

Park, M., Song, R., & Jeong, J. O. (2017). Effect of goal attainment theory based education program on cardiovascular risks, behavioral modification, and quality of life among patients with first episode of acute myocardial infarction: Randomized study. *International Journal of Nursing Studies, 71*(1), 8–16.

Pickett, S., Peters, R., & Jarosz, P. (2014). Toward a middle-range theory of weight management. *Nursing Science Quarterly, 27*(3), 242–247.

Radloff, L. S. (1977). The CES-D Scale: A self-report depression scale for research in the general population. *Applied Psychological Measurement, 1*(3), 385–401.

Reed, P. (1991). Toward a nursing theory of self-transcendence: Deductive reformulation using developmental theories. *Advances in Nursing Science, 13*(4), 64–77.

Reinoso, H. (2016). Uncertainty and the treatment experience of individuals with chronic hepatitis C. *Journal of Nurse Practitioners, 12*(7), 445–451.

Riegel, B., Dickson, V., & Faulkner, K. (2016). The situation-specific theory of heart failure self-care: Revised and updated. *Journal of Cardiovascular Nursing, 31*(3), 226–235.

Rogers, M. E. (1970). *An introduction to the theoretical basis of nursing*. Philadelphia, PA: F. A. Davis.

Roux, G., Dingley, C., & Bush, H. (2002). Inner strength in women: Metasynthesis of qualitative findings in theory development. *Journal of Theory Construction and Testing, 6*(1), 86–93.

Roy, C. (2011). Research based on the Roy Adaptation Model: Last 25 years. *Nursing Science Quarterly, 24*(4), 312–320.

Roy, C., & Andrews, H. A. (2008). *Roy Adaptation Model* (3rd ed.). Upper Saddle River, NJ: Prentice Hall Health.

Schaffer, M., Sandau, K., & Missal, B. (2017). Demystifying nursing theory: A Christian nursing perspective. *Journal of Christian Nursing, 34*(2), 102–107.

Sherwood, G., & Barnsteiner, J. (2017). *Quality and safety in nursing: A competency approach to improving outcomes* (2nd ed.). Ames, IA: Wiley-Blackwell.

Swanson, K. M. (1991). Empirical development of a middle range theory of caring. *Nursing Research, 40*(3), 161–166.

Thomas, S. (1991). Toward a new conceptualization of women's anger. *Issues in Mental Health Nursing, 12*(1), 31–49.

Toulouse, C., & Kodadek, M. (2016). Continuous access to medications and health outcomes in uninsured adults with type 2 diabetes. *Journal of the American Association of Nurse Practitioners, 28*(6), 327–334.

van Manen, M. (2017). Phenomenology in its original sense. *Qualitative Health Research, 27*(6), 810–825.

Ware, J. E., & Sherbourne, C. D. (1992). The MOS 36-item Short-Form Health Survey (SF-36): I. Conceptual framework and item selection. *Medical Care, 30*(6), 473–483.

Wilson, J., & Cleary, P. (1995). Linking clinical variables with health-related quality of life: A conceptual model of patient outcomes. *The Journal of the American Medical Association, 273*(1), 59–65.

Because of funding changes, the Agency for Healthcare Research and Quality (AHRQ) National Guideline Clearinghouse website was scheduled for decommissioning as of July 16, 2018. For more information, go to https://www.ahrq.gov/.

CHAPTER

8

Clarifying Quantitative Research Designs

Susan K. Grove

CHAPTER OVERVIEW

LEARNING OUTCOMES

After completing this chapter, you should be able to:

1. Identify the noninterventional or nonexperimental designs (descriptive and correlational) and intervention or experimental designs (quasi-experimental and experimental) commonly used in quantitative nursing studies.
2. Describe the concepts relevant to quantitative research designs.
3. Examine study designs for strengths and threats to design validity.
4. Critically appraise descriptive and correlational designs in studies.
5. Describe the elements of designs that examine causality.
6. Critically appraise the interventions implemented in studies.
7. Critically appraise the quasi-experimental and experimental designs in studies.
8. Examine the quality of randomized controlled trials conducted in nursing.

A **research design** is a blueprint for conducting a study. Over the years, several quantitative research designs have been developed for conducting descriptive, correlational, quasi-experimental, and experimental studies. Descriptive and correlational designs are focused on describing and examining relationships of variables in natural settings. Quasi-experimental and experimental designs have been developed to examine causality, or the cause and effect relationships between interventions and outcomes. The designs focused on causality were developed to maximize control over factors that could interfere with or threaten the validity of the study design. The strengths of the design validity increase the probability that the study findings are an accurate reflection of reality. Well-designed studies, especially those focused on testing the effects of nursing interventions, are essential for generating sound research evidence for practice (Melnyk, Gallagher-Ford, & Fineout-Overholt, 2017).

Being able to identify a study design and evaluate its strengths and weaknesses are an important part of critically appraising studies. Therefore, this chapter introduces you to the different types of quantitative study designs and provides an algorithm for determining whether a study design is descriptive, correlational, quasi-experimental, or experimental. Algorithms are also provided so that you can identify specific types of designs in published studies. The concepts relevant for understanding quantitative research designs are defined. The different types of validity—construct, internal, external, and statistical conclusion—are described. Guidelines are provided for critically appraising designs in quantitative studies. The chapter concludes with an introduction to randomized controlled trials (RCTs), with a flow diagram provided to examine the quality of these trials conducted in nursing.

IDENTIFYING QUANTITATIVE RESEARCH DESIGNS IN NURSING STUDIES

A variety of quantitative research designs are implemented in nursing studies; the four most common types are descriptive, correlational, quasi-experimental, and experimental. These designs are categorized in different ways in textbooks (Kerlinger & Lee, 2000; Shadish, Cook, & Campbell, 2002). Sometimes, descriptive and correlational designs are referred to as **noninterventional** or **nonexperimental designs** because the focus is on examining variables as they naturally occur in environments and not on the implementation of an intervention by the researcher.

Some of the noninterventional designs include a time element, such as the **cross-sectional design,** which involves data collection on variables at one point in time. For example, cross-sectional designs might involve examining a group of study participants simultaneously in various stages of development, levels of education, severity of illness, or stages of recovery to describe changes in a phenomenon across stages. The assumption is that the stages are part of a process that will progress over time. Selecting participants at various points in the process provides important information about the totality of the process, even though the same subjects are not monitored throughout the entire process (Gray, Grove, & Sutherland, 2017). For example, researchers might describe the depression levels of three different groups of women with breast cancer who are prechemotherapy, receiving chemotherapy, or postchemotherapy treatment to understand depression levels based on the phase of treatment. **Longitudinal design** involves collecting data from the same study participants at multiple points in time and might also be referred to as repeated measures. Repeated measures might be included in descriptive, correlational, quasi-experimental, or experimental study designs. With a longitudinal design, a sample of women with breast cancer could be monitored for depression before, during, and after their chemotherapy treatment.

Quasi-experimental and experimental studies are designed to examine causality or the cause and effect relationship between a researcher-implemented intervention and selected study outcomes. The designs for these studies are sometimes referred to as interventional or experimental because the focus is on examining the differences in dependent variables thought to be caused by independent variables or interventions. For example, the researcher-implemented intervention might be a home monitoring program for patients initially diagnosed with hypertension, and the dependent or outcome variables could be systolic and diastolic blood pressure values measured at 1 week, 1 month, and 6 months. This chapter introduces you to selected interventional designs and provides examples of these designs from published nursing studies. Details on other study designs can be found in a variety of methodology sources (Campbell & Stanley, 1963; Creswell, 2014; Gray et al., 2017; Kerlinger & Lee, 2000; Shadish et al., 2002).

The algorithm shown in Fig. 8.1 may be used to determine the type of design (e.g., descriptive, correlational, quasi-experimental, experimental) used in a study. This algorithm includes a series of yes or no responses to specific questions about the design. The algorithm starts with the question, "Is there an intervention?" The answer leads to the next question, with the four types of designs being identified in the algorithm. For example, if researchers conducted a study to identify the characteristics of nurses who either passed or failed their registered nurse (RN) licensure on the first try, Fig. 8.1 indicates that a descriptive design would be used. If the researchers examined the relationships among the nurses' characteristics and their score on the RN licensure examination, a correlational design would be implemented. If researchers tested the effectiveness of a relaxation intervention on graduates' RN licensure examination scores, either a quasi-experimental or experimental design would be implemented. Experimental designs have the greatest control because (1) a tightly controlled intervention is implemented and (2) study participants are randomly assigned to either the intervention or control group (see Fig. 8.1).

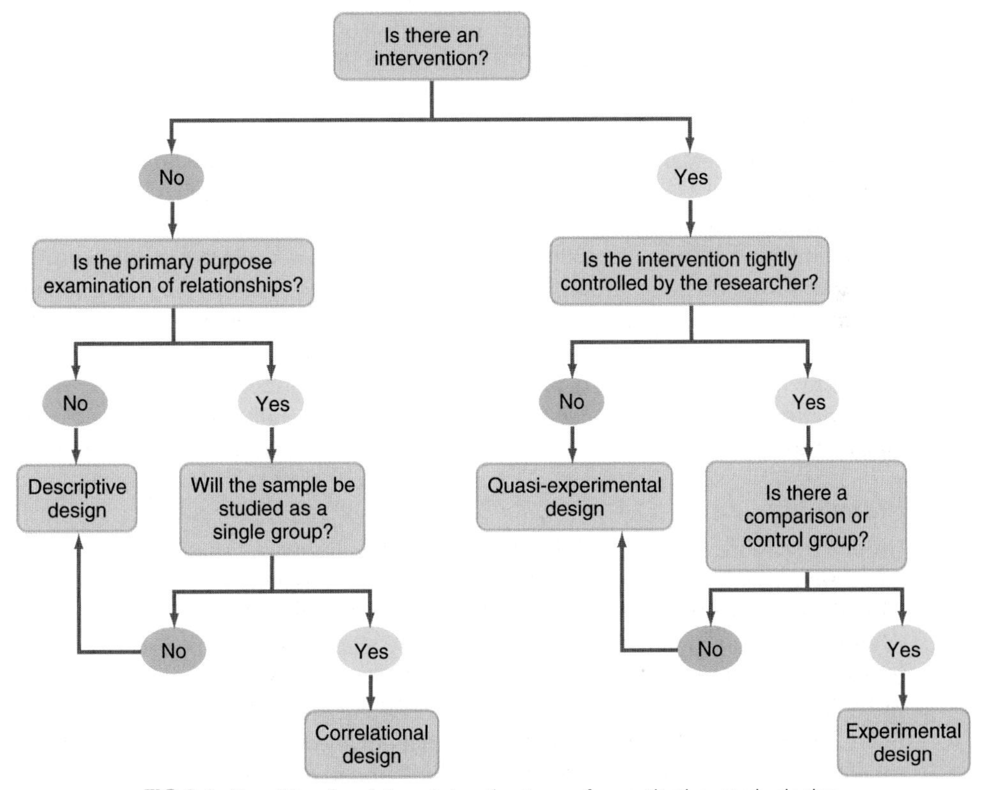

FIG 8.1 Algorithm for determining the type of quantitative study design.

UNDERSTANDING CONCEPTS RELEVANT TO QUANTITATIVE RESEARCH DESIGNS

Concepts relevant to quantitative research designs include causality, multicausality, probability, bias, prospective, retrospective, control, and manipulation. These concepts are described to provide a background for understanding noninterventional and interventional research designs.

Causality

Causality basically means that things have causes, and causes lead to effects. In a critical appraisal, you need to determine whether the purpose of the study is to examine causality, examine relationships among variables (correlational designs), or describe variables (descriptive designs). You may be able to determine whether the purpose of a study is to examine causality by reading the purpose statement and propositions within the framework (see Chapter 7). For example, the purpose of a causal study may be to examine the effect of an early ambulation program after surgery on the length of hospital stay. The framework proposition may state that early physical activity following surgery improves recovery time. However, the early ambulation program is not the only factor affecting the length of hospital stay. Other important factors or extraneous variables that affect the length of hospital stay include the diagnosis, type of surgery, patient's age, physical condition of the patient before surgery, and complications that occurred after surgery. Researchers usually design quasi-experimental and experimental studies to examine causality or the effect of an intervention (independent variable) on a selected outcome (dependent variable), using a design that controls for relevant extraneous variables.

Multicausality

Very few phenomena in nursing can be clearly linked to a single cause and a single effect. A number of interrelating variables can be involved in producing a particular effect. Therefore studies developed from a multicausal perspective will include more variables than those using a strict causal orientation. The presence of multiple causes for an effect is referred to as multicausality. For example, patient diagnosis, age, presurgical condition, and complications after surgery are interrelated causes of the length of a patient's hospital stay. Because of the complexity of causal relationships, a theory is unlikely to identify every element involved in causing a particular outcome. However, the greater the proportion of causal factors that can be identified and examined or controlled in a single study, the clearer the understanding will be of the overall phenomenon. This greater understanding is expected to increase the ability to predict and control the effects of study interventions.

Probability

Probability addresses relative rather than absolute causality. A cause may not produce a specific effect each time that a particular cause occurs, and researchers recognize that a particular cause *probably* will result in a specific effect. Using a probability orientation, researchers design studies to examine the probability that a given effect will occur under a defined set of circumstances. The circumstances may be variations in multiple variables. For example, while assessing the effect of multiple variables on length of hospital stay, researchers may choose to examine the probability of a given length of hospital stay under a variety of specific sets of circumstances. One specific set of circumstances may be that the patient had undergone a knee replacement, had no chronic illnesses, and experienced no complications after surgery. Sampling criteria could be developed to control most of these extraneous variables. The probability of a given length of hospital stay could be expected to vary as the set of circumstances are varied or controlled in the design of the study.

Bias

The term *bias* means a slant or deviation from the true or expected. Bias in a study distorts the findings from what the results would have been without the bias. Because studies are conducted to determine the real and the true, quantitative researchers place great value on identifying and removing sources of bias in their study and controlling their effects on the study findings. Any component of a study that deviates or causes a deviation from a true measurement of the study variables contributes to distorted findings. Many factors related to research can be biased; these include attitudes or motivations of the researcher (conscious or unconscious), components of the environment in which the study is conducted, selection of the study participants, composition of the sample, groups formed, measurement methods, data collection process, and statistical analyses (Gray et al., 2017; Grove & Cipher, 2017). For example, some of the participants for the study might be taken from a unit of the hospital in which the patients are participating in another study involving quality nursing care or a nurse, selecting patients for a study, might include only those who showed an interest in the study (Gray et al., 2017). Researchers might use a scale with limited reliability and validity to measure a study variable (Waltz, Strickland, & Lenz, 2017). Each of these situations introduces bias to nonintervention and intervention studies.

An important focus in critically appraising a study is to identify possible sources of bias. This requires careful examination of the methods section in the research report, including the strategies for obtaining study participants, methods of measurement, implementation of a study intervention, and data collection process. However, not all biases can be identified from the published study report. The article may not provide sufficient detail about the methods of the study to detect possible biases.

Prospective Versus Retrospective

Prospective is a term that means looking forward, whereas the term *retrospective* means looking backward, usually in relation to time. In research, these terms are used most frequently to refer to the timing of data collection. Are the data obtained in real time, with measurements being obtained by the research team, or are the study's data obtained from information collected at a prior time? Data collection in noninterventional research can be either prospective or retrospective because, by definition, it lacks researcher intervention. Many noninterventional studies in health care use retrospective data obtained from national electronic databases and clinical and administrative databases of healthcare agencies. Secondary analysis of data from a previous study to address a newly developed study purpose is also considered retrospective. However, prospective data collection is usually more accurate than retrospective data collection, especially when researchers are passionate about their phenomenon of study and are rigorous in the measurement of study variables and the implementation of the data collection process.

Data collection in interventional research, however, must be prospective because the researcher enacts an intervention in real time. This is not to say that the research team does not access current data from the health record for real-time studies. A researcher collecting arterial blood pressure data in critically ill infants might collect data over a 24-hour period for several days. Nurses on the various shifts would record arterial blood pressure at least hourly, as is common practice, and the research team would retrieve that information during daily data collection. Although information retrieval of the infants' electronic chart data does look back in time over the preceding 24-hour period, this study would be considered prospective because data are generated and recorded at the same time that the infants are hospitalized.

Control

One method of reducing bias is to increase the amount of control in the design of a study. **Control** means having the power to direct or manipulate factors to achieve a desired outcome. For example, in a study of an early ambulation program, study participants may be randomly selected and then randomly assigned to the intervention group or control group. The researcher would control the duration of and the assistance during the ambulation program or intervention. The time that the ambulation occurred in relation to surgery would also be controlled, as well as the environment in which the patient ambulated. Measurement of the length of hospital stay could be controlled by ensuring that the number of days, hours, and minutes of the hospital stay is calculated exactly the same way for each participant. Limiting the characteristics of the study participants, such as diagnosis, age, type of surgery, and incidence of complications, would also be a form of control. The greater the researcher's control over the study situation, the more credible (or valid) the study findings.

Manipulation

Manipulation is a form of control generally used in quasi-experimental and experimental studies. Controlling an intervention is the most common manipulation in these studies. In descriptive and correlational studies, little or no effort is made to manipulate factors regarding the circumstances of the study. Instead, the purpose is to examine the phenomenon and its characteristics as they exist in a natural environment or setting. However, when quasi-experimental and experimental designs are implemented, researchers must manipulate the intervention under study. Researchers need to develop quality interventions that are implemented in consistent ways by trained individuals (Eymard & Altmiller, 2016). This controlled manipulation of a study's intervention decreases the potential for bias and increases the validity of the study findings.

EXAMINING THE DESIGN VALIDITY OF QUANTITATIVE STUDIES

Study validity is a measure of the truth or accuracy of the findings obtained from a study. The validity of a study's design is central to obtaining accurate trustworthy results and findings from a study. **Design validity** encompasses the strengths and threats to the quality of a study design. Critical appraisal of studies requires that you identify the design strengths and think through the **threats to validity** or the possible weaknesses in a study's design. Four types of design validity relevant to nursing research include construct validity, internal validity, external validity, and statistical conclusion validity (Gray et al., 2017; Kerlinger & Lee, 2000; Shadish et al., 2002). Table 8.1 describes these four types of design validity and summarizes the threats common to each. Understanding these types of validity and their possible threats are important in critically appraising quantitative study designs.

Construct Validity

Construct validity examines the fit between the conceptual and operational definitions of variables. Theoretical constructs or concepts are defined within the study framework when a framework is identified. When the researchers do not identify a specific study framework, the variables may be defined according to how they have been defined in other studies. These abstract statements about the variables are the conceptual definitions, which provide the basis for the operational definitions of the variables. Operational definitions (methods of measurement) must accurately reflect the theoretical constructs or concepts. Construct validity is the extent of the congruence or

TABLE 8.1 **TYPES OF DESIGN VALIDITY CRITICALLY APPRAISED IN STUDIES**

TYPES OF DESIGN VALIDITY	DESCRIPTION	THREATS TO DESIGN VALIDITY
Construct validity	Validity is concerned with the fit between the conceptual and operational definitions of variables and that the instrument measures what it is supposed to in the study.	**Inadequate definitions of constructs:** Constructs or concepts examined in a study lack adequate conceptual or operational definitions, so the measurement method is not accurately capturing what it is supposed to in a study. **Mono-operation bias:** Only one measurement method is used to measure the study variable. **Experimenter expectancies (Rosenthal effect):** Researchers' expectations or bias might influence study outcomes, which could be controlled by researchers designating research assistants to collect study data. Another option is blinding researchers and data collectors to the group receiving the study intervention.
Internal validity	Validity is focused on determining if study findings are accurate or are the result of extraneous variables.	**Participant selection and assignment to group concerns:** The participants are selected by nonrandom sampling methods and are not randomly assigned to groups. **Participant attrition:** The percentage of participants withdrawing from the study is high or more than 25%, which can affect the findings of any quantitative study. **History:** An event not related to the planned study occurs during the study and could have an impact on the findings. **Maturation:** Changes in participants, such as growing wiser, more experienced, or tired, which might affect study results.
External validity	Validity is concerned with the extent to which study findings can be generalized beyond the sample used in the study.	**Interaction of selection and intervention:** The participants included in the study might be different than those who decline participation. If the refusal to participate is high, this might alter the study results. **Interaction of setting and intervention:** Bias exists in study settings and organizations that might influence implementation of a study intervention and data collection process. For example, some settings are more supportive and assist with a study, and others are less supportive and might encourage patients not to participate in a study. **Interaction of history and intervention:** An event, such as closing a hospital unit, changing leadership, or high nursing staff attrition, might affect the implementation of the intervention and the measurement of study outcomes, which would decrease generalization of findings.

Continued

TABLE 8.1 TYPES OF DESIGN VALIDITY CRITICALLY APPRAISED IN STUDIES—cont'd

TYPES OF DESIGN VALIDITY	DESCRIPTION	THREATS TO DESIGN VALIDITY
Statistical conclusion validity	Validity is concerned with whether the conclusions about relationships or differences drawn from statistical analysis are an accurate reflection of the real world.	**Low statistical power:** This refers to concluding that there are no differences between samples when one exists (Type II error), which is usually caused by small sample size. **Unreliable measurement methods:** Scales or physiological measures used in a study are not consistently measuring study variables. Reliability or consistency of scales is determined using the Cronbach alpha, which should be greater than 0.70 in a study (see Chapter 10). **Intervention fidelity concerns:** The intervention in a study is not consistently implemented because of lack of study protocol or training of individuals implementing the intervention. **Extraneous variances in study setting:** Extraneous variables in the study setting influence the scores on the dependent variables, making it difficult to detect group differences.

consistency between the conceptual definitions and operational definitions (see Chapter 5). The process of developing construct validity for an instrument often requires years of scientific work, and researchers need to discuss the construct validity of the instruments that they used in their study (see Chapter 10; Shadish et al., 2002; Waltz et al., 2017). The threats to construct validity are related to previous instrument development and to the development of measurement techniques as part of the methodology of a particular study. Threats to construct validity are described here and summarized in Table 8.1.

Inadequate Definitions of Constructs

Measurement of a construct stems logically from a concept analysis of the construct by the theorist who developed the construct or by the researcher. Ideally, the conceptual definition should emerge from the concept analysis, which is an in-depth study of the meanings of a construct or concept provided by theorists and researchers. The method of measurement (operational definition) should clearly reflect both the framework concept and study variable. A deficiency in the conceptual or operational definition leads to low construct validity.

Mono-Operation Bias

Mono-operation bias occurs when only one method of measurement is used to assess a construct. When only one method of measurement is used, fewer dimensions of the construct are measured. Construct validity greatly improves if the researcher uses more than one instrument (Waltz et al., 2017). For example, if pain were a dependent variable, more than one measure of pain could be used, such as a pain rating scale, verbal reports of pain, physical responses (e.g., increased pulse, blood pressure, respirations), and observations of behaviors that reflect pain (e.g., crying, grimacing, guarding of painful area, pulling away). It is sometimes possible to apply more than one measurement of the dependent variable with little increase in time, effort, or cost. Using multiple methods of measuring a construct increases the construct validity (see Chapter 10).

Experimenter Expectancies (Rosenthal Effect)

The expectancies of the researcher can bias the data. For example, **experimenter expectancy** occurs if a researcher expects a particular intervention to relieve pain. The data that he or she collects may be biased to reflect this expectation. If another researcher who does not believe that the intervention would be effective had collected the data, results could have been different. The extent to which this effect actually influences studies is not known. Because of their concern about experimenter expectancy, some researchers choose not to be involved in the data collection process. In other studies, data collectors do not know which study participants were assigned to the intervention and control groups, which means that they were blinded to group assignment. Using nonbiased data collectors or those who are blinded to group assignment increases the construct design validity of a study.

Internal Validity

Internal validity is the extent to which the effects detected in the study are a true reflection of reality, rather than the result of extraneous variables. Internal validity is a concern in all studies, but is a major focus in studies examining causality. When examining causality, the researcher must determine whether the dependent variables may have been influenced by a third, often unmeasured, variable (an extraneous variable). The possibility of an alternative explanation of cause is sometimes referred to as a *rival hypothesis* (Shadish et al., 2002). Any study can contain threats to internal design validity, and these validity threats can lead to false-positive or false-negative conclusions (see Table 8.1). The researcher must ask, "Is there another reasonable (valid) explanation (rival hypothesis) for the finding other than the one I have proposed?" Some of the common threats to internal validity, such as study participant selection and assignment to groups, participant attrition, history, and maturation, are discussed in this section.

Participant Selection and Assignment to Groups

Selection addresses the process whereby participants are chosen to take part in a study and how they are grouped within a study. A selection threat is more likely to occur in studies in which randomization is not possible (Gray et al., 2017; Shadish et al., 2002). In some studies, people selected for the study may differ in some important way from people not selected for the study. In other studies, the threat is a result of the differences in participants selected for study groups. For example, people assigned to the control group could be different in some important way from people assigned to the intervention group. This difference in selection could cause the two groups to react differently to the intervention; in this case, the groups' outcomes would not be due to the intervention, but to the differences in the individuals selected for the two groups. Random selection of participants for nursing studies is often not possible, and the number of participants available for studies is limited. The random assignment of participants to groups decreases the possibility of their selection being a threat to internal validity.

Participant Attrition

Attrition involves participants dropping out of a study before it is completed. Participant attrition becomes a threat (1) when those who drop out of a study are a different type of person from those who remain in the study or (2) there is a difference in the number and types of people who drop out of the intervention group and the people who drop out of the control or comparison group (see Chapter 9). If the attrition in a study is high (>25%), this could affect the accuracy of the study results (Cohen, 1988; Gray et al., 2017).

History

History is an event that is not related to the planned study but that occurs during the time of the study. History could influence a participant's response to the intervention or to the variables being measured and alter the outcome of the study. For example, if researchers studied the effect of an emotional support intervention on a participant's completion of his or her cardiac rehabilitation program, and several nurses quit their job at the rehabilitation center during the study, this historical event would create a threat to the study's internal design validity. Study participants who had worked closely with the nurses who quit may decide to stop participating in the study or working with different nurses might change the study outcomes.

Maturation

In research, maturation is defined as growing older, wiser, stronger, hungrier, more tired, or more experienced during the study. Such unplanned and unrecognized changes are a threat to the study's internal validity and can influence the findings of the study. Maturation is more likely to occur in longitudinal studies with repeated measures of study variables.

External Validity

External validity is concerned with the extent to which study findings can be generalized beyond the sample used in the study (Gray et al., 2017). With the most serious threat, the findings would be meaningful only for the group studied. To some extent, the significance of the study depends on the number or types of people and situations to which the findings can be applied. Sometimes, the factors influencing external validity are subtle and may not be reported in research reports; however, the researcher must be responsible for these factors. Generalization is usually narrower for a single study than for multiple replications of a study using different samples, perhaps from different populations in different settings. Some of the threats to the ability to generalize the findings (external validity) in terms of study design are described here and summarized in Table 8.1.

Interaction of Selection and Intervention

Finding individuals who are willing to participate in a study can be difficult, particularly if the study requires extensive amounts of time and energy. Researchers must report the number of persons who were approached and refused to participate in the study (refusal rate) so those examining the study can identify any threat to external validity. If the refusal rate for a study is high, there is a greater potential for threats to the external design validity. For example if 39% of the persons approached to participate in a study declined, the sample actually selected will be limited in ways that might not be evident at first glance to the researchers. Only the researcher knows the participants well. They might be volunteers, "do-gooders," or those with nothing better to do. In this case, generalizing the findings to all members of a population, such as all nurses, all hospitalized patients, or all persons experiencing diabetes, is not easy to justify.

Studies should be planned to limit the demands on people and increase their interest in participation. For example, researchers might select instruments that are valid and reliable but have fewer items to decrease participant burden. The study intervention must be skillfully developed and clearly communicated to individuals to increase their participation in the study. Sufficient data need to be collected on the participants to allow researchers to be familiar with their characteristics and, to the greatest extent possible, the characteristics of those who decline to participate (see Chapter 9).

Interaction of Setting and Intervention

Bias exists in regard to the types of settings and organizations that agree to participate in studies. This bias has been particularly evident in nursing studies. For example, some hospitals, such as those seeking Magnet designation, welcome nursing studies and encourage employed nurses to conduct studies. Others are resistant to the conduct of nursing research. These two types of hospitals may be different in important ways; thus there might be an interaction of setting and intervention that limits the generalizability of the findings.

Different settings may also serve different types of patients or potential study participants. For example, a low-income clinic may have patients with lower health literacy, whereas a clinic that only accepts patients with insurance might have a larger portion of college-educated patients. The intervention and measurement methods to be implemented may interact with the ability to read and comprehend written materials by the patients in different settings and cause variations in the study outcomes. Researchers must consider the characteristics of the settings and patients they serve when making statements about the population to which their findings can be generalized.

Interaction of History and Intervention

The circumstances occurring when a study is conducted might influence the intervention implemented or the outcomes measured, which could affect the generalization of the findings. For example, study participants receiving a supportive intervention to facilitate their dialysis process would probably have altered outcomes if three patients suddenly died as a result of dialysis equipment failure (historical event) during the study. Logically, one can never generalize to the future; however, replicating the study during various time periods strengthens the usefulness of findings over time. In critically appraising studies, you need to consider the effects of nursing practice and societal events that occurred during the period of the reported findings.

Statistical Conclusion Validity

The first step in inferring cause is to determine whether the independent and dependent variables are related. You can determine this relationship through statistical analysis. **Statistical conclusion validity** is concerned with whether the conclusions about relationships or differences drawn from statistical analysis are an accurate reflection of the real world (Grove & Cipher, 2017). The second step is to identify differences between and among groups. There are reasons why false conclusions can be drawn about the presence or absence of a relationship or difference. The reasons for the false conclusions are called threats to statistical conclusion validity (see Table 8.1). This text discusses some of the more common threats to statistical conclusion validity that you might identify in studies, such as low statistical power, unreliable measurement methods, limited intervention fidelity, and extraneous variances in the study setting. Shadish et al. (2002) have provided a more detailed discussion of statistical conclusion validity.

Low Statistical Power

Low statistical power increases the probability of concluding that there is no significant relationship between variables or significant difference between groups when actually there is one, a Type II error. A Type II error is most likely to occur when the sample size is small or when the power of the statistical test to determine differences is low (Cohen, 1988; Grove & Cipher, 2017). You need to ensure that the study has adequate sample size and power to detect relationships and differences. The concepts of sample size, statistical power, and Type II error are discussed in detail in Chapters 9 and 11.

Reliability or Precision of Measurement Methods

The technique of measuring variables must be reliable to reveal true differences. A measure is reliable if it gives the same result each time that the same situation or variable is measured. If a scale used to measure depression is reliable, it should give similar scores when depression is repeatedly measured over a short time period (Waltz et al., 2017). Physiological measures that consistently measure physiological variables are considered precise. For example, a thermometer would be precise if it showed the same reading when tested repeatedly on the same patient within a limited time (see Chapter 10). You need to examine the measurement methods in a study and determine if they are reliable.

Fidelity of the Intervention Implementation

Intervention fidelity ensures that the research intervention is standardized by a protocol and is applied consistently each time it is implemented in a study (Bova et al., 2017; Eymard & Altmiller, 2016). If the method of administering a research intervention varies from one person to another, the chance of detecting a true difference decreases. For example, one data collector might implement the study intervention to the first 20 participants and spend more time with them than was designated by intervention protocol; another data collector might then implement the intervention protocol exactly as was planned to the next 20 participants. Data collectors must be trained to ensure consistent or reliable implementation of a study intervention to prevent threats to the statistical conclusion validity.

Extraneous Variances in the Study Setting

Extraneous variables in complex settings (e.g., clinical units) can influence scores on the dependent variable. These variables increase the difficulty of detecting differences between the experimental and control groups. Consider the activities that occur on a nursing unit. The numbers and variety of staff, patients, health crises, and work patterns merge into a complex arena for the implementation of a study. Any of the dynamics of the unit can influence manipulation of the independent variable or measurement of the dependent variable. You might review the methods section of the study and determine how extraneous variables were controlled in the study setting. This discussion of design validity was presented to assist you in critically appraising the designs in the quantitative studies presented as examples in the next sections.

DESCRIPTIVE DESIGNS

Descriptive studies are designed to gain more information about concepts, variables, or elements in a particular field of study. The purpose of these studies is to provide a picture of a situation as it naturally happens. A descriptive design may be used to develop theories, identify problems with current practice, make judgments about practice, or identify trends of illnesses, illness prevention, and health promotion in selected groups. No manipulation of variables is involved in a descriptive design. Protection against bias in a descriptive design is achieved through: (1) conceptual and operational definitions of variables; (2) sample selection and size; (3) valid and reliable measurement methods; and (4) data collection procedures that might partially control the environment or setting. Descriptive studies differ in level of complexity. Some contain only two variables; others may include multiple variables that are studied over time. You can use the algorithm shown in Fig. 8.2 to determine the type of descriptive design used in a published study. Simple descriptive and comparative descriptive designs are discussed in this chapter. Gray and colleagues (2017) have provided details about additional descriptive designs.

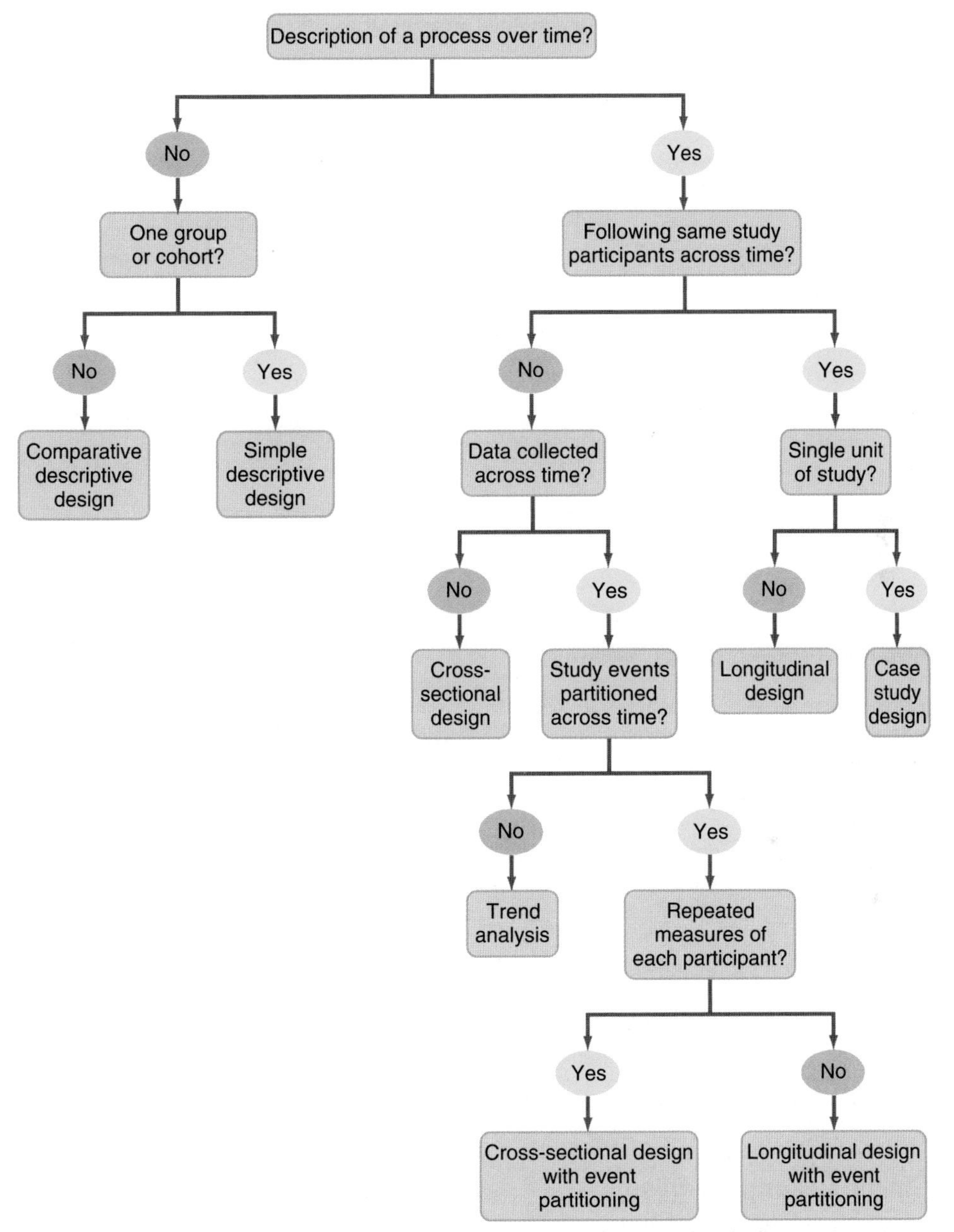

FIG 8.2 Algorithm for determining the type of descriptive design.

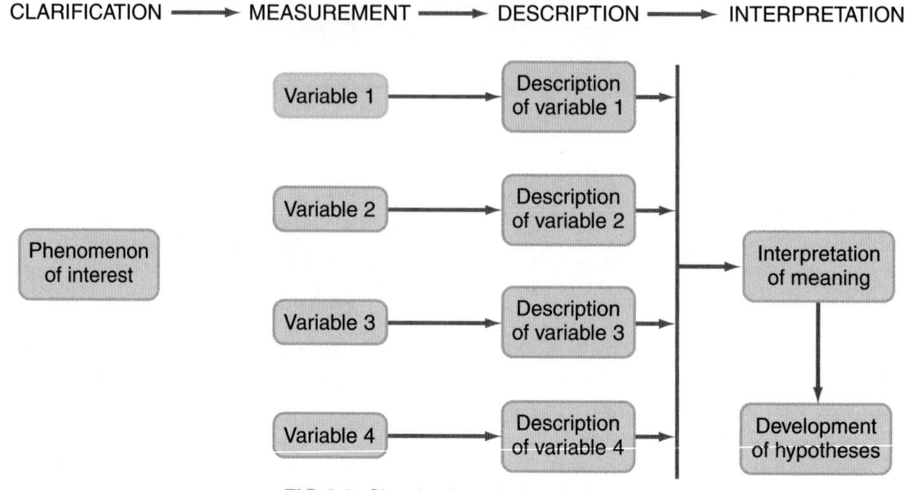

FIG 8.3 Simple descriptive design.

CRITICAL APPRAISAL GUIDELINES

Descriptive and Correlational Designs

The critical appraisal guidelines presented in this section will be applied to the designs from example descriptive and correlational studies. You need to address the following questions when critically appraising descriptive and correlational study designs:

1. Is the study design descriptive or correlational? Review the algorithm in Fig. 8.1 to determine the type of study design.
2. If the study design is descriptive, use the algorithm in Fig. 8.2 to identify the specific type of descriptive design implemented in the study.
3. If the study design is correlational, use the algorithm in Fig. 8.5 to identify the specific type of correlational design implemented in the study.
4. Does the study design address the study purpose and/or objectives or questions?
5. Was the sample appropriate for the study?
6. Were the study variables measured with quality (reliable and valid) measurement methods (see Chapter 10)?
7. Was the data collection process implemented consistently and without bias?

Simple Descriptive Design

A simple descriptive design is used to examine variables in a single sample (Fig. 8.3). This descriptive design includes identifying the variables within a phenomenon of interest, measuring these variables, and describing them. The description of the variables leads to an interpretation of the theoretical meaning of the findings and the development of possible relationships or hypotheses that might guide future correlational or quasi-experimental studies.

Spratling (2017, p. 62) conducted a descriptive study to expand the understanding of healthcare utilization by children with tracheostomies who required medical technology. This study included a simple descriptive design; key aspects of this study's design are presented in Research Example 8.1.

RESEARCH EXAMPLE 8.1

Simple Descriptive Design

Research Study Excerpt

Methods

In this study, a retrospective electronic health record (EHR) review was completed to identify common health problems that led to ED [emergency department] visits and hospitalization, and to create a data abstraction form... Charts were reviewed by the researcher and two trained Graduate Research Assistants [GRAs]...; all had experience with EHRs and medical terminology. The structured data abstraction form was created for the EHR review, and this was reviewed by an expert in technology dependent children and an expert in measurement prior to use (Spratling & Powers, 2017)....

The study sample included the EHRs on 171 children who require medical technology at an outpatient technology dependent pulmonary clinic that were reviewed over a three year period (January 2010–December 2012). Inclusion criteria were active clinic patients (newborn to age 21) who had at least one clinic visit since discharge from the hospital with a tracheostomy...

The study identified common health problems that led to ED visits and hospitalizations, used expert review to categorize these ED visits and hospitalizations as avoidable or unavoidable by expert review, and examined sociodemographic and clinical characteristics that affected the children's ED visits and hospitalizations. Expert review included... a clinic nurse practitioner [NP] with 15 years of experience, and the researcher who has both clinical and research expertise with children who require medical technology. (Spratling, 2017, p. 63)

Critical Appraisal

Spratling (2017) accurately identified their study as descriptive, with a retrospective design that involved EHR review. This simple descriptive design was appropriate to address the purpose and research questions of this study. The sample criteria were relevant to reduce the influence of extraneous variables. The sample size obtained over 3 years was strong (n = 171 children) and without attrition, which increases the representativeness of the sample and internal design validity. However, the setting was limited to only one pulmonary clinic in the South, which decreases the ability to generalize the findings. Consistency in data collection was facilitated by training the GRAs who used a quality data abstraction form developed and reviewed by experts. The structured unbiased collection of data strengthened the construct and statistical conclusion design validity of this study. Determining if ED visits and hospitalizations were avoidable or unavoidable was operationalized by experts in research and in the care of children who required medical technology, strengthening construct design validity (Shadish et al., 2002).

"The findings from this study noted an increased utilization of health care by these children, and identified common symptoms and medical technologies for which caregivers may need interventions, focusing on education in managing symptoms and medical technology prior to presentation to the ED or hospital" (Spratling, 2017, p. 62).

Comparative Descriptive Design

A comparative descriptive design is used to describe variables and examine differences in variables in two or more groups that occur naturally in a setting. The groups might be formed using gender, age, ethnicity and race, educational level, medical diagnosis, and/or severity of illness (Gray et al., 2017). Fig. 8.4 presents a comparative descriptive design's structure.

Mosleh, Eshah, and Almalik (2017, p. 418) conducted a descriptive study "to identify the differences in perceived learning needs between cardiac patients who have undergone major coronary interventions and their nurses." The study participants were obtained by a sample of convenience and included 365 cardiac patients who had either a percutaneous coronary angioplasty (PTCA) or coronary artery bypass graft (CABG) and 166 cardiac nurses. Research Example 8.2 includes key elements of this comparative descriptive design.

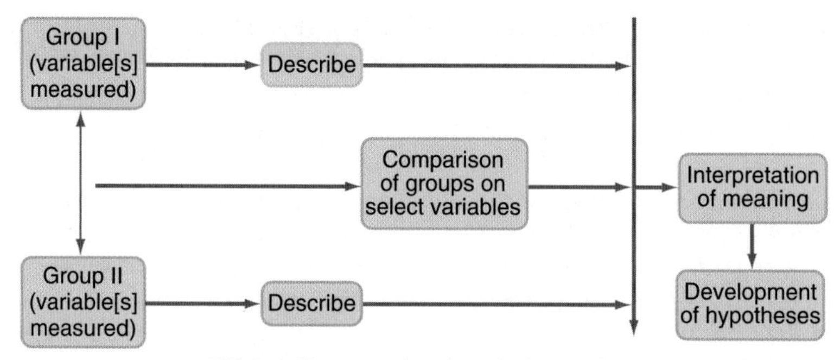

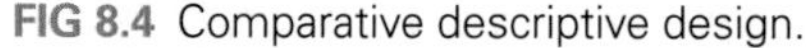
FIG 8.4 Comparative descriptive design.

RESEARCH EXAMPLE 8.2

Comparative Descriptive Design

Research Study Excerpt

Methods

A descriptive comparative design was used to examine the difference in perceived learning needs between cardiac patients who underwent major coronary interventional procedures and the nurses who provided care for them. The survey data were collected from three major hospitals...

Research assistants provided the self-report questionnaire along with verbal information about the study purpose... To ensure accuracy and consistency among the six research assistants, a workshop was held by the main researchers, wherein a full explanation of the study was provided. The steps of data collection were discussed with the assistants and they were trained in dealing with patients' inquiries during the data collection process...

The Patient Learning Needs Scale (PLNS) was used to identify the learning needs of patients who have undergone PTCA or CABG... The PLNS comprises 40 items rated on a five-point Likert scale ranging from 1 (not important) to 5 (extremely important). This scale comprises several subscales corresponding to different types of learning needs, including wound care, medications, daily physical activities, diet, postintervention complications, postintervention care, and risk-factor management... The Cronbach's alpha for PLNS in this study was 0.85; and the Cronbach's alpha for the subscales ranged from 0.72-0.94... A pilot study including 10 patients and five cardiac nurses was conducted to confirm the stability and clarity of the scale's items. (Mosleh et al., 2017, pp. 420–421)

Critical Appraisal

Mosleh and colleagues (2017) clearly identified their study design, which addressed their research purpose and questions. The sample sizes were strong for both patients and nurses and included relevant sample criteria for these populations. The researchers chose to have research assistants collect the data, which reduced the potential for bias and strengthened construct validity (Shadish et al., 2002). The training of the research assistants improved the consistency of the data collected, strengthening the statistical conclusion validity. The learning needs were measured with the PLNS, which was reported as valid from previous research and was reliable for this study population, supporting statistical conclusion validity (Gray et al., 2017). In addition, the pilot study supported the use of this scale with these study participants. In summary, this comparative descriptive design included several strengths that promoted the trustworthiness of the study results and findings.

Mosleh et al. (2017) did find a disparity between the perceptions of patients and nurses on essential learning needs following a cardiac intervention. The researchers recommended that the nurses focus on information about wound care, medications, and postintervention complications before discharge because these were the priority needs of the patients. Education on diet and physical activity needs to be presented later in the patients' recovery process.

CORRELATIONAL DESIGNS

The purpose of a **correlational design** is to examine relationships between or among two or more variables in a single group in a study. This examination can occur at any of several levels—descriptive correlational, in which the researcher can seek to describe a relationship; predictive correlational, in which the researcher can predict relationships among variables; or the model testing design, in which the relationships proposed by a theory are tested simultaneously.

In correlational designs, a large range in the variable scores is necessary to determine the existence of a relationship. Therefore the sample should be large to reflect the full range of scores possible on the variables being measured (Grove & Cipher, 2017). Some study participants should have very high scores and others very low scores, and the scores of the rest should be distributed throughout the possible range.

The algorithm in Fig. 8.5 can be used to identify the specific correlational design included in a study. Sometimes, researchers combine elements of different designs to accomplish their study purpose. For example, researchers might conduct a cross-sectional, descriptive, correlational study design to examine the relationship of body mass index (BMI) to blood lipid levels in early adolescence (ages 13–16 years) and late adolescence (ages 17–19 years). It is important that researchers clearly identify the specific design that they are using in their research report. More details on correlational designs in this algorithm are available from other research sources (Gray et al., 2017; Kerlinger & Lee, 2000).

Descriptive Correlational Design

The purpose of a descriptive correlational design is to describe variables and examine relationships among these variables. Using this design facilitates the identification of many interrelationships in a situation. The study may examine variables in a situation that has already occurred or is currently occurring. Researchers make no attempt to control or manipulate the situation. As with descriptive studies, variables must be clearly identified and defined conceptually and operationally (see Chapter 5). As shown in Fig. 8.6, the variables are measured, described, and examined for relationships. The findings from descriptive correlational studies are interpreted and provide the basis for further research.

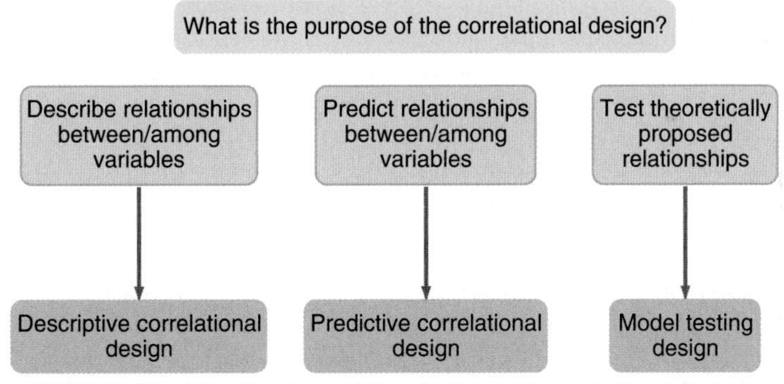

FIG 8.5 Algorithm for determining the type of correlational design.

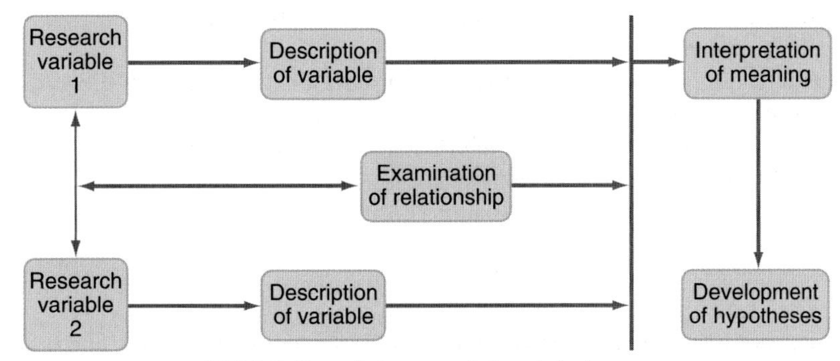

FIG 8.6 Descriptive correlational design.

Branson, Loftin, Hadley, Hartin, and Devkota (2016, p. 185) conducted a correlational study to "explore the relationship between attendance and course grade in a prenursing course." The sample included 445 prenursing students' records for those enrolled in a required skills and safety course in a Texas university. Research Example 8.3 includes key aspects of this descriptive correlational design.

RESEARCH EXAMPLE 8.3

Descriptive Correlational Design

Research Study Excerpt

Methods

For this project, a descriptive-correlational design was used. A retrospective analysis of prenursing student sign-in-sheets collected over a 4-year period was accomplished, allowing us to explore the relationship between the final course outcome and attendance. For the purposes of this study, course outcome was operationalized as the final course grade, and course attendance was operationalized as the percentage of classes attended during the semester that course content was presented. At this university, each semester consists of 15 weeks, and course content was delivered via a variety of means during 13 of the 15 weeks. The first week of each semester was generally considered an introductory week with no course content presented, and the final week was devoted to the final course examination... Thus, there were 13 course sign-in sheets analyzed per class for each semester and included in this study... This course is available to sophomore-level prenursing students. Neither attendance nor participation during class was considered mandatory for this course, and neither was considered for grading purposes. (Branson et al., 2016, p.186)

Critical Appraisal

Branson and colleagues (2016) identified their specific study design, which was relevant for their study purpose and research questions. A nonrandom sample of convenience (students in a prenursing course) was used, which is common for descriptive and correlational studies (Gray et al., 2017). Nonrandom sampling methods decrease the sample's representativeness of the population; however, the sample size was strong (n = 445) and produced significant results (no Type II error; Grove & Cipher, 2017). The variables of final grade and course attendance were clearly operationalized, promoting construct design validity (Shadish et al., 2002). The course grade came from the student record, and the process for obtaining course attendance was consistently implemented for one course over 4 years, supporting statistical conclusion validity. The study was limited to one setting, but data collection over several years increased the internal validity of the design. The potential for bias was decreased by not requiring course attendance or including it as part of the student's grade. The design of this study was strong, and the results and findings generated seem to be representative of the study population.

Branson and colleagues (2016) found a significant positive relationship between course grade and class attendance (r_{443} = 0.54; $p < 0.001$; Grove & Cipher, 2017). These study results support the long-held faculty belief that class attendance has a positive impact on final course grades. These researchers recommended that nursing advisors and faculty stress the importance of class attendance on final course grades and on successful program progression.

Predictive Correlational Design

The purpose of a **predictive correlational design** is to predict the value of one variable based on the values obtained for another variable or variables. Prediction is one approach for examining causal relationships between variables. Because causal phenomena are being examined, the terms *dependent* and *independent* are used to describe the variables. The variable to be predicted is classified as the dependent variable, and all other variables are independent or predictor variables. A predictive correlational design study attempts to predict the level of a dependent variable from the measured values of the independent variables. For example, the dependent variable of medication adherence could be predicted using the independent variables of age, number of medications, and medication knowledge of patients with heart failure. The independent variables that are most effective in prediction are significantly correlated with the dependent variable but are not highly correlated with other independent variables used in the study (Grove & Cipher, 2017). The predictive correlational design structure is presented in Fig. 8.7. Predictive designs require the development of a theory-based hypothesis proposing variables expected to predict the dependent variable effectively. Researchers then use regression analysis to test the hypothesis (see Chapter 11).

De Santis, Hauglum, Deleon, Provencio-Vasquez, and Rodriguez (2017) conducted a correlational study to determine if human immunodeficiency virus (HIV) risk perception and HIV knowledge are predictive of sexual risk behaviors in transgender women. Research Example 8.4 includes major elements of this predictive correlational design.

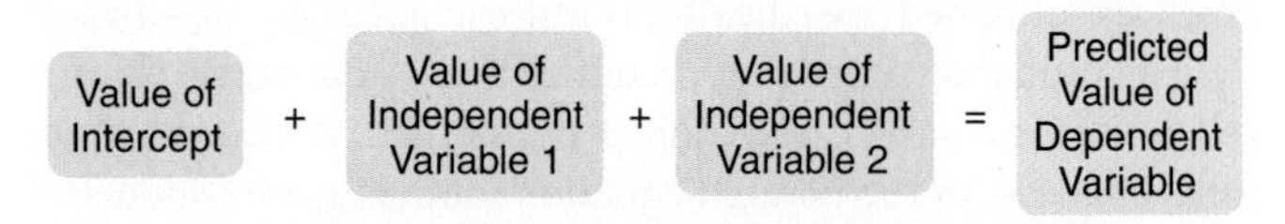

FIG 8.7 Predictive correlational design.

RESEARCH EXAMPLE 8.4

Predictive Correlational Design

Research Study Excerpt

Methods

Design and Sample

This pilot study used a descriptive correlation design to study health issues among a sample of MTF [male-to-female] transgender women living in South Florida (n = 50), an area with a large lesbian, gay, bisexual, and transgender (LGBT) population... Participants were recruited from agencies that serve transgender women such as HIV testing and counseling centers, mental health counseling centers, and a university-based gender reassignment surgery clinic.... After obtaining informed consent, participants were given the study's self-administered instruments to complete on paper...

Measures

HIV risk perception was measured using the four-item Perceived Risk for HIV Infection scale... While the instrument has not been previously used with transgender women, it has an overall reliability coefficient of .78... HIV knowledge was measured using the 18-item HIV knowledge Questionnaire-18... Although the instrument has not been previously used with transgender women, reliability coefficients of .76 to .94 have been reported... Sexual risk behaviors were measured using Behavior Risk Assessment Tool (BRAT), a clinical tool that assesses an individual's risk of HIV infection... This instrument has not been used in research with transgender women...

Analytic Strategy

Correlation coefficients were used to examine the relationship among the continuous variables of HIV risk perception, HIV knowledge, and sexual risk behaviors. A regression analysis was used to determine variables associated with sexual risk behaviors. (De Santis et al., 2017, pp. 211–212)

Critical Appraisal

De Santis and colleagues (2017) did not identify their study design as predictive correlational. However, the focus of this study was to predict the sexual risk behaviors of transgender women, and the results were generated by regression analysis (Grove & Cipher, 2017). The sample size was small for a correlational study, which resulted in low statistical power and contributed to the nonsignificant findings (Type II error; Gray et al., 2017). Because sample size is often smaller in pilot studies, additional research is needed for this understudied population. The measurement methods were a threat to construct validity because they had not been used with a transgender population

Continued

RESEARCH EXAMPLE 8.4—cont'd

and a threat to statistical conclusion validity because the researchers did not provide the reliability coefficients for the scales in this study. Consistency in data collection is unknown because participants self-administered the study questionnaires, threatening construct validity. De Santis et al. (2017) found that HIV risk perception and HIV knowledge were neither significantly correlated with nor predictive of sexual risk behaviors in transgender women. The researchers recommended further study with a larger sample size to examine factors contributing to sexual risk behaviors in this population. The design validity needs to be strengthened in future studies.

Model Testing Design

Some studies are designed specifically to test the accuracy of a hypothesized causal model (see Chapter 7). The model testing design requires that all concepts relevant to the model be measured and the relationships among these concepts examined. A large heterogeneous sample is required. Correlational analyses and structured equation modeling are conducted to determine the relationships among the model concepts, and the results are presented in the framework model for the study. This type of design is very complex; this text provides only an introduction to a model testing design implemented by Battistelli, Portoghese, Galletta, and Pohl (2013).

Battistelli and colleagues (2013) developed and tested a theoretical model to examine turnover intentions of nurses working in hospitals. The concepts of work-family conflict, job satisfaction, community embeddedness, and organizational affective commitment were identified as predictive of nurse turnover intention. The researchers collected data on these concepts using a sample of 440 nurses from a public hospital. The analysis of study data identified significant relationships among all concepts in the model. The results of this study are presented in Fig. 8.8 and indicate the importance of these concepts in predicting nurse turnover intention.

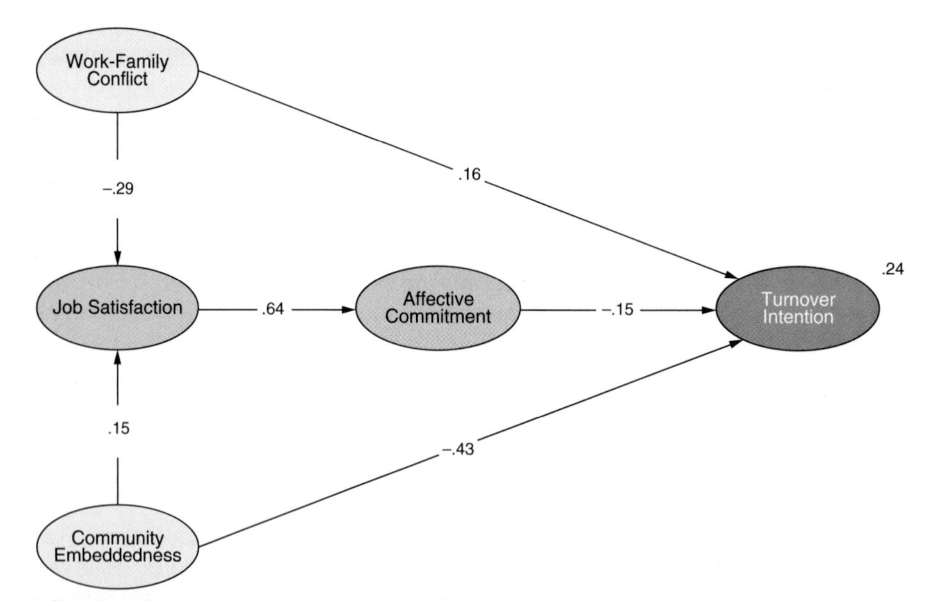

FIG 8.8 Results of the structural equation modeling analysis of the hypothesized model of turnover intention on the cross-validation sample (n = 440, standardized path loadings; P <0.05; two-tailed). (From Battistelli, A., Portoghese, I., Galletta, M., & Pohl, S. [2013]. Beyond the tradition: Test of an integrative conceptual model on nurse turnover. *International Nursing Review, 60*[1], 109.)

ELEMENTS OF DESIGNS EXAMINING CAUSALITY

Quasi-experimental and experimental designs are implemented in studies to obtain an accurate representation of cause and effect by the most efficient means. That is, the design should provide the greatest amount of control, with the least error possible. The effects of some extraneous variables are controlled in a study by using specific sampling criteria, a structured independent variable or intervention, and a highly controlled setting. An RCT is a type of experimental design often considered to be one of the strongest designs to examine cause and effect (Schulz, Altman, & Moher, 2010). RCTs are discussed later in this chapter. The essential elements of research to examine causality are:

- Random assignment of study participants to groups
- Precisely defined independent variable or intervention
- Researcher-controlled manipulation of the intervention
- Researcher control of the experimental situation and setting
- Inclusion of a control or comparison group in the study
- Clearly identified sampling criteria (see Chapter 9)
- Carefully measured dependent or outcome variables (see Chapter 10; Waltz et al., 2017)

Examining Interventions in Nursing Studies

In studies examining causality, investigators develop an **intervention** that is expected to result in differences in posttest measures between the treatment and control groups. Interventions may be physiological, psychosocial, educational, or a combination of these. The therapeutic intervention implemented in a nursing study needs to be carefully designed, clearly described, and appropriately linked to the outcomes (dependent variables) in the study. The intervention needs to be provided consistently to all study participants. The research report should document **intervention fidelity,** which includes a detailed description of the essential elements of the intervention and its consistent implementation during the study (Bova et al., 2017; Eymard & Altmiller, 2016). Sometimes, researchers provide a table of the intervention content and/or the protocol used to implement the intervention to each participant consistently. Researchers should indicate who implemented the intervention and what training was conducted to ensure consistent intervention implementation. Some studies document the monitoring of intervention fidelity (completeness and consistency of the intervention implementation) during the conduct of the study (Carpenter et al., 2013). For example, Bova et al. (2017, p. 54) examined the intervention fidelity for their study of 191 parents of young children newly diagnosed with type 2 diabetes, as indicated in the following quote: "Intervention fidelity was measured for both the intervention and control condition by direct observation, self-report of interventionist delivery, and parent participant receipt of educational information. Intervention fidelity data were analyzed after 50%, 75%, and 100% of the participants had been recruited and compared by group (treatment and control) and research site." This intervention monitoring allowed Bova et al., 2017 to make corrections as needed in their multisite study.

Spiva and colleagues (2017) conducted a quasi-experimental study to examine the effectiveness of an evidence-based practice (EBP) nurse mentor training program on clinical nurses' delivery of EBP. These researchers implemented a multifaceted intervention to train the EBP nurse mentors to prepare clinical nurses to incorporate research into their clinical practice. The components of their formal educational program (intervention) are detailed in Research Example 8.5.

RESEARCH EXAMPLE 8.5

Nursing Intervention

Research Study Excerpt

Interventions

A project charter and education curriculum were created by the study researchers, chief nursing officer (CNO) and a chief learning officer all knowledgeable in the principles of EBP and leadership development... Clinical nurse leaders, clinical nurse specialists, and educators received training to prepare them to serve as EBP mentors. Mentor training included didactic instruction and discussion, in-person training, and online interactive webinars (Table 1) to prepare a foundation to support and foster EBP... Clinical nurses training included four 30-minute online modules designed to equip nurses with the tools and resources to translate evidence to practice and implement an EBP project (Table 2). (Spiva et al., 2017, pp. 186–187)

TABLE 1 Educational Intervention Objectives for Nurse Mentor Training

- Introduction to EBP
  - Define and discuss the origins of EBP, QI, and research.
- Guidelines for implementation
  - Describe the Johns Hopkins EBP model and PET (practice question, evidence, and translation).
  - Describe how to develop an answerable practice (EBP) question.
- Search for evidence
  - Describe how to search for evidence and available resources.
- Appraisal of evidence
  - Review tools to critically appraise evidence (both research and nonresearch).
  - Discuss essential components of a research article.
  - Evaluate research and nonresearch articles using appraisal tools (independent study).
- Summarizing the evidence and beyond
  - Provide an overview of frameworks to conduct EBP, QI, and research.
  - Describe how to create a plan for translation, secure resources, and common evaluation methods.
- Evaluate outcomes
  - Provide an EBP project example from start to finish, including dissemination.
  - Describe how to move a project from practice to abstract to presentation to publication.
  - Identify the steps needed for poster and podium presentation development.
  - List components of an abstract, poster, and podium presentation.
  - Identify publication options.

EBP, Evidence-based practice; *QI*, quality improvement.

From Spiva, L., Hart, P. L., Patrick, S., Waggoner, J., Jackson, C., & Threatt, J. L. (2017). Effectiveness of an evidence-based practice nurse mentor training program. *Worldviews on Evidence-Based Nursing, 14*(3), 185.

TABLE 2 Computer-based learning module intervention objectives for clinical nurse training

Computer-Based Learning Module I (January 2015)
• Overview of EBP • How to develop an EBP question
Computer-Based Learning Module II (March 2015) • Overview of frameworks to conduct EBP, QI, and research • An overview of available evidence resources, how to search for evidence, and how to demonstrate appraisal and translation of evidence
Computer-Based Learning Module III (April 2015) • An overview of frameworks to conduct EBP, QI, and research • How to create a plan for translation, secure resources, and review common evaluation methods to evaluate outcomes • Review of a completed EBP project
Computer-Based Learning Module IV (May 2015) • How to move an EBP project from practice to abstract to presentation

EBP, Evidence-based practice; *QI*, quality improvement.
From Spiva, L., Hart, P. L., Patrick, S., Waggoner, J., Jackson, C., & Threatt, J. L. (2017). Effectiveness of an evidence-based practice nurse mentor training program. *Worldviews on Evidence-Based Nursing, 14*(3), 185.

Critical Appraisal

The educational programs were developed and implemented by experts in the area of EBP and leadership. Tables 1 and 2 detailed the content and protocol for training the nurse mentors and clinical nurses. The implementation of the educational programs was structured and consistently implemented by experts. The structure of the nurse mentor training and the computer-based modules for the clinical nurses promoted intervention fidelity. Spiva et al. (2017) used a quasi-experimental design, which is presented as an example later in this chapter.

Experimental and Control or Comparison Groups

The group of participants who received the study intervention is referred to as the **intervention, treatment,** or **experimental group**. The group that is not exposed to the intervention is referred to as the **control** or **comparison group**. In some disciplines, the control groups receive no care or action, but this is not possible in most nursing studies because patients must receive care. For example, it would be unethical not to provide preoperative education to a patient in the control group of a study. Furthermore, in many studies, just spending time with patients or having them participate in activities that they consider beneficial may cause a change in the dependent variable. Therefore nursing studies often include a comparison group receiving a nursing action so that both groups (intervention and comparison) receive time and attention. This design structure allows the researchers to differentiate between the effect of time and attention and the effect of the intervention (Gray et al., 2017).

The standard nursing action is the care that the patients would receive if a study were not being conducted. Researchers should describe in detail the standard nursing care that the control or comparison group receives so that the study can be adequately appraised. Because the quality of this standard care is likely to vary considerably among study participants, variance in the control or comparison group is likely to be high and needs to be considered in the discussion of findings. Some researchers provide the experimental group with both the intervention and standard nursing care to control the effect of standard care in the study.

QUASI-EXPERIMENTAL DESIGNS

Use of a **quasi-experimental design** facilitates the search for knowledge and examination of causality in situations in which complete control is not possible. This type of design was developed to control as many threats to validity (see Table 8.1) as possible in a situation in which some of the components of true experimental design were lacking (Shadish et al., 2002). Most studies with quasi-experimental designs have samples that were not selected randomly, and there is less control of the study intervention, extraneous variables, and setting. Most quasi-experimental studies include a sample of convenience, in which the participants are included in the study because they are in the right place at the right time (see Chapter 9). The participants selected are usually randomly assigned to receive the experimental intervention or standard care. The group that receives standard care is usually referred to as a comparison group versus a control group, which would receive no treatment or standard care (Shadish et al., 2002). However, the terms *control group* and *comparison group* are frequently used interchangeably in nursing studies.

Random assignment of participants from the original sample to either the intervention or comparison group promotes internal design validity. Occasionally, comparison and interventional groups may evolve naturally. For example, groups may include study participants who choose to be in the intervention group and those who choose not to receive the intervention as the comparison group. These groups cannot be considered equivalent because the participants who choose to be in the comparison group probably differ in important ways from those who select to be in the intervention group. For example, if researchers were implementing an intervention of a structured exercise program to promote weight loss, the participants should not be allowed to select whether they are in the intervention group receiving the exercise program or the comparison group receiving standard care. Participants' self-selecting to be in the intervention or comparison group is a threat to the internal design validity of a study.

Quasi-experimental designs have varying levels of control of the sampling process, group assignment, intervention, setting, and extraneous variables. The algorithm in Fig. 8.9 identifies a variety of quasi-experimental designs so you can identify the type of quasi-experimental design in a study. More details about specific designs identified in this algorithm are available from other sources (Gray et al., 2017; Shadish et al., 2002).

Pretest and Posttest Designs With Comparison Group

Quasi-experimental study designs vary widely. The most frequently used design in social science research is the untreated comparison group design, with a pretest and posttest (Fig. 8.10). With this design, the researchers have a group of participants who received the experimental intervention and a comparison group of participants who received standard care.

Another commonly used design is the posttest-only design with a comparison group, shown in Fig. 8.11. This design is used in situations in which a pretest is not possible. For example, if the researcher is examining differences in the amount of pain that a study participant feels during a painful procedure, and a nursing intervention is used to reduce pain for participants in the experimental group, it might not be possible (or meaningful) to pretest the amount of pain before the procedure. This design has a number of threats to validity because of the lack of a pretest (Shadish et al., 2002).

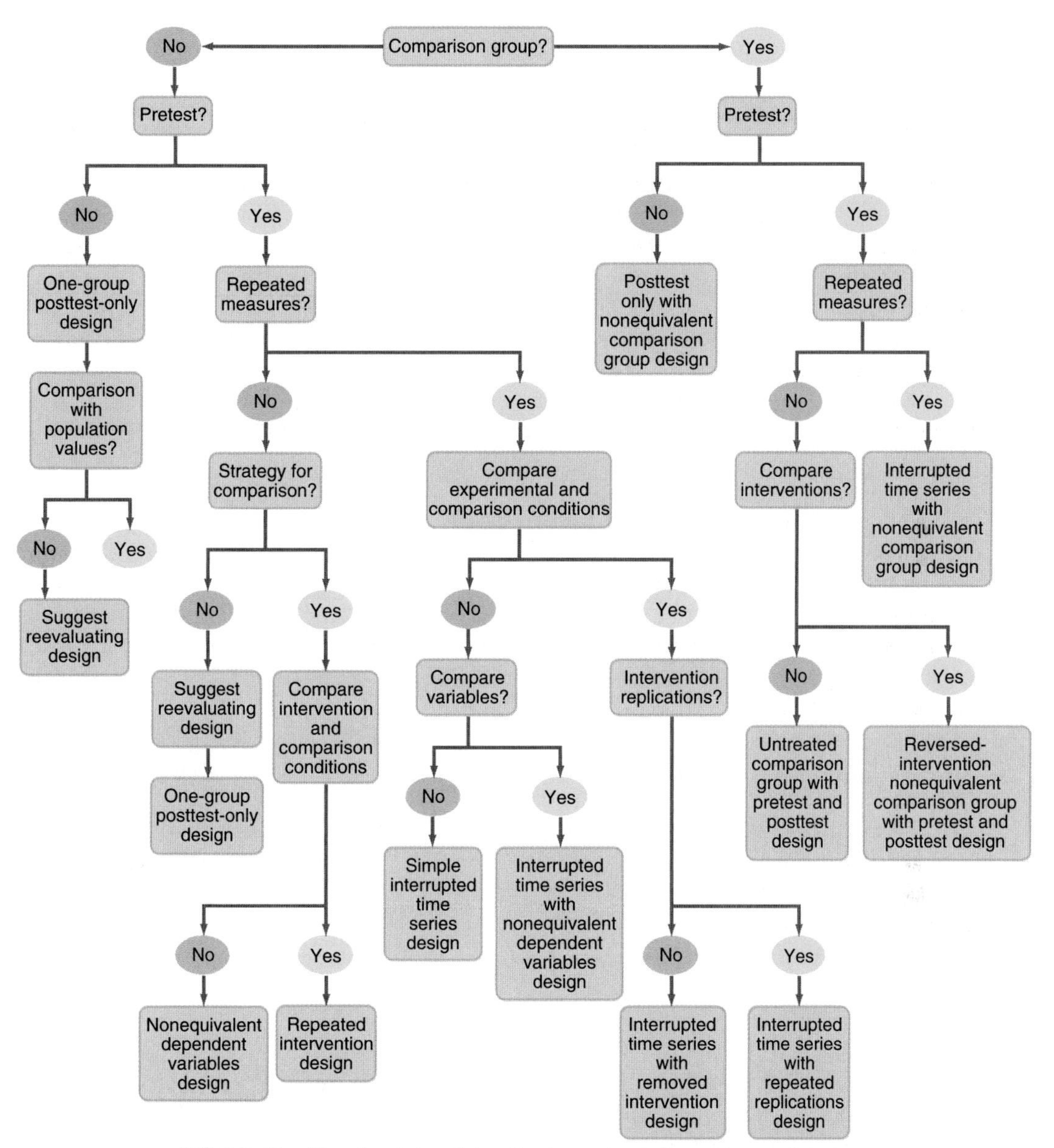

FIG 8.9 Algorithm for determining the type of quasi-experimental design.

Spiva and colleagues (2017) conducted a quasi-experimental study to examine the effects of an EBP nurse mentor training program (see Table 1) and clinical nurse module intervention (see Table 2) on the outcomes related to EBP. These two interventions were introduced in the previous section, and we encourage you to locate this article on the website for this text and critically appraise the design of this study. The critical appraisal of this study was conducted using the Guidelines for Critically Appraising Quasi-Experimental and Experimental Designs.

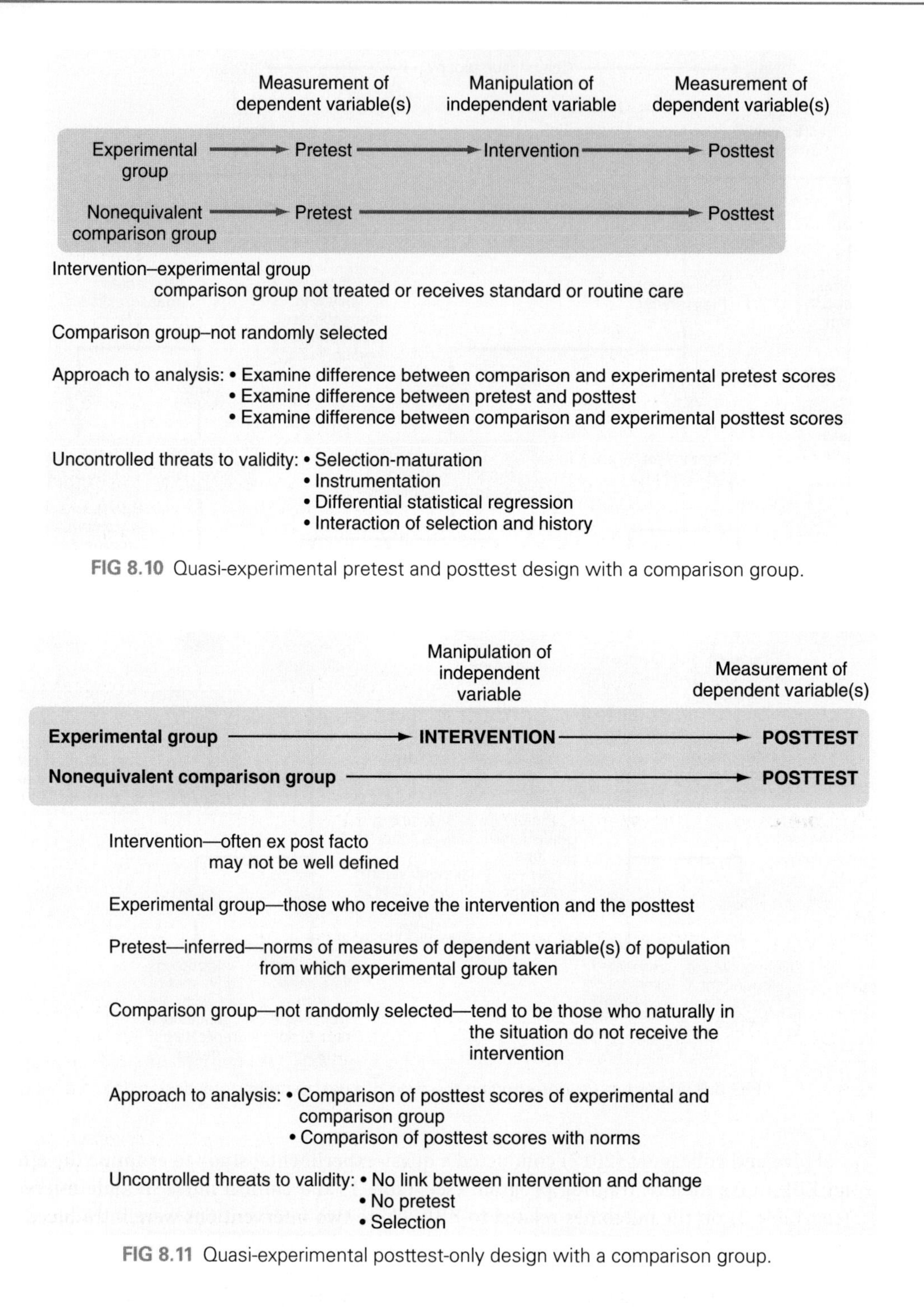

FIG 8.11 Quasi-experimental posttest-only design with a comparison group.

CRITICAL APPRAISAL GUIDELINES

Quasi-Experimental and Experimental Designs

When critically appraising the design of a quasi-experimental or experimental study, you need to address the following questions:

1. Is the study design quasi-experimental or experimental? Review the algorithm in Fig. 8.1 to determine the type of study design.
2. Identify the specific type of quasi-experimental or experimental design used in the study. Review the algorithm in Fig. 8.9 for the types of quasi-experimental study designs and the algorithm in Fig. 8.12 for the types of experimental designs.
3. What were the strengths and threats to validity (construct validity, internal validity, external validity, and statistical conclusion validity) in the study (see Table 8.1)? Review the methods section and limitations identified in the discussion section of the study report for ideas.
4. Which elements were controlled and which elements could have been controlled to improve the study design? Review the sampling criteria, sample size, assignment of participants to groups, and study setting.
5. Was the study intervention described in detail? Was a protocol developed to ensure consistent or reliable implementation of the intervention with each participant throughout the study? Did the study report indicate who implemented the intervention? If more than one person implemented the intervention, how were they trained to ensure consistency in the delivery of the treatment? Was intervention fidelity achieved in the study (Bova et al., 2017; Eymard & Altmiller, 2016; Murphy & Gutman, 2012)?
6. Were the study dependent variables measured with reliable and valid measurement methods (Waltz et al., 2017)?

The study design of Spiva et al. (2017) was very complex, so only selected content from the methods section of their study is presented in Research Example 8.6.

RESEARCH EXAMPLE 8.6

Quasi-Experimental Pretest-Posttest Design With a Comparison Group

Research Study Excerpt

Methods

Design

A two-group, pretest-posttest, quasi-experimental, interventional design was used...

Measures

The Evidence-Based Nursing Questionnaire was used to measure conditions that impede or sustain evidence-based nursing. The questionnaire has undergone validity and reliability testing. In our sample, subscales used included Cronbach's alpha coefficients of .87 total scale, .80 for organizational support (readiness), .92 nurses' beliefs and attitudes of research evidence, .79 EBP skills, and .80 nurses' knowledge of research language and statistics...

Confidence scale was used... to measure nurses' perceived confidence in their knowledge and ability to implement EBP. Higher mean scores indicate a higher perception of confidence. Content validity was established by five expert nurses knowledgeable in the field of EBP and staff education... The content validity index was .90. In a previous pilot study, the Cronbach's alpha coefficient was .94 and in this sample .96.....

The 29-item Barriers to Research Utilization Scale was used to measure perceived barriers to research utilization... This scale has undergone extensive testing and is deemed reliable and valid. In our study, Cronbach's alpha coefficients were total scale .96, .85 communication, .90 adopter, .89 organization, and .87 innovation. (Spiva et al., 2017, p. 184)

Continued

RESEARCH EXAMPLE 8.4—cont'd

Sample and Recruitment

A convenience sample of registered nurses and nurse mentors working in a five-hospital integrated nonprofit healthcare system located in the Southeast were recruited. Recruitment pool included 1,916 nurses... Sixty-six (66) mentors participated and completed the surveys... Initially, 793 [clinical nurses] completed the presurvey and module one. The final sample included 367 who completed the pre- and post-surveys and all modules. (Spiva et al., 2017, p. 187)

Critical Appraisal

Spiva and colleagues (2017) identified the specific quasi-experimental design used in their study, which addressed the study aims. However, the study would have been stronger if hypotheses had been developed to direct the study. The sample of convenience decreased the representativeness of the population but the setting included five hospitals, which increased representativeness. The sampling criteria were not clearly addressed in the study, and the nurses were not randomized into groups, resulting in threats to internal design validity. No attrition occurred from the nurse mentor group, but 426 (54%) of the clinical nurses dropped out of the study after the first module, resulting in possible threats to internal and statistical conclusion validity.

The instruments used in this study had reliability and validity from previous research and had strong reliability (most Cronbach alphas were >0.8) in this study, resulting in construct and statistical conclusion design validity. The structured interventions for the nurse mentors and clinical nurses were developed by experts and documented in the research report (see Tables 1 and 2). A historical event of implementing a new electronic medical record during the study delayed the training of the nurse mentors, which in turn delayed the training of the clinical nurses. Spiva et al. (2017) thought this delay probably caused the high attrition for the clinical nurses. The researchers noted that the threats to design validity might have altered the true effects of the interventions, and further study is needed. However, Spiva et al. (2017, p. 183) concluded that "EBP mentors are effective in educating and supporting nurses in evidence-based care. Leaders should use a multifaceted approach to build and sustain EBP, including developing a critical mass of EBP mentors to work with point of care staff." This type of study promotes EBP in nursing to ensure quality and safe care (Quality and Safety Education for Nurses [QSEN, 2014]; Sherwood & Barnsteiner, 2017).

EXPERIMENTAL DESIGNS

A variety of experimental designs, some relatively simple and others very complex, have been developed for studies focused on examining causality. In some cases, researchers may combine characteristics of more than one design to meet the needs of their study. Names of designs vary from one text to another. When reading and critically appraising a published study, determine the author's name for the design (some authors do not name the specific design used), and/or read the description of the design to determine the type of design used in the study. Use the algorithm shown in Fig. 8.12 to determine the type of experimental design used in a study. More details about the specific designs identified in Fig. 8.12 are available from other sources (Gray et al., 2017; Shadish et al., 2002).

Classic Experimental Pretest and Posttest Designs With Experimental and Control Groups

A common experimental design used in healthcare studies is the pretest-posttest design with experimental and control groups (Campbell & Stanley, 1963; Shadish et al., 2002). This design is shown in Fig. 8.13; it is similar to the quasi-experimental design in Fig. 8.10, except that the experimental

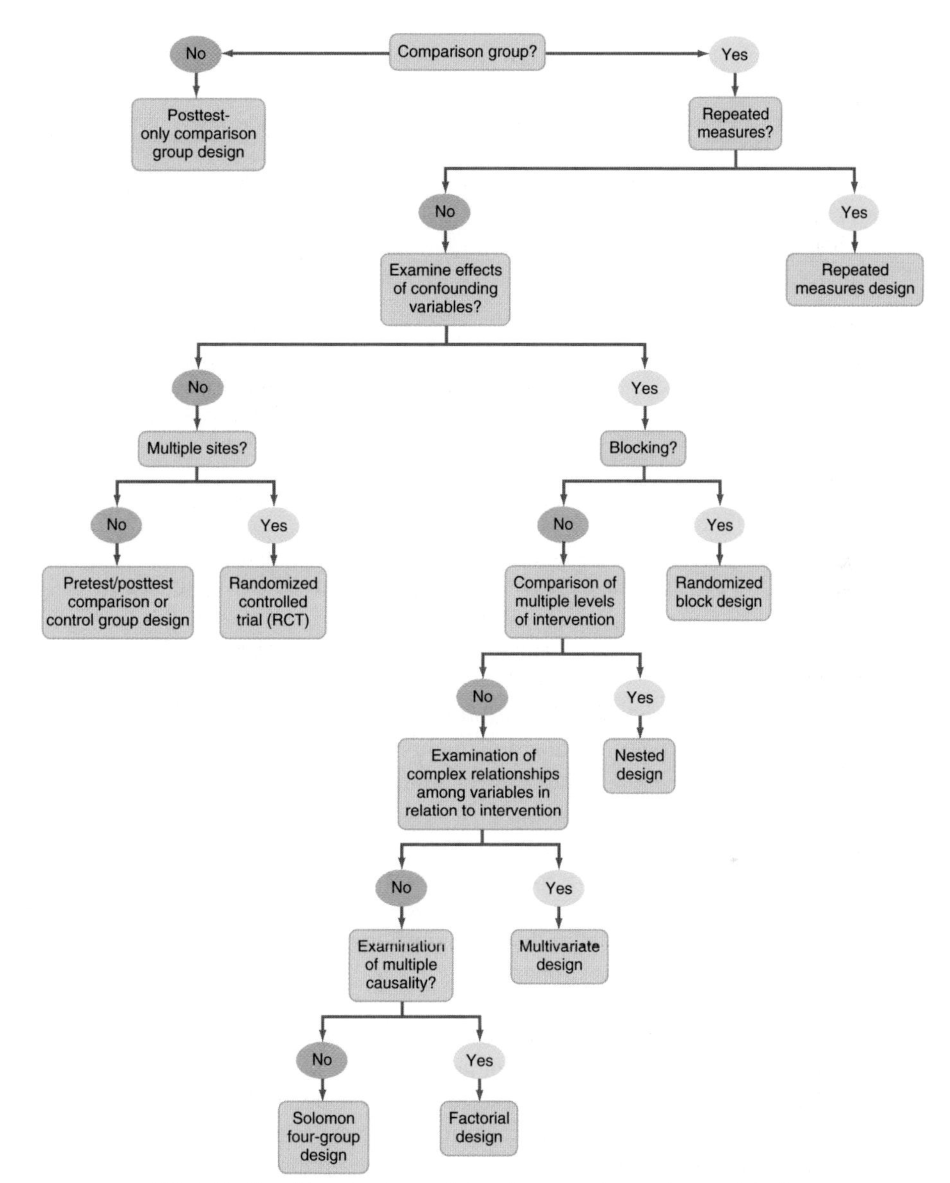

FIG 8.12 Algorithm for determining the type of experimental design.

study is more tightly controlled in the areas of intervention, setting, measurement, and/or extraneous variables, resulting in fewer threats to design validity. The experimental design is stronger if the initial sample is randomly selected; however, most healthcare studies do not include a random sample but do randomly assign participants to the experimental and control groups. Most studies in nursing use the quasi-experimental designs shown in Fig. 8.9 because of the inability to control selected extraneous and environmental variables.

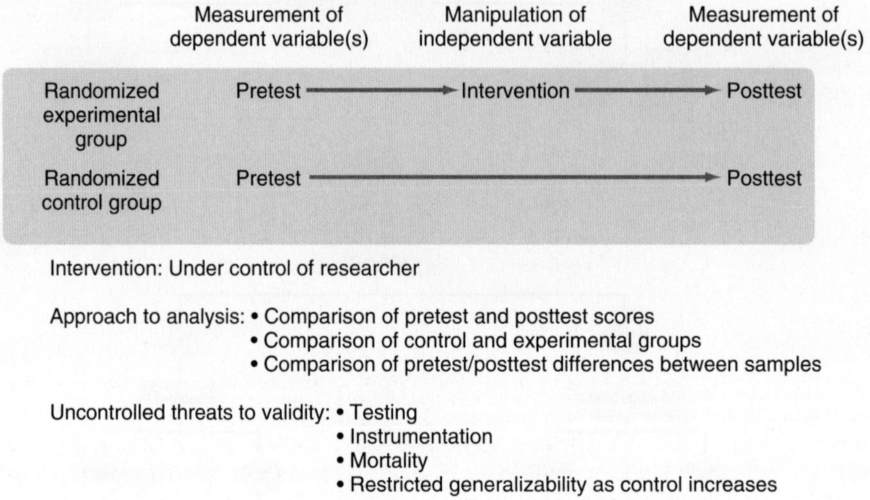

	Measurement of dependent variable(s)	Manipulation of independent variable	Measurement of dependent variable(s)
Randomized experimental group	Pretest →	Intervention →	Posttest
Randomized control group	Pretest →	→	Posttest

Intervention: Under control of researcher

Approach to analysis:
- Comparison of pretest and posttest scores
- Comparison of control and experimental groups
- Comparison of pretest/posttest differences between samples

Uncontrolled threats to validity:
- Testing
- Instrumentation
- Mortality
- Restricted generalizability as control increases

FIG 8.13 Experimental pretest-posttest control group design.

Multiple groups (both intervention and control) can be used to great advantage in experimental designs. For example, one control group might receive no treatment, another control group might receive standard care, and another control group might receive a placebo or intervention with no effect, like a sugar pill in a drug study. Each one of multiple experimental groups can receive a variation of the intervention, such as a different frequency, intensity, or duration of nursing care actions. For example, a different frequency, intensity, or duration of massage treatments might be implemented in a study to determine their effect(s) on patients' back pain. These additions greatly increase the generalizability of study findings when the sample is representative of the target population and the sample size is strong.

Posttest-Only With Control Group Design

The experimental posttest-only control group design is also frequently used in healthcare studies when a pretest is not possible or appropriate. This design is similar to the design in Fig. 8.13, with the pretest omitted. The characteristics of the experimental and control groups are usually examined at the start of the study to ensure that the groups are similar. The lack of a pretest does, however, increase the potential for error that might affect the findings. Additional research is recommended before generalization of findings.

McWilliams, Malecha, Langford, and Clutter (2017, p. 154) conducted an experimental study to examine "the effectiveness of cooperative team learning compared with independent learning when used with nursing students who are learning intravenous (IV) catheter insertion using a haptic IV simulator." Two convenience samples ($n = 180$) of junior-level nursing students attending the fall and spring semester (2015–2016) at a university in southeast Texas were randomized into four groups (A, B, C, and D). Participants from groups A, B, and C were used to make up each cooperative learning team, and group D participants included the independent learners. The study attrition was small ($n = 6$; 3.3%). The researchers conducted their study with a posttest-only experimental design that is presented in Research Example 8.7.

RESEARCH EXAMPLE 8.7

Experimental Posttest-Only Control Group Design

Research Study Excerpt

Methodology

A posttest-only experimental research design was used to evaluate the effectiveness of cooperative team learning compared with independent learning with nursing students while using the haptic IV simulator. The initial performance score and the number of attempts to earn a passing performance score on the haptic IV simulator (score of 85 or better) were used to examine differences between the four-student group assignments.

To increase the reliability of the study, a researcher-designed procedural checklist, including a script, was utilized. The goal of the checklist was to ensure that the primary investigator (PI) was consistent with all interactions with the students from random assignment and sequencing to instructions regarding procedures, use of assigned usernames/passwords, reiterating that grades earned on the simulator were not connected to their course, and the language needed to describe how the cooperative learning teams were to work together.

The Virtual Intravenous Simulator by Laerdal Corporation was designed to support learning of IV catheter insertion. The simulator includes an IV catheter/hub assembly and an interface that allows students to palpate a vein, stretch the skin, and feel resistance during venipuncture. Additionally, during the simulated cannulation, a computer screen provides immediate feedback related to bleeding, bruising, and swelling. (McWilliams et al., 2017, p. 156)

Procedure

On the day of their haptic IV simulation, the IV simulation cluster arrived in the nursing skills laboratory, and each learner was given an envelope with a group assignment (A, B, C, or D) listed on the outside... An independent learner (group assignment D) was brought to the first haptic IV simulator. After signing into the IV simulator, the independent learner was instructed to follow the instructions in his/hers envelope and to view the IV tutorial. The tutorial informed the learner how to use the IV simulator... The cooperative team of learners (group assignments A, B, C) was escorted to the second haptic IV simulator. The PI reviewed the instructions in the team's envelope and presented information on how the team must work together on the IV simulator until all team members completed the task...

For this study, the initial performance score earned by each learner on the haptic IV simulator, and the number of attempts to earn a passing performance score were recorded as the dependent variables. The initial performance scores were obtained from the haptic IV simulator's computer printout. The number of attempts to earn a passing performance score was obtained by logging into the computer system of the simulator and counting the number of attempts required by each learner. (McWilliams et al., 2017, p. 157)

Critical Appraisal

McWilliams and colleagues (2017) identified their specific experimental design which addressed the study purpose and hypotheses. The sample of convenience and the use of only one university for the study setting decreased the sample's representativeness of the nursing student population. However, the sample size was strong, attrition was low (3.3%), and the results were significant, indicating strength in internal and statistical conclusion validity. The random assignment of participants to the cooperative and independent learning groups was presented in detail, strengthening internal and external design validity (see Table 8.1; Shadish et al., 2002).

The researchers promoted intervention fidelity by using a procedural checklist and script (statistical conclusion validity; Eymard & Altmiller, 2016), and implemented the intervention using a quality IV simulator (external validity). McWilliams et al. (2017) clearly operationalized their study dependent variables—performance score earned and number of attempts to earn a passing score—that were measured using the simulator's computer. These computer-generated measures ensured the accuracy of the data collected and the construct validity of the design. The detailed control of the intervention, setting, and data collection process are consistent with implementing a quality, experimental study design (Gray et al., 2017; Shadish et al., 2002).

McWilliams and colleagues (2017, p. 154) found that the "cooperative team members performed better with fewer attempts than independent learners when using an IV simulator.... This study provided empirical evidence that supports the efficacy of simulation as a means of learning a psychometric skill."

Randomized Controlled Trials

Currently, in nursing and medicine, the randomized controlled trial (RCT) is noted to be the strongest methodology for testing the effectiveness of an intervention because of the elements of the experimental design that limit the potential for bias and error. Participants are randomized to the intervention and control groups to reduce selection bias (Carpenter et al., 2013; Schulz et al., 2010). In addition, blinding or withholding of study information from data collectors, participants, and their healthcare providers can reduce the potential for bias. RCTs, when appropriately conducted, are considered the gold standard for determining the effectiveness of healthcare interventions. RCTs may be carried out in a single setting or in multiple geographic locations to increase sample size and obtain a more representative sample.

The initial RCTs conducted in medicine demonstrated inconsistencies and biases. Consequently, a panel of experts—clinical trial researchers, medical journal editors, epidemiologists, and methodologists—developed guidelines to assess the quality of RCT reports. This group initiated the Standardized Reporting of Trials (SORT) statement that was revised and became the CONsolidated Standards for Reporting Trials (CONSORT). This current guideline includes a checklist and flow diagram that might be used to develop, report, and critically appraise published RCTs (CONSORT, 2010). Nurse researchers should follow the CONSORT 2010 statement recommendations in conducting and reporting RCTs (Schulz et al., 2010). You might use the flow diagram in Fig. 8.14 to critically appraise the RCTs reported in nursing journals. An RCT needs to include the following elements:

1. The study was designed to be a definitive test of the hypothesis that the intervention caused the defined dependent variables or outcomes.
2. The intervention is clearly described and consistently implemented to ensure intervention fidelity (Bova et al., 2017; CONSORT, 2010; Schulz et al., 2010; Yamada, Stevens, Sidani, Watt-Watson, & De Silva, 2010).
3. The study is conducted in a clinical setting, not in a laboratory.
4. The design meets the criteria of an experimental study (Schulz et al., 2010).
5. Study participants are drawn from a reference population through the use of clearly defined criteria. Baseline values are comparable in all groups included in the study. Selected participants are then randomly assigned to treatment and comparison groups (see Fig. 8.14), hence the term *randomized controlled trial* (CONSORT, 2010; Schulz et al., 2010).
6. The study has high internal validity. The design is rigorous and involves a high level of control of potential sources of bias that will rule out possible alternative causes of the effect (Shadish et al., 2002). The design may include blinding to accomplish this purpose. With blinding, the patient, those providing care to the patient, and/or the data collectors are unaware of whether the patient is in the experimental group or in the control group.
7. Dependent variables or outcomes are measured consistently with quality measurement methods (Waltz et al., 2017).
8. The intervention is defined in sufficient detail so that clinical application can be achieved (Schulz et al., 2010).
9. The participants lost to follow-up are identified with their rationale for not continuing the study. The attrition from the experimental and control groups needs to be addressed, as well as the overall sample attrition.
10. The study has received external funding sufficient to allow a rigorous design with a sample size adequate to provide a definitive test of the intervention.

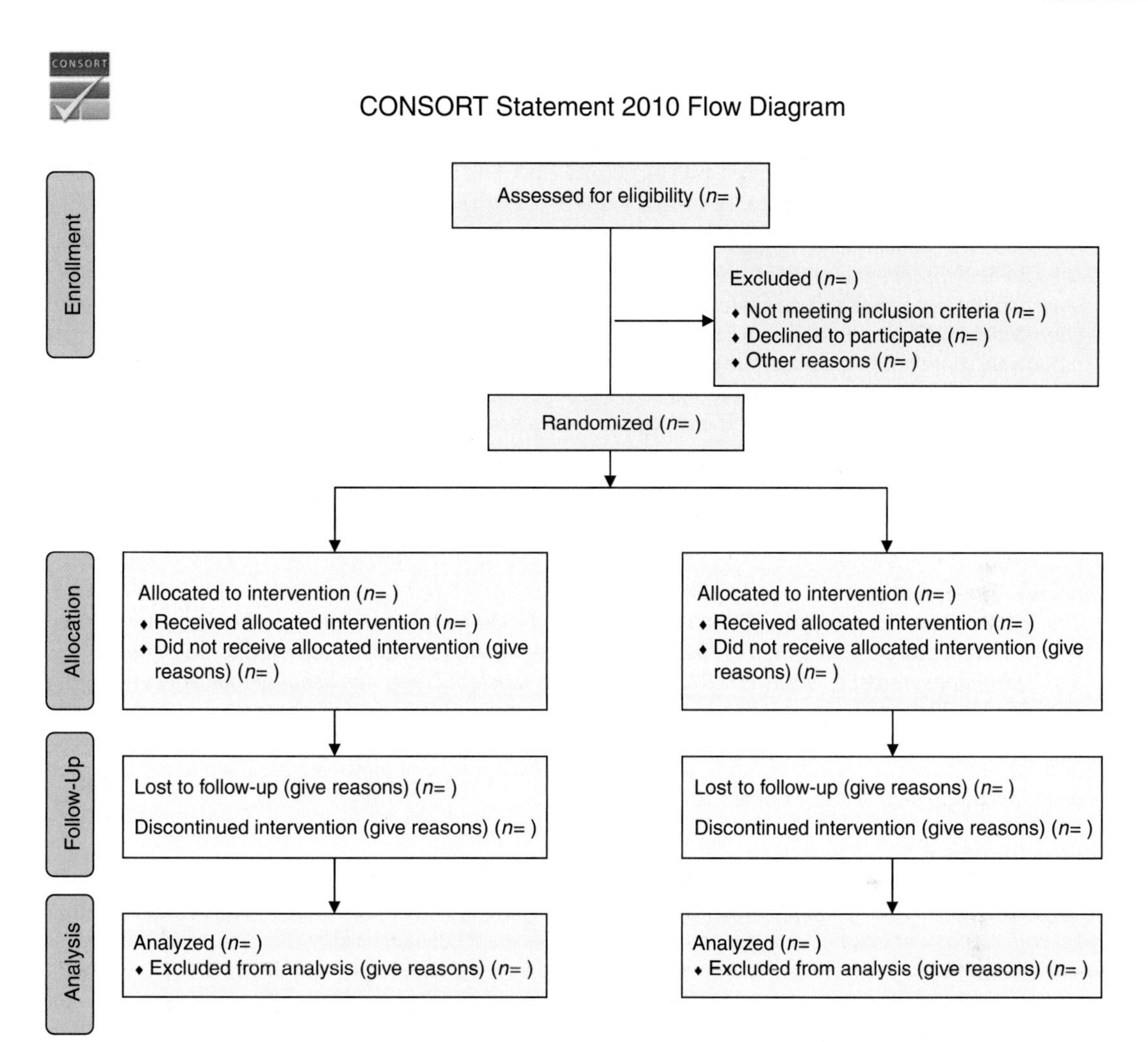

FIG 8.14 CONSORT 2010 statement showing a flow diagram of the progress through the phases of a parallel randomized trial of two groups: enrollment, intervention allocation, follow-up, and data analysis. (From CONSORT. [2010]. The CONSORT flow diagram. Retrieved June 26, 2017, from http://www.consort-statement.org/consort-statement/flow-diagram; and Schulz, K. F., Altman, D. G., & Moher, D. [2010]. CONSORT 2010 statement: Updated guidelines for reporting parallel group randomized trials. *Annals of Internal Medicine, 152*[11], 726–733.)

Hallas, Koslap-Petraco, and Fletcher (2017, p. 33) conducted an RCT "to examine the effectiveness of an office-based educational program to improve maternal confidence and social-emotional development of toddlers." The sample of convenience included mother and toddler dyads obtained from five pediatric primary healthcare offices and clinics in New York. The details of the sample size, randomization to groups, and attrition are presented in Fig. 4 in Research Example 8.8. This study was funded by a grant from the New York University Research Fund. Research Example 8.8 briefly presents the experimental design of this study.

RESEARCH EXAMPLE 8.8

Randomized Controlled Trial (RCT)

Research Study Excerpt

Methods

Trial Design

A prospective, double blind, randomized controlled trial using pretest/posttest experimental design was used to test the effectiveness of a videotape (DVD) parenting skills intervention on the social-emotional development of toddles and on maternal confidence of mothers caring for their toddlers... Two treatment intervention DVDs were designed: one for teenage mothers and one for all other mothers... The control group intervention was a standardized DVD on toddler nutrition.... The DVDs were available in English and Spanish. The wrapping for the DVD was the same as the one for the intervention DVD, thus the identification of the DVD contents (treatment and control) were concealed from the mothers, the RNs, and research assistants (RAs)....

After enrollment, each mother-toddler dyad was given a folder that had been randomized into either the treatment or control group using a computer-generated random numbers list... All RNs and RAs were blinded to the folder contents, as all folders were identical and the DVDs were all labeled with a code...

Outcome Assessments...

The Toddler Care Questionnaire (TCQ) is a measure of maternal confidence for all mothers of toddlers between the ages of 12 and 36 months... The TCQ instrument reliability is reported to be between 0.91 and 0.96 and test-retest reliability is 0.87... The Brigance Toddler Screen was used for toddlers between the ages of 12 to 33 months old... to measure their social-emotional skills... All participants completed the same study instruments, thus no information about the group assignments was known to the RNs or RAs. Since all participants watched a DVD privately, the participants did not know if they were assigned to the treatment or control group (Fig. 4). (Hallas et al., 2017, pp. 35–36)

Critical Appraisal

Hallas and colleagues (2017) identified the specific RCT design they used to address their study purpose and hypotheses. The sampling process, randomization to groups, and limited attrition are detailed in Fig. 4, indicating support for internal, external, and statistical conclusion design validity (Shadish et al., 2002). The researchers detailed their study intervention (DVDs of parenting skills) and controlled its implementation using checklists and scripts (Bova et al., 2017; Yamada et al., 2010). The steps taken to promote intervention fidelity by blinding mothers, RNs, and RAs to group assignment reduced the potential for bias and added to the internal and external design validity. The scales used to collect data were reliable in previous research and consistently administered in this study. However, no reliability values were provided for the scales in this study, causing a threat to statistical conclusion validity. In summary, Hallas et al. (2017) closely followed the CONSORT (2010) guidelines in conducting and reporting their RCT, which reduced the potential for bias and promoted trustworthy study results. The researchers concluded that the DVDs were a significant and efficient way to educate mothers of toddlers in office waiting rooms in order to improve their toddlers' social-emotional development.

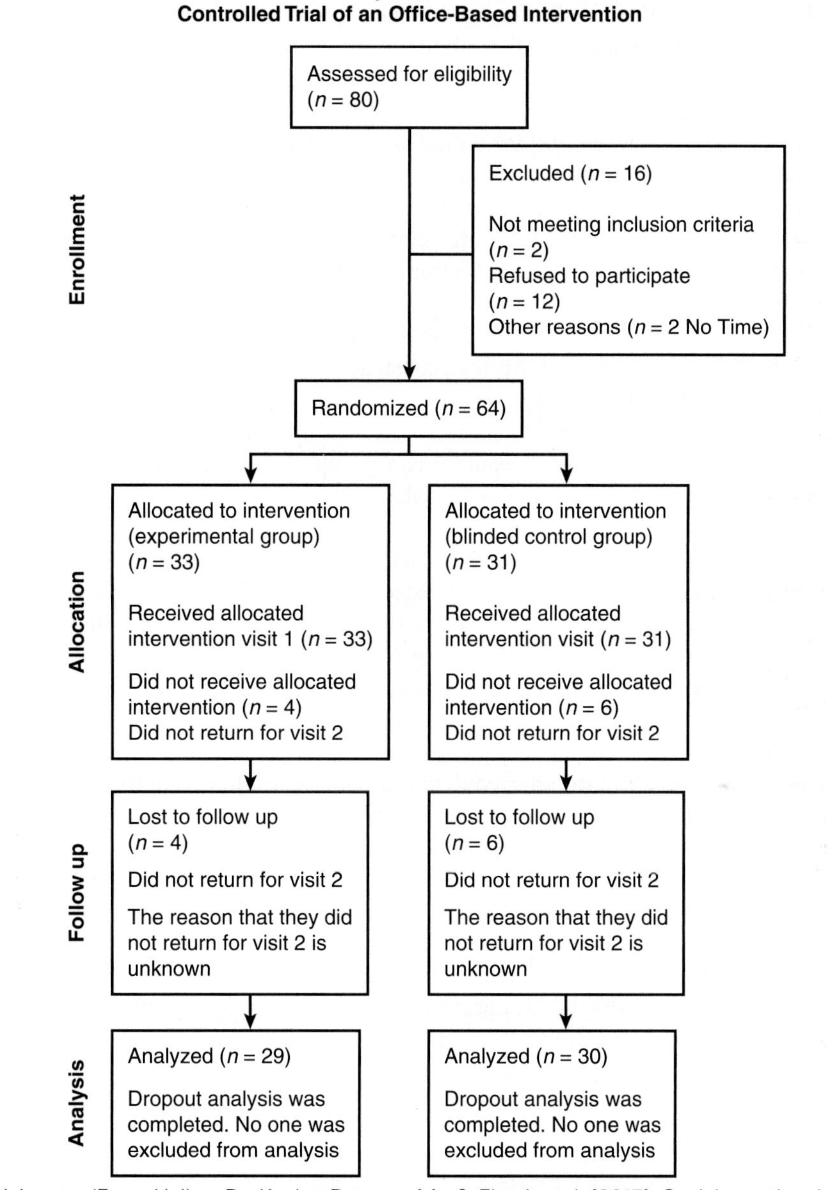

FIG. 4 Participants. (From Hallas, D., Koslap-Petraco, M., & Fletcher, J. [2017]. Social-emotional development of toddlers: Randomized controlled trial of an office-based intervention. *Journal of Pediatric Nursing, 33*[1], 37.)

KEY POINTS

- A research design is a blueprint for conducting a quantitative study that maximizes control over factors that could interfere with the validity of the findings.
- Four common types of quantitative designs conducted in nursing include descriptive, correlational, quasi-experimental, and experimental designs.
- The concepts important in understanding quantitative research designs include causality, multicausality, probability, bias, prospective, retrospective, control, and manipulation.
- Elements central to the study design include the presence or absence of an intervention, method of sampling, number of groups in the sample, number and timing of measurements to be performed, time frame for data collection, planned comparisons, and control of extraneous variables.
- Study validity is a measure of the truth or accuracy of the findings obtained from a study. Four types of validity are covered in this text: construct, internal, external, and statistical conclusion.
- Descriptive and correlational designs, called nonexperimental or noninterventional designs, focus on the description and examination of relationships among variables.
- Cross-sectional design involves examining a group of participants simultaneously in various stages of development, levels of educational, severity of illness, or stages of recovery to describe changes in a phenomenon across stages.
- Longitudinal design involves collecting data from the same participants at different points in time and might also be referred to as repeated measures.
- Correlational designs are of three different types: (1) descriptive correlational, in which the researcher can seek to describe a relationship; (2) predictive correlational, in which the researcher can predict relationships among variables; and (3) model testing design, in which all the relationships proposed by a theory are tested simultaneously.
- Interventions or treatments are implemented in quasi-experimental and experimental studies to determine their effect on selected dependent variables. Interventions may be physiological, psychosocial, educational, or a combination of these.
- The essential elements of experimental research are: (1) the random assignment of participants to groups; (2) the researcher's manipulation of the independent variable; and (3) the researcher's control of the experimental situation and setting, including a control or comparison group.
- Critically appraising a design involves examining the study setting, sample, intervention, measurement of variables, and data collection procedures.
- RCT design is noted to be the strongest methodology for testing the effectiveness of an intervention because the elements of the design limit the potential for bias.

REFERENCES

Battistelli, A., Portoghese, I., Galletta, M., & Pohl, S. (2013). Beyond the tradition: Test of an integrative conceptual model on nurse turnover. *International Nursing Review*, *60*(1), 103–111.

Bova, C., Jaffarian, C., Crawford, S., Quintos, J. B., Lee, M., & Sullivan-Bolyal, S. (2017). Intervention fidelity: Monitoring drift, providing feedback, and assessing the control condition. *Nursing Research*, *66*(1), 54–59.

Branson, M., Loftin, C., Hadley, L., Hartin, V., & Devkota, S. (2016). Impact of attendance on academic performance in prenursing students. *Nurse Educator*, *41*(4), 185–188.

Campbell, D. T., & Stanley, J. C. (1963). *Experimental and quasi-experimental designs for research*. Chicago, IL: Rand McNally.

Carpenter, J. S., Burns, D. S., Wu, J., Yu, M., Ryker, K., Tallman, E., et al. (2013). Methods: Strategies used and data obtained during treatment fidelity monitoring. *Nursing Research, 62*(1), 59–65.

Cohen, J. (1988). *Statistical power analysis for the behavioral sciences* (2nd ed.). New York, NY: Academic Press.

CONSORT. (2010). *The CONSORT statement*. Retrieved June 26, 2017, from http://www.consort-statement.org/consort-2010.

Creswell, J. W. (2014). *Research design: Qualitative, quantitative and mixed methods approaches* (4th ed.). Thousand Oaks, CA: Sage.

De Santis, J. P., Hauglum, S. D., Deleon, D. A., Provencio-Vasquez, E., & Rodriguez, A. E. (2017). HIV risk perception, HIV knowledge, and sexual risk behaviors among transgender women in south Florida. *Public Health Nursing, 34*(3), 210–218.

Eymard, A. S., & Altmiller, G. (2016). Teaching nursing students the importance of treatment fidelity in intervention research: Students as interventionists. *Journal of Nursing Education, 55*(5), 288–291.

Gray, J. R., Grove, S. K., & Sutherland, S. (2017). *The practice of nursing research: Appraisal, synthesis, and generation of evidence* (8th ed.). St. Louis, MO: Elsevier.

Grove, S. K., & Cipher, D. J. (2017). *Statistics for nursing research: A workbook for evidence-based practice* (2nd ed.). St. Louis, MO: Elsevier.

Hallas, D., Koslap-Petraco, M., & Fletcher, J. (2017). Social-emotional development of toddlers: Randomized controlled trial of an office-based intervention. *Journal of Pediatric Nursing, 33*(1), 33–40.

Kerlinger, F. N., & Lee, H. B. (2000). *Foundations of behavioral research* (4th ed.). Fort Worth, TX: Harcourt College Publishers.

McWilliams, L. A., Malecha, A., Langford, R., & Clutter, P. (2017). Comparisons of cooperative-based versus independent learning while using a haptic intravenous simulator. *Clinical Simulation in Nursing, 13*(4), 154–160.

Melnyk, B. M., Gallagher-Ford, E., & Fineout-Overholt, L. E. (2017). *Implementing evidence-based practice competencies in healthcare: A practical guide for improving quality, safety, & outcomes*. Indianapolis, IN: Sigma Theta Tau International.

Mosleh, S. M., Eshah, N. F., & Almalik, M. (2017). Perceived learning needs according to patients who have undergone major coronary interventions and their nurses. *Journal of Clinical Nursing, 26*(3/4), 418–426.

Murphy, S. L., & Gutman, S. A. (2012). Intervention fidelity: A necessary aspect of intervention effectiveness studies. *American Journal of Occupational Therapy, 66*(4), 387–388.

Quality and Safety Education for Nurses (QSEN). (2014). *Pre-licensure knowledge, skills, and attitudes (KSAs)*. Retrieved May 15, 2017, from http://qsen.org/competencies/pre-licensure-sas/.

Schulz, K. F., Altman, D. G., & Moher, D. (2010). CONSORT 2010 statement: Updated guidelines for reporting parallel group randomized trials. *Annals of Internal Medicine, 152*(11), 726–733.

Shadish, W. R., Cook, T. D., & Campbell, D. T. (2002). *Experimental and quasi-experimental designs for generalized causal inference*. Chicago, IL: Rand McNally.

Sherwood, G., & Barnsteiner, J. (2017). *Quality and safety in nursing: A competency approach to improving outcomes* (2nd ed.). Ames, IA: Wiley-Blackwell.

Spiva, L., Hart, P. L., Patrick, S., Waggoner, J., Jackson, C., & Threatt, J. L. (2017). Effectiveness of an evidence-based practice nurse mentor training program. *Worldviews on Evidence-Based Nursing, 14*(3), 183–191.

Spratling, R. (2017). Understanding the health care utilization of children who require medical technology: A descriptive study of children who require tracheostomies. *Applied Nursing Research, 34*(1), 62–65.

Spratling, R., & Powers, E. (2017). Development of a data abstraction form: Getting what you need from the electronic health record. *Journal of Pediatric Health Care, 31*(1), 126–130.

Waltz, C. F., Strickland, O. L., & Lenz, E. R. (2017). *Measurement in nursing and health research* (5th ed.). New York, NY: Springer Publishing Company.

Yamada, J., Stevens, B., Sidani, S., Watt-Watson, J., & De Silva, N. (2010). Content validity of a process evaluation checklist to measure intervention implementation fidelity of the EPIC Intervention. *Worldviews of Evidence- Based Nursing, 7*(3), 158–164.

Because of funding changes, the Agency for Healthcare Research and Quality (AHRQ) National Guideline Clearinghouse website was scheduled for decommissioning as of July 16, 2018. For more information, go to https://www.ahrq.gov/.

CHAPTER

9

Examining Populations and Samples in Research

Susan K. Grove

CHAPTER OVERVIEW

LEARNING OUTCOMES

After completing this chapter, you should be able to:

1. Describe sampling theory with its relevant concepts.
2. Critically appraise the sampling criteria in published studies.
3. Identify the specific type(s) of probability and nonprobability sampling methods implemented in quantitative and qualitative studies.
4. Describe the aspects of power analysis used to determine sample size in selected studies.
5. Critically appraise the sample size of quantitative and qualitative studies.
6. Critically appraise the sampling processes implemented in quantitative and qualitative studies.
7. Critically appraise the settings used for quantitative and qualitative studies.

Many of us have preconceived notions about samples and sampling, which we acquired from television commercials, polls of public opinion, Internet surveys, and reports of research findings. The advertiser boasts that four of five doctors recommend a particular medication, a newscaster predicts John Jones will win his senate seat by a 5% majority, an online survey identifies patient satisfaction with nurses, and researchers conclude that aggressive treatment of high blood pressure significantly reduces the risk for coronary artery disease and stroke.

All these examples include a sampling technique or method. Some of the outcomes from these sampling methods are more valid than others, based on the sampling method used and the sample size achieved. This chapter was developed to assist you in understanding and critically appraising the sampling processes implemented in quantitative and qualitative studies. Initially, the concepts of sampling theory are introduced, followed by a description of nonprobability and probability sampling methods commonly used in nursing studies. The sample sizes for quantitative and qualitative studies are detailed; and the chapter concludes with a discussion of the natural, partially controlled, and highly controlled settings used in conducting research.

UNDERSTANDING THE KEY CONCEPTS OF SAMPLING THEORY

Sampling involves selecting a group of people, events, objects, or other elements with which to conduct a study. A sampling method or plan defines the selection process, and the sample defines the selected group of people (or elements). A sample selected in a study should represent an identified population of people. The population might be people who have type 2 diabetes, patients who were hospitalized with pneumonia, or persons who received care from a registered nurse (RN). In most cases, however, it would be impossible for researchers to study an entire population. Sampling theory was developed to determine the most effective way to acquire a sample that accurately reflects the population under study. The key concepts of sampling theory are described in the following sections, including relevant examples from published studies.

Populations and Elements

The population is a particular group of individuals or elements, such as patients with heart failure or intravenous catheters, to be studied. The target population is the entire set of individuals or elements who meet the sampling criteria (defined in the next section), such as adult males, 18 years of age or older, diagnosed with type 2 diabetes, and hospitalized with a lower extremity infection. Fig. 9.1 demonstrates the link of the population, target population, and accessible population in a study. An accessible population is the portion of the target population to which the researcher has reasonable access. The accessible population might include individuals within a state, city, hospital, or nursing units, such as patients with diabetes who are in an acute care hospital in Dallas, Texas. Researchers obtain the sample from the

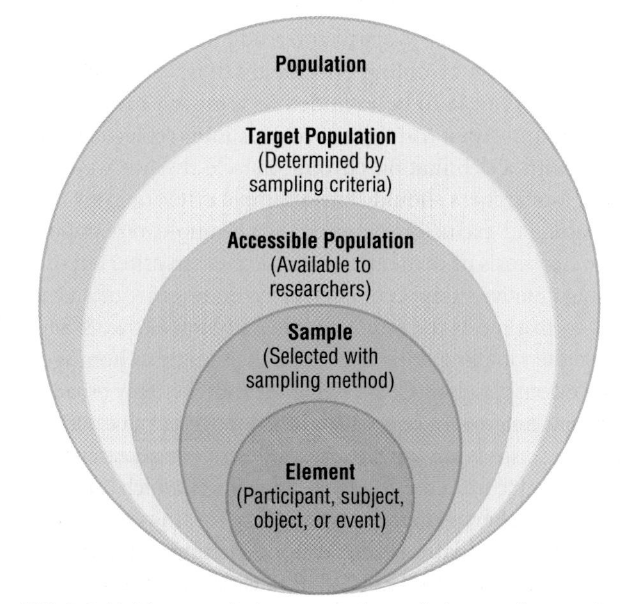

FIG 9.1 Linking populations, sample, and element in a study.

accessible population by using a particular sampling method or plan, such as simple random sampling. The individual units of the population and sample are called elements. An element can be a person, event, object, or any other single unit of study. When elements in a study are persons, they are referred to as participants or subjects. The term *participant* is commonly used in nursing research.

Generalization extends the findings from the sample under study to the larger population. In quantitative studies, researchers obtain a sample from the accessible population with the goal of generalizing the findings from the sample to the accessible population and then, more abstractly, to the target population (see Fig. 9.1). The quality of the study and consistency of the study's findings with the findings from previous research in this area influence the extent of the generalization. If a study is of high quality and has findings consistent with previous research, then researchers can be more confident in generalizing their findings to the target population. For example, the findings from the study of male patients, diagnosed with type 2 diabetes, and hospitalized with an infection in Dallas, may be generalized to the target population of males with type 2 diabetes hospitalized in Texas urban hospitals or, more broadly, to urban hospitals in the southern United States. With this information, you can decide whether it is appropriate to use this evidence in caring for the same type of patients in your practice, with the goal of moving toward evidence-based practice (EBP; Brown, 2018; Melnyk, Gallagher-Ford, & Fineout-Overholt, 2017).

Sampling or Eligibility Criteria

Sampling or eligibility criteria include the list of characteristics essential for eligibility or membership in the target population. For example, researchers may choose to study the effect of preoperative teaching about early ambulation on the outcome of length of hospital stay for older adults having knee joint replacement surgery. In this study, the sampling criteria may include adults 60 years of age or older, able to speak and read English, and undergoing surgical replacement of one knee joint. Those patients with a history of previous joint replacement surgery, diagnosis of dementia, or diagnosed with a debilitating chronic muscle disease will be excluded.

Inclusion sampling criteria are the characteristics that the study participant or element must possess to be part of the target population. In the previous example, the inclusion criteria are adults 60 years of age or older, ability to speak and read English, and undergoing a surgical replacement of one knee joint. Exclusion sampling criteria are those characteristics that can cause a person who meets the inclusion criteria to be excluded or removed from the target population. For example, any study participant with a history of previous joint replacement surgery, diagnosis of dementia, and diagnosed with a debilitating chronic muscle disease were excluded from the preoperative teaching study. Researchers should state a sample criterion only once and should not include it as both an inclusion and exclusion criterion. For example, researchers should *not* have an inclusion criterion of no diagnosis of dementia *and* an exclusion criterion of diagnosis of dementia.

When the quantitative study is completed, the findings are often generalized from the sample to the target population that meets the sampling criteria (Gray, Grove, & Sutherland, 2017). Researchers may narrowly define the sampling criteria to make the sample as homogeneous (or similar) as possible to control for extraneous variables. Conversely, the researcher may broadly define the criteria to ensure that the study sample is heterogeneous, with a broad range of values or scores on the variables being studied. If the sampling criteria are too narrow and restrictive, researchers may have difficulty obtaining an adequately sized sample from the accessible population, which can limit the generalization of findings.

Sometimes researchers generalize their study findings beyond the sampling criteria. Using the example of the early ambulation preoperative teaching study, the sample may need to be limited to participants who speak and read English because the preoperative teaching is in English, and one of the measurement instruments requires that they be able to read English. However, the researchers may believe that the findings can be generalized to non–English-speaking persons. When reading studies, you need to consider carefully the implications of using these findings with a non–English-speaking population. Perhaps non–English-speaking persons, because they come from another culture, do not respond to the teaching in the same way as observed in the study population. When critically appraising a study, examine the sample inclusion and exclusion criteria to determine whether the generalization of the study findings is appropriate based on these criteria.

REPRESENTATIVENESS OF A SAMPLE IN QUANTITATIVE RESEARCH

Representativeness means that the sample, accessible population, and target population are alike in as many ways as possible (see Fig. 9.1). In quantitative research, you need to evaluate representativeness in terms of the setting, characteristics of the participants, and distribution of values on variables measured in the study. Persons seeking care in a particular setting may be different from those who seek care for the same problem in another setting or those who choose to use self-care to manage their problems. Studies conducted in private hospitals are less likely to recruit participants with low incomes. Other settings may have few older adults or fewer adults with less education. People who do not have access to care are usually excluded from studies. Participants in research centers and the care that they receive are different from patients and the care that they receive in community hospitals, public hospitals, veterans' hospitals, or rural hospitals. People living in rural settings may respond differently to a health situation than those who live in urban settings. Thus the setting identified in a study does influence the representativeness of the sample. Researchers who gather data from participants across a variety of settings have a more representative sample of the target population than those limiting the study to a single setting.

A sample must be representative in terms of characteristics such as age, gender, ethnicity, income, and education, which often influence study variables. These are examples of demographic or attribute variables that might be selected by researchers for examination in their study. Researchers analyze data collected on the demographic variables to produce the sample characteristics—characteristics used to provide a picture of the sample. These sample characteristics must be reasonably representative of the characteristics of the population. If the study includes groups, the participants in the groups must have comparable demographic characteristics. Chapter 5 includes more details on demographic variables and sample characteristics.

Studies that obtain data from large databases have more representative samples. For example, Muroi, Shen, and Angosta (2017, p. 180) were concerned about nurses' errors related to medications and examined the "association of medication errors with drug classifications, clinical units, and consequences of errors." The sample included medical error (ME) incidence reports that were extracted from an existing database developed during previous research. The research database included data from "five hospitals from the southwest region of the United States (U.S.) in November 2011 through July 2014… A total of 2336 observations were collected (n = 1276 ME case group, n =1060 control group). Our study focused on the 1276 ME cases in the case group and excluded the control group that was not related to MEs" (Muroi et al., 2017, p. 181).

This study included an extremely large sample (n = 1276 ME observations) from a number of hospitals throughout the southwest United States. This study sample was representative of the accessible population (ME reports from five hospitals) and seemed representative of the target population of ME incident reports in the southwestern US region. Muroi and colleagues (2017) found that MEs were associated with drug classifications, clinical units, and consequence of errors. The greatest number of MEs occurred with anticoagulants, and the second most common source of errors was antimicrobials. Medical-surgical and intensive care units had the highest incidence of MEs, and 10% of the errors resulted in patient harm.

Random and Systematic Variation of Study Participants' Values

Measurement values also need to be representative. Measurement values in a study often vary randomly among participants. Random variation is the expected difference in values that occurs when different participants from the same sample are examined. The difference is random because some values will be higher and others lower than the average (mean) population value. As sample size increases, random variation decreases resulting in more values closer to the mean, which improves representativeness.

Systematic variation, or systematic bias—a serious concern in sampling—is a consequence of selecting study participants whose measurement values differ in some specific way from those of the population. This difference usually is expressed as a difference in the average (or mean) values between the sample and population. Because the participants have something in common, their values tend to be similar to those of others in the sample but different in some way from those of the population as a whole. These values do not vary randomly around the population mean. Most of the variation from the mean is in the same direction—it is systematic. Thus the sample mean may be higher than or lower than the mean of the target population. Increasing the sample size has no effect on systematic variation. For example, if all the participants in a study examining some type of knowledge level have an intelligence quotient (IQ) above 120, then all their test scores in the study are likely to be higher than those of the population mean, which includes people with a wide variation in IQ scores (but with a mean IQ of 100). The IQs of the study participants will introduce a systematic bias. When systematic bias occurs in quasi-experimental or experimental studies, it can lead the researcher to conclude that the treatment has made a difference, when in actuality the values would have been different, even without the treatment.

Acceptance and Refusal Rates in Studies

The probability of systematic variation increases when the sampling process is not random. Even in a random sample, however, systematic variation can occur when a large number of the potential participants declines participation. As the number of individuals declining participation increases, the possibility of a systematic bias in the study becomes greater. In published studies, researchers may identify a refusal rate, which is the percentage of subjects who declined to participate in the study, and their reasons for not participating (Grove & Cipher, 2017). The formula for calculating the refusal rate in a study is as follows:

$$\textbf{Refusal rate} = (\text{number refusing participation} \div \text{number meeting sampling criteria approached}) \times 100\%$$

For example, if 80 potential participants meeting sampling criteria are approached to participate in the hypothetical study about the effects of early ambulation preoperative teaching on the length of hospital stay, and four patients refuse, then the refusal rate would be as follows:

$$\textbf{Refusal rate} = (4 \div 80) \times 100\% = 0.05 \times 100\% = 5\%$$

Other studies record an acceptance rate, which is the percentage of participants meeting sampling criteria who consent to be in a study. However, researchers will report the refusal or acceptance rate, but not both. The formula for calculating the acceptance rate in a study is as follows:

$$\textbf{Acceptance rate} = (\text{number accepting participation} \div \text{number meeting sampling criteria approached}) \times 100\%$$

In the hypothetical preoperative teaching study, 4 of 80 potential participants refused to participate—so 80 − 4 = 76 accepted. Plugging the following numbers into the stated formula gives the following:

$$\textbf{Acceptance rate} = (76 \div 80) \times 100\% = 0.95 \times 100\% = 95\%$$

You can also calculate the acceptance and refusal rates as follows:

$$\textbf{Acceptance rate} = 100\% - \text{refusal rate}$$

or

$$\textbf{Refusal rate} = 100\% - \text{acceptance rate}$$

In this example, the acceptance rate was 100% − 5% (refusal rate) = 95%, which is a study strength. In studies with a high acceptance rate or a low refusal rate reported, the chance for systematic variation is less, and the sample is more likely to be representative of the target population. Researchers usually report the refusal rate, and it is best to provide rationales for the individuals refusing to participate.

Sample Attrition and Retention Rates in Studies

Systematic variation also may occur in studies with high sample attrition. **Sample attrition** is the withdrawal or loss of participants from a study that can be expressed as the number of participants withdrawing or a percentage. The percentage is the sample attrition rate, and it is best if researchers include both the number of participants withdrawing and the attrition rate. The formula for calculating the sample attrition rate in a study is as follows:

$$\textbf{Sample attrition rate} = (\text{number of participants withdrawing from a study} \div \text{sample size of study}) \times 100\%$$

For example, in the hypothetical study of preoperative teaching ($n = 76$), 31 subjects (12 from the treatment group and 19 from the comparison group) withdrew, for various reasons. Loss of 31 subjects means a 41% attrition rate:

$$\textbf{Sample attrition rate} = (31 \div 76) \times 100\% = 0.408 \times 100\% = 40.8\% = 41\%$$

In this example, the overall sample attrition rate was considerable (41%), and the rates differed for the two groups to which the participants were assigned. You can also calculate the attrition rates for the groups. If the two groups were equal at the start of the study and each included 38 subjects, then the attrition rate for the treatment group was $(12 \div 38) \times 100\% = 0.316 \times 100\% = 31.6\% = 32\%$. The attrition for the comparison group was $(19 \div 38) \times 100\% = 0.50 \times 100\% = 50\%$. Systematic variation is greatest when a large number of participants withdraws from the study before data collection is completed or when a large number of participants withdraws from one group but not the other(s) in the study. In studies involving a treatment, participants in the comparison group who do not receive the treatment may be more likely to withdraw from the study. However, sometimes the attrition is higher for the treatment group if the intervention is complex and/or time-consuming (Gray et al., 2017). In the early ambulation preoperative teaching example, there is a strong potential for systematic variation because the sample attrition rate was large (41%), and the attrition rate in the comparison group (50%) was larger than the attrition rate in the treatment group (32%). The increased potential for systematic variation results in a sample that is less representative of the target population.

The opposite of sample attrition is **sample retention**, which is the number of participants who remain in and complete a study. You can calculate the sample retention rate in two ways:

$$\textbf{Sample retention rate} = (\text{number of participants completing the study} \div \text{sample size}) \times 100\%$$

or

$$\textbf{Sample retention rate} = 100\% - \text{sample attrition rate}$$

In the example, early ambulation preoperative teaching study, 45 participants were retained in the study that had an original sample of 76 participants:

$$\textbf{Sample retention rate} = (45 \div 76) \times 100\% = 0.592 \times 100\% = 59.2\% = 59\%$$

or

$$\textbf{Sample retention rate} = 100\% - 41\% = 59\%$$

The higher the retention rate the more representative the sample is of the target population, and the more likely the study results are an accurate reflection of reality. Often, researchers will identify the attrition rate or retention rate, but not both. It is best to provide a rate as well as the number of participants withdrawing from a study. In addition, researchers need to provide rationales for the participants withdrawing to determine the impact on the study findings.

CRITICAL APPRAISAL GUIDELINES

Adequacy of the Populations, Sampling Criteria, Refusal Rates, and Attrition Rates in Quantitative Studies

When conducting an initial critical appraisal of the sampling process in quantitative studies, you need to address the following questions:

1. Did the researchers define the target and accessible populations for the study?
2. Are the sampling inclusion criteria, sampling exclusion criteria, or both clearly identified and appropriate for the study?
3. Is the refusal or acceptance rate identified? Is the sample attrition or retention rate addressed? Are reasons provided for the refusal and attrition rates?

Newnam and colleagues (2015) implemented a randomized experimental study design to identify differences in frequency and severity of nasal injuries in extremely low birth weight (BW) neonates on nasal continuous positive airway pressure (CPAP) treatments. The study included 78 neonates (sample size) in a 70-bed, level III neonatal intensive care unit (NICU) receiving nasal CPAP who were "randomized into three groups: continuous nasal prong, continuous nasal mask, or alternating mask/prongs every 4 hours" (Newnam et al., 2015, p. 37). These researchers provided a description of their study sampling criteria and documented the participants enrolled in their study using a flow diagram (see Fig. 1 in Research Example 9.1). This flow diagram is based on the CONsolidated Standards of Reporting Trials (CONSORT) Statement that is the international standard for reporting the sampling process in randomized controlled trials (RCTs; CONSORT Group, 2010). The population, inclusion and exclusion sampling criteria, refusal and attrition rates, and representativeness of this sample are described in Research Example 9.1. Particular aspects of the sample have been identified in [brackets] for clarity. The sampling method, sample size, and setting for the Newnam et al. (2015) study are described later in this chapter.

RESEARCH EXAMPLE 9.1

Adequacy of the Sampling Process in Quantitative Studies

Research Study Excerpt

Each infant admitted to the NICU between April, 2012 and January, 2013 was screened for inclusion criteria. Inclusion criteria included preterm infants with birth weight (BW) 500 to 1500 grams that required nasal CPAP treatment. Exclusion criteria included infants born with airway or physical anomalies that influenced their ability to extubate to nasal CPAP, infants not consented within 8 hours of nasal CPAP initiation, infants not treated with nasal CPAP or infants who had nasal skin breakdown at enrollment [target population]....

A total of 377 admissions [accessible population] to the NICU [setting] were screened for eligibility during the study period. Of these, 140 patients met BW criteria of 500-1500 g. Two patients were diagnosed with airway deformities that were eliminated. Parental consent was obtained on 90 infants (65%). Two parents refused study participation for their infant (1%). Fourteen (10%) expired prior to obtaining study consent, and 32 (23%) were missed. Typically these were infants who were admitted on nasal CPAP or quickly extubated with limited ability to obtain consent within the 8 hour time limit (see Fig. 1). (Newnam et al., 2015, p. 37–38)

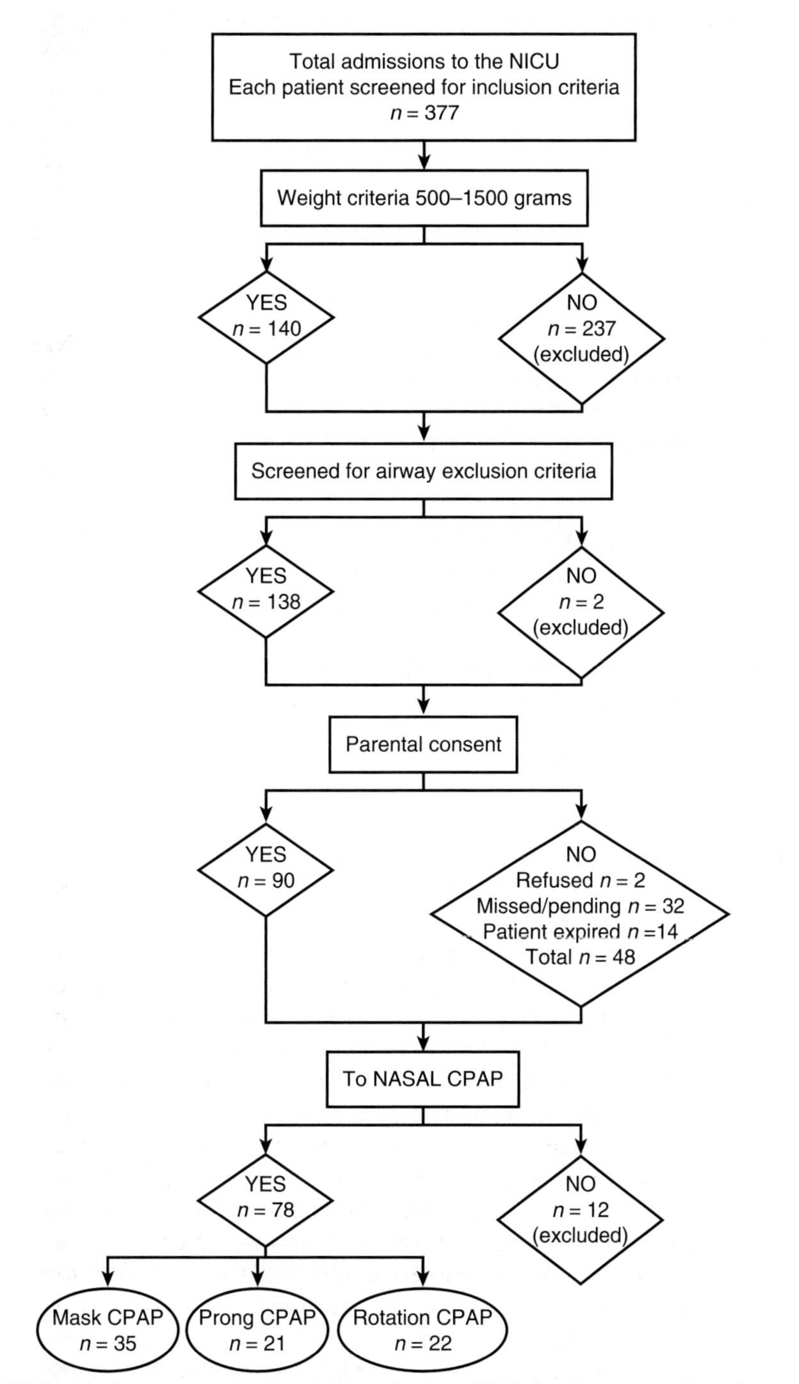

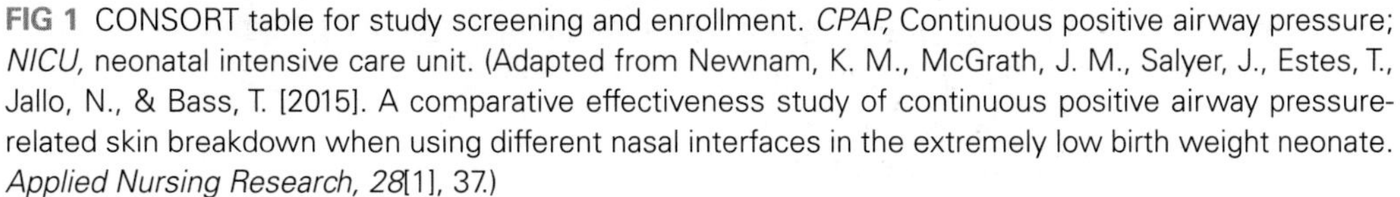

FIG 1 CONSORT table for study screening and enrollment. *CPAP,* Continuous positive airway pressure; *NICU,* neonatal intensive care unit. (Adapted from Newnam, K. M., McGrath, J. M., Salyer, J., Estes, T., Jallo, N., & Bass, T. [2015]. A comparative effectiveness study of continuous positive airway pressure-related skin breakdown when using different nasal interfaces in the extremely low birth weight neonate. *Applied Nursing Research, 28*[1], 37.)

Continued

RESEARCH EXAMPLE 9-1—cont'd

Critical Appraisal

Newnam and colleagues (2015) clearly presented the inclusion and exclusion sampling criteria used to identify the target population of this study. The screening of neonates with these sampling criteria is detailed in Fig. 1. A large number of neonates (n = 377) were screened, and an adequate number of neonates (n = 138) met the inclusion and exclusion criteria. The sampling criteria were appropriate for the purpose of this study to reduce the effects of possible extraneous variables that might have had an impact on the CPAP treatment delivery methods (nasal mask or prong) and the measurement of the dependent variables (frequency and severity of nasal injuries). The increased controls imposed by the sampling criteria strengthened the likelihood that the study results were caused by the treatment and not by extraneous variables or sampling error.

The refusal rate was minimal (1%), and the other reasons for not including neonates in the study were clearly described and appropriate. The final sample included 78 neonates who were randomized into the mask group (n = 35), prong group (n = 21), and rotation mask and prong group (n = 22; see Fig. 1). The study had no attrition of participants because the group sizes did not change throughout the study. The strong sample criteria and limited refusal and attrition rates increased the representativeness of this sample. Newnam and colleagues (2015) found that the neonates in the group with alternating CPAP by nasal mask and prongs had significantly fewer incidences of skin injury than those receiving CPAP by mask or prongs only.

Sampling Frames

From a sampling theory perspective, each person or element in the population should have an opportunity to be selected for the sample. One method of providing this opportunity is referred to as **random sampling**. For everyone in the accessible population to have an opportunity for selection in the sample, each person in the population must be identified. To accomplish this, the researcher must acquire a list of every member of the population, using the sampling criteria to define eligibility. This list is referred to as the **sampling frame**. In some studies, the complete sampling frame cannot be identified because it is not possible to list all members of the population. The Health Insurance Portability and Accountability Act (HIPAA) has also increased the difficulty in obtaining a complete sampling frame for several studies because of its requirements to protect individuals' health information (see Chapter 4 for more information on HIPAA). Once a sampling frame has been identified, researchers select participants for their studies using a sampling plan or method.

Sampling Methods or Plans

Sampling methods or **plans** outline strategies used to obtain samples for studies. Like a design, a sampling plan is not specific to a study. The sampling plan may include probability (random) or nonprobability (nonrandom) sampling methods. Probability sampling methods are designed to increase representativeness and decrease systematic variation or bias in quantitative studies. When critically appraising a study, identify the study sampling plan as probability or nonprobability, and determine the specific method or methods used to select the sample. The different types of probability and nonprobability sampling methods are introduced next.

PROBABILITY SAMPLING METHODS

In probability sampling, each person or element in a population has an opportunity to be selected for a sample, which is achieved through random sampling. Probability or random sampling methods increase the sample's representativeness of the target population. All the subsets of the population, which may differ from each other but contribute to the parameters (e.g., the means and standard deviations) of the population, have a chance to be represented in the sample. The opportunity for systematic bias is less when participants are selected randomly, although it is possible for a systematic bias to occur.

Without random sampling strategies, researchers, who have a vested interest in the study, might tend (consciously or unconsciously) to select individuals whose conditions or behaviors are consistent with the study hypotheses. For example, researchers may exclude potential participants because they are too sick, not sick enough, coping too well, not coping adequately, uncooperative, or noncompliant. By using random sampling, however, researchers leave the selection to chance, thereby increasing the validity of their study findings.

There are four sampling designs that achieve probability sampling presented in this text: simple random sampling, stratified random sampling, cluster sampling, and systematic sampling. Table 9.1 identifies the common probability and nonprobability sampling methods used in nursing studies, their applications, and their representativeness for the study. Probability and nonprobability sampling methods are used in quantitative studies (Kerlinger & Lee, 2000), and nonprobability sampling methods are used in qualitative studies (Creswell & Poth, 2018).

Simple Random Sampling

Simple random sampling is the most basic of the probability sampling plans. It is achieved by randomly selecting elements from the sampling frame. Researchers can accomplish random selection in a variety of ways; it is limited only by the imagination of the researcher. If the sampling frame is small, researchers can write names on slips of paper, place them into a container, mix them well, and then draw them out one at a time until they have reached the desired sample size. A computer program is the most common method for randomly selecting study participants. The researcher can enter the sampling frame (list of potential participants) into a computer, which randomly selects participants until the desired sample size is achieved.

Another method for randomly selecting a study sample is the use of a table of random numbers. Table 9.2 displays a section from a random numbers table. To use a table of random numbers, the researcher places a pencil or finger on the table with his or her eyes closed. That number is the starting place. Then, by moving the pencil or finger up, down, right, or left, numbers are identified in order until the desired sample size has been obtained. For example, if you want to select five participants from a population of 100, and the number 58 is initially selected as a starting point (fourth column from the left, fourth row down), your participants' numbers would be 58, 25, 15, 55, and 38. Table 9.2 is useful only when the population number is less than 100. Tables of random numbers can be created online with an option to select a random sample from the table using a program such as QuickCalcs (see http://graphpad.com/quickcalcs/ randomN2/).

Lee, Faucett, Gillen, Krause, and Landry (2013) conducted a predictive correlational study to determine critical care nurses' perception of the risk of musculoskeletal (MSK) injury. The researchers randomly selected 1000 critical care nurses from the 2005 American Association of Critical Care (AACN) membership list (sampling frame). The researchers described their sampling method in Research Example 9.2.

TABLE 9.1 PROBABILITY AND NONPROBABILITY SAMPLING METHODS

SAMPLING METHOD	COMMON APPLICATION(S)	REPRESENTATIVENESS OF SAMPLE OR IN-DEPTH RICHNESS OF FINDINGS TO PROMOTE UNDERSTANDING
Probability		
Simple random sampling	Quantitative research	Provides strong representativeness of the target population that increases with sample size.
Stratified random	Quantitative research	Provides strong representativeness of the target population that increases with control of stratified variable(s).
Cluster	Quantitative research	This method is less representative of the target population than simple random sampling and stratified random sampling, but representativeness increases with sample size.
Systematic	Quantitative research	This method is less representative of the target population than simple random sampling and stratified random sampling methods, but representativeness increases with sample size.
Nonprobability		
Convenience sampling	Quantitative and qualitative research	There is questionable representativeness of the target population, which improves with increasing sample size; it is used in qualitative research so that an adequate number of participants might be found to promote understanding of the study area.
Quota	Quantitative research; rarely, qualitative research	Use of stratification for selected variables in quantitative research makes the sample more representative than convenience sampling. In qualitative research, participants of different ages or ethnic groups might be selected to increase the depth and richness of the study findings.
Purposeful or purposive	Qualitative and sometimes quantitative research	Focus is on insight, description, and understanding of a phenomenon, situation, process, or cultural element with participants selected who have the potential to provide in-depth, rich data.
Network or snowball	Qualitative and sometimes quantitative research	Focus is on insight, description, and understanding of a phenomenon, situation, process, or cultural element in a difficult-to-access population.
Theoretical	Qualitative research	Focus is on developing a theory in a selected area with participants selected for their different perspectives.

TABLE 9.2 SECTION FROM A RANDOM NUMBERS TABLE

06	84	10	22	56	72	25	70	69	43
07	63	10	34	66	39	54	02	33	85
03	19	63	93	72	52	13	30	44	40
77	32	69	58	25	15	55	38	19	62
20	01	94	54	66	88	43	91	34	28

RESEARCH EXAMPLE 9.2

Simple Random Sampling

Research Study Excerpt

A total of 412 nurses returned completed questionnaires (response rate = 41.5%, excluding eight for whom mailing addresses were incorrect). Of these, 47 nurses who did not meet the inclusion criteria were excluded: not currently employed (n = 5); not employed in a hospital (n = 1); not employed in critical care (n = 8); not a staff or charge nurse (n = 28); or not performing patient-handling tasks (n = 5). In addition, four nurses employed in a neonatal ICU (NICU) were excluded because of the different nature of their physical workload. The final sample for data analysis comprised 361 [sample size] critical care nurses. (Lee et al., 2013, p. 38)

Critical Appraisal

Lee and associates (2013) clearly identified that a random sampling method was used to select study participants from a population of critical care nurses. The 41.5% response rate for mailed questionnaires is considered adequate because the response rate to questionnaires averages 25%–50% (Gray et al., 2017). The 47 nurses who did not meet sample criteria and the four nurses working in an NICU were excluded, ensuring a more homogeneous sample and decreasing the potential effect of extraneous variables. These sampling activities limit the potential for systematic variation or bias and increase the likelihood that the study sample is representative of the accessible and target populations. The study would have been strengthened if the researchers had indicated how the nurses were randomly selected from the AACN membership list, but this was probably a random selection by a computer.

Lee and coworkers (2013, p. 43) identified the following findings from their study: "Improving the physical and psychosocial work environment may make nursing jobs safer, reduce the risk of MSK injury, and improve nurses' perceptions of job safety. Ultimately, these efforts would contribute to enhancing safety in nursing settings and to maintaining a healthy nursing workforce."

Stratified Random Sampling

Stratified random sampling is used in situations in which the researcher knows some of the variables in the population that are critical for achieving representativeness. Variables commonly used for stratification include age, gender, race and ethnicity, socioeconomic status, diagnosis, geographic region, type of nursing care, and site of care. Stratification ensures that all levels of the identified variables are adequately represented in the sample. With stratification, researchers can use a smaller sample size to achieve the same degree of representativeness, relative to the stratified variable, that is derived from using a larger sample acquired through simple random sampling.

If researchers have used stratification, they must define categories (strata) of the variables selected for stratification in the published report. For example, using race and ethnicity for stratification, the researcher may define four strata: white non-Hispanic, black non-Hispanic, Hispanic, and other. The population may be 60% white non-Hispanic, 20% black non-Hispanic, 15% Hispanic, and 5% other. Researchers may select a random sample for each stratum equivalent to the target population proportions of that stratum. Thus a sample of 100 participants would need to include approximately 60 white non-Hispanic, 20 black non-Hispanic, 15 Hispanic, and 5 other. Alternatively, equal numbers of study participants may be randomly selected for each stratum. For example, if age is used to stratify a sample of 100 adult participants, the researcher may obtain 25 subjects 18 to 34 years, 25 subjects 35 to 50 years, 25 subjects 51 to 66 years, and 25 subjects older than 66 years of age. With equal numbers of study participants in each group, the smaller groups are overrepresented, which can create sampling error.

Lee and colleagues (2016, p. 84) conducted a predictive correlation study "to clarify the association of the combination of eating quickly (EQ), late evening meals (LEM), and skipping breakfast

(SB) with being overweight." The independent variables of EQ, LEM, and SB were used to predict the dependent variable of being overweight. This study included a stratified random sample that is described in Research Example 9.3.

RESEARCH EXAMPLE 9.3

Stratified Random Sampling

Research Study Excerpt

A cross-sectional survey was conducted in October 2011.... Using a stratified random sampling method among residents aged 20 to 80 years by gender and a 5-year age strata, 5002 residents (5.0%) were selected on the basis of the Basic Resident Register on March 31, 2010.... A cover letter and a questionnaire were mailed to the residents. Introduction of the study and its aims, assurance of anonymity, and encouragement for participation were included in the cover letter. After 2 weeks, volunteers visited each home to collect the sealed envelopes; 4570 (91.4%) returned the questionnaires. (Lee et al., 2016, p. 85)

Critical Appraisal

Lee and colleagues (2016) clearly identified their population as individuals from a Basic Resident Register, which was a national database. The study included a large sample (n = 5002), and the questionnaire used to measure the variables had an extremely high return rate (91.4%). Stratification by gender and 5-year age groups seemed important in this study to control extraneous variables that could affect individuals' weight. However, the researchers needed to provide more details about the stratification process and the numbers of participants in the gender and age strata. A cross-sectional survey also increased the representativeness of the sample (see Chapter 8 on design). In summary, this study included a strong stratified random sampling method, large sample size, and high return rate of questionnaires, which increased the representativeness of the sample and decreased the potential for systematic error or bias.

Lee et al. (2016) found that only EQ, or EQ in combination with LEM, and SB was predictive of being overweight. LEM and SB alone did not increase the risk of being overweight. Additional research is needed in this area, but patients might benefit from education about eating slowly to reduce their risk of being overweight.

Cluster Sampling

In **cluster sampling**, a researcher develops a sampling frame that includes a list of all the states, cities, institutions, or clinicians with which elements of the identified population can be linked. A randomized sample of these states, cities, institutions, or clinicians can then be used in the study. In some cases, this randomized selection continues through several stages and is then referred to as multistage sampling. For example, the researcher may first randomly select states and then randomly select cities within the sampled states. Next, the researcher may randomly select hospitals within the randomly selected cities. Within the hospitals, nursing units may be randomly selected. At this level, all patients on the nursing unit who fit the criteria for the study may be included or patients can be randomly selected.

Cluster sampling is commonly used in two types of research situations. In the first situation, the researcher considers it necessary to obtain a geographically dispersed sample but recognizes that obtaining a simple random sample will require too much travel time and expense. In the second, the researcher cannot identify the individual elements making up the population and therefore cannot develop a sampling frame. For example, a complete list of all people in the United States who have had open heart surgery does not exist. Nevertheless, it is often possible to obtain lists of institutions or organizations with which the elements of interest are associated—in this example, perhaps large medical centers, university hospitals with cardiac surgery departments, and large cardiac surgery practices—and then randomly select institutions from which the researcher can acquire study participants.

Reinke and colleagues (2017, p. 30) used cluster sampling in their study of the "long term impact of an end-of-life communication intervention among veterans with COPD [chronic obstructive pulmonary disease]." These researchers described their sampling method in Research Example 9.4 and the particular aspects of the sample have been identified in [brackets].

RESEARCH EXAMPLE 9.4

Cluster Sampling

Research Study Excerpt

*We conducted a clustered randomized trial to test an intervention to promote discussions about advanced care planning and goals of care... The unit of randomization was at the clinician level with patients clustered by clinician [cluster sampling]... The study was conducted at the VA Puget Sound Health Care System [setting]... Subjects included patients with COPD [population]... who participated in the End-of-Life Communication trial and died after study completion (*n *= 157) [sample size]... We examined whether the communication intervention lead to more conversations and advance care planning documentation in the medical record prior to death.* (Reinke et al., 2017, p. 31)

Critical Appraisal

Reinke and colleagues (2017) stated they used a randomized cluster sampling method to identify study participants. The population of veterans with COPD was appropriate for the purpose of this study. The study was conducted in a Veterans' Administration (VA) healthcare system, indicating more than one site for the study. The sample size might have been inadequate because the findings were not significant. The researchers found that the intervention did not increase the documentation of additional end-of-life conversations, "nor did it improve the documentation of advanced directives" (Reinke et al., 2017, p. 30). Additional research is needed in this area with larger, more representative samples to determine the effectiveness of this end-of-life intervention.

Systematic Sampling

Systematic sampling is used when an ordered list of all members of the population is available. The process involves selecting every kth individual on the list, using a starting point selected randomly. If the initial starting point is not random, the sample is a nonprobability or nonrandom sample. To use this design, the researcher must know the number of elements in the population and the size of the sample desired. The population size is divided by the desired sample size, giving k, the size of the gap between elements selected from the list. For example, if the population size is $N = 1200$ and the desired sample size is $n = 100$, then $k = 12$. Thus the researcher would include every 12th person on the list in the sample. You can obtain this value by using the following formula:

$$\boldsymbol{k} = \text{population size} \div \text{the desired sample size}$$

For example,

$$\boldsymbol{k} = 1200 \text{ participants in the population} \div 100 \text{ desired sample size} = 12$$

Some have argued that this procedure does not actually give each element of a population an opportunity to be included in the sample and does not provide as representative a sample as simple random sampling and stratified random sampling. Systematic sampling provides a random but not equal chance for inclusion of participants in a study (see Table 9.1; Kerlinger & Lee, 2000).

De Silva, Hanwella, and de Silva (2012) used systematic sampling in their study of the direct and indirect costs of care incurred by patients with schizophrenia (population) in a tertiary care psychiatric unit. Research Example 9.5 describes their sampling process.

RESEARCH EXAMPLE 9.5

Systematic Sampling

Research Study Excerpt

Systematic sampling [sampling method] selected every second patient with an ICD-10 [International Classification of Diseases-10] clinical diagnosis of schizophrenia [target population] presenting to the clinic during a two-month period [sampling frame].... Sample consisted of 91 patients [sample size]. Direct cost was defined as cost incurred by the patient (out-of-pocket expenditure) for outpatient care. (De Silva, et al., 2012, p. 14)

Critical Appraisal

De Silva and colleagues (2012) identified their sampling process as systematic. The population and target population were appropriate for this study. Using systematic sampling increased the representativeness of the sample, and the sample size of 91 schizophrenic patients seemed adequate for the focus of this study. However, the sampling frame was identified as only the patients presenting over 2 months, and *k* was small (every second patient) in this study, which limit the representativeness of the sample. The researchers might have provided more details on how they implemented the systematic sampling method to ensure that the start of the sampling process was random (Gray et al., 2017).

De Silva and colleagues (2012, p. 14) concluded that "despite low direct cost of care, indirect cost and cost of informal treatment results in substantial economic impact on patients and their families. It is recommended that economic support should be provided for patients with disabling illnesses such as schizophrenia, especially when patients are unable to engage in full-time employment."

NONPROBABILITY SAMPLING METHODS COMMONLY USED IN QUANTITATIVE RESEARCH

In **nonprobability sampling,** not every element of a population has an opportunity to be selected for a study sample. Although this approach decreases a sample's representativeness of a target population, it is commonly used in nursing studies because of the limited number of patients available for research. You need to be able to identify the common nonprobability sampling methods used in nursing studies, which include convenience sampling, quota sampling, purposive or purposeful sampling, network sampling, and theoretical sampling. Convenience sampling is most frequently used in both quantitative and qualitative studies. Quota sampling is occasionally used in quantitative studies. Purposive, network, and theoretical sampling are used more frequently in qualitative research and are discussed later in this chapter. Table 9.1 provides a list of the common applications of these sampling methods, the representativeness achieved in quantitative studies, and the depth and richness of findings in qualitative studies.

Convenience Sampling

Convenience sampling, also called accidental sampling, is a relatively weak approach because it provides little opportunity to control for biases; participants are included in the study merely because they happen to be in the right place at the right time (Gray et al., 2017). A classroom of students, patients attending a specific clinic, individuals in a support group, and patients hospitalized with a particular medical diagnosis are examples of convenience samples. The researcher simply enters available participants into the study until the desired sample size is reached. Multiple biases may exist in the sample, some of which may be subtle and unrecognized. However, serious biases are not always present in convenience samples. According to Kerlinger and Lee (2000), a convenience sample is acceptable when it is used with reasonable knowledge and care in implementing a study.

Convenience samples are inexpensive, accessible, and usually less time-consuming to obtain than other types of samples. This type of sampling provides a means to conduct studies on nursing interventions when researchers cannot use probability sampling methods. Probability or random sampling is not possible when the pool of potential patients is limited. Researchers often think it best to include all patients who meet sample criteria to increase the sample size.

Many researchers are conducting quasi-experimental studies and RCTs in nursing and medicine that include a convenience sampling method. The study design is strengthened when the participants obtained by convenience sampling are randomly assigned to groups (see Chapter 8). Random assignment to groups, which is not a sampling method but a design strategy, does not alter the risk of biases resulting from convenience sampling but does strengthen the equivalence of the study groups. To strengthen the representativeness of a sample, researchers often increase the sample size for clinical trials (Ruffano, Dinnes, Sitch, Hyde, & Deeks, 2017).

Rew, Powell, Brown, Becker, and Slesnick (2017) conducted a quasi-experimental study to determine the effects of a brief, street-based intervention on psychological capital (self-efficacy, hope, and resilience) and health outcomes (risky sexual behavior and substance use) in homeless young women. The study lasted for 2 months, with 4 weeks of intervention and 4 weeks of follow-up. Research Example 9.6 describes their sampling process with key sampling elements in [brackets].

RESEARCH EXAMPLE 9.6

Convenience Sampling

Research Study Excerpt

The setting for this study was a street outreach drop-in-center and a temporary housing facility for homeless pregnant or new mothers and their babies in Central Texas [sampling criteria]. The sample consisted of 80 women [sample size] between the ages of 18 and 23… years who received services from these facilities [sample criteria]. Personnel employed in the drop-in center and the new mothers' housing facility informed young women of the study. Interested youths were then directed to the members of the research team [sample of convenience]. (Rew et al., 2017, p. 359)

Critical Appraisal

Rew and colleagues (2017) described sampling criteria that were appropriate for the study purpose. The initial sample size of 80 young women seemed adequate. The researchers indicated that only 40 women attended the last intervention session, the data analyses indicated that the intervention group sizes ranged from 17 to 27 women based on the variable being analyzed, and the control group sizes ranged from 11 to 20 women. The researchers did acknowledge sample attrition as a study limitation and noted that in previous studies attrition was high for this population of young, pregnant, homeless women. The study lasted 2 months, which also increased the attrition rate. The sampling method was not clearly identified but appeared to be convenience sampling because the women in the designated settings were asked to participate and were enrolled in the study if they consented. The sample section would have been stronger if the researchers had clearly identified the refusal and attrition rates and the sampling method. The final sample size was small (<47 women), with a high attrition rate, which decreased the representativeness of the sample and increased the potential for bias.

Rew et al. (2017, p. 356) found that the street-based intervention was feasible and effective because the "intervention participants had significant improvements in psychological capital, hope, resilience, and self-efficacy to refuse alcohol, social connectedness, and substance use." However, they did recommend further research with the intervention, over a longer period of time, with additional adolescent women.

Quota Sampling

Quota sampling uses a convenience sampling technique with an added feature—a strategy to ensure the inclusion of participant types likely to be underrepresented in the convenience sample, such as females, minority groups, older adults, and the poor, rich, and undereducated. The goal of quota sampling is to replicate the proportions of subgroups present in the target population. This technique is similar to that used in stratified random sampling. Quota sampling requires that the researcher be able to identify subgroups and their proportions in the target population in order to achieve representativeness for the problem being studied. Quota sampling offers an improvement in representativeness over convenience sampling (see Table 9.1).

Campbell, Kero, and Templin (2017, p. 14) used quota sampling to determine the "mild, moderate, and severe intensity cut-points for the Respiratory Distress Observational Scale [RDOS]." RDOS is a means of assessing respiratory distress in patients, but cut points for mild, moderate, and severe distress are needed to guide the use of this scale in clinical practice. Research Example 9.7 describes their sampling process.

RESEARCH EXAMPLE 9.7

Quota Sampling

Research Study Excerpt

... Patients were stratified by level of estimated respiratory distress [stratified sampling] by two expert palliative care nurse practitioners [NPs]... Four levels of respiratory distress were used—none, mild, moderate, and severe....

Adult inpatients were recruited from an urban hospital in Midwest U.S. [setting]. Spontaneously breathing patients at risk for dyspnea with one or more of the following diagnoses: lung cancer, heart failure, chronic obstructive lung disease (COPD), or pneumonia [accessible population] were enrolled until the desired sample size was achieved [convenience sampling]... The NP and RA [nurse research assistant] simultaneously observed the patient; the NPs were blinded to [or unaware of] the recruitment stratification and the RDOS score to minimize bias; the RA was blinded to the NP ranking... Participants included 84 adult inpatients [sample size] ranging from 21 to 102 years. (Campbell et al., 2017, p. 15)

Critical Appraisal

Campbell and colleagues' (2017) original sample was one of convenience because the inpatients were recruited until the sample size was achieved. The researchers clearly identified how the patients were stratified by respiratory distress, which was essential to determine the intensity cut points for the RDOS. Quota sampling increased the representativeness of this sample. The setting for the study was appropriate and provided adequate participants for the study. The researchers used blinding for certain aspects of the study for the NP and RA to decrease the potential for bias. The sampling section would have been stronger if Campbell et al. (2017) had clearly identified their sampling methods as convenience and quota.

Campbell et al. (2017) found that the NP rankings of respiratory distress in these adult inpatients were significantly correlated with the RDOS values. The mild, moderate, and severe intensity cut points were clearly identified for the RDOS, enhancing its usefulness in practice.

SAMPLE SIZE IN QUANTITATIVE STUDIES

One of the most troublesome questions that arises during the critical appraisal of a study is whether the sample size was adequate. If the study was designed to make comparisons and significant differences were found, the sample size, or number of individuals participating in the study, was adequate. Questions about the adequacy of the sample size occur only when *no* significance is found.

When critically appraising a quantitative study in which no significance was found for at least one of the hypotheses or research questions, be sure to evaluate the adequacy of the sample size. Is there really no difference? Or was an actual difference not found because of inadequacies in the research methods, such as small sample size?

Currently, the adequacy of the sample size in quantitative studies is evaluated using a power analysis (Grove & Cipher, 2017). Power is the ability of the study to detect differences or relationships that actually exist in the population. Expressed another way, it is the ability to reject a null hypothesis correctly (see Chapter 5). The minimum acceptable level of power for a study is 0.8, or 80% (Aberson, 2010; Cohen, 1988). This power level results in a 20% chance of a Type II error, in which the study fails to detect existing effects (differences or relationships). The alpha (α) or level of significance is frequently set at 0.05 in nursing studies. The power analysis results should be included in the sample section of the study. Researchers also need to perform a power analysis to evaluate the adequacy of their sample size for all nonsignificant findings, and this should be included in the discussion section of their study.

Ruffano and colleagues (2017) conducted a review of the methodological quality of 103 RCTs. Power analyses were reported for 81 (79%) of the RCTs, but 24 (30%) of these studies did not include the required number of participants indicated by the power calculations. Inadequate sample size is of particular concern in RCTs because these studies are designed to test the effectiveness of interventions. Samples that are too small can result in studies that lack power to identify significant relationships among variables or differences among groups. Low-powered studies increase the risk of a Type II error—saying something is not significant when it is actually significant (Grove & Cipher, 2017).

Factors that influence the adequacy of sample size (because they affect power) include effect size, type of quantitative study, number of variables studied, sensitivity of the measurement methods, and data analysis techniques. When critically appraising the adequacy of the sample size, consider the influence of these factors that are discussed in the next sections.

Effect Size

The effect is the presence of the phenomenon examined in a study. The effect size is the extent to which the null or statistical hypothesis is false or, stated another way, the strength of the expected relationship between two variables or differences between two groups. In a study in which the researchers are comparing two populations, the null hypothesis states that the difference between the two populations is zero. However, if the null hypothesis is false, an identifiable effect is present—a difference between the two groups does exist. If the null hypothesis is false, it is false to some degree; this is the effect size (Cohen, 1988). The statistical test tells you whether there is a difference between groups, or whether variables are significantly related. The effect size tells you the size of the difference between the groups or the strength of the relationship between two variables (Grove & Cipher, 2017).

When the effect size is large (e.g., considerable difference between groups or very strong relationship between two variables), detecting it is easier and can be done with a smaller sample. When the effect size is small (e.g., only a small difference between groups or a weak relationship between two variables), detecting it is more difficult and requires a larger sample. There are different types of effect size measures, and each corresponds to the type of statistic computed. Effect sizes can be positive or negative based on the type of relationship (positive or negative) between two variables or the differences between groups (dependent variable increases or decreases). The following are guidelines for categorizing the quality of the effect size for Pearson product-moment correlation coefficient (*r*; Grove & Cipher, 2017):

Small effect size < 0.30 or < -0.30

Medium effect size $= 0.30$ to 0.50 or -0.30 to -0.50

Large effect size > 0.50 or > -0.50

Effect size is smaller with a small sample, so effects are more difficult to detect. Increasing the sample size also increases the effect size, making it more likely that the effect will be detected, and the study findings will be significant. When critically appraising a study, determine whether the study sample size was adequate by noting whether a power analysis was conducted and what power was achieved. Examine the attrition rate for the study to determine the final sample size for data analysis. Was the final sample greater than the minimal sample size recommended by the power analysis? Also, check to see if the researchers calculated the power level of the study again when findings were not significant. When there is a post priori calculation of power, you can determine more accurately whether the sample size was adequate (Grove & Cipher, 2017).

Types of Quantitative Studies

Descriptive studies (particularly those using survey questionnaires) and correlational studies often require very large samples. In these studies, researchers may examine multiple variables, and extraneous variables are likely to affect participant response(s) to the variables under study. Researchers often make statistical comparisons on multiple subgroups in a sample, such as groups formed by gender, age, or ethnicity, requiring that an adequate sample be available for each subgroup being analyzed. Quasi-experimental and experimental studies use smaller samples more often than descriptive and correlational studies. As control in the study increases, the sample size can be decreased and still approximate the target population. Instruments in these studies tend to be more refined, with stronger reliability and validity. The type of study design can influence sample size, such as using matched pairs of subjects, which increases the power to identify group difference and decreases the sample size needed (see Chapter 8).

Number of Variables

As the number of variables under study increases, the sample size needed may increase. For example, the inclusion of multiple dependent variables in a study increases the sample size needed. When variables such as age, gender, ethnicity, and education are included in the data analyses, to answer the research questions or test the hypotheses, the sample size must be increased to detect differences between groups. Using demographic variables only to describe the sample does not cause a problem in terms of power.

Measurement Sensitivity

Quality physiological instruments measure phenomena with accuracy and precision. A thermometer, for example, measures body temperature accurately and precisely. Tools measuring psychosocial variables tend to be less precise. However, a tool that is reliable and valid measures more precisely than a tool that is less well developed. Variance tends to be higher with a less well-developed tool than with one that is well developed (Waltz, Strickland, & Lenz, 2017). For example, if you are measuring anxiety, and the actual anxiety score of several participants is 80, you may obtain measures ranging from 70 to 90 with a less well-developed tool. Much more variation from the true score occurs with new or less developed scales than when a well-developed scale is used, which will tend to show a score closer to the actual score of 80 for each participant. As variance in instrument scores increases, the sample size needed to obtain significance increases (see Chapter 10).

Data Analysis Techniques

Data analysis techniques vary in their capability to detect differences in the data. Statisticians refer to this as the "power of the statistical analysis." An interaction also occurs between the measurement sensitivity and power of the data analysis technique. The power of the analysis technique increases as precision in measurement increases. Because of this, techniques for analyzing variables measured at interval and ratio levels are more powerful in detecting relationships and differences than those used to analyze variables measured at nominal and ordinal levels (see Chapter 10 for more details on levels of measurement). Larger samples are needed when the power of the planned statistical analysis is weak.

For some statistical procedures, such as the *t*-test and analysis of variance (ANOVA), equal group sizes will increase power because the effect size is maximized with equal groups. The more unbalanced the group sizes, the smaller is the effect size. Therefore in unbalanced groups, the total sample size must be larger (Kraemer & Theimann, 1987). The chi-square test is the weakest of the statistical tests and requires large sample sizes to achieve acceptable levels of power (see Chapter 11 for more details on statistical analysis techniques).

CRITICAL APPRAISAL GUIDELINES

Adequacy of the Sample Size and Sampling Method, and Representativeness of the Sample in Quantitative Studies

The initial critical appraisal guidelines for the sampling processes used in quantitative studies were introduced earlier in this chapter. This section will focus only on the questions about the adequacy of sample size and sampling method, and the representativeness of the sample.

1. Is the sampling method probability or nonprobability? Is the specific sampling method used in the study to obtain the sample identified and appropriate (Gray et al., 2017)?
2. Is the sample size identified? Is a power analysis reported? Was the sample size appropriate, as indicated by the power analysis? If groups were included in the study, is the sample size for each group equal and appropriate (Grove & Cipher, 2017)?
3. Is the sampling process adequate to achieve a representative sample? Is the sample representative of the accessible and target populations?

Newnam and colleagues' (2015) study, which was critically appraised earlier for sample criteria and refusal and attrition rates, is presented as an example in discussing sample size, sampling method, and representativeness of the sample. These researchers conducted a RCT to identify differences in frequency and severity of nasal injuries in extremely low BW neonates on nasal CPAP treatments. Research Example 9.8 describes the power analysis conducted to determine sample and groups sizes and the sampling method.

RESEARCH EXAMPLE 9.8

Quantitative Study Sample

Research Study Excerpt

An a priori sample size estimation was calculated using 80% power, $\alpha = 0.05$ with F *tests as the statistical basis of the calculation using G*Power 3.0™. The calculated group size of 72 total subjects, 24 subjects in each of the three groups was deemed adequate to determine significant difference between groups...*

The neonates [population] were extubated to nasal CPAP. They were randomized into one of the three groups, (1) continuous nasal prongs, (2) continuous nasal mask, or (3) alternating mask/prongs every 4 hours. The specific timing of extubation was based on demonstrated clinical readiness... Participants were block stratified according to BW into four categories: <750 g; 750-1000 g; 1001-1250 g; and 1251-1500 g [quota sampling]. Known differences in skin integrity have been demonstrated with the lowest BW infants considered the most vulnerable; thus, stratification was used to keep the groups more homogeneous since it was expected that the <750 g group would contain the fewest patients. (Newnam et al., 2015, pp. 37–38)

Continued

RESEARCH EXAMPLE 9-8—cont'd

Critical Appraisal

Newnam et al. (2015) detailed the power analysis conducted to determine their study sample size. Three elements of power analysis were included: (1) standard power of 80%; (2) alpha = 0.05; and (3) statistical test (*F* test for analysis of variance [ANOVA]). However, the researchers did not provide the effect size used in the calculation. The focus of the study was determining differences among the three groups of neonates receiving CPAP by the following methods: mask CPAP, *n* = 35; prong CPAP, *n* = 21; and rotation mask and prong CPAP, *n* = 22 (see Fig. 1). The total sample size was 78, which is larger than the 72 participants recommended by power analysis. However, the study would have been stronger if the group sizes were more equal and each group included at least 24 neonates, as indicated in the power analysis. Newnam et al. (2015) did find significantly less skin injury in the group that had rotation of mask and prong. The significant results indicate that the study had an adequate sample size to determine differences among the three groups using ANOVA. The neonates admitted to this NICU were screened, and those meeting sampling criteria were admitted with parental consent, which is convenience sampling. The quota sampling involved stratification of the sample based on BW, which reduced the potential for error from extraneous variables. The quota sampling and the limited refusal and attrition rates increased the sample's representativeness of the target population. However, the sample was selected from only one NICU, and the group sizes were small (*n* = 21, 22, and 35), which decrease the representativeness of the sample and increases the potential for bias.

SAMPLING IN QUALITATIVE RESEARCH

Qualitative research is conducted to gain insights and discover meaning about a particular phenomenon, situation, event, or cultural element (Creswell & Poth, 2018; Munhall, 2012). The intent is an in-depth understanding gained from a selected sample, not on the generalization of findings from a randomly selected sample to a target population, as in quantitative research. The sampling in qualitative research focuses more on experiences, events, incidents, and settings than on people. In ethnography studies, qualitative researchers often select the setting and site and then the population and phenomenon of interest (Marshall & Rossman, 2016). In phenomenological research, researchers often select the phenomenon or population of interest and identify potential participants for their studies. The participants selected need to have experience and be knowledgeable in the area of study and willing to share rich, in-depth information about the phenomenon, situation, culture, or event being studied. For example, if the goal of the study is to describe the phenomenon of living with chronic pain, the researcher will select individuals who are articulate and reflective, have a history of chronic pain, and are willing to share their chronic pain experience (Creswell 2014; Creswell & Poth, 2018).

Common sampling methods used in qualitative nursing research are purposeful sampling, network or snowball sampling, theoretical sampling, and convenience sampling (described earlier). These sampling methods, summarized in Table 9.1, enable researchers to select information-rich cases or participants who they believe will provide them with the best data for their studies. The sample selection process can have a profound effect on the quality of the study; researchers need to describe this in enough depth to promote interpretation of the findings.

Purposeful Sampling

With **purposeful or purposive sampling,** sometimes referred to as judgmental or selective sampling, the researcher consciously selects certain participants, elements, events, or incidents to include in the study. Researchers may try to include typical or atypical participants or similar or varied situations. Qualitative researchers may select participants who are of various age categories, those who have different diagnoses or illness severity, or those who received an ineffective rather than an effective treatment for their illness. For example, researchers describing grief following the loss of a child might include parents who lost a child in the previous 6, 12, and 24 months, and the children who were lost might be of varying ages (<5, 5–10, and >10 years old). The ultimate goal of purposeful sampling is selecting information-rich cases from which researchers can obtain in-depth information for their studies.

Some have criticized the purposeful sampling method because it is difficult to evaluate the accuracy or relevance of the researcher's judgment. To offset this perception, researchers must report the characteristics that they desire in study participants and provide a rationale for selecting these types of individuals to obtain essential data for their study. In qualitative studies, purposeful sampling seems the best way to gain insights into a new area of study; discover new meaning; and/or obtain in-depth understanding of a complex experience, situation, or event (Marshall & Rossman, 2016).

Sadeghi, Hasanpour, Heidarzadeh, Alamolhoda, and Waldman (2016) conducted an exploratory-descriptive qualitative study to explore the spiritual needs of families who experienced the loss of an infant in an NICU. The researchers implemented purposeful sampling in five medical centers to recruit their study participants, as described in Research Example 9.9.

RESEARCH EXAMPLE 9.9

Purposeful Sampling

Research Study Excerpt

The research environment was the NICUs in five educational and noneducational medical centers... Sampling was done with a purposeful sampling method and considering maximal variation. In this method, the researcher for diversity selects a small number of units or cases with maximum variation relevant to the research question. In maximum variation, heterogeneity in cases is important... Inclusion criteria for families, nurses, and physicians were having experienced at least one newborn death in the last six months in the NICU. The study data were collected from June 2013 to March 2014 with face-to-face, semi-structured, in-depth interviews... In this study, 24 participants (mother, father, grandmother, nurse, and doctor), who met the inclusion criteria, were interviewed. (Sadeghi et al., 2016, pp. 36–37)

Critical Appraisal

Sadeghi et al. (2016) used purposeful sampling to select their 24 study participants. The participants were a variety of family members, nurses, and physicians from multiple, varied settings, five educational and noneducational medical centers. The participants were selected with maximum variations in age, education, and employment to obtain in-depth, rich data. The participants had to have experienced a neonate's death, with data gathered over a significant time period. In addition, the sample size seemed adequate to provide rich quality data for this study. Sadeghi and colleagues (2016, p. 35) stated that "data analysis revealed three main themes: spiritual belief in a supernatural power, the need for comfort of the soul, and human dignity for the newborn."

Network Sampling

Network sampling, sometimes referred to as snowball, chain, or nominated sampling, holds promise for locating participants who would be difficult or impossible to obtain in other ways or who had not been previously identified for study (Marshall & Rossman, 2016; Munhall, 2012). Network sampling takes advantage of social networks and the fact that friends tend to have characteristics in common. This strategy is also particularly useful for finding participants in socially devalued populations, such as persons who are dependent on alcohol, abuse children, commit sexual offenses, are addicted to drugs, or commit criminal acts. These persons seldom are willing to make themselves known.

Other groups, such as widows, grieving siblings, or persons successful at lifestyle changes, also may be located using network sampling. They are typically outside the existing healthcare system and are otherwise difficult to find. When researchers find a few participants who meet the sampling criteria, they ask for their assistance in finding others with similar characteristics.

Researchers often obtain the first few study participants through a purposeful or convenience sampling method and expand the sample size using network sampling. In qualitative research, network sampling is an effective strategy for identifying participants who can provide the greatest insight and essential information about an experience or event that is being studied. For example, if a study were being conducted to describe the lives of adolescents who are abusing substances, network sampling would enable researchers to find participants who have a prolonged history of substance abuse and who could provide rich information about their lives in an interview.

Quinn (2016) conducted a grounded theory study to explore how US nurses integrated pregnancy and full-time employment. The sample included 20 nurses "who were pregnant and delivered their first baby while employed full time on 12-hour work shifts" (Quinn, 2016, p. 170). Convenience and snowball (network) sampling methods were used to recruit study participants as described in Research Example 9.10 with key sampling elements in [brackets].

RESEARCH EXAMPLE 9.10

Network Sampling

Research Study Excerpt

The research design included recruitment of study participants from two acute care hospitals [settings] serving the tri-state area surrounding New York City. A recruitment flyer was created that invited nurses who were RNs [sample of convenience]; were employed full-time on a medical-surgical, progressive care/step-down, or critical care unit; and had recently given birth to their first babies [sampling criteria] to contact the researcher via e-mail or telephone… A second recruitment strategy relied on the network of nurses working in the tri-state area who responded to the recruitment flyer and could refer friends, coworkers, or peers [network sampling] who met the study criteria to the researcher for possible inclusion in the study. Thus, convenience and network sampling approaches were used. (Quinn, 2016, p. 172)

Critical Appraisal

Quinn (2016) clearly identified that convenience and network sampling methods used to recruit study participants. The sampling methods seemed appropriate to obtain the data needed to address the study purpose. A sufficient sample of 20 nurses from multiple units within two acute care hospitals was obtained. The participants were knowledgeable and could provide in-depth, first-hand information about being pregnant and employed full time. This study demonstrates a quality sampling process for selecting appropriate study participants who provided rich study data. Quinn (2016) described the social process of the nurses as "becoming someone different" when integrating pregnancy and full-time work. The four core categories that emerged were "(a) 'looking different, feeling different', (b) 'expectations while expecting', (c) 'connecting differently', and (d) 'transitioning labor'" (Quinn, 2016, p. 170).

Theoretical Sampling

Theoretical sampling is used in qualitative research to develop a selected theory or model through the research process. This type of sampling strategy is used most frequently with grounded theory research. The researcher gathers data from any person or group who is able to provide relevant, varied, and rich information for theory generation. The data are considered relevant and rich if they include information that generates, delimits, and saturates the theoretical codes in the study needed for theory generation (Charmaz, 2014; Creswell & Poth, 2018). A code is saturated if it is complete and the researcher can see how it fits in the theory. When a code or concept is unclear, the researcher continues to seek participants and gather data. The process continues until the codes are saturated, and the theory evolves from the codes and data. Diversity in the sample is encouraged so that the theory developed covers a wide range of behaviors in varied situations and settings.

Chase, McMahon, and Winch (2016, p. 116) conducted a grounded theory study "to understand facilitators and barriers to care seeking among blast-exposed veterans and service members who served before the implementation of systematic screening for traumatic brain injury [TBI]." The theoretical and snowball sampling methods used to recruit study participants are described in Research Example 9.11.

RESEARCH EXAMPLE 9.11

Theoretical Sampling

Research Study Excerpt

This study drew upon Grounded Theory methodology. Specifically, we used concurrent data collection and analysis, constant comparison, theoretical sampling, and a delayed literature review to understand the concepts and processes most salient to veterans and their families regarding care seeking in the years following a high-intensity combat deployment... We employed broad eligibility criteria for this study (namely, being deployed to Iraq or Afghanistan with the U.S. Army and being exposed to potentially injurious combat) and snowball sampling to capture the perspectives of veterans with a rich set of experiences related to combat exposure, postdeployment adjustment, and care seeking potentially related to TBI. (Chase et al., 2016, pp. 116–117)

Critical Appraisal

Chase and colleagues' (2016) sampling methods were appropriate for a study conducted with grounded theory methodology. Both snowball and theoretical sampling methods were applied because the researchers wanted an adequate number of veterans and family members with varied experiences to participate in the study. The sampling methods provided a quality sample of 15 veterans and 10 family members. The number of participants allowed a broader view of the facilitators and barriers to seeking care in military health systems. More details on this study are presented in the next section in the discussion of sample size in qualitative studies.

SAMPLE SIZE IN QUALITATIVE STUDIES

In quantitative research, the sample size must be large enough to identify relationships among variables or determine differences between groups. The larger the sample size and effect size, the greater the power to detect relationships and differences in quantitative studies. However, qualitative research focuses on the quality of information obtained from the person, situation, or event sampled, rather than on the size of the sample (Creswell & Poth, 2018; Munhall, 2012).

The purpose of the study determines the sampling plan and initial sample size. The depth of information that is obtained and needed to gain insight into a phenomenon, describe a cultural element, develop a theory, or describe an important healthcare concept or issue determines the final number of people, sites, and artifacts sampled. Researchers continue to obtain additional participants during data collection and analysis to promote the development of quality study findings. The sample size can be too small when the data collected lack adequate depth or richness, and an inadequate sample size can reduce the quality and credibility of the study findings.

The number of participants in a qualitative study is adequate when saturation occurs. **Saturation** occurs when newly collected data begins to be the same as what has already been collected. Concepts are understandable and well described, details of culture are available, and patterns or themes of a theory emerge. The researcher has adequate data to answer the research question while appropriately implementing the study design (Gray et al., 2017). Important factors that need to be considered in determining sample size are: (1) scope of the study; (2) nature of the topic; (3) quality of the data; and (4) design of the study (Charmaz, 2014; Creswell & Poth, 2018; Munhall, 2012).

Scope of the Study

If the scope of the study is broad, researchers will need extensive data to address the study purpose, and it may take additional participants or observations to reach saturation. A study with a broad scope requires more sampling of participants than what is needed for a study with a narrow scope. For example, a qualitative study of the experience of living with chronic illness in older adulthood would require a large sample because of the broad scope of the problem. A study that has a clear purpose and provides focused data collection usually has richer, more credible findings. In contrast to the study of chronic illness experiences of older adults, researchers exploring the lived experience of adults older than 60 years who have Parkinson disease could obtain credible findings with a smaller sample. When critically appraising a qualitative study, determine whether the sample size was adequate for the identified scope of the study.

Nature of the Topic

If the topic of study is clear and easily discussed by the study participants, fewer participants are needed to obtain the essential data. If the topic is difficult to define and awkward for people to discuss, more participants are often needed to achieve data saturation (Creswell & Poth, 2018). Mansour (2011) conducted an exploratory-descriptive qualitative study of nurses' experiences with medication administration errors. Because of the sensitive and ethical challenges of reporting medication errors, the researcher noted the need to recruit a larger sample. Topics such as gender identity, loss of a child, and history of child sexual abuse are very sensitive, complex topics to investigate. These types of topics probably will require increased participants and interview time to collect essential data. When critically appraising published studies, be sure to consider whether the sample size was adequate based on the complexity and sensitivity of the topic studied.

Quality of the Information

The quality of information obtained from interviews or observations influences the sample size. When data quality is high, with rich content, few participants are needed to achieve saturation of data in the area of study. Quality data are best obtained from articulate, well-informed, and communicative participants (Creswell & Poth, 2018; Munhall, 2012). These participants are able to share richer data in a clear concise manner. In addition, participants who have more time to be interviewed usually provide data with greater depth and breadth. The researchers will continue sampling until saturation and verification of data have been achieved to produce the best study results.

Study Design

Some studies are designed to increase the number of interviews with each participant. When researchers conduct multiple interviews with a person, they probably will collect higher quality, richer data. For example, a study design that includes an interview before and after an event usually produces higher quality data than a single-interview design. In a design with multiple interviews of each participant, they may have considered the topic and had additional insights between interviews or be more open with the researcher in subsequent interviews. Designs that involve interviewing families usually produce richer data than designs with single-participant interviews (Marshall & Rossman, 2016).

CRITICAL APPRAISAL GUIDELINES

Adequacy of the Sampling Processes in Qualitative Studies

When critically appraising the sampling processes in qualitative studies, you need to address the following questions:

1. Is the sampling plan adequate to address the purpose of the study? If purposive sampling is used, does the researcher provide a rationale for the sample selection process? If network or snowball sampling is used, does the researcher identify the networks used to obtain the sample and provide a rationale for their selection? If theoretical sampling is used, does the researcher indicate how participants are selected to promote the generation of a theory?
2. Are the sampling criteria identified and appropriate for the study?
3. Does the researcher identify the study setting and describe the entry into the setting?
4. Does the researcher discuss the quality of the data provided by the study participants? Are the participants articulate, well informed, and willing to share information relevant to the study topic?
5. Does the sampling process produce saturation and verification of data in the area of the study?
6. Is the sample size adequate based on the scope of the study, nature of the topic, quality of the data, and study design?

Chase and colleagues (2016) conducted a grounded theory study that was introduced earlier in the discussion of theoretical sampling. This study focused on understanding U.S. veterans' and their family members' experiences with the healthcare system. Theoretical and snowball sampling methods were used to recruit a sample of 25 participants. Research Example 9.12 provides the researchers' rationale for the final sample size of their study.

RESEARCH EXAMPLE 9.12

Qualitative Study Sample

Research Study Excerpt

Ultimately, the sample included veterans with and without TBI diagnoses, those seeking and those not seeking care, and those who experienced both subconcussive and concussive blast exposure during combat. Family members of veterans were also eligible to participate if they were cited by a participant as playing a role in experiences pertinent to the study. A total of 15 veterans and 10 family members participated... Participants ranged in rank (enlisted and officer), age (20-50 among veterans, 20-70 among family members), and gender (male and female veterans and family members)... Three eligible veterans contacted for the study did not participate...

All interviews were guided by a semi-structured questionnaire... and followed by open-ended questions related to combat experiences, signs and symptoms, and care seeking. Most interview questions probed earlier responses (e.g., 'Can you tell me more about...?' and emerging themes... Open coding on a subset of information-rich transcripts informed future interviews... We sought to find variation in our final four interviews to challenge our understanding of themes, but these were consistent with prior findings. Data collection for this study concluded once saturation was reached. Near the end of data collection, authors engaged in a literature review, wherein results of the study were compared with others and relationships across codes were reassessed in light of existing findings and framework. (Chase et al., 2016, p. 117)

Critical Appraisal

Chase and colleagues' (2016) study has many strengths in the area of sampling, including quality sampling methods (theoretical and snowball); conscientious, information-rich participants; and a robust sample size (n = 25), which allowed for multiple, in-depth perspectives of veterans and family members on the facilitators and barriers to the healthcare system for veterans. The refusal rate for the study was limited ($[3 \div 25] = 0.12 \times 100\% = 12\%$) and no attrition of participants was indicated. The researchers provided extensive details of the theoretical sampling

Continued

RESEARCH EXAMPLE 9-12—cont'd

conducted to ensure that data saturation was achieved. Chase et al. (2016) provided a clear rationale for the final sample size because they conducted four final interviews to challenge their understanding of theoretical themes, found consistency in their findings, and concluded that data saturation was achieved with 25 participants. The study would have been strengthened by knowing how many study participants were obtained by each of the sampling methods (theoretical and snowball). In addition, the setting for this study was not clearly designated. The researchers reported that the interviews were conducted in person or by phone, so the setting might have been the study participants' homes. Knowing the study setting adds strength to the findings.

Chase et al. (2016) found that the study participants overwhelmingly described the veteran and military health systems as inadequate for meeting their needs. Most providers were generally dismissive or insensitive to the veterans' many health needs but others were exceptional in providing care. The authors hope that this research will provide direction for rebuilding the trust between struggling veterans and their healthcare system.

RESEARCH SETTINGS

The **research setting** is the site or location used to conduct a study. Three common settings for conducting nursing studies are natural, partially controlled, and highly controlled (Gray et al., 2017). Chapter 2 initially introduced the types of settings for quantitative research. Some studies are strengthened by having more than one setting, making the sample more representative of the target population. The selection of a setting in quantitative and qualitative research is based on the purpose of the study, accessibility of the setting or sites, and number and types of participants available in the setting. The setting needs to be clearly described in the research report, with a rationale for selecting it. If the setting is partially or highly controlled, researchers should include a discussion of how they controlled the setting. The following sections describe the three types of research settings, with examples provided from some of the studies discussed earlier.

Natural Setting

A **natural or field setting** is an uncontrolled, real-life situation or environment. Conducting a study in a natural setting means that the researcher does not manipulate or change the environment for the study. Descriptive and correlational quantitative studies and qualitative studies are often conducted in natural settings.

Quinn (2016) conducted a grounded theory study to promote understanding of how RNs integrate pregnancy and full-time employment. This study was introduced earlier in the section on snowball sampling, which described the recruitment of 20 RNs from two acute care hospitals in the area surrounding New York City. Quinn implemented his study in a natural setting, the participants' home, described in Research Example 9.13.

RESEARCH EXAMPLE 9.13

Natural Setting

Research Study Excerpt

The researcher sought to conduct individual, semistructured interviews with nurses who had recently given birth to their first babies and were currently on maternity leave... Once potential participants provided contact information to the investigator, information about the study and the informed consent document were mailed to their homes or sent electronically—depending on each participant's preference... Individual, semistructured, face-to-face interviews were used to collect the data... All participants were given a pseudonym known only to the researcher, and no identifying data about place of employment were collected or used. (Quinn, 2016, p. 172)

Critical Appraisal

Quinn (2016) conducted the study interviews during maternity leave in places convenient to the participants. This is a natural study setting because the study environment was not controlled or changed by the researcher during the implementation of the study. The participants' privacy was protected by assigning them a pseudonym and not collecting identifying data about their place of employment. Because of the sensitive nature of the topic, it was important to make the participants as comfortable as possible during the study in a convenient, natural setting.

Partially Controlled Setting

A partially controlled setting is an environment that is manipulated or modified in some way by the researcher. An increasing number of nursing studies, usually correlational, quasi-experimental, and experimental studies, are being conducted in partially controlled settings. Control of a study environment is very uncommon in qualitative research; however, qualitative researchers might adapt a setting to promote the most effective environment to obtain the information they need. For example, a qualitative researcher might collect data in a private conference room in a clinic, but schedule the interviews for weekends or after clinic hours to minimize interruptions and noise.

Campbell and colleagues (2017) conducted a descriptive study to determine the cut points for mild, moderate, and severe respiratory distress with the RDOS. This study was introduced earlier in the discussion of quota sampling. The study included 84 participants in a partially controlled setting of an urban hospital, described in Research Example 9.14.

RESEARCH EXAMPLE 9.14

Partially Controlled Setting

Research Study Excerpt

Adult inpatients were recruited from an urban hospital in the Midwest U.S... Patients were identified from a pool of inpatients who were estimated to be in the last 2 weeks of life using the Palliative Performance Scale... Eligible patients were identified by the RA [research assistant] in review of the palliative care nurse practitioner's caseload of referred patients and from hospital walking rounds. (Campbell et al., 2017, p. 15)

Critical Appraisal

This partially controlled hospital environment made it possible for the RA and NP to observe and rate the dyspnea of each of the patients in the study simultaneously. The patients' illness severity was controlled using the Palliative Performance Scale to identify patients in the last 2 weeks of life. This urban hospital provided a feasible and appropriate setting for conducting this study.

Highly Controlled Setting

A highly controlled setting is an environment structured for the purpose of conducting research. Laboratories, research or experimental centers, and test units in hospitals or other healthcare settings are highly controlled environments in which experimental studies often are conducted. This type of setting reduces the influence of extraneous variables, which enables researchers to examine the effects of independent variables on dependent variables accurately.

Newnam et al. (2015) conducted an experimental study to determine the effectiveness of CPAP on related skin breakdown when using different nasal interfaces in extremely low BW neonates. This study, introduced earlier, had strong inclusion and exclusion sampling criteria to ensure a homogenous sample was selected. The sample size was large (78 neonates), with a minimal refusal rate (1%) and no attrition (see Fig. 1). The highly controlled setting used in this study is described in Research Example 9.15.

RESEARCH EXAMPLE 9.15

Highly Controlled Setting

Research Study Excerpt

A three group prospective randomized experimental study design was conducted in a 70 bed level III neonatal intensive care unit (NICU) in the southeastern United States... A team of skin experts, described as the Core Research Team (CRT), was made up of the principal investigator and three advanced practice nurses. The CRT was responsible for obtaining parental consent and conducting serial skin care evaluations on enrolled subjects during routine care in an effort to protect the infant's quiet environment. The initial skin assessment was completed within 8 hours of extubation and at intervals of every 10-12 hours while receiving nasal CPAP. (Newnam et al., 2015, pp. 37–38)

Critical Appraisal

The setting for the study of Newnam et al. (2015) was highly controlled due to the structure of the NICU and the organization and type of care delivered in this setting. The researchers also ensured that the CPAP treatments were continuously implemented with a selected nasal device (mask, prongs, or mask and prongs). The nasal skin evaluations were done in a precise and accurate way by experts, the CRT. This controlled setting was appropriate for this study to reduce the effects of extraneous variables and increase the credibility of the findings.

KEY POINTS

- Sampling involves selecting a group of people, events, behaviors, or other elements to study.
- Sampling theory was developed to determine the most effective way of acquiring a sample that accurately reflects the population under study.
- Important sampling theory concepts include population, sampling criteria, target population, accessible population, study elements, representativeness, randomization, sampling frame, and sampling method or plan.
- In quantitative research, a sampling plan is developed to increase the representativeness of the target population and decrease systematic bias and sampling error.
- In qualitative research, a sampling plan is developed to increase the depth and richness of the findings related to the phenomenon, situation, processes, or cultural elements being studied.
- The two main types of sampling plans are probability and nonprobability.
- The common probability sampling methods used in nursing research include simple random sampling, stratified random sampling, cluster sampling, and systematic sampling.
- The five nonprobability sampling methods discussed in this chapter are convenience sampling, quota sampling, purposeful sampling, network sampling, and theoretical sampling.
- Convenience sampling and quota sampling are used frequently in quantitative studies.
- Purposeful, network, and theoretical sampling are used more often in qualitative research.
- Factors to consider in making decisions about sample size in quantitative studies include the type of study, number of variables studied, sensitivity of measurement methods, data analysis techniques, and expected effect size.
- Power analysis is an effective way to determine an adequate sample size for quantitative and outcomes studies. In power analysis, effect size, level of significance ($\alpha = 0.05$), and standard power (0.8 or 80%) are used to determine sample size for a prospective study and evaluate the sample size of a completed study.

- The number of participants in a qualitative study is adequate when saturation and verification of data are achieved on the study topic.
- Important factors to consider in determining sample size for qualitative studies include: (1) scope of the study; (2) nature of the topic; (3) quality of the data collected; and (4) design of the study.
- Three common settings for conducting nursing research are natural, partially controlled, and highly controlled.

REFERENCES

Aberson, C. L. (2010). *Applied power analysis for the behavioral sciences*. New York, NY: Routledge Taylor & Francis Group.

Brown, S. J. (2018). *Evidence-based nursing: The research-practice connection* (4th ed.). Sudbury, MA: Jones & Bartlett.

Campbell, M. L., Kero, K. K., & Templin, T. N. (2017). Mild, moderate, and severe intensity cut-points for the Respiratory Distress Observation Scale. *Heart & Lung, 46*(1), 14–17.

Charmaz, K. (2014). *Constructing grounded theory* (2nd ed.). Los Angeles, CA: Sage.

Chase, R. P., McMahon, S. A., & Winch, P. J. (2016). "Tell me what you don't remember"; Care-seeking facilitators and barriers in the decade following repetitive blast exposure among army combat veterans. *Military Medicine, 181*(2), 116–122.

Cohen, J. (1988). *Statistical power analysis for the behavioral sciences* (2nd ed.). New York, NY: Academic Press.

CONSORT Group. (2010). *Welcome to the CONSORT Website*. Retrieved March 20, 2017, from http://www.consort-statement.org.

Creswell, J. W. (2014). *Research design: Qualitative, quantitative and mixed methods approaches* (4th ed.). Thousand Oaks, CA: Sage.

Creswell, J. W., & Poth, C. N. (2018). *Qualitative inquiry & research design: Choosing among five approaches* (4th ed.). Thousand Oaks, CA: Sage.

De Silva, J., Hanwella, R., & de Silva, V. A. (2012). Direct and indirect cost of schizophrenia in outpatients treated in a tertiary care psychiatry unit. *Ceylon Medical Journal, 57*(1), 14–18.

Gray, J. R., Grove, S. K., & Sutherland, S. (2017). *The practice of nursing research: Appraisal, synthesis, and generation of evidence* (8th ed.). St. Louis, MO: Elsevier Saunders.

Grove, S. K., & Cipher, D. J. (2017). *Statistics for nursing research: A workbook for evidence-based practice* (2nd ed.). St. Louis: MO: Elsevier.

Kerlinger, F. N., & Lee, H. B. (2000). *Foundations of behavioral research*. New York, NY: Harcourt Brace.

Kraemer, H. C., & Theimann, S. (1987). *How many subjects? Statistical power analysis in research*. Newbury Park, CA: Sage.

Lee, J. S., Mishra, G., Hayashi, K., Watanabe, E., Mori, K., & Kawakubo, K. (2016). Combined eating behaviors and overweight: Eating quickly, late evening meals, and skipping breakfast. *Eating Behaviors, 21*(1), 84–88.

Lee, S., Faucett, J., Gillen, M., Krause, N., & Landry, L. (2013). Risk perception of musculoskeletal injury among critical care nurses. *Nursing Research, 62*(1), 36–44.

Mansour, M. (2011). Methodological and ethical challenges in investigating the safety of medication administration. *Nurse Researcher, 18*(4), 28–32.

Marshall, C., & Rossman, G. B. (2016). *Designing qualitative research* (6th ed.). Thousand Oaks, CA: Sage.

Melnyk, B. M., Gallagher-Ford, E., Fineout-Overholt. (2017). *Implementing evidence-based practice competencies in healthcare: A practical guide for improving quality, safety, & outcomes*. Indianapolis, IN: Sigma Theta Tau International.

Munhall, P. L. (2012). *Nursing research: A qualitative perspective* (5th ed.). Sudbury, MA: Jones & Bartlett Learning.

Muroi, M., Shen, J. J., & Angosta, A. (2017). Association of medication errors with drug classifications, clinical units, and consequence of errors: Are they related? *Applied Nursing Research, 33*(1), 180–185.

Newnam, K. M., McGrath, J. M., Salyer, J., Estes, T., Jallo, N., & Bass, T. (2015). A comparative effectiveness study of continuous positive airway pressure-related skin breakdown when using different nasal interfaces in the extremely low birth weight neonate. *Applied Nursing Research, 28*(1), 36–41.

Quinn, P. (2016). A grounded theory study of how nurses integrate pregnancy and full-time employment. *Nursing Research, 65*(3), 170–178.

Reinke, L. F., Feemster, L. C., McDowell, J., Gunnink, E., Tartaglione, E. V., Udris, E., et al. (2017). The long term impact of an end-of-life communication intervention among veterans with COPD. *Heart & Lung, 46*(1), 30–34.

Rew, L., Powell, T., Brown, A., Becker, H., & Slesnick, N. (2017). An intervention to enhance psychological capital and health outcomes in homeless female youths. *Western Journal of Nursing Research, 39*(3), 356–373.

Ruffano, L. F., Dinnes, J., Sitch, A. J., Hyde, C., & Deeks, J. H. (2017). Test-treatment RCTs are susceptible to bias: A review of the methodological quality of randomized trials that evaluate diagnostic tests. *BMC Medical Research Methodology, 17*(1), 1–12.

Sadeghi, N., Hasanpour, M., Heidarzadeh, M., Alamolhoda, A., & Waldman, E. (2016). Spiritual needs of families with bereavement and loss of an infant in the neonatal intensive care unit: A qualitative study. *Journal of Pain and Symptom Management, 52*(1), 35–42.

Waltz, C. F., Strickland, O. L., & Lenz, E. R. (2017). *Measurement in nursing and health research* (5th ed.). New York, NY: Springer Publishing Company.

Because of funding changes, the Agency for Healthcare Research and Quality (AHRQ) National Guideline Clearinghouse website was scheduled for decommissioning as of July 16, 2018. For more information, go to https://www.ahrq.gov/.

CHAPTER

10

Clarifying Measurement and Data Collection in Quantitative Research

Susan K. Grove

CHAPTER OVERVIEW

LEARNING OUTCOMES

After completing this chapter, you should be able to:

1. Describe measurement theory and its relevant concepts of directness of measurement, levels of measurement, measurement error, reliability, and validity.
2. Determine the levels of measurement—nominal, ordinal, interval, and ratio—achieved by measurement methods in studies.
3. Critically appraise the reliability and validity of measurement methods in studies.
4. Critically appraise the accuracy, precision, and error of physiological measures used in studies.
5. Critically appraise the sensitivity, specificity, negative predictive value, and likelihood ratios of diagnostic tests implemented in research and clinical practice.
6. Critically appraise the measurement strategies—physiological measures, observations, interviews, questionnaires, and scales—used in quantitative studies.
7. Critically appraise the quality of the data collection section in quantitative studies.

Quality measurement of human functions and emotions is essential in research and clinical practice. **Measurement** is the process of assigning numbers or values to concepts, objects, events, or situations using a set of rules (Kaplan, 1963). The rules of measurement established for research are similar to those used in nursing practice. For example, a patient's blood pressure (BP) is measured with physiological instruments (e.g., stethoscope, cuff, sphygmomanometer). Measuring a BP requires that the patient be allowed to rest for 5 minutes and then sit with his or her legs uncrossed and arm relaxed on a table at heart level. The BP cuff must be of accurate size and placed correctly on the upper arm that is free of restrictive clothing. In addition, the stethoscope must be correctly placed over the brachial artery at the elbow (Weber et al., 2014). Following these rules ensures that the patient's BP is accurately and precisely measured and that any change in the BP reading can be attributed to a change in BP, rather than to an inadvertent error in the measurement technique. In research, variables are measured with the highest quality measurement method available to produce trustworthy data for statistical analysis. Trustworthy data are essential if a study is to produce credible findings to guide nursing practice (Waltz, Strickland, & Lenz, 2017).

Understanding the logic of measurement is important for critically appraising the adequacy of measurement methods in nursing studies. This chapter includes a discussion of the key concepts of measurement theory, with examples from nursing studies. The critical appraisals of the accuracy and precision of physiological measures and sensitivity and specificity of diagnostic tests are addressed. The most common measurement methods or strategies used in nursing research are briefly described. The chapter concludes with guidelines for critically appraising the data collection process in studies.

CONCEPTS OF MEASUREMENT THEORY

Measurement theory was developed many years ago by mathematicians, statisticians, and other scholars to guide how things are measured (Kaplan, 1963). The rules of measurement promote consistency in how individuals perform measurements, so that a measurement method used by one person will consistently produce similar results when used by another person. This section discusses some of the basic concepts and rules of measurement theory, including directness of measurement, levels of measurement, measurement error, reliability, and validity.

Directness of Measurement

Researchers must first identify the object, characteristic, element, event, or situation to be measured in their study. In some cases, identifying the object to measure and determining how to measure it are quite simple, such as measuring a person's weight and height. These are referred to as direct measures. **Direct measures** involve determining the value of concrete factors such as weight, waist circumference, temperature, heart rate, and BP. Technology is available to measure many bodily functions, biological indicators, and chemical characteristics (Stone & Frazier, 2017). The focus of measurement in these cases is on the accuracy of the measurement method and the precision of the measurement process. If a patient's BP is to be accurate, it must be measured with a quality stethoscope, cuff, and sphygmomanometer and must be precisely or consistently measured, as discussed earlier. In research, three BP measurements are usually taken and averaged to determine the most accurate and precise BP reading (Weber et al., 2014). Nurse researchers are also experienced in gathering direct measures of demographic variables such as age, educational level, number of surgeries, and days of hospitalization.

In nursing, often what is to be measured is not a concrete object but an abstract idea, characteristic, or concept, such as pain, coping, depression, or adherence. Researchers cannot directly measure an abstract idea, but they can capture some of its elements in their measurements, which are referred to as **indirect measures** or **indicators** of the concept. Rarely, if ever, can a single measurement strategy measure all aspects of an abstract concept. Therefore multiple measurement methods or indicators are needed, and even then they cannot be expected to measure all elements of an abstract concept. For example, multiple measurement methods might be used to describe pain in a study, which decreases the measurement error and increases the understanding of pain. The measurement methods of pain might include the FACES® Pain Rating Scale (presented later),

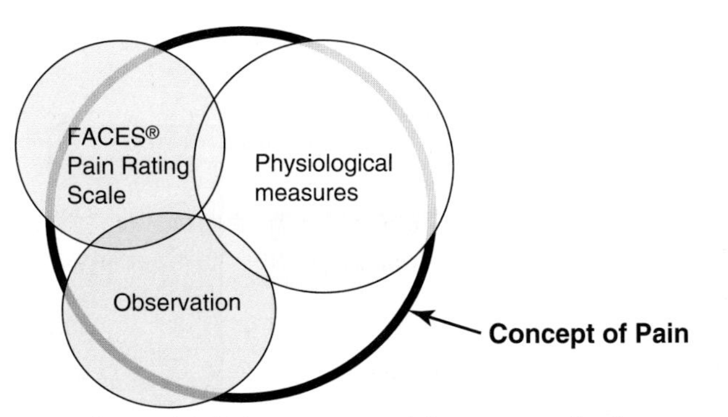

FIG 10.1 Multiple measures of the concept of pain.

observation (rubbing and/or guarding the area that hurts, facial grimacing, and crying), and physiological measures, such as pulse, BP, and respiration.

Fig. 10.1 demonstrates how multiple measures of pain increase the understanding of the concept. The bold, black-rimmed largest circle represents the concept of pain, and the colored smaller circles represent the measurement methods. A larger circle is represented by physiological measures (pulse, BP, and respirations) that provide a more objective measurement of pain. Even with three different types of measurement methods being used, the entire concept of pain is not completely measured, as indicated by the white areas within the black-rimmed circle.

Levels of Measurement

Various instruments and scales produce data that are at different levels of measurement. The traditional levels of measurement were developed by Stevens (1946), who organized the rules for assigning numbers to objects, so that a hierarchy in measurement was established. The levels of measurement, from low to high, are nominal, ordinal, interval, and ratio.

Nominal-Level Measurement

Nominal-level measurement is the lowest of the four measurement categories. It is used when data can be organized into categories of a defined property but the categories cannot be rank-ordered. For example, researchers sometimes categorize study participants by medical diagnosis. However, the category of kidney stone cannot be rated higher than the category of gastric ulcer; similarly, across categories, ovarian cyst is no closer to kidney stone than to gastric ulcer. The categories differ in quality but not quantity. Therefore it is not possible to say that study participant A possesses more of the property being categorized than participant B. (**Rule:** The categories must not be orderable.) Categories must be established in such a way that each datum will fit into only one of the categories. (**Rule:** The categories must be exclusive.) For example, a study participant may have been widowed in the past, but has remarried. If the demographic questionnaire included "Martial Status" and the categories of "Widowed" and "Married," which would the individual select? In this situation, the researcher would need to redefine the variable to be "Current Marital Status" so that the categories are exclusive. All the data must fit into the established categories. (**Rule:** The categories must be exhaustive.) The demographic questionnaire may include a variable called "Cardiac Medical Diagnoses," with the options of "Hypertension," "Heart Failure," and "Myocardial Infarction." These options are not exhaustive because individuals with cardiomyopathy would not know what to mark. Researchers might add an "Other" category, making the "Cardiac Medical Diagnoses" options exhaustive, but these data are difficult to analyze and interpret. Data such as

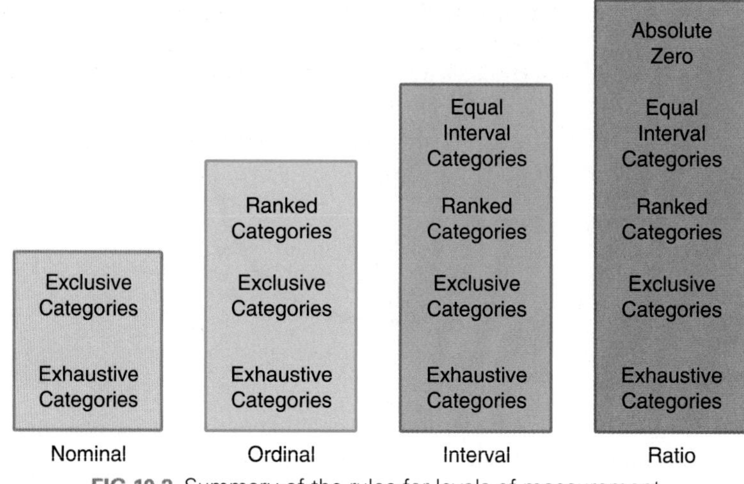

FIG 10.2 Summary of the rules for levels of measurement.

gender, race and ethnicity, marital status, and diagnoses are examples of nominal data. The rules for the four levels of measurement are summarized in Fig. 10.2 (Grove & Cipher, 2017).

Ordinal-Level Measurement

With **ordinal-level measurement,** data are assigned to categories that can be ranked. (**Rule:** The categories can be ranked.) To rank data, one category is judged to be (or is ranked) higher or lower, or better or worse, than another category. Rules govern how the data are ranked. As with nominal data, the categories must be exclusive (each datum fits into only one category) and exhaustive (all data fit into at least one category; see Fig. 10.2). With ordinal data, the quantity also can be identified (Stevens, 1946). For example, if you are measuring intensity of pain, you may identify different levels of pain. You probably will develop categories that rank these different levels of pain, such as excruciating, severe, moderate, mild, and no pain. However, in using categories of ordinal measurement, you cannot know with certainty that the intervals between the ranked categories are equal. A greater difference may exist between mild and moderate pain, for example, than between excruciating and severe pain. Therefore ordinal data are considered to have unequal intervals.

Many scales used in nursing research are ordinal levels of measurement. For example, it is possible to rank levels of mobility, ability to provide self-care, or levels of dyspnea on an ordinal scale. For dyspnea with activities of daily living (ADLs), the scale could be:

0 = no shortness of breath with ADLs
1 = minimal shortness of breaths with ADLs
2 = moderate shortness of breath with ADLs
3 = extreme shortness of breath with ADLs
4 = shortness of breath so severe that the person is unable to perform ADLs without assistance

The measurement is ordinal because it is not possible to claim that equal distances exist between the rankings. A smaller difference may exist between the ranks of 1 and 2 than between the ranks of 3 and 4.

Interval-Level Measurement

Interval-level measurement uses scales, which have equal numerical distances between the intervals. These scales follow the rules of mutually exclusive, exhaustive, and ranked categories and are assumed to represent a continuum of values. (**Rule:** The categories must have equal intervals between them.) Therefore the magnitude of the attribute can be more precisely defined. However, it is not possible to provide the absolute amount of the attribute because the interval scale lacks a zero point. Temperature is the most commonly used example of an interval scale. The difference between the temperatures of 70° F and 80° F is 10° F and is the same as the difference between the temperatures of 30° F and 40° F. Changes in temperature can be measured precisely. However, a temperature of 0° F does not indicate the absence of temperature.

Ratio-Level Measurement

Ratio-level measurement is the highest form of measurement and meets all the rules of other forms of measurement: mutually exclusive categories, exhaustive categories, ordered ranks, equally spaced intervals, and a continuum of values. Interval- and ratio-level data can be added, subtracted, multiplied, and divided because of the equal intervals and continuum of values of these data. Thus interval and ratio data can be analyzed with statistical techniques of greater strength to determine significant relationships and differences in studies (Grove & Cipher, 2017). In addition, ratio-level measures have absolute zero points. (**RULE:** The data must have absolute zero [see Fig. 10.2].) Weight, length, and volume are commonly used as examples of ratio scales. All three have absolute zeros, at which a value of zero indicates the absence of the property being measured; zero weight means the absence of weight. Because of the absolute zero point, such statements as "Participant A weighs 25 more pounds than participant B" or "Medication container A holds twice as much as container B" can be justified (Stevens, 1946). In critically appraising a study, you need to determine the level of measurement achieved for each measurement method.

Measurement Error

The ideal perfect measure is referred to as the true measure or score. However, some error is always present in any measurement strategy. Measurement error is the difference between the true measure and what is actually measured (Gray, Grove, & Sutherland, 2017). The amount of error in a measure varies from considerable error in one measurement to very little in another. Direct measures, which generally are expected to be highly accurate, are subject to error. For example, a weight scale may be inaccurate for 0.5 pound, precisely calibrated BP equipment might decrease in accuracy with use, or a tape measure may not be held at exactly the same tension in measuring the waist of each patient. A study participant in a study may be 65 years old but may write illegibly on the demographic form. As a result, the age may be entered inaccurately into the study database.

With indirect measures, the element being measured cannot be seen directly. For example, you cannot see pain. You may observe behaviors or hear words that you think represent pain, but pain is a sensation that is not always clearly recognized or expressed by the person experiencing it. The measurement of pain is usually conducted with a scale but can also include observation and physiological measures. Sometimes measures may identify some aspects of the concept but may include other elements that are not part of the concept. In Fig. 10.1, the measurement methods of scale, observation, and physiological measures include factors other than pain, as indicated by the parts of the colored circles that are outside the black-rimmed circle of the concept pain. For example, measurement methods for pain might be measuring aspects of anxiety and fear in addition to pain. However, measuring a concept with multiple methods usually decreases the measurement error and increases the understanding of the concept being measured.

Two types of error are of concern in measurement: random error and systematic error. The difference between random and systematic error is in the direction of the error. In random measurement error, the difference between the measured value and the true value is without pattern or direction (random). In one measurement, the actual value obtained may be lower than the true value, whereas in the next measurement, the actual value obtained may be higher than the true value. A number of chance situations or factors can occur during the measurement process that can result in random error (Waltz et al., 2017). For example, the person taking the measurements may not use the same procedure every time, a study participant completing a paper and pencil scale may accidentally mark the wrong column, or the person entering the data into a computer may punch the wrong key. The purpose of measuring is to estimate the true value, usually by combining a number of values and calculating an average. An average value, such as the mean, is a closer estimate of the true measurement. As the number of random errors increases, the precision of the estimate decreases.

Measurement error that is not random is referred to as systematic error. In **systematic measurement error,** the variation in measurement values from the calculated average is primarily in the same direction. For example, most of the variation may be higher or lower than the average that was calculated. Systematic error occurs because something else is being measured in addition to the concept. For example, a paper and pencil rating scale designed to measure hope may actually also be measuring perceived support. When measuring participants' weights, a scale that shows weights that are 2 pounds over the true weights will give measures with systematic error. All the measured weights will be high, and as a result the mean will be higher than if an accurate weight scale were used.

In critically appraising a study, you will not be able to judge the extent of measurement error directly. However, you may find clues about the amount of measurement error in the published report. For example, if the researchers have described the method of measurement in great detail and have provided evidence of accuracy and precision of the measurement, then the probability of error typically is reduced. The measurement errors for BP readings can be minimized by checking the BP sphygmomanometer for accuracy and recalibrating it periodically during data collection, obtaining three BP readings and averaging them to determine one BP reading for each participant, and having a trained nurse using a protocol to take the BP readings. If a checklist of pain behaviors is developed for observation, less error occurs than if the observations for pain are unstructured. Measurement will also be more precise if researchers describe using a well-developed, reliable, and valid scale, such as the FACES® Pain Rating Scale, instead of developing a new pain scale for their study. You need to critically appraise the steps researchers have taken to decrease measurement error in their studies.

Reliability

Reliability focuses on the consistency of a measurement method. For example, if you are using a multiple-item scale to measure depression, the scale should indicate similar depression scores each time an individual completes it within a short period of time. A scale that does not produce similar scores with repeat testing of this individual is considered unreliable, resulting in increased measurement error (Waltz et al., 2017). For example, the Center for Epidemiologic Studies Depression Scale (CES-D) was developed through research to diagnose depression in mental health patients (Radloff, 1977). The CES-D has been used over the last 40 years and proven to be a quality measure of depression in clinical practice and research. Fig. 10.3 illustrates this 20-item Likert scale. If the items on this scale consistently measure what it was developed to measure, depression, then this scale is considered to be both reliable and valid. The different types of reliability and validity testing outlined in Table 10.1 are discussed in the next sections.

Reliability Testing

Reliability testing determines the measurement error in an instrument or scale used in a study (Waltz et al., 2017). Because all measurement methods contain some error, reliability exists in degrees and is usually expressed as a correlation coefficient. *Estimates of reliability are specific to the sample being tested.* High reliability values reported for an established instrument do not guarantee

Center for Epidemiologic Studies Depression Scale DEPA					
THESE QUESTIONS ARE ABOUT HOW YOU HAVE BEEN FEELING LATELY. AS I READ THE FOLLOWING STATEMENTS, PLEASE TELL ME HOW OFTEN YOU FELT OR BEHAVED THIS WAY IN THE LAST WEEK. [*Hand card*]. **FOR EACH STATEMENT, DID YOU FEEL THIS WAY:** [Interviewer: You may help respondent focus on the whichever "style" answer is easier] 0 = **R**arely or none of the time (or less than 1 day)? 1 = **S**ome or a little of the time (or 1–2 days)? 2 = **O**ccasionally or a moderate amount of time (or 3–4 days)? 3 = **M**ost or all of the time (or 5–7 days)?					
	R	S	O	M	NR
1. I WAS BOTHERED BY THINGS THAT USUALLY DON'T BOTHER ME.	0	1	2	3	--
2. I DID NOT FEEL LIKE EATING; MY APPETITE WAS POOR.	0	1	2	3	--
3. I FELT THAT I COULD NOT SHAKE OFF THE BLUES EVEN WITH HELP FROM MY FAMILY AND FRIENDS.	0	1	2	3	--
4. I FELT THAT I WAS JUST AS GOOD AS OTHER PEOPLE.	0	1	2	3	--
5. I HAD TROUBLE KEEPING MY MIND ON WHAT I WAS DOING.	0	1	2	3	--
6. I FELT DEPRESSED.	0	1	2	3	--
7. I FELT THAT EVERYTHING I DID WAS AN EFFORT.	0	1	2	3	--
8. I FELT HOPEFUL ABOUT THE FUTURE.	0	1	2	3	--
9. I THOUGHT MY LIFE HAD BEEN A FAILURE.	0	1	2	3	--
10. I FELT FEARFUL.	0	1	2	3	--
11. MY SLEEP WAS RESTLESS.	0	1	2	3	--
12. I WAS HAPPY.	0	1	2	3	--
13. I TALKED LESS THAN USUAL.	0	1	2	3	--
14. I FELT LONELY.	0	1	2	3	--
15. PEOPLE WERE UNFRIENDLY.	0	1	2	3	--
16. I ENJOYED LIFE.	0	1	2	3	--
17. I HAD CRYING SPELLS.	0	1	2	3	--
18. I FELT SAD.	0	1	2	3	--
19. I FELT PEOPLE DISLIKED ME.	0	1	2	3	--
20. I COULD NOT GET GOING.	0	1	2	3	--

FIG 10.3 Center of Epidemiologic Studies Depression Scale (CES-D). (Adapted from Radloff, L. S. [1977]. The CES-D scale: A self-report depression scale for research in the general population. *Applied Psychological Measures, 1*[3], 385–394.)

that reliability will be satisfactory in another sample or with a different population. Researchers need to perform reliability testing on each instrument used in a study to ensure that it is reliable for that study (Bialocerkowski, Klupp, & Bragge, 2010; DeVon et al., 2007).

Reliability testing focuses on the following aspects of reliability: stability, equivalence, and internal consistency (see Table 10.1). **Stability reliability** is concerned with the reproducibility of scores with repeated measures of the same concept or attribute with a scale or instrument over time. Instrument stability is usually determined using **test-retest reliability**. This measure of reliability

TABLE 10.1 **DETERMINING THE QUALITY OF MEASUREMENT METHODS**

QUALITY INDICATOR	DESCRIPTION
Reliability	**Stability reliability** – concerned with the reproducibility of scores with repeated measures of the same concept or attribute with an instrument or scale over time. Stability is usually examined with **test-retest reliability.** **Equivalence reliability** **Interrater reliability** – comparison of two observers or judges in a study to determine their equivalence in making observations or judging events. **Alternate forms reliability** – comparison of two paper and pencil instruments to determine their equivalence in measuring a concept. **Internal consistency** – also known as homogeneity reliability testing; used primarily with multi-item scales where each item on the scale is correlated with all other items to determine the consistency of the scale in measuring a concept.
Validity	**Content validity** – examines the extent to which a measurement method includes all the major elements relevant to the construct being measured. **Construct validity** – focuses on determining whether the instrument actually measures the theoretical construct that it purports to measure, which involves examining the fit between the conceptual and operational definitions of a variable. **Validity from contrasting (known) groups** – instrument or scale given to two groups expected to have opposite or contrasting scores, therefore one group scores high on the scale and the other scores low. **Convergent validity** – two scales measuring the same concept are administered to a group at the same time, and the participants' scores on the scales should be positively correlated. For example, participants completing two scales to measure depression should have positively correlated scores. **Divergent validity** – two scales that measure opposite concepts, such as hope and hopelessness, are administered to participants at the same time and should result in negatively correlated scores on the scales. **Criterion-related validity** – validity that is strengthened when a study participant's score on an instrument can be used to infer his or her performance on another variable or criterion. **Predictive validity** – extent to which an individual's score on a scale or instrument can be used to predict future performance or behavior on a criterion. **Concurrent validity** – focuses on the extent to which an individual's score on an instrument or scale can be used to estimate her or his present or concurrent performance on another variable or criterion.
Readability	**Readability level** – conducted to determine the participants' ability to read and comprehend the items on an instrument. Researchers should report the level of education needed to read the instrument. Readability must be appropriate to promote the reliability and validity of an instrument.
Precision	**Precision of physiological measure** – degree of consistency or reproducibility of the measurements made with physiological instruments or equipment; comparable to reliability for multi-item scales.
Accuracy	**Accuracy of physiological measure** – addresses the extent to which the physiological instrument or equipment measures what it is supposed to measure in a study; comparable to validity for multi-item scales.

is generally used with physical measures, technological measures, and scales. An assumption of test-retest reliability is that the attribute to be measured remains the same at the two testing times and that any change in the value or score is a consequence of random error. For example, a physiological measure such as BP equipment can be tested and then immediately retested, or the equipment can be used for a time and then retested to determine the necessary frequency of recalibration. Researchers need to include test-retest reliability results in their published studies to document the reliability of their measurement methods. For example, the CES-D (see Fig. 10.3) has been used frequently in nursing studies and has demonstrated test-retest reliability values ranging from $r = 0.51$ to $r = 0.67$ in 2- to 8-week intervals. This is very solid test-retest reliability for the CES-D, indicating that it is consistently measuring depression with repeat testing and recognizing that subjects' levels of depression vary somewhat over time (Armenta, Hartshorn, Whitbeck, Crawford, & Hoyt, 2014; Sharp & Lipsky, 2002).

Reliability testing also includes **equivalence**, which involves the comparison of two versions of the same paper and pencil instrument or of two observers measuring the same event. Comparison of two observers or two judges in a study is referred to as **interrater reliability** (Polit & Yang, 2016). Studies that include collecting observational data or the making of judgments by two or more data gatherers require the reporting of interrater reliability. There is no absolute value below which interrater reliability is unacceptable. However, any value below 0.80 should generate serious concern about the reliability of the data, data gatherer, or both. The interrater reliability value is best at a value of 0.90 or 90% or higher, which means that the data collectors are equivalent during the study.

Comparison of two paper and pencil instruments or scales is referred to as **alternate forms reliability**, or parallel forms reliability (Waltz et al., 2017). Alternative forms of instruments are of concern in the development of normative knowledge testing, such as the Scholastic Aptitude Test (SAT), which is used as a college entrance requirement. The SAT has been used for decades, and there are many forms of this test, with a variety of items included on each. These alternate forms of the SAT were developed to measure students' knowledge consistently and to protect the integrity of the test.

Internal consistency is also known as homogeneity reliability testing that is used primarily with multi-item scales, in which each item on a scale is correlated with all other items on the scale to determine consistency (see Table 10.1). The principle is that each item should be consistently measuring a concept such as depression and therefore should be highly correlated with the other items on the scale. The Cronbach alpha coefficient is the most commonly used measure of internal reliability for scales with multiple items. The Cronbach alpha coefficient can only be calculated for interval- and ratio-level data. A coefficient of 1.00 indicates perfect reliability, and a coefficient of 0.00 indicates no reliability (Waltz et al., 2017). A reliability of 0.80 is usually considered a strong coefficient for a scale that has been used in several studies. For example, the CES-D has strong internal consistency reliability, with Cronbach alpha values ranging from 0.84 to 0.90 in field studies (Armenta et al., 2014; Locke & Putnam, 2002; Sharp & Lipsky, 2002). For relatively new scales, a reliability of 0.70 is considered acceptable because the scale is being refined and used with a variety of samples. The stronger correlation coefficients, which are closer to 1.0, indicate less random error and a more reliable scale. If the data are dichotomous (yes or no responses), the Kuder-Richardson formula (K-R 20) is used to estimate internal consistency (Waltz et al., 2017). A research report should include the results from stability, equivalence, and/or homogeneity reliability testing done on a measurement method from previous research and in the present study (Gray et al., 2017).

Validity

The **validity** of an instrument is a determination of how well the instrument measures the abstract concept being examined. Validity, like reliability, is not an all-or-nothing phenomenon; it is measured on a continuum. No instrument is completely valid, so researchers determine the degree of validity of an instrument rather than whether validity exists (DeVon et al., 2007; Waltz et al., 2017). Validity will vary from one sample to another and one situation to another; therefore validity testing evaluates the use of an instrument for a specific group or purpose, rather than the instrument itself. An instrument may be valid in one situation but not another. For example, the CES-D was developed to measure the depression of patients in mental health settings. Will the same scale be valid as a measure of the depression of cancer patients? Researchers determine this by pilot-testing the scale to examine the validity of the instrument in a new population. The original CES-D (see Fig. 10.3) was developed for adults, but different versions of the scale have been tested on young children (4–6 years of age), school-age children, adolescents, and older adults. These versions of the CES-D were found to be valid in these different age groups (Armenta et al., 2014; Locke & Putnam, 2002; Sharp & Lipsky, 2002).

Many types of validity exist, but this chapter will focus on the types most commonly reported in nursing studies, which include content validity, construct validity, and criterion validity (see Table 10.1; Bannigan & Watson, 2009; Polit & Yang, 2016). **Content validity** examines the extent to which the measurement method or scale includes all the major elements or items relevant to the construct being measured. The evidence for content validity of a scale includes the following: (1) how well the items of the scale reflect the description of the concept in the literature (or face validity); (2) the content experts' evaluation of the relevance of items on the scale that might be reported as an index; and (3) the study participants' responses to scale items (Gray et al., 2017).

Construct validity focuses on determining whether the instrument actually measures the theoretical construct that it purports to measure, which involves examining the fit between the conceptual and operational definitions of a variable (see Chapter 5). Three common types of construct validity presented in published studies include evidence of validity from (1) contrasting groups, (2) convergence, and (3) divergence. An instrument's **evidence of validity from contrasting groups** can be tested by identifying groups that are expected (or known) to have contrasting scores on an instrument. For example, researchers select samples from a group of individuals with a diagnosis of depression and from a group that does not have this diagnosis. You would expect these two groups of individuals to have contrasting scores on the CES-D. The group with the diagnosis of depression would be expected to have higher scores than those without the depression diagnosis, which supports the construct validity of this scale.

Evidence of validity from convergence is determined when a relatively new instrument is compared with an existing instrument(s) that measures the same construct. The instruments—new and existing—are administered to a sample at the same time, and the results are evaluated with correlational analyses. If the measures are strongly positively correlated, the validity of each instrument is strengthened. For example, the CES-D has shown positive correlations ranging from 0.40 to 0.80 with the Hamilton Rating Scale for Depression, which supports the convergent validity of both scales (Locke & Putnam, 2002; Sharp & Lipsky, 2002).

Sometimes instruments can be located that measure a concept opposite to the concept measured by the newly developed instrument. For example, if the newly developed instrument is a measure of hope, you could search for an instrument that measures hopelessness or despair. Having study participants complete these scales, which measure opposite concepts, at the same time is a way to examine **evidence of validity from divergence**. Correlational procedures are performed with the measures of the two concepts. If the divergent measure (hopelessness scale) is negatively correlated (e.g., −0.4 to −0.8) with the other instrument (hope scale), the construct validity of the instruments is supported (Waltz et al., 2017).

Criterion-related validity is strengthened when a study participant's score on an instrument can be used to infer his or her performance on another variable or criterion. The two types of criterion-related validity are predictive and concurrent validity. Predictive validity is the extent to which an individual's score on a scale or instrument can be used to predict future performance or behavior on a criterion (Waltz et al., 2017). For example, nurse researchers might want to determine the ability of a scale developed to measure health promotion behaviors to predict the future BP, body mass index, and minutes of exercise per day of individuals.

Concurrent validity focuses on the extent to which an individual's score on an instrument or scale can be used to estimate her or his present or concurrent performance on another variable or criterion. For example, concurrent validity could be examined if you measured an individual's self-esteem and used the score to estimate his or her score on a coping with illness scale. Individuals with high scores on self-esteem would also be expected to have high coping scores. The difference between concurrent validity and predictive validity is the timing of the measurement of the other criterion. Concurrent validity is examined within a short period of time, and predictive validity is examined in terms of future performance.

The evidence of an instrument's validity from previous research and the current study should be included in the published report. In critically appraising a study, you need to judge the validity of the measurement methods that were used. However, you cannot consider validity apart from reliability (see Table 10.1). If a measurement method does not have acceptable reliability, then it is not valid.

Readability Level of Measurement Methods

Readability level focuses on the study participants' ability to read and comprehend the content of an instrument or scale. Readability is essential if an instrument is to be considered valid and reliable for a sample (see Table 10.1). Assessing the level of readability of an instrument is relatively simple and takes about 10 to 15 minutes. More than 30 readability formulas are available. These formulas use counts of language elements to provide an index of the probable degree of difficulty of comprehending a scale's items (Gray et al., 2017). Readability formulas are now a standard part of word processing software. Researchers should report the reading level or level of education study participants need to complete an instrument.

ACCURACY, PRECISION, AND ERROR OF PHYSIOLOGICAL MEASURES

Physiological measures are measurement methods used to quantify the level of functioning of human beings (Ryan-Wenger, 2017). Laboratory tests and biomedical devices are used to measure biophysical constructs such as cardiac status in research and practice. The precision, accuracy, and error of physiological and biochemical measures tend not to be reported or are minimally covered in published studies. These routine physiological measures are assumed to be accurate and precise, an assumption that is not always correct. Some of the most common physiological measures used in nursing studies include BP, heart rate, weight, body mass index, and laboratory values. Sometimes researchers obtain these measures from the patient's record, with no consideration given to their accuracy. For example, how many times have you heard a nurse ask a patient his or her height or weight, rather than measuring or weighing the patient? Researchers using physiological measures should provide evidence of the measure's accuracy, precision, and potential for error (see Table 10.1; Gift & Soeken, 1988; Ryan-Wenger, 2017).

Accuracy

Accuracy is comparable to validity in that it addresses the extent to which the instrument measures what it is supposed to measure in a study (Ryan-Wenger, 2017). For example, oxygen saturation measurements with pulse oximetry are considered comparable with measures of oxygen saturation with arterial blood gases. Because pulse oximetry is an accurate measure of oxygen saturation, it has been used in studies because it is easier, less expensive, less painful, and less invasive for research participants. Researchers need to document that previous research has been conducted to determine the accuracy of pulse oximetry for the measurement of an individual's oxygen saturation level in their study.

Precision

Precision is the degree of consistency or reproducibility of measurements made with physiological instruments. Precision is comparable to reliability. The precision of most physiological equipment depends on following the manufacturer's instructions for care and routine testing of the equipment. Test-retest reliability is appropriate for physiological variables that have minimal fluctuations, such as lipid levels, bone mineral density, or weight of adults (Ryan-Wenger, 2017). Test-retest reliability can be inappropriate if the variables' values frequently fluctuate with various activities, such as with pulse, respirations, and BP. However, test-retest is a good measure of precision if the measurements are taken in rapid succession. For example, national BP guidelines encourage taking three BP readings 1 to 2 minutes apart and then averaging them to obtain the most precise and accurate measure of BP (Weber et al., 2014).

Error

Sources of error in physiological measures can be grouped into the five categories—environment, user, subject, equipment, and interpretation. The environment affects the equipment and study participant. Environmental factors might include temperature, barometric pressure, and static electricity. User errors are caused by the person using the equipment and may be associated with variations by the same user, different users, or changes in supplies or procedures used to operate the equipment. Subject errors occur when the participant alters the equipment, or the equipment alters the participant. In some cases, the equipment may not be used to its full capacity. Equipment error may be related to calibration or the stability of the equipment. Signals transmitted from the equipment are also a source of error and can result in misinterpretation. Researchers need to report the

CRITICAL APPRAISAL GUIDELINES

Reliability and Validity of Scales, and Accuracy, Precision, and Error of Physiological Measures

In critically appraising a study, you need to determine the directness and level of measurement, reliability and validity of scales, accuracy and precision of physiological measures, and potential measurement errors for the different measurement methods used in a study. In most studies, the methods section includes a discussion of measurement methods, and you can use the following questions to evaluate them:

1. What measurement method(s) were used to measure each study variable?
2. Was the type of measurement direct or indirect?
3. What level of measurement was achieved for each of the study variables?
4. Was reliability information provided from previous studies and for this study?
5. Was the validity of each measurement method adequately described? In some studies, researchers simply state that the measurement method has acceptable validity based on previous research. This statement provides insufficient information for you to judge the validity of an instrument.
6. Did the researchers address the accuracy, precision, and potential for errors with the physiological measures?
7. Was the process for obtaining, scoring, and/or recording data described?
8. Did the researchers provide adequate description of the measurement methods to judge the extent of measurement error?

protocols followed or steps taken to prevent errors in their physiological and biochemical measures in their published studies (Ryan-Wenger, 2017; Stone & Frazier, 2017).

Schmitt and colleagues (2017) studied the relationships among the concepts of depression, self-management, and hyperglycemia in 430 adults with diabetes (57.7%, type 1, 42.3%, type 2). Research Example 10.1 describes some of the measurement methods used in this study.

RESEARCH EXAMPLE 10.1

Reliability and Validity of Scales, and Accuracy, Precision, and Error of Physiological Measures

Research Study Excerpt

Depressive Symptoms

Depressive symptoms were measured using the Center for Epidemiologic Studies Depression Scale (CES-D). The CES-D assesses the frequencies of 20 common symptoms of depression during the previous week. Responses are given on a four-point Likert scale ranging from 0—'rarely or never' to 3—'most of the time'. Total scores range between 0 and 60, with higher values indicating more depressive symptoms. The CES-D has very good reliability and validity in assessing depression... which was also confirmed for people with diabetes.... In the present study, Cronbach's α [alpha] amounted to 0.88, indicating adequate reliability...

Glycemic Control

To estimate glycemic control, glycosylated hemoglobin (HbA_{1c}) was assessed. All blood samples were analyzed in one central laboratory at the same time as the psychometric assessments were conducted. HbA_{1c} values were determined using high performance liquid chromatography, performed with the Bio-ad Variant II Turbo analyzer (meeting the current standards of HbA_{1c} measurement; DCCT standard). The laboratory normal range is 4.3-6.1% (24-43 mmol/mol). (Schmitt et al., 2017, pp. 18–19)

Critical Appraisal

Schmitt and colleagues (2017) described the CES-D structure and scoring process. This scale is an indirect measure of depression producing interval-level data. A CES-D score of 16 or higher is associated with depression. The CES-D has been widely used in various types of studies and with diabetic patients, which adds to the construct validity of the scale. The researchers also identified the 20-item scale that was measuring depressive symptoms, which addresses the scale's content validity. The scale was reported to have "very good reliability and validity in assessing depression," but no specific information was provided to support this statement. The Cronbach α for this study was $r = 0.88$, which indicates acceptable internal consistency of the scale in this study. The researchers should have discussed the reliability and validity information from previous studies to support the use of the CES-D in this study (Gray et al., 2017).

The participants' glycemic control was measured directly with the HbA_{1c} laboratory test, which provides an average blood sugar level for each individual over the last 90 days. The blood samples were collected at the same point in the study for all participants and analyzed at one central laboratory. Current standards were followed in analyzing the blood, and the normal results were identified for HbA_{1c}. These actions increased the precision and accuracy of the HbA_{1c} measurements. However, the researchers should have provided more details about the collection, storage, and transmission of the blood samples to the laboratory. They also needed to discuss the certification of the laboratory and the process for providing the results to the researchers. This information is needed for you determine the potential for measurement error in this study (Ryan-Wenger, 2017).

Schmitt et al. (2017) found that depression was related to hyperglycemia for people with both types 1 and 2 diabetes. These researchers concluded that the treatment of depression might decrease hyperglycemia and promote improved self-management by patients with diabetes.

USE OF SENSITIVITY, SPECIFICITY, AND LIKELIHOOD RATIOS TO DETERMINE THE QUALITY OF DIAGNOSTIC TESTS

Sensitivity, Specificity, and Predictive Values of Diagnostic Tests

An important part of evidence-based practice (EBP) is the use of quality diagnostic tests or screening tools to determine the presence or absence of disease (Straus, Glasziou, Richardson, Rosenberg, & Haynes, 2011). Nurses need to know which laboratory test or imaging study is best for diagnosing specific diseases. When the test is conducted, are the results accurate? The **accuracy of a screening test** or a test used to confirm a diagnosis is evaluated in terms of its ability to assess the presence or absence of a disease or condition correctly as compared with the criterion standard. The **criterion standard** is the most accurate means of currently diagnosing a particular disease or current best practice (Umberger, Hatfield, & Speck, 2017). This standard serves as a basis for comparison with newly developed diagnostic or screening tests. If the test is positive, what is the probability that the disease is present? If the test is negative, what is the probability that the disease is not present? When nurses, nurse practitioners, and physicians talk to their patients about the results of their tests, how sure are they that the patient does or does not have the disease? Sensitivity and specificity are terms commonly used to describe the accuracy of a diagnostic test (Grove & Cipher, 2017). You will see these terms used in studies and other healthcare literature, and we want you to be able to understand them and their usefulness for practice and research.

The possible outcomes of a screening test for a disease include: (1) ***true-positive***, which is an accurate identification of the presence of a disease; (2) ***false-positive***, which indicates that a disease is present when it is not; (3) ***false-negative***, which indicates that a disease is not present when it is; or (4) ***true-negative***, which indicates accurately that a disease is not present. Table 10.2 is commonly used to visualize these four outcomes (Grove & Cipher, 2017; Straus et al., 2011).

You can calculate sensitivity and specificity based on research findings and clinical practice outcomes to determine the most accurate diagnostic or screening tool to use when identifying the presence or absence of a disease for a population of patients. More recently, Umberger and colleagues (2017, p. 22) recommended calculating the negative predictive value (NPV) for "preventing, detecting, and ruling out disease, where the positive predictive value (PPV) may not be relevant for that purpose." A high NPV test means that the patient probably does not have the

TABLE 10.2 POSSIBLE OUTCOMES FOR DIAGNOSTIC OR SCREENING TESTS

DIAGNOSTIC TEST RESULT	DISEASE PRESENT	DISEASE ABSENT	TOTAL
Positive test	a (true-positive)	b (false-positive)	a + b
Negative test	c (false-negative)	d (true-negative)	c + d
Total	a + c	b + d	a + b + c + d

a, Number of people who have the disease and the test is positive (*true-positive*).
b, Number of people who do not have the disease and the test is positive (*false-positive*).
c, Number of people who have the disease and the test is negative (*false-negative*).
d, Number of people who do not have the disease and the test is negative (*true-negative*).
From Grove, S. K., & Cipher, D. J. (2017). *Statistics for nursing research: A workbook for evidence-based practice* (2nd ed.) (p. 393). St. Louis, MO: Elsevier.

disease, which reduces the number of uncomfortable, costly treatments that the patient might have to undergo. The formulas for calculating sensitivity, specificity, NPV, and PPV are provided as follows:

$$\textbf{Sensitivity calculation} = \text{probability of disease} = \frac{a}{(a+c)} \times 100\% = \text{true-positive rate}$$

$$\textbf{Specificity calculation} = \text{probability of no disease} = \frac{d}{(b+d)} \times 100\% = \text{true-negative rate}$$

$$\textbf{Negative Predictive Value (NPV)} = \text{percentage of true-negatives among all who test negative} = d/(c+d) \times 100\%$$

$$\textbf{Positive Predictive Value (PPV)} = \text{percentage of true-positives among all who test positive} = a/(a+b) \times 100\%$$

Sensitivity is the proportion of patients with the disease who have a positive test result, or true-positive rate. The CES-D (see Fig. 10.3) with a score of 15 or higher has 89% sensitivity for diagnosing depression in adults and 92% sensitivity in older adults. The researcher or clinician might refer to the test sensitivity in the following ways:

- A highly sensitive test is very good at identifying the disease in a patient.
- If a test is highly sensitive, it has a low percentage of false negatives, which vary based on the focus of the test and participants' scores on the test.

Specificity is the proportion of patients without the disease who have a negative test result, or true-negative rate. You need to know that as a test becomes more sensitive, it usually becomes less specific (Umberger et al., 2017). The CES-D with a score of 15 or higher has 70% specificity for diagnosing depression in adults and 87% specificity in older adults. The researcher or clinician might refer to the test specificity in the following ways:

- A highly specific test is very good at identifying the patients without a disease.
- If a test is very specific, it has a low percentage of false-positives.

CRITICAL APPRAISAL GUIDELINES

Sensitivity, Specificity, and Predictive Values of Diagnostic Tests

When critically appraising a study, you need to judge the sensitivity, specificity, and NPV of the diagnostic tests used in the study.

1. Was a diagnostic test used in a study?
2. Are the sensitivity and specificity values provided for the diagnostic test from previous studies and for this study's population (Grove & Cipher, 2017)?
3. Did the researchers discuss the NPV and what it means for the accuracy of the test (Umberger et al., 2017)?

Ballard and colleagues (2017) conducted a study to determine the sensitivity and specificity of the Ask Suicide Screening Questions (ASQ) in a pediatric emergency department (ED). Suicide is now the second leading cause of death in children and adolescents aged 10 to 19 years. Research Example 10.2 describes the accuracy of the ASQ in research.

RESEARCH EXAMPLE 10.2

Sensitivity, Specificity, and Negative Predictive Value

Research Study Excerpt

The Ask Suicide Screening Questions *(ASQ) is a four-item non-proprietary suicide screening instrument that can be administered to patients in the ED for psychiatric or non-psychiatric reasons, aged 10 to 21 years, by nurses regardless of psychiatric training (Horowitz et al., 2012). All questions are asked to the patient, and a 'yes' response to any of the four items is considered a positive screen. The four items are the following: 'In the past few weeks, have you wished you were dead?' 'In the past few weeks, have you felt that you or your family would be better off if you were dead?', 'In the past week, have you been having thoughts about killing yourself?' and 'Have you ever tried to kill yourself?' The ASQ was developed from a study of 524 patients across three pediatric EDs using the* Suicide Ideation Questionnaire *(SIQ) as the criterion standard... In the initial development study, for psychiatric patients, the ASQ was found to have a sensitivity of 97.6%, a specificity of 65.6%, and a negative predictive value of 96.9% compared with the SIQ.*

The ASQ was implemented with a compliance rate of 79%. Fifty-three percent of the patients who screened positive (237/448) did not present to the ED with suicide-related complaints. These identified patients were more likely to be male, African American, and have externalizing behavior diagnoses. The ASQ demonstrated a sensitivity of 93% and specificity of 43% to predict return ED visits with suicide-related presenting complaints within 6 months of the index visit. (Ballard et al., 2017, pp. 174–176)

The results of the study by Ballard and colleagues (2017) are shown in Table 10.3, so you can understand the calculations of sensitivity, specificity, and NPV for this study.

TABLE 10.3 Outcomes of the ASQ for repeat emergency department visits by 6-month follow-up

Diagnostic Test Result	Visit with Suicide Presenting Complaint	No Visit with Suicide Presenting Complaint	Total
ASQ Positive	28 (a)	250 (b)	278 (a + b)
ASQ Negative	2 (c)	194 (d)	196 (c + d)
Total	30 (a + c)	444 (b + d)	474 (a + b + c + d)

a, Number of individuals with repeat ED visit with suicide-presenting complaint who had positive ASQ (*true-positive*).
b, Number of individuals with no repeat ED visit with suicide-presenting complaint who had a positive ASQ (*false-positive*).
c, Number of individuals with repeat ED visit with suicide-presenting complaint who had a negative ASQ (*false-negative*).
d, Number of individuals with no repeat ED visit with suicide-presenting complaint who had a negative ASQ (*true-negative*).
ASQ, Ask Suicide Screening Questions; *ED*, emergency department.
Data from Ballard, E. D., Cwik, M., Van Eck, K., Goldstein, M., Alfes, C., Wilson, M. E., et al. (2017). Identification of at-risk youth by suicide screening in a pediatric emergency department. *Prevention Science, 18*(2), 174–182.

$$\textbf{Sensitivity calculation} = \textbf{probability of disease} = \frac{\textbf{a}}{\textbf{(a + c)}} \times \textbf{100\%} = \text{true-positive rate}$$

$$\text{Sensitivity} = \text{probability of suicidal complaint} = \frac{28}{(28+2)} \times 100\% = \frac{28}{30} \times 100\% = 0.933 \times 100\% = 93.3\%$$

$$\textbf{Specificity calculation} = \textbf{probability of no disease} = \frac{\mathbf{d}}{(\mathbf{b+d})} \times \mathbf{100\%} = \textbf{true-negative rate}$$

$$\text{Specificity} = \text{probability no suicidal complaint} = \frac{194}{(250+194)} \times 100\% = \frac{194}{444} \times 100\%$$
$$= 0.437 \times 100\% = 43.7\%$$

$$\textbf{Negative Predictive Value (NPV)} = \textbf{percentage of people who probably do not have the disease when the test is negative} = \mathbf{d/(c+d) \times 100\%}$$

$$\text{NPV} = 194/(2+194) \times 100\% = 0.9898 \times 100\% = 98.98\%$$

The sensitivity of 93.3% indicates the percentage of patients with a positive ASQ who presented to the ED with suicidal complaint(s) (true-positive rate) within 6 months. The specificity of 43.3% indicates the percentage of the patients with a negative ASQ who did not present to the ED with suicidal complaint(s) (true-negative rate) within 6 months. NPV was extremely strong (98.98%) in identifying children and adolescents with a negative ASQ, who probably did not have suicidal complaints. These children and adolescents would not need additional assessment or treatment for suicidal intentions.

Critical Appraisal

Ballard and colleagues (2017) described the process for developing the ASQ from the SIQ, which had been considered the criterion standard. The scoring for the ASQ was described and easily accomplished by nurses. The ASQ had strong sensitivity (97.6%), specificity (65.6%), and NPR (96.9%) when compared with the SIQ during development. In this study, the ASQ also presented strong sensitivity (93.3%) and specificity (43.7%), as presented in the calculations related to Table 10.3 data. The NPV was not noted in the study but was calculated to be 98.98%, which is very strong in determining children and adolescents who did not have suicidal intentions.

Ballard et al. (2017) encouraged nurses to incorporate the ASQ into the standard care of pediatric ED settings. This brief screening instrument "can identify patients who do not directly report suicide-related presenting complaints at triage and who may be at particular risk for future suicidal behaviors" (Ballard et al., 2017, p. 174).

Likelihood Ratios

Likelihood ratios (LRs) are additional calculations that can help researchers determine the accuracy of diagnostic or screening tests, which are based on the sensitivity and specificity results. The LRs are calculated to determine the likelihood that a positive test result is a true-positive and that a negative test result is a true-negative. The ratio of the true-positive results to false-positive results is known as the positive LR (Campo, Shiyko, & Lichtman, 2010; Straus et al., 2011). The positive LR is calculated as follows, using the data from the study by Ballard et al. (2017):

$$\textbf{Positive LR} = \text{sensitivity} \div (100\% - \text{specificity})$$

$$\text{Positive LR for suicide complaints} = 93.3\% \div (100\% - 43.7\%) = 93.3\% \div 56.3\% = 1.657 = 1.66$$

The negative LR is the ratio of true-negative results to false-negative results and is calculated as follows:

$$\textbf{Negative LR} = (100\% - \text{sensitivity}) \div \text{specificity}$$

$$\text{Negative LR suicide complaints} = (100\% - 93.3\%) \div 43.7\% = 6.7\% \div 43.7\% = 0.153 = 0.15$$

The very high LRs (or those that are >10) rule in the disease or indicate that the patient has the disease. The very low LRs (or those that are <0.1) almost rule out the chance that the patient has the disease (Campo et al., 2010; Straus et al., 2011). Understanding sensitivity, specificity, NPV, and LR increases your ability to read clinical studies and determine the most accurate diagnostic test to use in clinical practice (Straus et al., 2011; Umberger et al., 2017).

MEASUREMENT STRATEGIES IN NURSING

Because nursing studies examine a wide variety of phenomena, an extensive array of measurement methods are needed to conduct these studies. Some nursing phenomena have not been examined because no one has thought of a way to measure them, which has implications for clinical practice and research. This section describes some of the most common measurement methods used in nursing research, including physiological measures, observational measurements, interviews, questionnaires, and scales.

Physiological Measures

A variety of approaches for obtaining physiological measures is possible. Some measurements are relatively easy to obtain and are an extension of the measurement methods used in nursing practice, such as those used to obtain weight and BP. Other measurements are more complex, expensive, and sometimes require an imaginative approach. For example, some physiological measures are obtained by using self-report with diaries, scales, or observation checklists, and other physiological measures are obtained using laboratory tests and electronic monitoring.

The availability of electronic monitoring equipment has greatly increased the possibilities of physiological measurement in nursing studies, particularly in critical care environments (Stone & Frazier, 2017). Electronic monitoring requires placing sensors on or within the study participant, such as electrocardiographic leads and arterial lines. The sensors measure changes in bodily functions as electrical energy. Some electronic equipment provides simultaneous recording of multiple physiological measures that are displayed on a monitor, such as equipment that records the pulse, heart rhythm, and arterial pressure. The equipment is often linked to a computer, which allows retrieval, review, and analysis of the complex data.

Lu, Lin, Chen, Tsang, and Su (2013) conducted a quasi-experimental study to determine the effect of acupressure on the sleep quality of psychogeriatric inpatients. Acupressure was performed for each study participant in the psychiatric hospital's examination room. Sleep quality was measured by the patients' self-report of their sleep and by using actigraphy, a method that uses an electronic device to detect and record movement. Research Example 10.3 describes these two physiological measures that were critically appraised using the guidelines presented earlier.

RESEARCH EXAMPLE 10.3

Physiological Measures

Research Study Excerpt

Sleep quality was assessed subjectively and objectively. Subjective data were measured by the PSQI [Pittsburg Sleep Quality Index] developed by Buysse, Reynolds, Monk, Berman, and Kupfer (1989). The PSQI is a 19-item questionnaire used to measure sleep quality and disturbances for the previous 4 weeks leading up to administration. Seven component scores (sleep latency, sleep duration, habitual sleep efficiency, sleep disturbances, the use of sleeping medications, daytime dysfunction, and perceived sleep quality) are generated and are summed to yield one global score. The higher the score is, the worse the sleep quality. The sensitivity and specificity of a global score over 5 (poor sleeper) is 90% and 87%, respectively (Buysse et al., 1989).

Objective data were measured using actigraphy (Lenience No. 019678), a standardized, noninvasive, ambulatory device equipped with a sensor (piezoelectric accelerometer) that is worn by participants to monitor and record gross motor activities continuously over an extended period of time. Actigraphy is useful to assess sleep-wake cycles and circadian rhythms and offers reliable results with an average accuracy over 90%, which approximates that of the polysomnography... Participants wore the device all day, every day for 4 weeks, except when showering. The participant elected to wear the device on either the nondominant wrist or ankle. To enhance the data accuracy and prevent the device from being incidentally dislodged, an external wrapper was used during the wearing. Data were read, transferred, stored, and analyzed using ActiWeb software.... [T]he actigraphical data were translated into meaningful information used to assess the participants' sleep latency, total sleep time, sleep efficiency, number of sleep interruptions (wake episodes), and minutes of wake time after the onset of sleep. (Lu et al., 2013, pp. 132–133)

Critical Appraisal

Lu and colleagues (2013) used two strong physiological measures of self-report (PSQI) and electronic monitoring (actigraphy) to measure their dependent variable of sleep quality. The PSQI has strong sensitivity (90%) and specificity (87%) in determining sleep problems and was reliable in this sample (Cronbach $\alpha = 0.87$). The discussion of this scale would have been strengthened by providing reliability and validity information from previous studies (Waltz et al., 2017). The actigraphy used to electronically monitor sleep activities was described in detail. The researchers compared this device with polysomnography and indicated that it was 90% as accurate. When wearing the device, the participants took actions to promote the accuracy and precision of the data. The processes for transferring and analyzing the data were also detailed, indicating that the results were strong in describing sleep quality, with limited potential for measurement error.

Lu and associates (2013) found that sleep quality was significantly improved after acupressure, as measured by PSQI and actigraphy. Because acupressure is a noninvasive, low-risk, and low-cost tool, the researchers recommended that it might be an effective intervention to treat insomnia in this population.

Observational Measurement

Observational measurement involves an interaction between the study participants and observer(s), in which the observer has the opportunity to watch the participant perform in a specific setting (Waltz et al., 2017). Unstructured observation is often used to collect data in qualitative studies (see Chapter 3). **Unstructured observations** involve spontaneously observing and recording what is seen in words. The analysis of these data may lead to a more structured observation and the development of an observational checklist (Creswell, 2014; Creswell & Poth, 2018; Marshall & Rossman, 2016).

In **structured observational measurement,** the researcher carefully defines what he or she will observe and how the observations are to be made, recorded, and coded as numbers (Waltz et al., 2017).

For observations to be structured, researchers will develop a category system for organizing and sorting the behaviors or events being observed. Checklists are often used to indicate whether a behavior occurred. Rating scales allow the observer to rate the behavior or event. This provides more information for analysis than dichotomous data, which indicate only whether or not the behavior occurred. Because observation tends to be more subjective than other types of measurement, it is often considered less credible. In many cases, observation may be the only approach for obtaining important data for nursing's body of knowledge. As with any means of measurement, consistency is very important. As a result, reporting interrater reliability of those doing the observations is essential.

CRITICAL APPRAISAL GUIDELINES

Observational Measurement

When critically appraising observational measures, consider the following questions:

1. Is the object of observation clearly identified and defined?
2. Are the techniques for recording observations described?
3. Is interrater reliability for the observers described?

McLellan, Gauvreau, and Connor (2017) conducted a study to validate the newly developed Children's Hospital Early Warning Score (CHEWS) with the previously validated Brighton Pediatric Early Warning Score (PEWS). The PEWS was originally developed for early detection of critical deterioration of all noncardiac pediatric patients. The CHEWS was a modified version of the PEWS observational tool that was developed to identify pediatric cardiac patients at risk for critical deterioration, enabling clinicians to intervene early and prevent further deterioration. Research Example 10.4 includes part of the researchers' description of their observational tool's validity and reliability.

RESEARCH EXAMPLE 10.4

Observational Measurement

Research Study Excerpt

The final revised tool (Fig. 2, called the Cardiac Children's Hospital Earl Warning Score (C-CHEWS)... was successfully piloted, fully implemented and then formally validated (... sensitivity 95.3%, specificity 76.2%) in the pediatric cardiac population in a previous study (McLellan, Gauvreau, & Connor, 2014). In this study, the tool demonstrated excellent discrimination in identifying critical deterioration in children with cardiac disease and performed significantly better than the PEWS in identifying critical deterioration (McLellan et al., 2014). To optimize safety and to improve clarity, the hospital leadership decided to implement the cardiac tool throughout all inpatients area rather than having similar but different tools operating in the same institution. The C-CHEWS was renamed the Children's Hospital early Warning Score (CHEWS) and incorporated into the electronic health record....

...Inter-rater reliability between staff nurses of all experience levels had previously been established for the CHEWS tool (100% score ≥ 3, kappa statistic 1.00) during the initial validation study and was not repeated. (McLellan et al., 2017, pp. 53–54)

Children's Hospital Early Warning Score					
	0	1	2	3	Score
Behavior/Neuro	• Playing/sleeping appropriately • Alert, at patient's baseline	• Sleepy, somnolent when not disturbed	• Irritable, difficult to console • Increase in patient's baseline seizure activity	• Lethargic, confused, floppy • Reduced response to pain • Prolonged or frequent seizures • Pupils asymmetric or sluggish	
Cardiovascular	• Skin tone appropriate for patient • Capillary refill ≤2 seconds	• Pale • Capillary refill 3–4 seconds • Mild* tachycardia • Intermittent ectopy or irregular HR (not new)	• Grey • Capillary refill 4–5 seconds • Moderate* tachycardia	• Grey and mottled • Capillary refill >5 seconds • Severe* tachycardia • New onset bradycardia • New onset/increase in ectopy, irregular HR or heart block	
Respiratory	• Within normal parameters • No retractions	• Mild* tachypnea/ increased WOB (flaring, retracting) • Up to 40% supplemental oxygen • Up to 1L NC > patient's baseline need • Mild desaturations < patient's baseline • Intermittent apnea self-resolving	• Moderate* tachypnea/increased WOB (flaring, retracting, grunting, use of accessory muscles) • 40–60% oxygen via mask • 1–2 L NC > patient's baseline need • Nebs q 1–2 hr • Moderate desaturations < patient's baseline • Apnea requiring repositioning or stimulation	• Severe* tachypnea • RR < normal for age • Severe increased WOB (i.e. head bobbing, paradoxical breathing) • >60% oxygen via mask • >2 L NC > patient's baseline need • Nebs q 30 minutes – 1 hr • Severe desaturations < patient's baseline • Apnea requiring interventions other than repositioning or stimulation	
Staff Concern		Concerned			
Family Concern		Concerned or absent			
					Total

	Mild*	Moderate*	Severe*
Infant	≥10% ↑ for age	≥15% ↑ for age	≥25% ↑ for age
Toddler and Older	≥10% ↑ for age	≥25% ↑ for age	≥50% ↑ for age

FIG 2 The Children's Hospital Early Warning Score. *HR*, Heart rate; *L*, liters; *NC*, nasal cannula; *WOB*, work of breathing. (From McLellan, M. C., Gauvreau, K., & Connor, J. A. [2017]. Validation of the Children's Hospital Early Warning System for critical deterioration recognition. *Journal of Pediatric Nursing, 32*[1], p. 54.)

Sensitivity for scores ≥ 3 was 91.4% for CHEWS and 73.6% for PEWS with specificity of 67.8% for CHEWS and 88.5% for PEWS. Sensitivity scores ≥ 5 was 75.6% for CHEWS and 38.9% for PEWS with specificity of 88.5% for CHEWS and 93.9% for PEWS. The early warning time from critical score (≥ 5) to critical deterioration was 3.8h for CHEWS versus 0.6h for PEWS (p < 0.001)... The CHEWS system demonstrated higher discrimination, higher sensitivity, and longer early warning time than the PEWS for identifying children at risk for critical deterioration. (McLellan et al., 2017, p. 52)

Critical Appraisal

McLellan and colleagues (2017) provide extensive information about the development of the CHEWS from the PEWS. Fig. 2 details the behaviors to be observed, the scoring process, and the critical score indicating potential deterioration. The validity and interrater reliability of the CHEWS from previous research (McLellan et al., 2014) were strong. However, the interrater reliability needed to be provided for this study because many staff nurses of different levels were involved in the data collection process.

The CHEWS was found to be a significantly stronger tool for use in clinical practice than the PEWS, demonstrating convergent validity. The CHEWS also provided earlier prediction of critical deterioration in children than the PEWS, which indicated predictive criterion validity. The CHEWS had very strong sensitivity for identifying children at risk for critical deterioration and acceptable specificity in determining children who were not at risk for deterioration (Grove & Cipher, 2017).

Interviews

An interview involves verbal communication between the researcher and the study participant, during which information is provided to the researcher. Although this data collection strategy is most commonly used in qualitative and descriptive studies, it also can be used in other types of quantitative studies. You can use a variety of approaches to conduct an interview, ranging from a totally unstructured interview (see Chapter 3), in which the content is controlled by the study participant (Creswell & Poth, 2018), to a structured interview, in which the content is similar to that of a questionnaire, with the possible responses to questions carefully designed by the researcher (Waltz et al., 2017). During structured interviews, researchers use strategies to control the content of the interview. Usually, researchers ask specific questions and enter the participant's responses onto a rating scale or paper and pencil instrument during the interview. For example, researchers could use an in-person or telephone interview to obtain responses to an instrument. Researchers might also enter responses into an electronic database.

Because nurses frequently use interviewing techniques in nursing assessment, the dynamics of interviewing are familiar. However, using the technique for measurement in research requires greater sophistication and needs to be discussed in the study's methods section. The response rate for interviews is higher than for questionnaires, which usually allows a more representative sample to be obtained. Interviewing also allows collection of data from participants who are unable or unlikely to complete questionnaires, such as those who are very ill or may have limited ability to read, write, and express themselves. Interviews are a form of self-report, and it must be assumed that the information provided is accurate. Because of time and cost, sample size is usually limited. Participant bias is always a threat to the validity of the findings, as is inconsistency in data collection from one participant to another (Waltz et al., 2017).

CRITICAL APPRAISAL GUIDELINES

Structured Interviews

When critically appraising interviews conducted in studies, you need to consider the following questions:

1. For structured interviews, what guided the interview process?
2. Are the interview questions relevant for the research purpose?
3. Does the methods indicate the process for conducting the interviews?
4. If multiple interviewers are used to gather data, how were these individuals trained, to what extent, and was consistency achieved for the interview process?
5. Do the questions tend to bias study participants' responses?

Dickson, Buck, and Riegel (2013) used a structured interview format to determine the comorbid conditions of a sample of patients with heart failure (HF). The focus of the study was to examine how multiple comorbid conditions challenge HF patients' self-care. Research Example 10.5 describes the structured interview process used in this study.

RESEARCH EXAMPLE 10.5

Structured Interview

Research Study Excerpt

The interview format of the Charlson Comorbidity Index (CCI) was used to gather data about comorbid conditions (Charlson, Pompei, Ales, & MacKenzie, 1987). Participants were asked about preexisting diseases (e.g., diabetes), most of which are scored with 1 point, although some (e.g., cirrhosis) are assigned > 1 point. Scores on the CCI can range from 0 to 34, with each study participant having a score ≥ 1 because of the HF. Responses were summed, weighted, and indexed into one of three categories: 0-1 = low, *2-3 =*

moderate, *and* ≥ *4* = high, *according to the published methods.... The ability of the CCI to predict mortality, complications, acute care resource use, length of hospital stay, discharge disposition, and cost (Charlson et al., 1987) provide evidence for the criterion-related validity.* (Dickson et al., 2013, p. 4)

Critical Appraisal

Dickson and colleagues (2013) identified the CCI as the structure for their interviews and detailed the scoring process with HF patients. The CCI seemed to collect data that were relevant to the study purpose. The researchers needed to provide more detail on the process for implementing the CCI to indicate if the interviews were consistently conducted. The CCI had criterion-related validity and included nonbiased questions, but more information could have been provided about the content and construct validity of the CCI.

Dickson et al. (2013) found that multiple comorbid conditions decreased HF patients' self-efficacy, which reduced the patients' ability to provide self-care. The researchers stressed the importance of delivering self-care education that integrated the patients' comorbid conditions. In addition, studies are needed to develop and test interventions that foster self-efficacy and focus on self-care for patients across multiple chronic conditions.

Questionnaires

A **questionnaire** is a self-report form designed to elicit information through written, verbal, or electronic responses of the study participant. Questionnaires may be printed and distributed in person, mailed, available on a computer, or accessed online. Questionnaires are sometimes referred to as surveys, and a study using a questionnaire may be referred to as survey research. The information obtained from questionnaires is similar to that obtained by an interview, but the questions tend to have less depth. Study participants are not permitted to elaborate on responses or asked for clarification of comments, and the data collector cannot use probing strategies. However, questions are presented in a consistent manner to each participant, and the opportunity for bias is less than that in an interview.

Questionnaires often are used in descriptive studies to gather a broad spectrum of information from participants, such as facts about the participant or facts about persons, events, or situations known by the participant. It is also used to gather information about beliefs, attitudes, opinions, knowledge, or intentions of the study participants. Questionnaires are often developed for a particular study to enable researchers to gather data from a selected population in a new area of study. Like interviews, questionnaires can have various structures. Some questionnaires have open-ended questions, which require written responses (qualitative data) from the participant. Other questionnaires have closed-ended questions, which have limited options from which participants can select their answers.

Although you can distribute questionnaires to very large samples face to face, through the mail, or via the Internet, the response rate for questionnaires generally is lower than that for other forms of self-report, particularly if the questionnaires are mailed. If the response rate is lower than 50%, the representativeness of the sample is in question. The response rate for mailed questionnaires is usually small (25%–40%), so researchers frequently are unable to obtain a representative sample, even with random sampling methods. Questionnaires distributed via the Internet are more convenient for study participants, which may result in a higher response rate than questionnaires that are mailed. Many researchers are choosing the Internet format if they have access to the potential participants' e-mail addresses (Waltz et al., 2017).

Some respondents fail to mark responses to all the questions, especially on long questionnaires. The incomplete nature of the data can threaten the validity of the instrument. Therefore researchers need to describe how missing data were managed in their study report. With most questionnaires, researchers analyze data at the level of individual items, rather than adding the items together and analyzing the total scores. Responses to items are usually measured at the nominal or ordinal level.

CRITICAL APPRAISAL GUIDELINES

Questionnaires

When critically appraising a questionnaire in a published study, consider the following questions:

1. Does the questionnaire address the focus of the study outlined in the study purpose and/or objective, questions, or hypotheses?
2. Examine the description of the contents of the questionnaire in the measurement section of the study. Does the study provide information on content-related validity for the questionnaire?
3. Was the questionnaire pilot-tested or used in previous studies? What type of validity and reliability information was provided related to the questionnaire?
4. Was the questionnaire implemented consistently from one study participant to another?

Musiello and colleagues (2017) conducted a descriptive correlational study to examine the distress of individuals provided care in an outpatient oncology clinic. The National Comprehensive Cancer Network (NCCN) Distress Thermometer (DT) and Problem List (PL) questionnaire were used to collect data and are described in Research Example 10.6.

RESEARCH EXAMPLE 10.6

Questionnaires

Research Study Excerpt

The 2005 NCCN Distress Thermometer (DT) and Problem List (PL) questionnaire were used to screen patients for self-reported levels of distress and problems currently experienced. The DT measures distress on a score from 0 (no distress) to 10 (severe distress). Recommended cut-off scores to identify clinically significant distress, or 'caseness' on the DT vary according to setting and screening objectives... Boyes et al. (2013) suggest a cut-off score on the DT of ≥2 as best for clinical use, ≥3 for detecting cases of anxiety, depression and comorbid anxiety/depression, and ≥4 as best for research use. A cut-off score of ≥4 to identify significantly distressed patients was selected as appropriate. Scores ≤ 3 were considered to be a 'normal' level of destress for this study (Boyes et al., 2013). The PL includes physical (e.g. constipation, pain, fatigue); emotional (e.g. worry, sadness); practical (e.g. childcare, transport), family (e.g. dealing with family/children), and spiritual/existential problems. Under each problem domain is a list that patients can tick to identify which problems are contributing to their distress. (Musiello et al., 2017, p. 16)

Critical Appraisal

Musiello and colleagues (2017) noted that the DT was a national scale used to screen for distress in clinical and research settings. The NCCN DT cutoff scores for clinical practice and research were determined based on previous research (Boyes et al., 2013). The PL's content validity was addressed by listing the problems that patients could identify as contributing to their distress. The researchers needed to describe the construction and previous use of the PL in studies. In summary, additional information is needed to determine the reliability and validity of the DT and PL questionnaire used in this study.

Scales

The scale, a form of self-report, is a more precise means of measuring phenomena than a questionnaire. Most scales are developed to measure psychosocial variables, but researchers also use scaling techniques to obtain self-reports on physiological variables such as pain, nausea, or functional capacity. The various items on most scales are summed to obtain a single score. These are termed *summated scales.* Fewer random and systematic errors occur when the total score of a scale is used (Nunnally & Bernstein, 1994). The various items in a scale increase the dimensions of the concept that are measured by the instrument. The scales commonly used in nursing research include rating, Likert, and visual analog scales.

Rating Scales

Rating scales are the crudest form of measurement involving scaling techniques. A rating scale lists an ordered series of categories of a variable that are assumed to be based on an underlying continuum. A numerical value is assigned to each category, and the fineness of the distinctions between categories varies with the scale. Rating scales are commonly used by the general public. In conversations, one can hear statements such as "On a scale of 1 to 10, I would rank that…" Rating scales are fairly easy to develop, but researchers need to be careful to avoid end statements that are so extreme that no study participant will select them. You can use a rating scale to rate the degree of cooperativeness of the patient or the value placed by the study participant on nurse-patient interactions. Rating scales are also used in observational measurement to guide data collection (see Fig. 2 of the Children's Hospital Early Warning Score developed by McLellan et al., 2017).

Some rating scales are more valid than others because they were constructed in a structured way and used in a variety of studies with different populations. For example, the Wong-Baker FACES® Pain Rating Scale has documented reliability and validity through research and is commonly used to assess the pain of children in clinical practice (Fig. 10.4; Wong-Baker FACES Foundation, 2017). Nurses often assess pain in adults with a numeric rating scale (NRS), similar to the one in Fig. 10.5. Using the NRS is more valid and reliable than asking a patient to rate her or his pain on a scale from 1 to 10.

Likert Scale

The Likert scale is designed to determine the opinions or attitudes of study subjects. This scale contains a number of declarative statements, with a scale after each statement. The Likert scale is the most commonly used of the scaling techniques. The original version of the scale included five response categories. Each response category was assigned a value, with a value of 0 or 1 given to the most negative response and a value of 4 or 5 given to the most positive response (Ho, 2017; Nunnally & Bernstein, 1994). Response choices in a Likert scale usually address agreement, evaluation, or frequency. Agreement options may include statements such as *strongly disagree, disagree, neutral,*

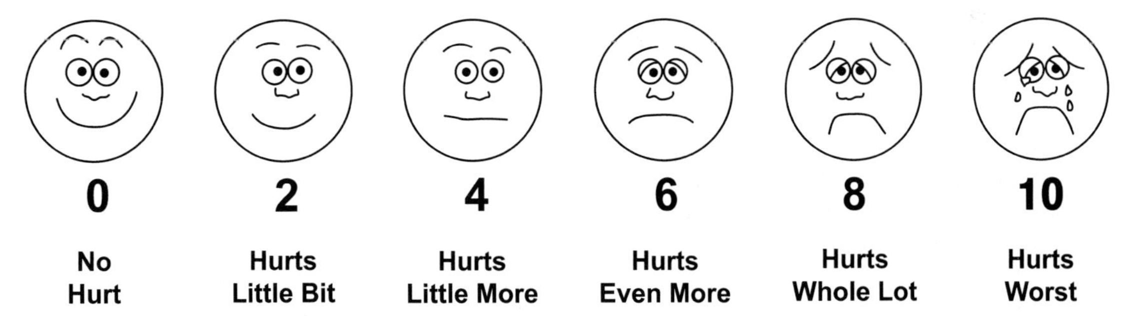

FIG 10.4 Wong-Baker FACES® Pain Rating Scale. Point to each face using the words to describe the pain intensity. Ask the child to choose the face that best describes the child's own pain, and record the appropriate number. (From Wong-Baker FACES Foundation [2017]. *Wong-Baker FACES® Pain Rating Scale*. Retrieved April 25, 2017, from http://www.wongbakerfaces.org.)

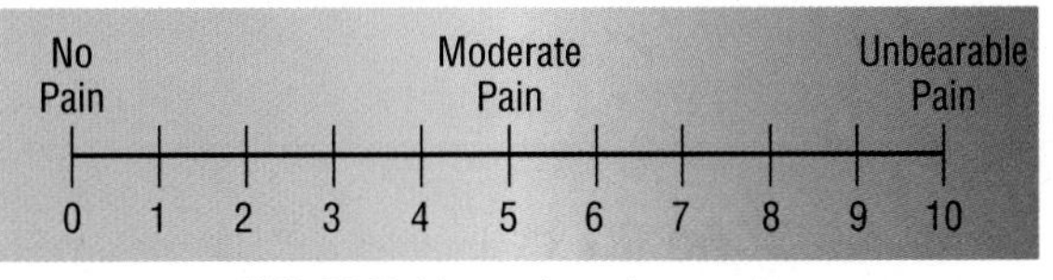

FIG 10.5 Numeric rating scale.

agree, and *strongly agree*. Evaluation responses ask the respondent for an evaluative rating along a bad-good dimension, such as negative to positive or terrible to excellent. Frequency responses may include statements such as *never, rarely, sometimes, frequently*, and *all the time*. The terms used are versatile and are selected based on the content of the questions or items in the scale. For example, an item such as "Describe the nursing care you received during your hospitalization" could have a response scale of *unsatisfactory, below average, average, above average*, and *excellent*.

Sometimes seven options are given on a response scale, sometimes only four. When the response scale has an odd number of options, the middle option is usually an uncertain or neutral category. Using a response scale with an odd number of options is controversial because it allows the study participant to avoid making a clear choice of positive or negative statements. To avoid this, researchers may choose to provide only four or six options, with no middle point or uncertain category. This type of scale is termed a *forced choice version* (Nunnally & Bernstein, 1994). Ho (2017) provided an excellent description of the strengths and limitations of Likert scales.

A Likert scale usually consists of 10 to 20 items, with each addressing an element of the concept being measured. Usually, the values obtained from each item in the instrument are summed to obtain a single score for each participant. Although the values of each item are technically ordinal-level data, the summed score is often analyzed as interval-level data. The CES-D is a Likert scale, introduced earlier and presented in Fig. 10.3, is used to assess the level of depression in patients in clinical practice and research. Schmitt and colleagues (2017) used the CES-D in their study presented earlier. Study participants are given the following instructions for using the scale: "Below is a list of the ways you might have felt or behaved. Please tell me how often you have felt this way during the past week" (see Fig. 10.3; Radloff, 1977). This scale has four response options: *Rarely or none of the time (less than 1 day)* = 0; *Some or a little of the time (1 to 2 days)* = 1; *Occasionally or a moderate amount of time (3 to 4 days)* = 2; and *Most or all of the time (5 to 7 days)* = 3. As discussed previously, the scores on the scale can range from 0 to 60, with the higher scores indicating more depressive symptoms. A score of 16 or higher has been used extensively as the cutoff point for depression. The scale has strong reliability, validity, sensitivity, and specificity (Armenta et al., 2014; Locke & Putnam, 2002; Sharp & Lipsky, 2002).

Visual Analog Scales

The visual analog scale (VAS) is typically used to measure strength, magnitude, or intensity of individuals' subjective feelings, sensations, or attitudes about symptoms or situations. The VAS is a line that is usually 100 mm long, with right angle "stops" at either end. Researchers can present the line horizontally or vertically, with bipolar anchors or descriptors beyond either end of the line (Waltz et al., 2017). These end anchors must include the entire range of sensations possible for the phenomenon being measured (e.g., all and none, best and worst, no pain and unbearable pain). An example of a VAS for measuring pain is presented in Fig. 10.6.

Participants are asked to place a mark through the line to indicate the intensity of the sensation or feeling. Then researchers use a ruler to measure the distance between the left end of the line (on a horizontal scale) and the participant's mark. This measure is the value of the sensation. The VAS has been used to measure pain, mood, anxiety, alertness, craving for cigarettes, quality of sleep, attitudes toward environmental conditions, functional abilities, and severity of clinical symptoms.

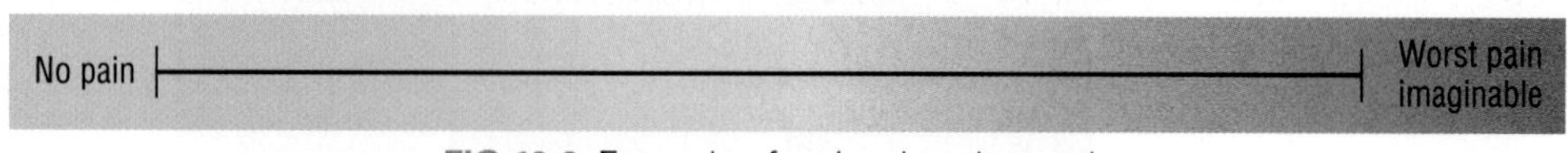

FIG 10.6 Example of a visual analog scale.

The reliability of the VAS is usually determined by the test-retest method. The correlations between the two administrations of the scale need to be moderate or strong to support the reliability of the scale (Wewers & Lowe, 1990). Because these scales are used to measure phenomena that are dynamic or changing over time, test-retest reliability is sometimes not appropriate because the low correlation is caused by the change in sensation versus a problem with the scale. Because the VAS contains a single item, other methods of determining reliability, such as homogeneity, cannot be used. The validity of the VAS is usually determined by correlating the VAS scores with other measures, such as rating or Likert scales, that measure the same phenomenon, such as pain (Waltz et al., 2017).

CRITICAL APPRAISAL GUIDELINES

Scales

When critically appraising a rating scale, Likert scale, or VAS in a study, ask the following questions:

1. Is the rating scale, Likert scale, or VAS clearly described in the research report?
2. Are the techniques used to administer and score the scale provided?
3. Is information about the validity and reliability of the scale described from previous studies and for this study?

Williams, Turner-Henson, Langhinrichsen-Rohling, and Azuero (2017) conducted a predictive correlational study to determine if stressful life events, perceived stress, and bullying were predictive of depressive symptoms in ninth graders. The measurement methods for depressive symptoms and bullying are presented in Research Example 10.7.

RESEARCH EXAMPLE 10.7

Scales

Research Study Excerpt

Depressive symptoms were measured with The Center for Epidemiologic Studies Depression Survey (CESD-10) that has been used to measure four factors related to depressive symptoms including: positive/negative affect, somatic symptoms, retarded activity, and interpersonal issues. CESD-10 scores range from 0 to 30 with scoring from 0 to 3: 0 (rarely), 1(some of the time), 2 (occasionally or moderate amount), 3 (all the time) for each item. A score of 10 or greater indicates need for referral (clinically meaningful). The CESD-10 was chosen due to the applicability for adolescent populations and the length of the measure (10 questions). In a study of n *= 156 adolescents, reliability of CESD-10 was found to be* $\alpha = 0.85$ *(Bradley, Bagnell, & Brannen, 2010). Reliability for the current study was* $\alpha = 0.86$*...*

Bullying was measured using The Personal Experiences Checklist (PECK), a 32-item Likert scale instrument that was previously used in adolescents ages 8 to 15 years (Hunt, Peters, & Rapee, 2012). This self-report instrument is scored from 0 to 4: 0 (never), 1 (rarely), 2 (sometimes), 3 (most days), and 4 (every day). Bullying behaviors included the following number of items, internal consistency, and test-retest coefficients: verbal/relational bullying (11 items, $\alpha = 0.90$, $r = 0.75$*); physical bullying (9 items,* $\alpha = 0.91$, $r = 0.61$*); cyberbullying (8 items,* $\alpha = 0.90$, $r = 0.86$*; and cultural bullying (4 items,* $\alpha = 0.78$, $r = 0.77$*). High scores indicate more bullying. Reliability for the overall scale was* $\alpha = 0.94$ *in the current study.* (Williams et al., 2017, p. 25)

Critical Appraisal

Williams and colleagues (2017) selected Likert scales (CESD-10 and PECK) that had been developed for adolescent populations and had been reliable in previous studies. The content and construct validity for both the CESD-10 and PECK were discussed, indicating the subscales for both scales. The items of both scales and the scoring processes were clearly described. The clinically meaningful score of 10 was identified for determining

Continued

RESEARCH EXAMPLE 10.7—cont'd

depression in adolescents. However, no critical score was noted for the PECK, only that high scores indicated more bullying. The scales had strong reliability in this study (CESD-10 had $\alpha = 0.86$ and PECK had $\alpha = 0.94$). The internal consistency alpha values and test-retest reliability values were also strong for the PECK subscales. The researchers documented the reliability of the CESD-10 and PECK from previous research and for this study but provided very limited information on the scales' validity.

Williams and colleagues (2017, p. 27) found that "9th graders' perception of stress, bullying, and sexual orientation explained 59% of the variance of depressive symptoms" in this sample of 143 adolescents. Clinically significant depressive symptoms (CESD-10 > 9) were self-reported in 39.2% of the adolescents. The self-reports of bullying were low (20%) in this sample as compared with the US rates of 26%–28% for adolescent bullying. Nurses are encouraged to screen adolescents for depressive symptoms and refer them as necessary for treatment.

DATA COLLECTION PROCESS

Data collection is the process of acquiring study participants and collecting the data for a study. The actual steps of collecting the data are specific to each study and depend on the research design, sample, and measurement techniques. During the data collection process, researchers initially train the data collectors, recruit study participants, implement the study intervention (if applicable), collect data in a consistent way, and protect the integrity (or validity) of the study.

Researchers need to describe their data collection process clearly in their research report. Often, the data collection process is addressed in the methods section of the report in a subsection entitled "Procedure." The strategies used to approach potential participants who meet the sampling criteria need to be described (see Chapter 9). Researchers should also specify the number and characteristics of individuals who decline to participate in the study. If the study includes an intervention, the details about the intervention and how it was implemented should be described (see Chapter 8). The approaches used to perform measurements and the time and setting for the measurements should also be described. The desired result is a step-by-step description of exactly how, where, and in what sequence the researchers collected the study data. The following sections discuss some of the common data collections tasks described in research reports, including recruitment of study participants, consistency of data collection, and control in implementing the study design. Nurse researchers are also conducting studies using data from existing databases, and it is important to critically appraise data obtained from these databases.

Recruitment of Study Participants

The research report needs to describe the study participant recruitment process. Study participants may be recruited only at the initiation of data collection or throughout the data collection period. The design of the study determines the method of selecting the participants. Recruiting the number of participants originally planned is critical because data analysis and interpretation of findings depend on having an adequate sample size.

Consistency in Data Collection

The key to accurate data collection in any study is consistency. Consistency involves maintaining the data collection pattern for each collection event as it was developed in the research plan. A good plan will facilitate consistency and maintain the validity of the study. Researchers should note deviations, even if they are minor, and report their impact on the interpretation of the findings in their final study report. If a study uses data collectors, researchers need to report the training process and the interrater reliability achieved during training and data collection.

Control in the Study Design

Researchers build controls into their study plan to minimize the influence of intervening forces on the findings. Control is very important in quasi-experimental and experimental studies to ensure that the intervention is consistently implemented (Shadish, Cook, & Campbell, 2002). The research report needs to reflect the controls implemented in a study and any problems that needed to be managed during the study. In addition to maintaining the controls identified in the plan, researchers continually look for previously unidentified, extraneous variables that might have an impact on the data being collected. An extraneous variable often is specific to a study, tends to become apparent during the data collection period, and needs to be discussed in the research report. For example, Lu and associates (2013) examined the effects of acupressure on sleep quality and controlled the environment in which the intervention was implemented to decrease the effects of any extraneous variables, such as noise, temperature, or lighting that might influence the study findings. The participants did not receive sleeping medications during this study to prevent the influence of this extraneous variable. Researchers need to consider the extraneous variables identified during data collection, data analysis, and interpretation. They should also note these variables in the research report so that future researchers can be aware of and attempt to control them.

Studies Obtaining Data From Existing Databases

Nurse researchers are using existing databases to address the research problem and purpose for their study. The reasons for obtaining data from existing databases for a study are varied. With the computerization of healthcare information, more databases have been developed internationally, nationally, regionally, at the state level, and within clinical agencies. These databases include large amounts of information that have relevance in developing research evidence needed for practice (Brown, 2018; Melnyk, Gallagher-Ford, & Fineout-Overholt, 2017). The costs and technology for storage of data have improved over the last 10 years, making these databases more reliable and accessible. Using existing databases makes it possible to conduct complex analyses to expand our understanding of healthcare outcomes. Another reason is that the primary collection of data in a study is limited by the availability of research participants and expense of the data collection process. By using existing databases, researchers are able to have larger samples, conduct more longitudinal studies, have lower costs during the data collection process, and limit the burdens placed on the study participants (Johantgen, 2010).

The existing healthcare data commonly used in research include: secondary and administrative. Data collected for a particular study are considered **primary data**. Data collected from previous research and stored in a database are considered **secondary data** when used by other researchers to address their study purposes. Because these data were collected as part of research, details can be obtained about the data collection and storage processes, including any previous publications based on the data. In the methodology section of their research report, researchers usually indicate when they used secondary data analyses in their study (Johantgen, 2010).

Data collected for reasons other than research are considered administrative data. **Administrative data** are collected within clinical agencies, obtained by national, state, and local professional organizations, and collected by federal, state, and local agencies. The processes for collection and storage of administrative data are more complex and often more unclear than the data collection process for research (Johantgen, 2010). The data in administrative databases are collected by different people in different sites using different methods. However, the data elements collected for most administrative databases include demographics, organizational characteristics, clinical diagnosis and treatment, and geographic information. These database elements have been standardized by the Health Insurance Portability and Accountability Act (HIPAA), which has improved the quality of the databases (see Chapter 4).

The type of database used in a study needs to be clearly described. The data in the database should address the researchers' study purpose and their objectives, questions, or hypotheses. The validity and reliability of the data in the existing database should be described in the research report.

CRITICAL APPRAISAL GUIDELINES

Data Collection

When critically appraising the data collection process, consider the following questions:

1. Were the recruitment and selection of study participants clearly described and appropriate?
2. Were the data collected in a consistent way?
3. Were the study controls maintained as indicated by the design? Did the design include an intervention that was consistently implemented?
4. Was the integrity of the study protected, and how were any problems resolved?
5. Did the researchers obtain data from an existing database? If so, did the data obtained address the study purpose and objectives, questions, or hypotheses? Were the reliability and validity of the database addressed in the research report?

Williams and colleagues' (2017) study (presented earlier) examined stress and bullying as predictive of depressive symptoms in adolescents. Elements of the data collection process for this study are presented in Research Example 10.8.

RESEARCH EXAMPLE 10.8

Data Collection

Research Study Excerpt

A nonprobability, convenience sampling method was used; the resulting sample consisted of 143 9th graders recruited from two public suburban southeastern U.S. high schools. Eligibility requirements included: (1) 9th grade students aged 14-16 years... and (5) having parental consent. Exclusion criteria included: (1) non-English speaking... and (5) physical illness with resulting self-report of elevated temperature...

The study was reviewed and approved by the university institutional review board [IRB] as well as the two school systems' superintendents, principals, and school nurses. The primary investigator explained the study to all 9th graders and provided packets with a letter to parents, a refusal form, and consent form to sign and return. Adolescents who were eligible to participate signed an assent form before the study began. Study participants were scheduled from 8am to 11am to complete the four self-report questionnaires (demographics, perceived stress, bullying, and depressive symptoms) during a 50-minute elective class in the school computer laboratory... At the completion of the study, each participant was provided with a $5.00 gift card to a local food establishment and information about mental health counselors who are available at low or no cost. Study measures were selected based on the conceptual framework, reliability, validity, and feasibility...

The Statistical Package for Social Sciences (SPSS), 2011, v20.0 for Windows, was used for all statistical analyses. (Williams et al., 2017, p. 25)

Critical Appraisal

Williams and colleagues (2017) implemented detailed sampling criteria to promote a homogenous sample and reduce the effects of extraneous variables. The sample size was strong (n = 143), and the findings were significant, indicating no Type II error. The researchers scheduled data collection during the students' elective classes so that their required courses were not disrupted. A small gift card was provided to increase participation but would probably not have biased students' responses on the measurement methods. The ethics of the study were documented with university IRB approval, approval at the schools, consent of the parents, and assent of the adolescents. The reliability values of the scales used were strong but the researchers might have expanded on the description of the scales' validity (see earlier discussion of instruments). The statistical analyses were appropriate for the study data, and the results indicated that 59% of the variance of depressive symptoms in the adolescents was predicted by perception of stress, bullying, and sexual orientation. The strong sampling criteria and sample size, the inclusion of two settings, the use of measurement methods appropriate for adolescents, and the structured data collection process increased the likelihood that the study findings were an accurate reflection of reality.

KEY POINTS

- The purpose of measurement is to obtain trustworthy data that can be used to address the quantitative study purpose and objectives, questions, or hypotheses.
- The rules of measurement ensure that the assignment of values or categories is performed consistently from one study participant (or situation) to another and, eventually, if the measurement strategy is found to be meaningful, from one study to another.
- The levels of measurement from low to high are nominal, ordinal, interval, and ratio.
- Reliability in measurement is concerned with the consistency of the measurement technique; reliability testing focuses on stability, equivalence, and internal consistency.
- The validity of an instrument is a determination of the extent to which the instrument reflects the abstract concept being examined. The types of validity described in this chapter include content validity, construct validity, and criterion validity
- Readability level focuses on the study participants' ability to read and comprehend the content of an instrument, which adds to the reliability and validity of the instrument.
- Physiological measures are examined for precision, accuracy, and error in research reports.
- Diagnostic and screening tests are examined for sensitivity, specificity, negative predictive value, and likelihood ratios.
- Common measurement approaches used in nursing research include physiological measures, observation, interviews, questionnaires, and scales.
- Rating, Likert, and visual analog scales are described for use in research and practice.
- If an existing database is used in conducting studies, the quality of the database should be addressed in the research report.
- The data collection tasks that should be critically appraised in a study include: (1) recruitment of study participants; (2) consistency of data collection; and (3) maintenance of controls in the study design.

REFERENCES

Armenta, B. E., Hartshorn, K. J., Whitbeck, L. B., Crawford, D. M., & Hoyt, D. R. (2014). A longitudinal examination of the measurement properties and predictive utility of the Center for Epidemiologic Studies Depression Scale among North American indigenous adolescents. *Psychological Assessment, 26*(4), 1347–1355.

Ballard, E. D., Cwik, M., Van Eck, K., Goldstein, M., Alfes, C., Wilson, M. E., et al. (2017). Identification of at-risk youth by suicide screening in a pediatric emergency department. *Prevention Science, 18*(2), 174–182.

Bannigan, K., & Watson, R. (2009). Reliability and validity in a nutshell. *Journal of Clinical Nursing, 18*(23), 3237–3243.

Bialocerkowski, A., Klupp, N., & Bragge, P. (2010). Research methodology series: How to read and critically appraise a reliability article. *International Journal of Therapy and Rehabilitation, 17*(3), 114–120.

Boyes, A. D., Carey, M., Lecathelinais, C., & Girgis, A. (2013). How does the Distress Thermometer compare to the Hospital Anxiety and Depression Scale for detecting possible cases of psychological morbidity among cancer survivors? *Supportive Care in Cancer, 21*(1), 119–127. https://www.ncbi.nlm.nih.gov/pubmed/22618735.

Bradley, K. L., Bagnell, A. L., & Brannen, C. L. (2010). Factorial validity of the Center for Epidemiological Studies Depression-10 in adolescents. *Issues in Mental Health Nursing, 31*(6), 408–412.

Brown, S. J. (2018). *Evidence-based nursing: The research-practice connection* (4th ed.). Sudbury, MA: Jones & Bartlett.

Buysse, D. L., Reynolds, C. F., 3rd., Monk, T. H., Berman, S. R., & Kupfer, D. J. (1989). The Pittsburgh Sleep Quality Index: A new instrument for psychiatric practice and research. *Psychiatry Research, 28*(2), 193–213.

Campo, M., Shiyko, M. P., & Lichtman, S. W. (2010). Sensitivity and specificity: A review of related statistics and controversies in the context of physical therapist education. *Journal of Physical Therapy Education, 24*(3), 69–78.

Charlson, M. E., Pompei, P., Ales, K. L., & MacKenzie, C. R. (1987). A new method of classifying prognostic comorbidity in longitudinal studies: Development and validation. *Journal of Chronic Diseases, 40*(5), 373–383.

Creswell, J. W. (2014). *Research design: Qualitative, quantitative and mixed methods approaches* (4th ed.). Thousand Oaks, CA: Sage.

Creswell, J. W., & Poth, C. N. (2018). *Qualitative inquiry & research design: Choosing among five approaches* (4th ed.). Thousand Oaks, CA: Sage.

DeVon, H. A., Block, M. E., Moyle-Wright, P., Ernst, D. M., Hayden, S. J., Lazzara, D. J., et al. (2007). A psychometric toolbox for testing validity and reliability. *Journal of Nursing Scholarship, 39*(2), 155–164.

Dickson, V. V., Buck, H., & Riegel, B. (2013). Multiple comorbid conditions challenge heart failure self-care by decreasing self-efficacy. *Nursing Research, 62*(1), 2–9.

Gift, A. G., & Soeken, K. L. (1988). Assessment of physiologic instruments. *Heart & Lung, 17*(2), 128–133.

Gray, J. R., Grove, S. K., & Sutherland, S. (2017). *The practice of nursing research: Appraisal, synthesis, and generation of evidence* (8th ed.). St. Louis, MO: Elsevier Saunders.

Grove, S. K., & Cipher, D. J. (2017). *Statistics for nursing research: A workbook for evidence-based practice* (2nd ed.). St. Louis, MO: Elsevier.

Ho, G. W. K. (2017). Examining perceptions and attitudes: A review of Likert-type scales versus Q-methodology. *Western Journal of Nursing Research, 39*(5), 674–689.

Horowitz, L. M., Bridge, J. A., Teach, S. J., Ballard, E., Klima, J., Rosenstein, D. L., et al. (2012). Ask Suicide-Screening Questions (ASQ); A brief instrument for the pediatric emergency department. *Achieves of Pediatric and Adolescent Medicine, 166*(12), 1170–1176.

Hunt, C., Peters, L., & Rapee, R. M. (2012). Development of a measure of being bullied in youth. *Psychological Assessment, 24*(1), 156–165.

Johantgen, M. (2010). Using existing administrative and national databases. In C. F. Waltz, O. L. Strickland, & E. R. Lenz (Eds.), *Measurement in nursing and health research.* (4th ed.) (pp. 241–250). New York, NY: Springer.

Kaplan, A. (1963). *The conduct of inquiry: Methodology for behavioral science.* New York, NY: Harper & Row.

Locke, B. Z., & Putnam, P. (2002). *Center for Epidemiologic Studies Depression Scale (CES-D Scale).* Bethesda, MD: National Institute of Mental Health.

Lu, M., Lin, S., Chen, K., Tsang, H., & Su, S. (2013). Acupressure improves sleep quality of psychogeriatric inpatients. *Nursing Research, 62*(2), 130–137.

Marshall, C., & Rossman, G. B. (2016). *Designing qualitative research* (6th ed.). Thousand Oaks, CA: Sage.

McLellan, M. C., Gauvreau, K., & Connor, J. A. (2014). Validation of the Cardiac Children's Hospital Early Warning Score: An early warning scoring tool to prevent cardiopulmonary arrests in children with heart disease. *Congenital Heart Disease*, *9*(3), 194–202.

McLellan, M. C., Gauvreau, K., & Connor, J. A. (2017). Validation of the Children's Hospital Early Warning System for critical deterioration recognition. *Journal of Pediatric Nursing*, *32*(1), 52–58.

Melnyk, B. M., Gallagher-Ford, E., & Fineout-Overholt. (2017). *Implementing evidence-based practice competencies in healthcare: A practical guide for improving quality, safety, & outcomes*. Indianapolis, IN: Sigma Theta Tau International.

Musiello, T., Dixon, G., O'Connor, M., Cook, D., Miller, L., Petterson, A., et al. (2017). A pilot study of routine screening for distress by a nurse and psychologist in an outpatient hematological oncology clinic. *Applied Nursing Research*, *33*(1), 15–18.

Nunnally, J. C., & Bernstein, I. H. (1994). *Psychometric theory* (3rd ed.). New York, NY: McGraw-Hill.

Polit, D. F., & Yang, F. M. (2016). *Measurement and the measurement of change*. Philadelphia, PA: Wolters Kluwer.

Radloff, L. S. (1977). The CES-D scale: A self-report depression scale for research in the general population. *Applied Psychological Measurement*, *1*, 385–394.

Ryan-Wenger, N. A. (2017). Precision, accuracy, and uncertainty of biophysical measurements for research and practice. In C. F. Waltz, O. L. Strickland, & E. R. Lenz (Eds.), *Measurement in nursing and health research*. (5th ed.) (pp. 427–445). New York, NY: Springer.

Schmitt, A., Reimer, A., Hermanns, N., Kulzer, B., Ehrmann, D., Krichbaum, M., et al. (2017). Depression is linked to hyperglycemia via suboptimal diabetes self-management: A cross-sectional mediation analysis. *Journal of Psychosomatic Research*, *94*(1), 17–23.

Shadish, W. R., Cook, T. D., & Campbell, D. T. (2002). *Experimental and quasi-experimental designs for generalized causal inference*. Chicago, IL: Rand McNally.

Sharp, L. K., & Lipsky, M. S. (2002). Screening for depression across the lifespan: A review of measures for use in primary care settings. *American Family Physician*, *66*(6), 1001–1008.

Stevens, S. S. (1946). On the theory of scales of measurement. *Science*, *103*(2684), 677–680.

Stone, K. S., & Frazier, S. K. (2017). Measurement of physiological variables using biomedical instrumentation. In C. F. Waltz, O. L. Strickland, & E. R. Lenz (Eds.), *Measurement in nursing and health research*. (5th ed.) (pp. 379–425). New York, NY: Springer.

Straus, S. E., Glasziou, P., Richardson, W. S., Rosenberg, W., & Haynes, R. B. (2011). *Evidence-based medicine: How to practice and teach EBM* (5th ed.). Edinburgh: Churchill Livingstone Elsevier.

Umberger, R. A., Hatfield, L. A., & Speck, P. M. (2017). Understanding negative predictive value of diagnostic tests used in clinical practice. *Dimensions of Critical care Nursing*, *36*(1), 22–29.

Waltz, C. F., Strickland, O. L., & Lenz, E. R. (2017). *Measurement in nursing and health research* (5th ed.). New York, NY: Springer Publishing Company.

Weber, M. A., Schiffrin, E. L., White, W. B., Mann, S., Lindholm, L. H., Kenerson, J. G., et al. (2014). Clinical practice guidelines for the management of hypertension in the community: A statement by the American Society of Hypertension and the International Society of Hypertension. *Journal of Hypertension*, *32*(1), 3–15.

Wewers, M. E., & Lowe, N. K. (1990). A critical review of visual analogue scales in the measurement of clinical phenomena. *Research in Nursing & Health*, *13*(4), 227–236.

Williams, S. G., Turner-Henson, A., Langhinrichsen-Rohling, J., & Azuero, A. (2017). Depressive symptoms in 9th graders: Stress and physiological contributors. *Applied Nursing Research*, *34*(1), 24–28.

Wong-Baker FACES Foundation. (2017). *Wong-Baker FACES® Pain Rating Scale*. Retrieved April 25, 2017, from http://www.wongbakerfaces.org/.

Because of funding changes, the Agency for Healthcare Research and Quality (AHRQ) National Guideline Clearinghouse website was scheduled for decommissioning as of July 16, 2018. For more information, go to https://www.ahrq.gov/.

CHAPTER

11

Understanding Statistics in Research

Susan K. Grove

CHAPTER OVERVIEW

LEARNING OUTCOMES

After completing this chapter, you should be able to:

1. Describe probability theory and decision theory, which guide the statistical analysis of data.
2. Describe the process of inferring from a sample to a population.
3. Compare and contrast Type I and Type II errors that can occur in studies.
4. Identify the steps of the data analysis process: (a) management of missing data; (b) description of the sample; (c) reliability of the measurement methods; (d) exploratory analysis of the data; and (e) use of inferential statistical analyses guided by study objectives, questions, or hypotheses.
5. Identify descriptive analyses, such as frequency distributions, percentages, measures of central tendency, and measures of dispersion, which are conducted to describe the sample and study variables in research reports.
6. Describe the results obtained from the inferential statistical analyses conducted to examine relationships (Pearson product-moment correlation and factor analysis) and make predictions (linear regression analysis and multiple regression analysis).
7. Describe the results obtained from inferential statistical analyses conducted to examine differences, such as chi-square analysis, *t*-test, analysis of variance, and analysis of covariance.
8. Describe the five types of results obtained from quasi-experimental and experimental studies that are interpreted within a decision theory framework: (a) significant and predicted results; (b) nonsignificant results; (c) significant and unpredicted results; (d) mixed results; and (e) unexpected results.
9. Compare and contrast statistical significance and clinical importance of results.
10. Critically appraise statistical results, findings, limitations, conclusions, generalization of findings, nursing implications, and suggestions for further research in a published study.

The expectation that nursing practice should be based on research evidence has made it important for students and clinical nurses to acquire skills in reading and evaluating the results from statistical analyses (Gray, Grove, & Sutherland, 2017). Nurses probably have more anxiety about data analysis and statistical results than they do about any other aspect of the research process. We hope this chapter will dispel some of that anxiety and facilitate your critical appraisal of the results in research reports. The statistical information in this chapter is provided from the perspective of reading, understanding, and critically appraising the results sections in quantitative studies, rather than on selecting statistical procedures for data analysis or performing statistical analyses.

Relevant theories and concepts of statistical analysis are described to provide a background for understanding the results in research reports. The steps of data analysis are briefly introduced. Some of the common statistical procedures used to describe variables, examine relationships among variables, predict outcomes, and test causal hypotheses are discussed. Strategies are provided to determine the appropriateness of statistical analyses conducted to obtain study results, and guidelines are provided for critically appraising the results of studies. The chapter concludes with guidelines for critically appraising the following study outcomes: findings, limitations, conclusions, generalizations, implications for nursing practice, and recommendations for further study. Examples from current studies are provided throughout this chapter to promote your understanding of the content.

UNDERSTANDING THEORIES AND CONCEPTS OF THE STATISTICAL ANALYSIS PROCESS

One reason that nurses tend to avoid statistics is that many were taught only the mathematical procedures of calculating statistical equations, with little or no explanation of the logic behind those procedures or the meaning of the results. Computation is a mechanical process usually performed by a computer, and information about the calculation procedure is not necessary to begin understanding statistical results. We present an approach to data analysis that will enhance your understanding of the statistical analysis process. You can use this understanding to critically appraise the analysis techniques and the results in research reports.

A brief explanation of some of the theories and concepts important in understanding the statistical analysis process is provided. Probability theory and decision theory are discussed, and the concepts of hypothesis testing, level of significance, inference, generalization, normal curve, tailedness, Type I and Type II errors, power, and degrees of freedom are described. More extensive discussion of these topics can be found in other sources; and we recommend our own texts (Gray et al., 2017; Grove & Cipher, 2017) and other quality statistical texts (Plichta & Kelvin, 2013; Polit, 2010).

Probability Theory

Probability theory is used to explain the extent of a relationship, the probability that an event will occur in a given situation, or the probability that an event can be accurately predicted. The researcher might want to know the probability that a particular outcome will result from a nursing intervention. For example, the researcher may want to know how likely it is that urinary catheterization during hospitalization will lead to a urinary tract infection (UTI) after discharge from the hospital. The researcher also may want to know the probability that study participants in the experimental group are members of the same larger population from which the comparison or control group participants were obtained. Probability is expressed as a lower case letter p, with values expressed as percentages or as a decimal value, ranging from 0 to 1. For example, if the probability is 0.23, then it is expressed as $p = 0.23$. This means that there is a 23% probability that a particular outcome (e.g., a UTI) will occur. Probability values also can be stated as less than a specific value, such as 0.05, expressed as $p < 0.05$. A study may indicate the probability that the experimental group participants were members of the same larger population as the comparison group participants was less than or equal to 5% ($p \leq 0.05$). In other words, it is not very likely that the comparison group and the experimental group are from the same population. Put another way, you might say that there is a 5% chance that the two groups are from the same population, and a 95% chance that they are not from the same population. The inference is that the experimental group is different from the comparison group because of the effect of the intervention in the study. Probability values are often stated with the results of inferential statistical analyses.

Decision Theory, Hypothesis Testing, and Level of Significance

Decision theory assumes that all of the groups in a study (e.g., experimental and comparison groups) used to test a particular hypothesis are components of the same population relative to the variables under study. This expectation (or assumption) traditionally is expressed as a null hypothesis, which states that there is no difference between (or among) the groups in a study in terms of the variables included in the hypothesis (see Chapter 5 for more details about hypotheses). It is up to the researcher to provide evidence for a genuine difference between the groups. For example, the researcher may hypothesize that the frequency of UTIs that occur after discharge from the hospital in patients who were catheterized during hospitalization is no different from the frequency of such infections in those who were not catheterized. To test this null hypothesis, a cutoff point is selected before data collection. The cutoff point, referred to as alpha (α), or the **level of statistical significance,** is the probability level at which the results of statistical analysis are judged to indicate a statistically significant difference between the groups. The level of significance selected for most nursing studies is 0.05. If the p value found in the statistical analysis is ≤ 0.05, the experimental and comparison groups are considered to be significantly different (members of different populations).

Decision theory requires that the cutoff point selected for a study be absolute. Absolute means that even if the value obtained is only a fraction above the cutoff point, the samples are considered to be from the same population, and no meaning can be attributed to the differences. It is inappropriate when using decision theory to state that the findings approached significance at $p = 0.051$ if the alpha level was set at 0.05. Using decision theory rules, this finding indicates that the groups tested are not significantly different, and the null hypothesis is accepted. On the other hand, once the level of significance has been set at 0.05 by the researcher, if the analysis reveals a significant difference of 0.001, this result is not considered more significant than the 0.05 originally proposed (Slakter, Wu, & Suzaki-Slakter, 1991). The level of significance is dichotomous, which means that the difference is significant or not significant; there are no "degrees" of significance. However, some people, not realizing that their reasoning has shifted from decision theory to probability theory, indicate in their research report that the 0.001 result makes the findings more significant than if they had obtained a value of $p = 0.05$.

From the perspective of probability theory, there is considerable difference in the risk of occurrence of a Type I error—saying something is significant when it is not—when the probability is between 0.05 and 0.001. If $p = 0.001$, the probability that the two groups are components of the same population is 1 in 1000; if $p = 0.05$, the probability that the groups belong to the same population is 5 in 100. In other words, if $p = 0.05$, then in 5 times out of 100, groups with statistical values such as those found in the statistical analyses actually are members of the same population, and the conclusion that the groups are different is erroneous.

In computer analysis, the probability value obtained from each data analysis (e.g., $p = 0.03$ or $p = 0.07$) frequently is provided on the printout and is usually reported by the researcher in the published study, along with the level of significance that was set before data analysis was conducted. In summary, the probability (p) value reveals the risk of a Type I error in a particular study. The alpha (α) value, set before the study, usually at $\alpha = 0.05$, reveals whether the probability value for a particular analysis in a study met the cutoff point for a significant difference between groups or a significant relationship between variables.

Inference and Generalization

An inference is a conclusion or judgment based on evidence. Statistical inferences are made cautiously and with great care. The decision theory rules used to interpret the results of statistical procedures increase the probability that inferences are accurate. A generalization is the application of information that has been acquired from a specific instance to a general situation. Generalizing requires making an inference; both require the use of inductive reasoning. An inference is made from a specific case and extended to a general truth, from a part to the whole, from the concrete to the abstract, and from the known to the unknown. In research, an inference is made from the study findings obtained from a specific sample and applied to a more general target population, using the results from statistical analyses. For example, a researcher may conclude in a research report that a significant difference was found in the number of UTIs between two samples, one in which the participants had been catheterized during hospitalization and another in which the participants had not. The researcher also may conclude that this difference can be expected in all patients who have received care in hospitals. The findings are generalized from the sample in the study to all previously hospitalized patients. Statisticians and researchers can never prove something using inference; they can never be certain that their inferences and generalizations are correct. The researcher's generalization of the incidence of UTIs may not have been carefully thought out—the findings may have been generalized to a population that was overly broad. It is possible that in the more general population, there is no difference in the incidence of UTIs based on whether the patient was catheterized or not. Generalizing study findings are part of the discussion section of a research report presented later in this chapter.

Normal Curve

A normal curve is a theoretical frequency distribution of all possible values in a population; however, no real distribution exactly fits the normal curve (Fig. 11.1). The idea of the normal curve was developed by an 18-year-old mathematician, Johann Gauss, in 1795. He found that the results from the analysis of data from variables (e.g., the mean of each sample) determined repeatedly in many samples from the same population can be combined into one large sample. From this large sample, a more accurate representation can be developed of the pattern of the curve in that population than is possible with only one sample. Surprisingly, in most cases, the curve is similar, regardless of the specific variables examined or the population studied.

Levels of significance and probability are based on the logic of the normal curve. The normal curve in Fig. 11.1 shows the distribution of values for a single population. Note that 95.5% of the values are within two standard deviations (*SDs*) of the mean, ranging from −2 to +2 *SDs*. (*SD* is described later in this chapter.) There is approximately a 95% probability that a given measured value (e.g., the mean of a group) would fall within approximately two *SDs* of the mean of the population, and there is a 5% probability that the value would fall in the tails of the normal curve (Fig. 11.2). The tails are the extreme ends of the normal curve that include below −2 (−1.96 exactly) *SDs* (2.5%) or above +2 (+1.96 exactly) *SDs* (2.5%). If the groups being compared are from the same

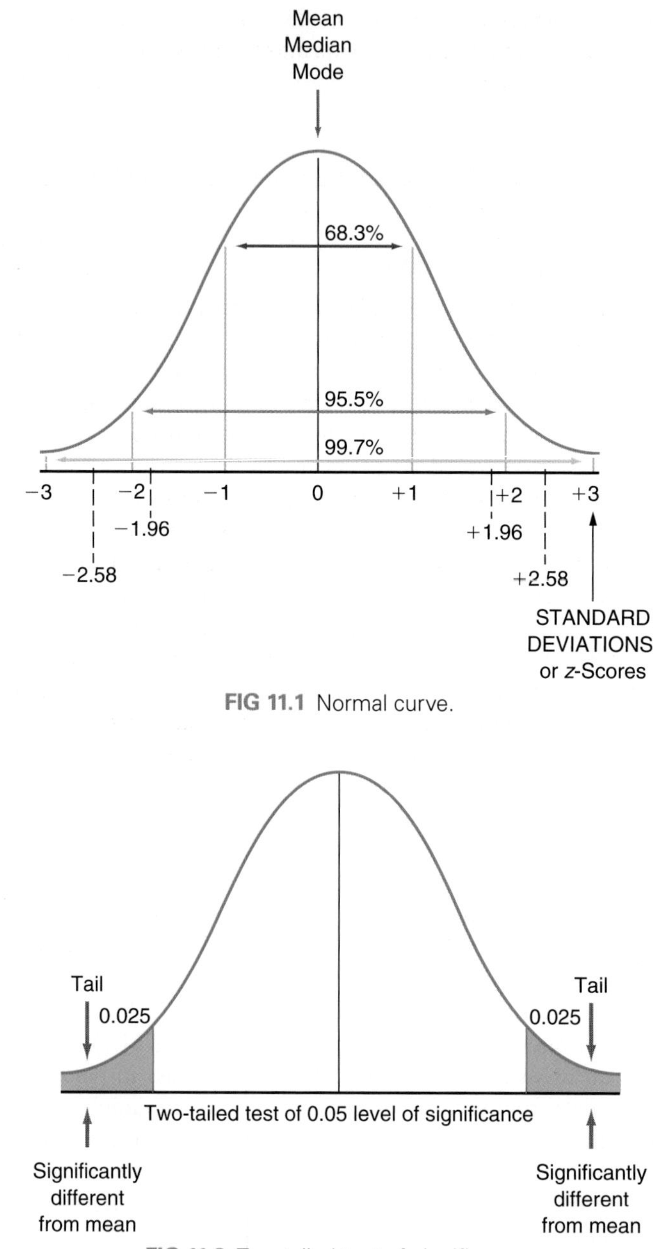

FIG 11.1 Normal curve.

FIG 11.2 Two-tailed test of significance.

population (not significantly different), you would expect the values (e.g., the means) of each group to fall within the 95% range of values on the normal curve. If the groups are from (significantly) different populations, you would expect one of the group values to be outside the 95% range of values. An inferential statistical analysis performed to determine differences between groups, using a level of significance (α) set at 0.05, would test that expectation. If the statistical test demonstrates a significant difference (the value of one group does not fall within the 95% range of values), the groups are considered to belong to different populations. However, in 5% of statistical tests, the value of one of the groups can be expected to fall outside the 95% range of values but still belong to the same population (a Type I error).

Tailedness

With nondirectional hypotheses, researchers assume that an extreme score (obtained because the group with the extreme score did not belong to the same population) can occur in either tail of the normal curve (see Fig. 11.2). The analysis of a nondirectional hypothesis is called a **two-tailed test of significance**. In a **one-tailed test of significance,** the hypothesis is directional, and extreme statistical values that occur in a single tail of the curve are of interest (see Chapter 5 for a discussion of directional and nondirectional hypotheses). The hypothesis states that the extreme score is higher or lower than that for 95% of the population, indicating that the sample with the extreme score is not a member of the same population. In this case, 5% of statistical values that are considered significant will be in one tail, rather than two. Extreme statistical values occurring in the other tail of the curve are not considered significantly different.

Fig. 11.3 shows a one-tailed test of significance, in which the statistical values considered for significance are in the right tail. Developing a one-tailed hypothesis requires that the researcher have sufficient knowledge of the variables to predict whether the difference will be in the tail above the mean or in the tail below the mean. For example, McKee, Long, Southward, Walker, and McCown (2016, p. 197) "hypothesized that children of overweight or obese parents are more likely to be obese." This directional hypothesis predicts that the area of significance is in the right tail of the normal curve as shown in Fig. 11.3. Researchers found that having an obese parent was a significant predictor of childhood obesity. One-tailed statistical tests are uniformly more powerful than two-tailed tests, decreasing the possibility of a Type II error.

Type I and Type II Errors

According to decision theory, two types of error can occur when a researcher is deciding what the result of a statistical test means, Type I and Type II errors (Table 11.1). A **Type I error** occurs when the null hypothesis is rejected when it is true (e.g., when the results indicate that there is a significant difference, when in reality there is not). The risk of a Type I error is indicated by the level of

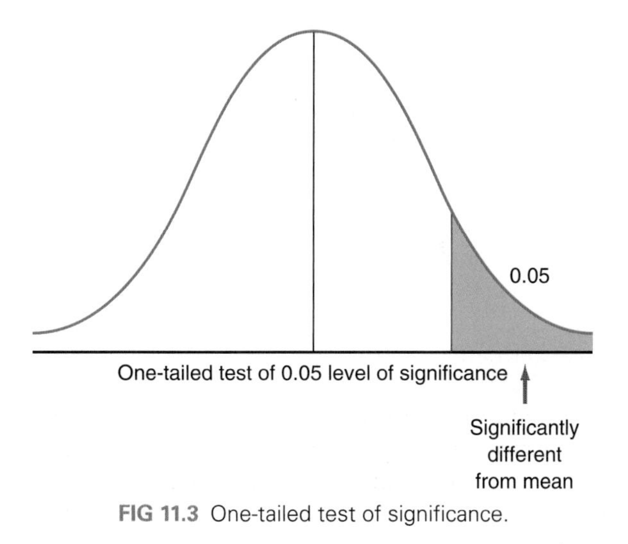

FIG 11.3 One-tailed test of significance.

TABLE 11.1 **TYPE I AND TYPE II ERRORS**

	DECISION	
	REJECT NULL[a]	ACCEPT NULL[a]
Null[a] is true.	Type I error: alpha (α)	Correct decision: 1 – α (power)
Null[a] is false.	Correct decision: 1 – β	Type II error: beta (β)

[a]The null hypothesis states that no difference or relationship exists in the study sample.

significance. There is a greater risk of a Type I error with a 0.05 level of significance (5 chances for error in 100) than with a 0.01 level of significance (1 chance for error in 100).

A **Type II error,** or beta (β), occurs when the null hypothesis is regarded as true but is in fact false. For example, statistical analyses may indicate no significant relationship between variables or difference between groups, but in reality there is a significant relationship or difference (see Table 11.1). There is a greater risk of a Type II error when the level of significance is 0.01 than when it is 0.05. However, Type II errors are often caused by flaws in the research methods. In nursing research, many studies are conducted with small samples and with instruments that do not accurately and precisely measure the variables under study (Gray et al., 2017; Polit & Yang, 2016; Waltz, Strickland, & Lenz, 2017). In many nursing situations, multiple variables interact to cause differences within populations. When only a few of the interacting variables are examined, small differences between groups may be overlooked. This leads to nonsignificant study results, which can cause researchers to conclude falsely that there are no differences between the samples when there actually are. Thus the risk of a Type II error is often high in nursing studies.

Power: Controlling the Risk of a Type II Error

Power is the probability that a statistical test will detect a significant difference that exists (see Table 11.1). The risk of a Type II error can be determined using **power analysis**. Cohen (1988) has identified the four parameters of a power analysis: (1) power, (2) level of significance, (3) effect size, and (4) sample size. If three of the four are known, the fourth can be calculated using power analysis formulas that vary for the type of analysis to be conducted. The minimum acceptable power level is 0.80 (80%). The researcher sets the level of significance (usually set at $\alpha = 0.05$; see Chapter 9). **Effect size** is "the degree to which the phenomenon is present in the population, or the degree to which the null hypothesis is false" (Cohen, 1988, pp. 9–10). The effect size can be calculated from previous study results. For example, if changes in anxiety level are measured in a group of patients just before surgery, the effect size will be large if a great change in anxiety occurs in the group before and after surgery. If the effect of a preoperative teaching program on the level of anxiety is measured, the effect size will be the difference in the posttest level of anxiety in the experimental group compared with that in the comparison group. If only a small change in the level of anxiety is expected, the effect size will be small. In many nursing studies, only small effect sizes can be expected. In such a study, a sample of 200 or more is often needed to detect a significant difference (Cohen, 1988). Small effect sizes occur in nursing studies with small samples, weak study designs, and instruments measuring only large changes. Researchers use the power value (80%), level of significance ($\alpha = 0.05$), and effect size to calculate the sample size needed for a study (Cohen, 1988; see Chapter 9). The power level should be discussed in studies that fail to reject the null hypothesis (nonsignificant findings). If the power level is below 0.80, you need to question the validity of the nonsignificant findings.

Degrees of Freedom

The concept of degrees of freedom (*df*) is important for calculating statistical analyses and interpreting the results. Degrees of freedom involve the freedom of a score value to vary given the other existing scores' values and the established sum of these scores (Gray et al., 2017). Degrees of freedom are often reported with statistical results.

IDENTIFYING THE STEPS OF THE DATA ANALYSIS PROCESS

The data analysis process in quantitative research involves the management of numerical data and the statistical analysis of these data to produce study results. Statistical analyses are techniques or procedures conducted to examine, reduce, and give meaning to the numerical data gathered in a study. In this text, statistics are divided into two major categories, descriptive and inferential. Descriptive statistics are summary statistics that allow the researcher to organize data in ways that give meaning and facilitate insight. Descriptive statistics are calculated to describe the sample and key study variables. Inferential statistics are designed to address objectives, questions, and hypotheses in studies to allow inference from the study sample to the target population. Inferential analyses are conducted to identify relationships, examine predictions, and determine group differences in studies.

When critically appraising a study, it is helpful to understand the following steps researchers implement during data analysis: (1) management of missing data; (2) description of the sample; (3) examination of the reliability of measurement methods; (4) performance of exploratory analyses of study data; and (5) performance of inferential analyses guided by the study hypotheses, questions, or objectives (Box 11.1). Although not all these steps are equally reflected in the final report of the study, they all contribute to the insights that can be gained from analysis of the study data.

Management of Missing Data

Except in very small studies, researchers almost always use computers for data analyses. The first step of the process is entering the data into the computer using a systematic plan designed to reduce errors. Missing data points are identified during data entry. If enough data are missing for certain variables, researchers may have to determine whether the data are sufficient to perform analyses using those variables. In some cases, study participants must be excluded from an analysis because data considered essential to that analysis are missing. In examining the results of a published study, you might note that the number of participants included in the final analyses is less than the original sample; this could be a result of attrition and/or participants with missing data being excluded from the analyses. It is important for researchers to discuss missing data and their management in the study.

BOX 11.1 STEPS OF THE DATA ANALYSIS PROCESS

1. Management of missing data
2. Description of the sample
3. Examination of the reliability of the measurement methods
4. Performance of exploratory analysis of the data
5. Performance of inferential statistical analyses guided by study objectives, questions, or hypotheses

Description of the Sample

Researchers present as complete a picture of the sample as possible in their research report. Variables relevant to the sample are called demographic variables, which might include age, gender, ethnicity, educational level, and diagnosis. Analysis of demographic variables produces the sample characteristics for the study participants (see Chapter 5). When a study includes more than one group (e.g., treatment group and control or comparison group), researchers often compare the groups in relation to the demographic variables. For example, it might be important to know whether the groups' distributions of age and educational levels were similar. When demographic variables are similar for the treatment (intervention) and comparison groups, the study is stronger because the results are more likely to be caused by the intervention rather than by group differences at the start of the study.

Reliability of Measurement Methods

Researchers need to report the reliability of the measurement methods used in their study. The reliability of observational or physiological measures is usually determined during the data collection phase and noted in the research report. If a multi-item scale was used to collect data in a study, the Cronbach alpha value should be included in the research report (Waltz et al., 2017). A value of 0.70 is considered acceptable, especially for newly developed scales. A Cronbach alpha coefficient value of 0.80 to 0.90 from previous research indicates that a scale is sufficiently reliable to use in a study. The *t*-test or Pearson correlation statistics may be used to determine test-retest reliability. In critically appraising a study, you need to examine the reliability of the measurement methods and the statistical procedures used to determine these values. Sometimes researchers examine the validity of the measurement methods used in their studies, and this content also needs to be included in the research report (see Chapter 10).

Exploratory Analyses

The next step, **exploratory analysis,** is used to examine all the data descriptively. This step is discussed in more detail later in this chapter. Data on each study variable are examined using measures of central tendency and dispersion to determine the nature of variation in the data and to identify outliers. **Outliers** are study participants or data points with extreme values (values that lie far from other plotted points on a graph) that seem unlike the rest of the sample. Researchers usually indicate whether outliers are identified during data analysis and how these were managed. In critically appraising a study's results, note any discussion of outliers and determine how they were managed and might have affected the study results.

Inferential Statistical Analyses

The final phase of data analysis involves conducting inferential statistical analyses for the purpose of generalizing findings from the study sample to appropriate accessible and target populations. To justify generalization of the results from inferential analyses, a rigorous research methodology is needed, including a strong research design (Shadish, Cook, & Campbell, 2002), reliable and valid measurement methods (Polit & Yang, 2016; Waltz et al., 2017), and a large sample size (Cohen, 1988).

Most researchers include a section in their research report that identifies the statistical analysis techniques conducted on the study data and the program used to calculate them. This discussion includes the inferential analysis techniques (e.g., those focused on relationships, prediction, and differences) and sometimes the descriptive analysis techniques (e.g., frequencies, percentages, and measures of central tendency and dispersion) conducted in the study. The data analysis techniques conducted in a study are usually presented just before the study's results section.

STATISTICS CONDUCTED TO DESCRIBE VARIABLES

Descriptive statistics, introduced earlier, allow researchers to organize numerical data in ways that give meaning and facilitate insight. In any study in which the data are numerical, data analysis begins with descriptive statistics. For some descriptive studies, researchers limit data analyses to descriptive statistics. For other studies, researchers use descriptive statistics primarily to describe the characteristics of the sample and the values obtained from the measurement of dependent or research variables. Descriptive statistics presented in this book include frequency distributions, percentages, measures of central tendency, measures of dispersion, and standardized scores.

Frequency Distributions

Frequency distribution describes the occurrence of scores or categories in a study. For example, the frequency distribution for gender in a study might be 42 males and 58 females. A frequency distribution usually is the first method used to organize the data for examination. There are two types of frequency distributions, ungrouped and grouped.

Ungrouped Frequency Distributions

Most studies have some categorical data that are presented in the form of an ungrouped frequency distribution, in which a table is developed to display all numerical values obtained for a particular variable. This approach is generally used on discrete rather than continuous data. Examples of data commonly organized in this manner are gender, ethnicity, marital status, diagnoses of study participants, and values obtained from the measurement of selected research and dependent variables. Table 11.2 is an example table developed for this text; it includes nine different scores obtained by 50 participants. This is an example of ungrouped frequencies because each score is represented in the table with the number of participants receiving this score.

Grouped Frequency Distributions

Grouped frequency distributions are used when continuous variables are being examined. Many measures taken during data collection, including body temperature, vital lung capacity, weight, age, scale scores, and time, are measured using a continuous scale. Any method of grouping

TABLE 11.2 EXAMPLE OF AN UNGROUPED FREQUENCY TABLE ($N = 50$)

SCORE	FREQUENCY	PERCENTAGE (%)	CUMULATIVE FREQUENCY (f)	CUMULATIVE PERCENTAGE (%)
1	4	8%	4	8%
3	6	12%	10	20%
4	8	16%	18	36%
5	14	28%	32	64%
7	8	16%	40	80%
8	6	12%	46	92%
9	4	8%	50	100%

TABLE 11.3 INCOME OF FULL-TIME REGISTERED NURSES (N = 100)

INCOME	FREQUENCY (–%)	CUMULATIVE PERCENTAGE (%)
Below $60,000	5 (5%)	5%
$60,000–$69,999	20 (20%)	25%
$70,000–$79,999	35 (35%)	60%
$80,000–$90,000	25 (25%)	85%
Above $90,000	15 (15%)	100%

results in loss of information. For example, if age is grouped, a breakdown into two groups, those younger than 65 years and those older than 65 years, provides less information about the data than groupings of 10-year age spans. As with levels of measurement, rules have been established to guide classification systems. There should be at least five but not more than 20 groups. The categories established must be exhaustive; each datum must fit into one of the identified categories. The categories must be exclusive; each datum must fit into only one (Grove & Cipher, 2017). A common mistake occurs when the ranges contain overlaps that would allow a datum to fit into more than one class. For example, a researcher may classify age ranges as 20 to 30, 30 to 40, 40 to 50, and so on. By this definition, participants aged 30, 40, and so on can be classified into more than one category. The range of each category must be equivalent. For example, if 10 years is the age range, each age category must include 10 years of ages. This rule is violated in some cases to allow the first and last categories to be open-ended and worded to include all scores above or below a specified point. Table 11.3 presents an example of a grouped frequency distribution for income for registered nurses (RNs), in which the categories are exhaustive and mutually exclusive.

Percentage Distributions

A **percentage distribution** indicates the percentage of study participants in a sample whose scores fall into a specific group and the number of scores in that group. Percentage distributions are particularly useful for comparing the present data with findings from other studies that have different sample sizes. A cumulative distribution is a type of percentage distribution in which the percentages and frequencies of scores are summed as one moves from the top to the bottom of the table. Consequently, the bottom category would have a cumulative frequency equivalent to the sample size and a cumulative percentage of 100 (see Table 11.2). Frequency distributions are also displayed using tables or graphs (e.g., pie chart, bar chart, line graph). Graphic displays of the frequency distribution of data from Table 11.2 are presented in Fig. 11.4. You might note in the bar and line graphs that the data distribution forms a normal curve.

Measures of Central Tendency

Measures of central tendency frequently are referred to as the midpoint in the data or as an average of the data. These measures are the most concise statement of the nature of the data in a study. The three measures of central tendency that are commonly used in statistical analyses are the mode, median, and mean. For a data set that has a perfect normal distribution, these values are equal (see Fig. 11.1); however, they usually are somewhat different for data obtained from real samples.

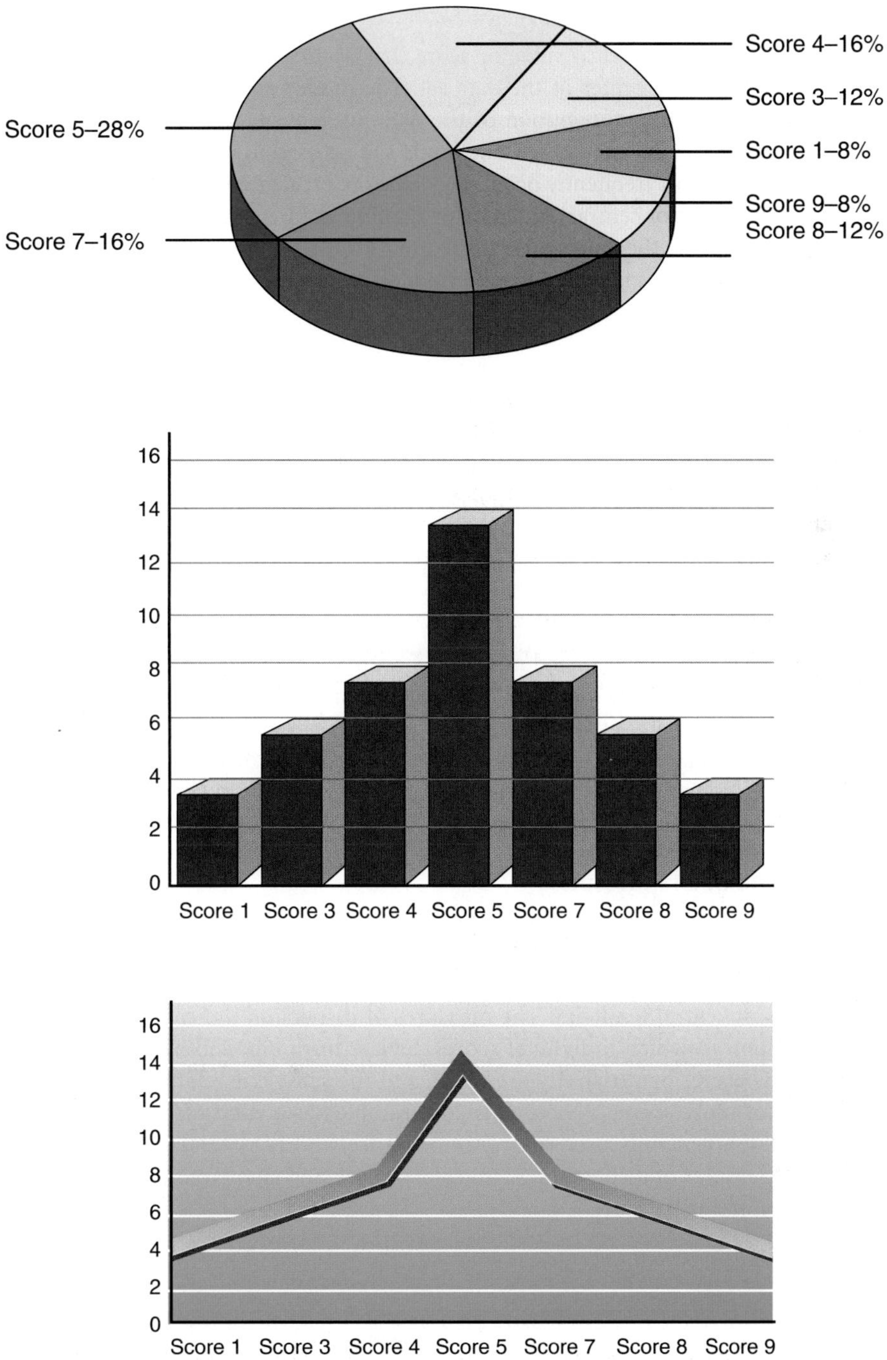

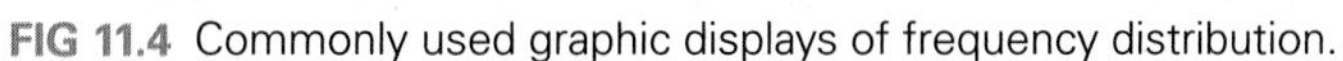

FIG 11.4 Commonly used graphic displays of frequency distribution.

Mode

The mode is the numerical value or score that occurs with greatest frequency; it does not necessarily indicate the center of the data set. The mode can be determined by examination of an ungrouped frequency distribution of the data. In Table 11.2, the mode is the score of 5, which occurred 14 times in the data set. The mode can be used to describe the typical study participant or identify the most frequently occurring value on a scale item (see Fig. 11.4). The mode is the appropriate measure of central tendency for nominal data. A data set can have more than one mode. If two modes exist, the data set is referred to as bimodal distribution (Fig. 11.5). A data set with more than two modes is said to be multimodal.

Median

The median is the midpoint or the score at the exact center of the ungrouped frequency distribution—the 50th percentile. The median is obtained by rank-ordering the scores. If the number of scores is uneven, exactly 50% of the scores are above the median, and 50% are below it. If the number of scores is even, the median is the average of the two middle scores; thus the median may not be one of the scores in the data set. Unlike the mean, the median is not affected by extreme scores or outliers in the data. The median is the most appropriate measure of central tendency for ordinal data. The median for the data in Table 11.2 is 5.

Mean

The most commonly conducted measure of central tendency is the mean. The mean is the sum of the scores divided by the number of scores being summed. Like the median, the mean may not be a member of the data set. The mean is the appropriate measure of central tendency for interval- and ratio-level data. However, if the study has outliers, the mean is most affected by these, and the median might be the measure of central tendency included in the research report. The mean for the data in Table 11.2 is 5.28.

Measures of Dispersion

Measures of dispersion, or variability, are measures of individual differences of the members of the sample. They give some indication of how scores in a sample are dispersed or spread around the mean. These measures provide information about the data that is not available from measures of central tendency. The measures of dispersion indicate how different the scores are or the extent to which individual scores deviate from one another. If the individual scores are similar, measures of variability are small, and the sample is relatively homogeneous, or similar, in terms of those scores. A heterogeneous sample has a wide variation in scores. The measures of dispersion generally used are range, variance, and *SD*. Standardized scores may be used to express measures of dispersion. Scatterplots (discussed later) frequently are used to illustrate the dispersion in the data.

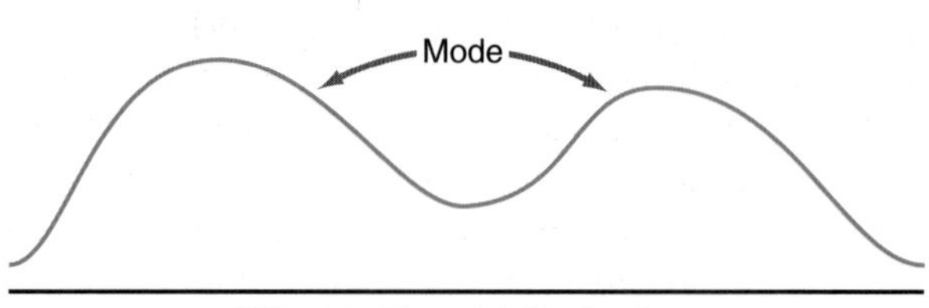

FIG 11.5 Bimodal distribution.

Range

The simplest measure of dispersion is the range, which is obtained by subtracting the lowest score from the highest score. The range for the scores in Table 11.2 is calculated as 9 – 1 = 8. The range is a difference score, which uses only the two extreme scores for the comparison. It is a very crude measure of dispersion but is sensitive to outliers. The range might also be expressed as the lowest to the highest scores. For the data in Table 11.2, the range might also be expressed as the scores from 1 to 9.

Variance

The variance for scores in a study is calculated with a mathematical equation and indicates the spread or dispersion of the scores (see Grove & Cipher, 2017, for the equation and calculation). The variance can only be calculated on data at the interval or ratio level of measurement. The numerical value obtained from the calculation depends on the measurement scale used, such as the laboratory measurement of fasting blood glucose values or the scale measurement of weights. The calculated variance value has no absolute value and can be compared only with data obtained using similar measures. Generally, however, the larger the variance value, the greater the dispersion of scores. The variance for the data in Table 11.2 is 4.94.

Standard Deviation

The *SD* is the square root of the variance. Just as the mean is the average value, the *SD* is the average difference (deviation) value. The *SD* provides a measure of the average deviation of a value from the mean in that particular sample. It indicates the degree of error that would result if the mean alone were used to interpret the data. In the normal curve, 68% of the values will be within 1 *SD* above or below the mean, 95% will be within 1.96 *SDs* above or below the mean, and 99% will be within 2.58 *SDs* above or below the mean (see Fig. 11.1; Grove & Cipher, 2017).

The *SD* for the example data presented in Table 11.2 is 2.22. The mean is 5.28, so the value of a study participant 1 *SD* below the mean would be 5.28 – 2.22, or 3.06. The value of a participant 1 *SD* above the mean would be 5.28 + 2.22, or 7.50. Therefore approximately 68% of the sample (and perhaps the population from which it was derived) can be expected to have values in the range of 3.06 to 7.50, which is expressed as (3.06, 7.50). Extending this calculation further, the value of a participant 2 *SDs* below the mean would be 5.28 – 2.22 – 2.22 = 0.84, and the value of a participant 2 *SDs* above the mean would be 5.28 + 2.22 + 2.22 = 9.72. The values for 2 *SDs* below and above the mean would be expressed as (0.84, 9.72). Using this strategy, the entire distribution of values can be estimated (Grove & Cipher, 2017). The value of a single individual can be compared with the value calculated for the total sample (e.g., mean, median, mode). *SD* is an important measure, both for understanding dispersion within a distribution and interpreting the relationship of a particular value to the distribution. In a published study, the *SD* is often written as the mean ± (plus or minus) the *SD*—for example 5.28 ± 2.22.

Confidence Interval

When the probability of including the value of the population within an interval estimate is known, it is referred to as a confidence interval (*CI*). Calculating a *CI* involves the use of two formulas to identify the upper and lower ends of the interval (see Grove & Cipher, 2017, for the formulas and calculations). For example, the *CI* for a study might include a lower value of 15.34 and an upper value of 20.56 and would be expressed as (15.34, 20.56). *CIs* are usually calculated for 95% and 99% intervals. The 95% *CI* indicates that 95% of the time, the population mean would fall within this interval. Theoretically, we can produce a *CI* for any population value or parameter of a distribution. It is a generic statistical procedure. For example, *CIs* can also be developed around correlation coefficients and *t*-test values. Estimation can be used for a single population or for multiple populations. You will see the use of *CIs* when reading the results section of studies.

Standardized Scores

Because of differences in the characteristics of various distributions, comparing a value in one distribution with a value in another is difficult. For example, perhaps you want to compare test scores from two classroom examinations. The highest possible score on one test is 100 and on the other it is 70; the scores will be difficult to compare. To facilitate this comparison, a mechanism was developed to transform raw scores into standardized scores. Numbers that make sense only within the framework of measurements used within a specific study are transformed into numbers (standardized scores) that have a more general meaning. Transformation into standardized scores allows an easy conceptual grasp of the meaning of the score. A common standardized score is the *z*-score. It expresses deviations from the mean (difference scores) in terms of *SD* units (see Fig. 11.1). A score that falls above the mean will have a positive *z*-score, whereas a score that falls below the mean will have a negative *z*-score. The mean expressed as a *z*-score is zero. The *SD* is equal to the *z*-score. Thus a *z*-score of 2 indicates that the score from which it was obtained is 2 *SDs* above the mean. A *z*-score of −0.5 indicates that the score is 0.5 *SD* below the mean.

Scatterplots

A scatterplot has two scales, horizontal and vertical. Each scale is referred to as an axis. The vertical scale is called the *Y*-axis; the horizontal scale is the *X*-axis. A scatterplot can be used to illustrate the dispersion of values on a variable. In this case, the *X*-axis represents the possible values of the variable. The *Y*-axis represents the number of times each value of the variable occurred in the sample. Scatterplots also can be used to illustrate the relationship between values on one variable and values on another. Then each axis will represent one variable. For example, if a graph is developed to illustrate the relationship between study participants' anxiety and depression scores measured with Likert scales, the horizontal axis could represent anxiety and the vertical axis could represent depression. For each unit or participant, there is a value for *X* and a value for *Y*. The point at which the values of *X* and *Y* for a single participant intersect is plotted on the graph (Fig. 11.6). When the values for each participant in the sample have been plotted, the degree of relationship between the variables is revealed (Fig. 11.7). If the scatterplot in Fig. 11.7 was an example of the relationship

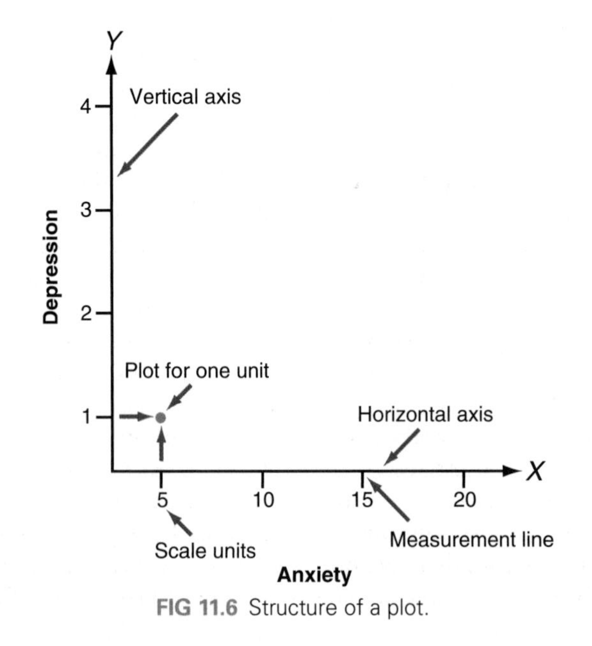

FIG 11.6 Structure of a plot.

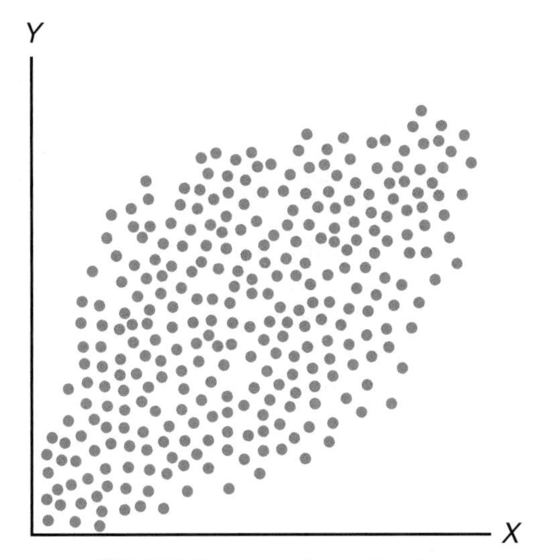

FIG 11.7 Example of a scatterplot.

between anxiety and depression, the plot is positive and indicates that as anxiety increases, so does depression in the study participants. The plotted points in a positive relationship extend from the lower left to the upper right corners of the scatterplot, as in Fig. 11.7. With a negative relationship, the plotted points extend from the upper left to lower right corners of the plot. The closer the plotted points are to a straight line, the stronger the relationship between the two variables.

Understanding Descriptive Statistical Results

Researchers report descriptive statistics in tables and in the narrative of the results section of their study. Descriptive statistics are conducted to describe the sample and study variables. Measures of central tendency (mode, median, and mean) and measures of dispersion (range and *SD*) are usually calculated to describe study variables. Also, descriptive and inferential statistics might be presented together to describe differences or similarities between groups at the start of a study. When a study is focused on determining if an intervention given to one group has made a difference, it is important to know if the groups were different from the beginning of the study. If the groups are different from the beginning, the effect of the intervention on the outcome may be exaggerated or attenuated. Inferential statistical procedures often used for this purpose include the chi-square test for nominal-level data and the *t*-test for interval- and ratio-level data (discussed later). From a perspective of descriptive analyses, the purpose is not to test for causality, but rather to describe the differences or similarities between or among the groups in a study.

Valiee, Razavi, Aghajani, and Bashiri (2017) conducted a randomized controlled trial (RCT) to examine the effectiveness of a psychoeducation program (PEP) on the quality of life (QOL) of patients with coronary heart disease (CHD). The study included an intervention group and control group, and the 70 participants were randomized equally into these groups. The PEP (intervention) consisted of eight sessions that are described in the article. QOL was measured with the MacNew Quality of Life Questionnaire in heart disease. This scale provided an overall QOL score for the study participants and scores for the three subscales—emotional health, physical health, and social functioning. The demographic and dependent variables (at baseline or pretest) for the intervention and control groups were described and examined for differences, as presented in Research Example 11.1.

RESEARCH EXAMPLE 11.1

Description of Study Variables

Research Study Excerpt

Data analysis was conducted using SPSS [Statistical Package for Social Sciences] version 13 (SPSS Inc., Chicago, IL, USA), and descriptive statistics were calculated. A Kolmogorov-Smirnov test was used to examine the normal distribution of variables, and the chi-square test was used to compare the distribution of sociodemographic variables within the two groups. An independent sample t*-test was used to examine the difference between the mean ages of the two groups. The independent sample* t*-test was also used to examine the differences between the overall QOL mean scores, and the subscale mean scores within the two groups at the beginning of the study… A* p*-value of < 0.05 was considered significant for all tests.*

Results

Of the 70 participants, three in the intervention group were excluded from analysis due to irregular attendance. In addition, two participants in the control group died during the course of the study and another was excluded from analysis due to incomplete answers on the post-test questionnaire. In total, the data of 64 patients were analyzed.

No significant differences were found between the two groups' clinical-demographic variables (Table 1). An independent sample t*-test was used to examine the differences between the two groups' mean QOL scores (96.34 ± 19.01 for the intervention group, and 94.75 ± 17.61 for the control group), and the mean QOL subscale scores at the beginning of the study, and no significant differences were observed in these scores* (p *> 0.05) (Table 2).* (Valiee et al., 2017, p. 39)

TABLE 1 Demographic Characteristic of Intervention and Control Groups

Variables	Intervention Group (n = 32)	Control Group (n = 32)	p Value
Age (mean ± *SD*)	50.12 ± 8.76	53.56 ± 8.41	0.35[a]
Sex			0.39[b]
Female	21 (65.6%	19 (59.4%)	
Male	11 (34.4%)	13 (40.6%)	
Inpatient history			0.1[b]
Yes	12 (37.5%)	18 (56.2%)	
No	20 (62.5%)	14 (43.8%)	
Underlying diseases			0.39[c]
None	13 (40.6%)	9 (28.1%)	
Diabetes	4 (12.5%)	6 (18.8%)	
Hypertension	5 (15.6%)	2 (6.2%)	
Hyperlipidemia	3 (9.4%)	7 (21.9%)	
All three cases	7 (21.9%)	8 (25%)	
Surgical history			0.14[b]
Yes	8 (25%)	13 (40.6%)	
No	24 (75%)	19 (59.4%)	
Smoking			1[b]
Yes	4 (12.5%)	3 (9.4%)	
No	28 (87.5%)	29 (90.6%)	

[a] *t*-test

[b] Fisher test.

[c] Chi-square test.

SD, Standard deviation.

From Valiee, S., Razavi, N. S., Aghajani, M., & Bashiri, Z. (2017). Effectiveness of a psychoeducation program on the quality of life in patients with coronary heart disease: A clinical trial. *Applied Nursing Research, 33*(1), 40.

TABLE 2 Comparison of Quality of Life at the Baseline Between Two Groups

GROUP	INTERVENTION GROUP		CONTROL GROUP			
Variables	**Mean**	***SD***	**Mean**	***SD***	***t***	***p* Value**
Emotional	35.94	6.61	33.84	7.19	1.21	0.23
Physical	34.78	6.79	34.12	8.33	0.34	0.73
Social	25.62	11.30	26.78	7.73	−0.47	0.63
Quality of life	96.34	19.01	94.75	17.61	0.34	0.72

SD, Standard deviation.

From Valiee, S., Razavi, N. S., Aghajani, M., & Bashiri, Z. (2017). Effectiveness of a psychoeducation program on the quality of life in patients with coronary heart disease: A clinical trial. *Applied Nursing Research, 33*(1), 40.

Critical Appraisal

Valiee and colleagues (2017) provided a clear concise presentation of their data analysis process and results. A rationale was provided for the study attrition, with the final analyses conducted on data from 64 participants (32 participants in each group). Most of the demographic variables were measured at the nominal level and were appropriately described with frequencies and percentages (see Table 1 from the study). The data were normally distributed (as indicated by the Kolmogorov-Smirnov test), so the conduct of means and *SDs* for the age data were appropriate. QOL was measured with a Likert-type scale and the totals of these scales and subscales are considered interval-level data (Grove & Cipher, 2017; Waltz et al., 2017). The descriptive results were appropriately presented in tables and discussed in the narrative of the results section. However, it would have been helpful to include the range for these variables to examine for outliers.

Differences between the groups were appropriately analyzed with chi-square or independent samples *t*-tests based on the variables' levels of measurement. Because the intervention and control groups had no significant differences for the demographic or dependent variables at the start of the study, these groups are considered homogeneous or similar for these variables. These results strengthened the study because the groups needed to be as similar as possible for these variables at the beginning of the study. Therefore significant differences noted at the end of the study are more likely to be a result of the study intervention than from error. More results from this study are presented in the section on *t*-tests.

DETERMINING THE APPROPRIATENESS OF INFERENTIAL STATISTICS IN STUDIES

Multiple factors are involved in determining the appropriateness or suitability of inferential statistical techniques conducted in a study. Inferential statistics are conducted to examine relationships, make predictions, and determine causality or differences in studies. Evaluating statistical procedures requires that you make a number of judgments about the nature of the data and what the researcher wanted to know. You need to determine: (1) The nature of the research question or hypothesis; (2) whether the data for analysis were treated as nominal, ordinal, or interval/ratio (see Fig. 10.2 in Chapter 10); (3) how many groups were in the study; and (4) whether the groups were paired (dependent) or independent.

You might see analysis techniques identified as parametric or nonparametric, based on the level of measurement of the study variables. If the variables are measured at the nominal and ordinal levels, nonparametric analyses are conducted. If variables are at the interval or ratio level of measurement, and the values of the study participants for the variable are normally distributed, parametric analyses are conducted (Grove & Cipher, 2017). Researchers run a computer program to determine if the data for variables are normally distributed and include the results in their study, as the result from the Kolmogorov-Smirnov test was included in the excerpt from the Valiee et al. (2017) study. Interval and ratio levels of data are often included together because the analysis techniques are the same whether the data are at the interval or ratio level of measurement.

In independent groups, the selection of one study participant is unrelated to the selection of other participants. For example, if participants are randomly assigned to treatment and control groups, the groups are independent. In paired groups (also called dependent groups), participants or observations selected for data collection are related in some way to the selection of other participants or observations. For example, if study participants serve as their own control by using the pretest as a control group, the measurements (and therefore the groups) are paired. Also, if matched pairs of participants are used for the comparison and intervention groups, the observations are paired (see Chapter 8). Researchers sometimes match groups according to age and severity of illness to control the effect of these demographic variables in a study. In a study of twins, for example, one twin may be placed in the control group and the other in the experimental group. Because they are twins, they are matched on several variables.

One approach for judging the appropriateness of an analysis technique in a study is to use a decision tree or algorithm. The algorithm directs you by gradually narrowing the number of appropriate analysis techniques as you make judgments about the nature of the study and the data. The algorithm in Fig. 11.8 identifies four factors related to the appropriateness of an analysis technique—nature of the research question or hypothesis, level of measurement of the dependent and research variables, number of groups in the study, and research design. To use the decision tree or algorithm in Fig. 11.8, you would: (1) determine whether the research question or hypothesis focused on differences or associations (relationships); (2) determine the level of measurement (nominal, ordinal, or interval/ratio) of the study variables; (3) select the number of groups that are included in the study; and (4) determine the design, with independent or paired (dependent) samples, that most closely fits the study you are critically appraising. The lines on the algorithm are followed through each selection to identify the appropriate analysis technique that is listed at the far right of the figure.

Critical Appraisal Guidelines for Data Analysis and Results Presented in Studies

To critically appraise the results section of quantitative studies, you need to be able to: (1) identify the statistical procedures conducted; (2) judge whether these procedures were appropriate for the purpose and the hypotheses, questions, or objectives of the study and the data collected; and (3) determine whether the researchers' presentation and interpretations of the results were accurate. When critically appraising the analysis techniques included in a study, you must not only be familiar with the analyses conducted, but you also must be able to compare those techniques with others that could have been conducted, perhaps to greater advantage.

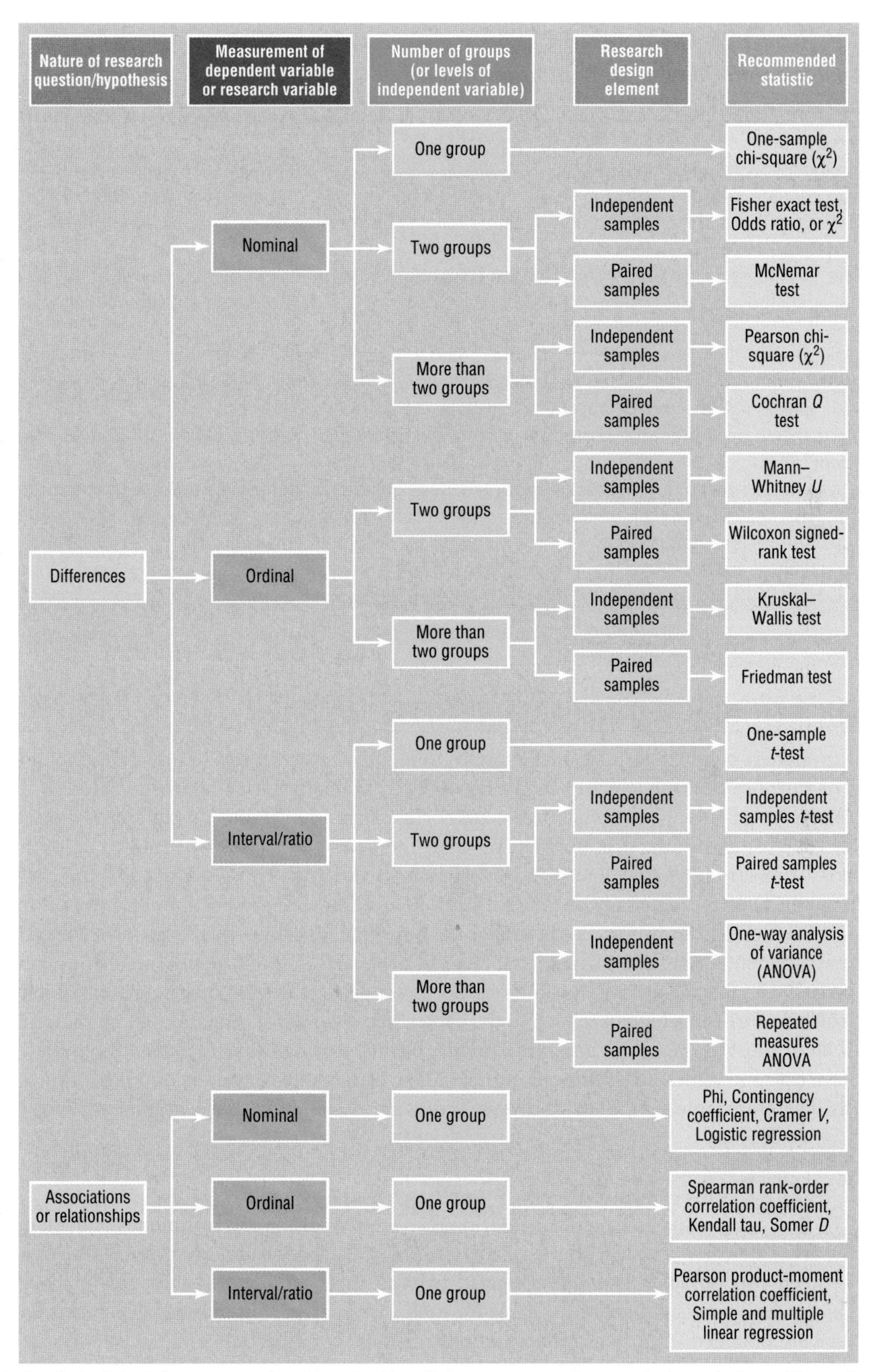

FIG 11.8 Statistical decision tree or algorithm for identifying an appropriate analysis technique. (From Gray, J. R., Grove, S. K., & Sutherland, S. [2017]. *The practice of nursing research: Appraisal, synthesis, and generation of evidence* [8th ed.]. St. Louis, MO: Elsevier; p. 532.)

CRITICAL APPRAISAL GUIDELINES

Data Analysis and Results Presented in Studies

The following critical appraisal guidelines will assist you in determining the quality of the data analysis and results presented in studies. The critical appraisals of analysis techniques presented later in this chapter are guided by the following questions:

1. Were appropriate analyses performed to address the study purpose and/or objectives, questions, or hypotheses? Was the focus of the study on examining relationships, making predictions, and/or determining group differences?
2. Was the analysis technique appropriate for the level of measurement of the data (nominal, ordinal, or interval/ratio) and study design? Use Fig. 11.8 to help you determine if the appropriate analyses techniques were conducted.
3. Were the results from the analyses clearly presented and appropriately interpreted? The American Psychological Association (APA, 2010) and Grove and Cipher (2017) have provided directions for reporting study results in tables, figures, and narrative.
4. Did the researchers identify the level of significance or α used in the study? Were the results statistically significant?
5. Were the effect size and power presented for any nonsignificant finding? Was the power adequate for the study, at least 0.80 or stronger, or was there a potential for a Type II error? (See earlier discussion of Type I and Type II errors and Table 11.1.)
6. Should additional analyses have been conducted? Provide a rationale for your answer (Grove & Cipher, 2017; Hoare & Hoe, 2013; Hoe & Hoare, 2012; Plichta & Kelvin, 2013; Polit, 2010).

STATISTICS CONDUCTED TO EXAMINE RELATIONSHIPS

Researchers conduct correlational analyses to identify relationships between or among variables. The purpose of these analyses might be to describe relationships between variables, clarify the relationships among theoretical concepts, or assist in identifying possible causal relationships by analyses examining group differences. All the data for the analysis need to be from a single population from which values are available for all variables to be examined in the correlational analysis. Data measured at the interval or ratio level provide the best information on the nature of a relationship. However, correlational analysis procedures are available for different levels of measurement. Data for a correlational analysis also need to span the full range of possible values on each variable included in the analysis. For example, if values for a particular variable can range from a low of 1 to a high of 9, each of the values from 1 to 9 will probably be found in the data set. If all or most of the values are in the middle of that scoring range (4, 5, and 6) and few or none have extreme values, a full understanding of the relationship cannot be obtained from the analysis. Therefore large samples with diverse scores are desirable for correlational analyses (Grove & Cipher, 2017).

Pearson Product-Moment Correlation

The Pearson product-moment correlation is an inferential analysis technique conducted to examine bivariate correlations in studies. Bivariate correlation measures the extent of the relationship between two variables. Data are collected from a single sample, and measures of the two variables to be examined must be available for each study participant in the data set. Less commonly, data are obtained from two related participants, such as breast cancer incidence in mothers and daughters. Correlational analysis provides two pieces of information about the data—the nature of a relationship (positive or negative) between the two variables and the magnitude (or strength) of the relationship. Scatterplots sometimes are presented to illustrate the relationship graphically (see Fig. 11.7). The outcomes of correlational analyses are symmetrical, rather than asymmetrical. Symmetrical means that the analysis gives no indication of the direction of the relationship. It is not possible to establish from correlational analysis whether variable A leads to or causes variable B, or that B causes A. The focus of correlational analysis techniques is examining relationships, *not determining cause and effect.*

Interpreting Pearson Product-Moment Correlation Analysis Results

The result of the Pearson correlation analysis is a correlation coefficient (r) with a value between -1 and $+1$. This r value indicates the degree of relationship between the two variables. A value of 0 indicates no relationship. A value of $r = -1$ indicates a perfect negative (inverse) correlation. In a negative relationship, a high score on one variable is correlated with a low score on the other variable. A value of $r = +1$ indicates a perfect positive relationship. In a positive relationship, a high score on one variable is correlated with a high score on the other variable. A positive correlation also exists when a low score on one variable is correlated with a low score on another variable. The variables vary or change in the same direction, either increasing or decreasing together. As the negative or positive values of r approach 0, the strength of the relationship decreases (Grove & Cipher, 2017).

Traditionally, an r value of less than 0.3 or -0.3 is considered a weak relationship, and a value between 0.3 and 0.5 or -0.3 and -0.5 indicates a moderate relationship; if the r value is above 0.5 or -0.5, it is considered a strong relationship (Gray et al., 2017). However, this interpretation of the r value depends to a great extent on the variables being examined and the situation in which they were measured. Therefore interpretation requires some judgment on the part of the researcher.

When a Pearson correlation coefficient is squared (r^2), the resulting number is the percentage of variance explained by the relationship. Even when two variables are related, values of the two variables will not be a perfect match. For example, if two variables show a strong positive relationship, a high score on one variable can be expected to be associated with a high score on the other variable. However, a study participant who has the highest score on one variable will not necessarily have the highest score on the other variable. The r^2 indicates the variance that is known by correlating two variables (Grove & Cipher, 2017).

There will be some variation in the relationship between values for the two variables for individual participants. Some of the variation in values is explained by the relationship between the two variables and is called explained variance, which is indicated by r^2 and is expressed as a percentage. For example, researchers may state that the relationship of the two variables anxiety and depression in their study was $r = 0.6$, and $r^2 = 0.36 \times 100\% = 36\%$. The explained variance is 36% for the variables anxiety and depression, which means that the patients' anxiety scores can explain 36% of the variance in their depression scores (Fig. 11.9). However, part of the variation is the result of factors other than the relationship and is called unexplained variance. In the example provided, 100% − 36% (explained variance) = 64% (unexplained variance; see Fig. 11.9). Therefore 64% of the variation in scores is a result of something other than the relationship studied, perhaps variables that were not examined in the study. A strong correlation has less unexplained variance than a weak correlation.

There has been a tendency to disregard weak correlations in nursing research. This approach can result in overlooking a relationship that may actually have some meaning within nursing knowledge if the relationship is examined in the context of other variables. Three common

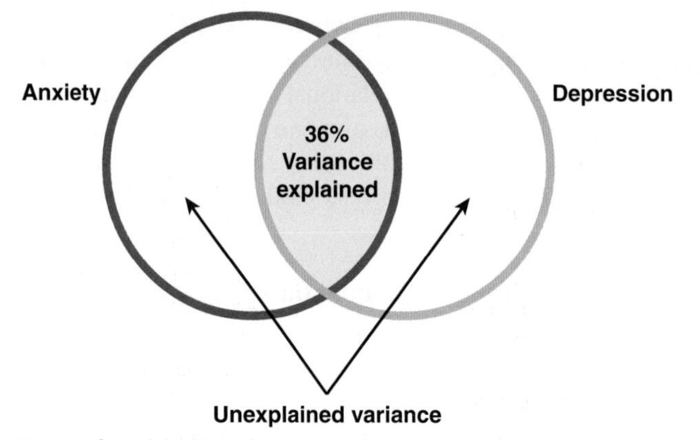

FIG 11.9 Percentages of explained and unexplained variances between anxiety and depression.

reasons for this situation, which is similar to that of a Type II error, have been recognized. First, many nursing measurements are not powerful enough to detect fine discriminations. Some instruments may not detect extreme scores, and a relationship may be stronger than that indicated by the crude measures available. Second, correlational studies must have a wide range of scores for relationships to be detected. If the study scores are homogeneous or the sample is small, relationships that exist in the population may not show up as clearly in the sample. Third, in many cases, bivariate analysis does not provide a clear picture of the dynamics in the situation. A number of variables can be linked through weak correlations, but together they provide increased insight into situations of interest. Statistical procedures (e.g., regression analysis [see later]) are available for examining the relationships among multiple variables simultaneously (Plichta & Kelvin, 2013).

Testing the Significance of a Correlation Coefficient

Before inferring that the sample correlation coefficient applies to the population from which the sample was taken, statistical analysis must be performed to determine whether the coefficient is significantly different from zero (no correlation). With a small sample, a strong correlation coefficient can be nonsignificant. With a very large sample, the correlation coefficient can be statistically significant when the degree of association is too small to be clinically important. Therefore in judging the significance of the coefficient, both the size of the coefficient and its statistical significance need to be considered.

Walker (2017) conducted a correlational study to examine the relationships among variables identified in the literature on school-age children's emotional responses to asthma. The study variables examined for relationships included child problem behaviors total, child problem behaviors internalizing subset, child problem behaviors externalizing subset, caregiver emotional functioning QOL, severity of asthma, and child emotional functioning QOL. Asthma severity was measured with the Severity of Chronic Asthma (SCA) scale, the child problem behaviors were measured with the Behavior Problem Index (BPI) scale, and caregiver and child emotional functioning QOL were measured with scales developed by Juniper and colleagues (1996). All these were Likert scales described in detail in the article. The data analysis and results from this study are presented in Research Example 11.2.

RESEARCH EXAMPLE 11.2

Pearson Product-Moment Correlation Results

Research Study Excerpt

Data Analysis

The Statistical Package for the Social Science (SPSS Statistic 20) was used to analyze the data collected in this study. The level of significance that was selected for this study was $\alpha = 0.05$*. Prior to performing the statistical analysis, data screening steps were taken to examine the data for entry errors, missing values, and outliers of undue influence. Entry errors were checked and corrected by returning to the original survey instruments if there was a questionable entry. Data screening checks included checking assumptions of linearity, normal distribution... Reliability checks of all survey instruments were run using Cronbach's* α*... Bivariate correlations were run using Pearson's* r *for all variables except for the dichotomous variable missed school days, which was run with Spearman rho (see Table 4)...*

Descriptive statistics for study measures are reported in Table 3. Asthma related child emotional functioning QOL was significantly and negatively correlated with asthma severity, externalizing child problem behaviors, and internalizing child problem behaviors. Greater asthma severity was associated with worse emotional functioning in children related to asthma, $r = -0.30$, $p < 0.01$*. More externalizing, and internalizing, child problem behaviors were reported when children reported more negative feelings regarding their asthma,* $r = -043$, $p < 0.001$ *and* $r = -0.26$, $p < 0.05$ *respectively [see Table 4]...*

Greater asthma severity was correlated with more caregiver negative feelings related to their children's asthma, $r = -0.39$, $p < 0.001$*. Greater externalizing and internalizing problem behaviors in children were associated with decreased caregiver emotional functioning QOL,* $r = -0.25$*;* $r = -0.22$, $p < 0.05$ *respectively [see Table 4].* (Walker, 2017, pp. 57–58)

TABLE 3 Descriptive Statistics of Variables

Variable	*n*	Range	Minimum	Maximum	Mean	*SD*	α
Child problem behaviors total (24 items)	85	29.00	24.00	53.00	31.36	6.407	0.889
Child problem behaviors internalizing subset (7 items)	85	6.00	7.00	13.00	8.40	1.575	0.529
Child problem behaviors externalizing subset (17 items)	85	25.00	17.00	42.00	22.96	5.384	0.889
QOL child emotional functioning (8 items)	84	20.00	20.00	40.00	34.15	5.861	0.790
QOL caregiver emotional functioning (9 items)	85	45.00	18.00	63.00	55.61	9.456	0.896

QOL, Quality of life; *SD*, standard deviation.

From Walker, V. G. (2017). Exploration of the influence of factors identified in the literature on school-aged children's emotional responses to asthma. *Journal of Pediatric Nursing, 33*(1), 58.

Continued

RESEARCH EXAMPLE 11-2—cont'd

TABLE 4 School-Age Children's Emotional Functioning Quality of Life

Variable	2	3	4	5	6
1. Child emotional functioning QOL	0.15	−0.30[b]	−0.43[c]	−0.26[a]	0.071
2. Caregiver emotional functioning QOL		−0.39[c]	−0.25[a]	−0.22[a]	0.105
3. Asthma severity			0.06	0.13	−0.17
4. Child problem behaviors externalizing				0.57[c]	−0.102
5. Child problem behaviors internalizing					0.004
6. Missed school days (yes, no)[d]					

NOTE: Pearson *r* used for all correlations except for *missed school days*.
[a]≤0.05.
[b]≤0.01.
[c]≤0.001.
[d]Spearman rho.
QOL, Quality of life.
From Walker, V. G. (2017). Exploration of the influence of factors identified in the literature on school-aged children's emotional responses to asthma. *Journal of Pediatric Nursing, 33*(1), 59.

Critical Appraisal

Walker (2017) detailed the steps of the data analysis process: (1) managing missing data and data entry errors; (2) exploring data for outliers; (3) setting the level of significance at $\alpha = 0.05$; (4) checking for linearity and normal distribution of the data; and (5) examining reliability (Cronbach alphas) of the Likert scales used for data collection. The summed Likert scales' scores provided interval level data that were appropriately described with means and *SDs*. The range and minimum and maximum scores for each variable enabled the researcher to examine for outliers. The ranges for variables indicated a wide spread of scores, which are important in examining relationships among variables. Pearson *r* was the appropriate statistic for correlating the variables measured by Likert scales, and the missed school days variable provided ordinal data that were correctly correlated with the Spearman rho, a nonparametric statistical test (see Fig. 11.8). The bivariate correlation values for the study variables were clearly presented in a correlation matrix table (see Table 4 from study). The significant correlation values were discussed in the study narrative and appropriately identified with asterisks in Table 4 (see the key below the table).

Factor Analysis

We wanted to provide you with some idea of the meaning of factor analysis when you see it in research reports. **Factor analysis** is commonly conducted to examine the interrelationships among large numbers of items on a scale and disentangles those relationships to identify clusters of items that are most closely linked. Intellectually, you might do this by identifying categories and sorting the items according to your judgment of the most appropriate category. Factor analysis sorts the items into categories according to how closely related they are to the other variables. Closely related items are grouped together into a **factor**. Several factors may be identified within a data set. Once the factors have been identified mathematically, the researcher must interpret the results by explaining why the analysis grouped the items in a specific way. Statistical results will indicate the amount of variance in the data set that can be explained by a particular factor and the amount of variance in the factor that can be explained by a particular item.

Factor analysis is frequently used in the process of developing measurement instruments, particularly those related to psychological variables, such as attitudes, beliefs, values, and opinions (Gray et al., 2017). Factor analysis aids in the identification of theoretical constructs; it is also conducted to confirm the accuracy of a theoretically developed construct. For example, a theorist may state that the concept of "hope" consists of the following elements: (1) anticipation of the future; (2) belief that things will work out for the best; and (3) optimism. Ways to measure these three elements can be developed, usually with a multi-item scale. The scale operationalizes the theoretical concept, such as hope, with items on it linked to one of the three subscales that measure the three elements of hope. A factor analysis can be conducted on the data to determine whether the participants' responses clustered into these three factors (subscales) identified for the concept of hope. In this way, factor analysis is being conducted to examine the construct validity of a scale for the population studied (see Chapter 10).

STATISTICS CONDUCTED TO PREDICT OUTCOMES

The ability to predict future events is becoming increasingly more important worldwide. People are interested in predicting who will win the football game, what the weather will be like next week, or which stocks are likely to increase in value in the near future. In nursing practice, as in the rest of society, the ability to predict is crucial. For example, nurse researchers would like to be able to predict the length of a hospital stay for patients with illnesses of different severity, as well as the responses of patients with a variety of characteristics (e.g., age, gender, level of education) to nursing interventions. Nurses need to know which variables play an important role in predicting health outcomes in patients and families. For example, variables of hours of sleep per night, minutes of exercise per week, calories consumed per day, and body mass index might be used to predict individuals' physical health scores on a QOL scale. Predictive analyses are based on probability theory, not on decision theory (see earlier discussion). Prediction is one approach for examining causal relationships between or among variables.

Regression Analysis

Regression analysis is used to predict the value of one variable when the value of one or more other variables is known. The variable to be predicted in a regression analysis is referred to as the *dependent* or *outcome variable*. The dependent variable is usually measured at the interval or ratio level. The goal of the analysis is to explain as much of the variance in the dependent variable as possible. In regression analysis, variables used to predict values of the dependent variable are referred to as independent variables. When one independent variable is used to predict a dependent variable, the analysis technique conducted is simple linear regression. For example, researchers might conduct simple linear regression to predict depression (dependent variable) by examining the influence of average hours of sleep per week (independent variables).

Multiple regression is conducted to analyze study data that include two or more independent variables. Using a multiple regression analysis, researchers might measure the influence of average hours of sleep per week, perceived social support, and family history of depression (independent variables) on depression (dependent variable). In regression analysis, the symbol for the dependent variable is Y, and the symbol for the independent variable(s) is X. Scatterplots and a bivariate correlation matrix are often developed before regression analysis is performed to examine the relationships that exist among the variables. The purpose of the regression analysis is to develop a line of best fit that will best reflect the values on the scatterplot. The line of best fit is often illustrated as an overlay on the scatterplot (Fig. 11.10). Many regression analysis techniques have been developed to analyze various types of data. One type, logistic regression, was developed to predict values of a dependent variable measured at the nominal level. Logistic regression is being used with increasing frequency in nursing studies. This type of regression can test whether a patient responds or did not respond to the intervention (Grove & Cipher, 2017; Plichta & Kelvin, 2013; Polit, 2010).

Interpreting Regression Analysis Results

The result of regression analysis is the regression coefficient, R. When R is squared (R^2), it indicates the amount of variance in the data that is explained by the equation (Grove & Cipher, 2017). When more than one independent variable is being used to predict values of the dependent variable, R^2

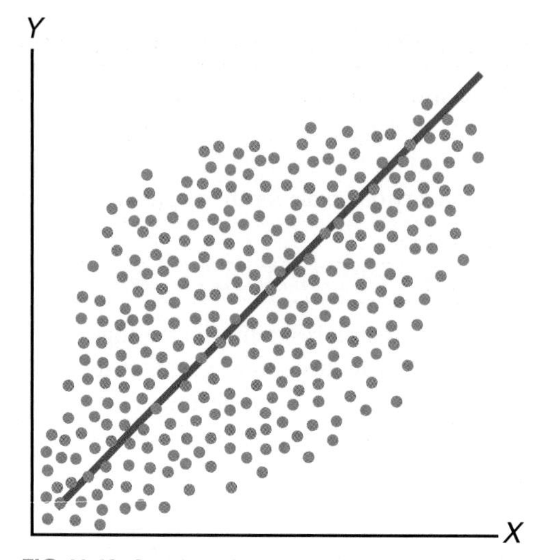

FIG 11.10 Overlay of scatterplot and best-fit line.

is sometimes referred to as the **coefficient of multiple determination**. The test statistic used to determine the significance of a regression coefficient may be t (from t-test) or F (from the analysis of variance [ANOVA]). Small sample sizes decrease the possibility of obtaining statistical significance. Values for R^2 and t or F are reported with the results of a regression analysis. Many studies using regression analysis are complex, including multiple independent variables and involving more than one regression procedure. Understanding the discussion of complex results requires reading each sentence carefully for comprehension, looking up unfamiliar terms, and determining the statistical significance of the results.

Walker's (2017) study was introduced earlier in the discussion of correlational analyses. We recommend that you review the correlation results presented in Table 4 of the study in Research Example 11.2. These results provided direction for the variables included in the regression analysis. The independent variables (caregiver emotional functioning QOL, severity of asthma, child problem behaviors externalizing, and child problem behaviors internalizing) were used to predict the dependent variable child emotional functioning QOL. Walker (2017) analyzed the study data with multiple regression analysis, and the results are presented in Research Example 11.3.

RESEARCH EXAMPLE 11.3

Regression Analysis

Research Study Excerpt

Multiple regression was run in order to address the second research question which examined the extent of influence of asthma severity, caregiver emotional functioning QOL, child internalizing and child externalizing behaviors, on asthma related child emotional functioning QOL. The variable that was removed from the model due to its non-significant relationships with all other variables in the model was missed school days. *The model accounted for 26% of the variance in asthma related child emotional functioning. The model fit was good,* $F(4,79) = 7.051$, $p < 0.001$*). Significant predictors of asthma related to child emotional functioning QOL were as follows: asthma severity,* $\beta = -0.31$, $p < 0.01$*; child externalizing problem behaviors,* $\beta = -0.43$, $p < 0.001$*. The results of the regression analyses are shown in Table 5.* (Walker, 2017, p. 58)

TABLE 5 School-Age Children's Emotional Functioning Quality of Life

Variables	*B*	*SE*	*β*	*p*	R^2
Constant	55.603	6.774		<0.001	
Asthma severity	−2.462	0.84	−0.31	0.004	
Caregiver emotional functioning QOL	−0.048	0.07	−0.08	0.48	
Child problem behaviors externalizing	−0.470	0.13	−0.43	<0.001	
Child problem behaviors internalizing	0.034	0.44	0.01	0.94	
					0.26

B, Unstandardized coefficient; *β*, standardized coefficient; *QOL*, quality of life; R^2, coefficient of determination or variance; *SE*, standard error.

From Walker, V. G. (2017). Exploration of the influence of factors identified in the literature on school-aged children's emotional responses to asthma. *Journal of Pediatric Nursing, 33*(1), 59.

Critical Appraisal

Walker (2017) appropriately conducted multiple regression analysis to answer the study research question. The Spearman rho values (presented earlier in Table 4 in Research Example 11.2) supported omitting the variable *missed school days* from the regression analysis because the correlation values were low and nonsignificant with all other variables. The Pearson *r* correlation values supported the inclusion of four independent variables in the analysis to predict the dependent variable, child emotional functioning QOL. The results of the multiple regression analysis were concisely presented in Table 5 and discussed in the article narrative. The study identified two independent variables, asthma severity and child externalizing problem behaviors (see the *p* values in Table 5) to be significant predictors of the dependent variable child emotional functioning QOL. Walker (2017) presented a correct but inconsistent *p* value for asthma severity in the narrative ($p < 0.01$) versus that in Table 5 ($p = 0.004$) that might be confusing to readers. Walker appropriately conducted an ANOVA ($F(4,79) = 7.051$, $p < 0.001$) to determine the significance of the regression model. The regression results explained 26% ($R^2 \times 100\% = 0.26 \times 100\%$) of the variance in the child emotional functioning QOL for children with asthma. Walker (2017. p. 54) "recommended that asthma research should consider problem behaviors of school-aged children when addressing asthma related emotional functioning QOL."

STATISTICS CONDUCTED TO EXAMINE DIFFERENCES

Inferential statistics are used to examine differences between groups, such as examining differences between intervention and control groups on selected demographic variables (see Table 1 in Research Example 11.1). Differences are also examined among other types of groups, such as examining differences of blood lipid values between males and females or differences in fasting blood sugar (FBS) and hemoglobin A1c (HbA1c) levels among white, black, Native American, and Hispanic racial and ethnic groups. Statistical techniques conducted to examine differences are also used to determine causality of the independent variable on the dependent variable. **Causality** is a way of knowing that one event leads to or causes another. Analysis techniques conducted to examine causality are essential for determining the effects of interventions on patient and family outcomes. These statistics examine causality by testing for significant differences in outcomes between the intervention and control groups. The statistical procedures used to examine differences included in this text are the chi-square test of independence, *t*-test, ANOVA, and **analysis of covariance** (ANCOVA). The *t*-test is used to examine differences between two groups and the chi-square test, ANOVA, and ANCOVA can be used to examine differences among three or more groups. The chi-square test is used to analyze nominal or ordinal levels of data, and the *t*-test, ANOVA, and ANCOVA are conducted to analyze interval and ratio levels of data (Grove & Cipher, 2017; Plichta & Kelvin, 2013).

When differences are examined among three groups, **post hoc analyses** are conducted to determine which of the groups are significantly different. The chi-square test and ANOVA indicate significant differences among the groups but do not specify which groups are different. For example, a study examined four occupational groups of workers who consume alcohol and determined that they were significantly different for the amount of alcohol consumed. Post hoc analyses are needed to identify which of the four groups is (are) significantly different. When post hoc analyses are conducted in a study, researchers usually identify the type of post hoc analysis and the results.

Chi-Square Test of Independence

The **chi-square test of independence** determines whether two variables are independent or related; the test can be used with nominal or ordinal data (see Fig. 11.8). The procedure examines the frequencies of observed values and compares them with the frequencies that would be expected if the data categories were independent of each other. The procedure is not very powerful; thus the risk of a Type II error is high—outcome of the study is nonsignificant when significant differences actually exist. Large sample sizes are needed to decrease the risk of a Type II error (Plichta & Kelvin, 2013). Most studies using this procedure place little importance on results in which no differences are found. Researchers frequently perform multiple chi-square tests in a sample. However, results generally are presented only when a chi-square analysis shows a significant difference.

Interpreting Chi-Square Results

Often, the first reaction to a sentence about "significant differences" by those unfamiliar with reading statistical results is panic. However, a sentence that looks dense with statistics provides a great deal of information in a small amount of space. For example, in the results χ^2 (1) = 18.10, $p = 0.001$, the author is using chi-square (χ^2) analysis to compare two groups on a selected variable, such as the presence or absence of chronic illness. The author provides the degrees of freedom ($df = 1$), so that the reader can validate the accuracy of the results using a statistical chi-square table (see the text by Grove & Cipher, 2017, p. 445, for a χ^2 statistical table). The numerical value 18.10 is the χ^2 value obtained from calculating the χ^2 equation (probably using a computer). SPSS and other data analysis programs automatically calculate and report the significance level of χ^2 results that can be validated using a χ^2 statistical table. As noted earlier, the symbol *p* is the abbreviation for probability. The groups were significantly different because $p = 0.001$, which is below the level of significance set at $\alpha = 0.05$. The phrase also indicates that the probability is 1 in 1000 that these groups come from the same population. The two groups are reported as significantly different because there is only 1 chance in 1000 that the study results are in error.

If a study variable has only two categories, such as the presence or absence of chronic illness, the researchers know what is significantly different. However, the exact location of specific differences among more than two categories of variables cannot be determined from chi-square analysis alone. Chi-square analysis identifies whether there is a significant difference, and post hoc analyses are conducted to identify the categories in which the significant differences occur.

Park and colleagues (2016) examined the effect of an intravenous (IV) infiltration management program on hospitalized children. The comparison group received routine care for preventing IV infiltrations, and the IV infiltration management program was applied to the experimental group. The sample included 2894 IV catheter insertions in the comparison group and 3651 IV catheter insertions in the experimental group. The study design was quasi-experimental because the comparison group data were obtained historically before the IV infiltration management program was implemented. IV infiltration was measured on a scale of 0 to 4, with 0 indicating no IV infiltration and 1 to 4 indicating the extent of the effusion of fluids. The data analysis and results of this study are presented in Research Example 11.4.

RESEARCH EXAMPLE 11.4

Chi-Square

Research Study Excerpt

Data Analysis

SPSS Win (version 18.0) was used for data analysis, and a two-tailed test with a significance level (α) of 0.05 was performed. 1) IV infiltration rate was calculated according to the standard method of the Infusion Nurses Society (2006). A chi-square or Fisher's exact test was performed to evaluate differences in IV infiltration rate between two groups. IV infiltration rate % = (number of IV infiltration occurrence/number of total IV insertions) x 100...

Results

IV Infiltration Rates

For the comparison group, the number of total IV insertions was 2894, the number of IV infiltration occurrences was 127, and the IV infiltration rate was 4.4%. For the experimental group, the number of total IV insertions was 3651, the number of occurrences of IV infiltration was 34, and the IV infiltration rate was 0.9%. A significant statistical difference in the IV infiltration rate was observed between the two groups (χ^2 = 80.42, p < .001; Table 2). (Park et al., 2016, pp. 174–175)

TABLE 2 Infiltration Incidence Rate Between Comparison and Experimental Groups

Variables	Comparison Group	Experimental Group	χ^2	*p*
Number of intravenous catheter insertions	2894	3651	80.42	<0.001
Number of infiltrations	127	34		
Infiltration incidence rate (%)	4.4	0.9		

From Park, S. M., Jeong, I. S., Kim, K. L., Park, K. J., Jung, M. J., & Jun, S. S. (2016). The effect of intravenous infiltration management program for hospitalized children. *Journal of Pediatric Nursing, 31*(2), 174.

Critical Appraisal

Chi-square analysis is appropriate to examine differences between the comparison and experimental groups in this study. The Fisher's exact test is the commonly conducted chi-square test in nursing research (Grove & Cipher, 2017). The data on IV infiltration were analyzed as though at the nominal level, with 0 indicating no infiltration and 1 to 4 indicating infiltration according to a designated standard. The numbers of IV catheter insertions in the groups were very robust, reducing the potential for a Type II error. Table 2 clearly presented the frequency and infiltration rate for both groups, as well as the chi-square results. Because the study only included two groups, no post hoc analyses were required. Because of the large sample and the significant findings, Park et al. (2016) recommended the wide use of this IV infiltration management program in clinical settings.

t-Test

One of the most common analyses conducted to test for significant differences between two samples is the *t*-test. The *t*-test is used to examine group differences when the variables are measured at the interval or ratio levels. A variety of *t*-tests have been developed for various types of samples. For example, when independent groups are being compared, the *t*-test for independent samples is conducted. For paired or dependent groups, the *t*-test for paired samples is conducted (see Fig. 11.8).

Sometimes researchers misuse the *t*-test by conducting multiple *t*-tests to examine differences in various aspects of data collected in a study. This misapplication will result in an escalation of significance that increases the risk of a Type I error—saying that something is significant when it is not. The Bonferroni procedure, which controls for the escalation of significance, may be used when multiple *t*-tests must be performed on different aspects of the same data set. This procedure makes the significance level more stringent based on the number of comparisons conducted. For example if five *t*-tests were conducted, the level of significance would need to be set at 0.01 ($0.05 \div 5 = 0.01$).

Interpreting *t*-Test Results

The result of the analysis is a *t* statistic, and the value and significance of this result are reported in studies. The *t*-test results in published studies can be validated by comparing them with the *t* values in a statistical table (see Grove & Cipher, 2017, pp. 439–440). The table is used to identify the critical value of *t*. If the computed statistic is greater than or equal to the critical value in the table, the groups are significantly different.

Valiee and colleagues' (2017) study, introduced earlier, was conducted to determine the effects of a psychoeducation program (PEP) on the emotional health, physical health, social functioning, and QOL of patients with CHD. These researchers conducted *t*-tests to determine differences between the intervention and control groups in their study. This study was an RCT that included an experimental pretest-posttest design (see Chapter 8). Study participants were randomly assigned to either the intervention or control group, resulting in independent groups. The two groups were not significantly different on the pretest, indicating that the groups were similar for the dependent variables at the start of the study (see Table 2 in Research Example 11.1). The intervention group underwent eight group sessions of the PEP, and then the posttests were conducted. The results of the *t*-tests were presented in tables and the narrative, as indicated in Research Example 11.5.

RESEARCH EXAMPLE 11.5

t-Test Results

Research Study Excerpt

An independent sample t*-test was used to examine the differences between the two groups' mean QOL scores (96.34 ± 19.01 for the intervention group, and 94.75 ± 17.61 for the control group), and the mean QOL subscale scores at the beginning of the study, and no significant differences were observed in these scores (p < 0.05) (Table 2 [in Research Example 11.1]). However, both the mean overall QOL scores (157.97 ± 25.51 for the intervention group, and 105.03 ± 8.38 for the control group), and the mean QOL subscale scores were significantly increased post-intervention for the intervention group. The differences between the two groups were statistically significant in both the overall QOL scores and across all of the subscales (p < 0.05) (Table 3).*

...Using the paired t*-test, a significant difference was observed between the mean overall QOL scores of the intervention group prior to and after the PEP intervention (96.34 ± 19.01 versus 157.97 ± 25.51) (p < 0.0001). However, no significant changes were observed in the control group's scores when comparing them before and after the study (94.75 ± 17.61 versus 105.03 ± 8.38) (p = 0.07) (Table 4).* (Valiee et al., 2017, p. 39)

TABLE 3 Comparison of Quality of Life at The End of Study Between Two Groups

GROUP	INTERVENTION GROUP		CONTROL GROUP			
Variables	**Mean**	***SD***	**Mean**	***SD***	***t***	***p* Value**
Emotional	54.09	8.16	39.41	4.26	9.01	0.0001
Physical	54.22	8.16	33.78	3.79	12.84	0.0001
Social	49.39	10.08	31.84	2.91	9.44	0.0001
Quality of life	157.97	25.51	105.03	8.38	11.14	0.0001

SD, Standard deviation.

From Valiee, S., Razavi, N. S., Aghajani, M., & Bashiri, Z. (2017). Effectiveness of a psychoeducation program on the quality of life in patients with coronary heart disease: A clinical trial. *Applied Nursing Research, 33*(1), 40.

TABLE 4 Comparison of Quality of Life Pretest and Posttest Between Two Groups

	MEAN ± *SD*		
QOL Group	**Baseline**	**After Intervention**	**Paired *t*-Test**
Intervention group	96.34 ± 19.01	157.97 ± 25.51	$p = 0.001$
Control group	94.75 ± 17.61	105.03 ± 8.38	$p = 0.07$
Independent *t*-test	$p = 0.72$	$p = 0.0001$	

QOL, Quality of life; *SD,* standard deviation.
From Valiee, S., Razavi, N. S., Aghajani, M., & Bashiri, Z. (2017). Effectiveness of a psychoeducation program on the quality of life in patients with coronary heart disease: A clinical trial. *Applied Nursing Research, 33*(1), 40.

Critical Appraisal

Valiee and colleagues (2017) conducted *t*-tests for independent samples to determine differences between the intervention and the control groups on the posttests for the dependent variables (emotional health, physical health, social functioning, and QOL; see Table 3). The independent *t*-test analysis technique was appropriate because the focus of the study was to determine differences between the randomly assigned intervention and control groups for dependent variables measured at the interval or ratio level (Grove & Cipher, 2017). There were significant differences between the two groups for all dependent variables, as indicated by $p < 0.0001$, which are less than $\alpha = 0.05$. The significant findings indicated adequate power to detect group differences—no Type II errors. The significant findings support the effectiveness of the PEP on QOL of patients with CHD. However, conducting multiple *t*-tests without the Bonferroni procedure or another post hoc test raises a concern about an increased risk for a Type I error. The study results would have been strengthened by including the Bonferroni correction for multiple *t*-tests.

Valiee et al. (2017) also examined differences in QOL from pretest to posttest for both the intervention and control groups. The paired or dependent *t*-tests were appropriate because the differences were examined in the same group using pretest and posttest scores (served as their own control). The intervention group had a significant difference from pretest to posttest, indicating that the PEP significantly changed the participants' QOL scores. As expected, the control group that received standard care had nonsignificant results from pretest to posttest. Valiee et al. (2017, p. 36) concluded that "Based on the findings, PEPs helped CHD patients improve their quality of life through reducing tension, relieving their negative emotions, and improving their social relationships."

Analysis of Variance

Analysis of variance (ANOVA) is a parametric statistical technique conducted to examine differences among three or more groups. Because this is a parametric analysis, the variables must be measured at the interval or ratio level. There are many types of ANOVA; some are developed for analysis of data from complex experimental designs (Grove & Cipher, 2017; Plichta & Kelvin, 2013). Rather than focusing just on differences between means, ANOVA tests for differences in variance. One source of variance is the variance within each group because individual scores in the group will vary from the group mean. This variance is referred to as the within-group variance. Another source of variance is the variation of the group means around the grand mean, referred to as the between-group variance. The assumption is that if all the samples are taken from the same population, these two sources of variance will exhibit little difference. When these two types of variance are combined, they are referred to as the total variance.

Interpreting Analysis of Variance Results

The results of an ANOVA are reported as an *F* statistic. The *F* distribution table can be used to validate the significance of the *F* values reported in studies (see Grove & Cipher, 2017, pp. 443–444). If the *F* value is equal to or greater than the appropriate table value, there is a statistically significant difference between the groups. If only two groups are being examined, the location of a significant difference is clear. However, if more than two groups are under study, it is not possible to determine from the ANOVA where the significant differences occur. Therefore post hoc analyses are conducted to determine the location of the differences among groups. The frequently used post hoc tests are the Bonferroni correction and the Newman-Keuls, Tukey honestly significantly difference (HSD), Scheffé, and Dunnett tests (Grove & Cipher, 2017; Plichta & Kelvin, 2013).

Yektatalab, Oskouee, and Sodani (2017) conducted an RCT to determine the effectiveness of a counseling intervention based on the Bowen system theory of marital conflict of couples in a family nursing practice. Marital conflict was measured with a 42-item Likert scale that had a Cronbach's alpha = 0.95 for this study. The couples were sorted into either the intervention or control group using a table of random numbers. The intervention group received the eight sessions of family counseling and the control group received standard care. The design included measurement of marital conflict at pretest and two posttests, one immediately after the intervention and the other 1 month later. Power analysis indicated that a sample of 24 couples was needed, but the researchers used 42 couples because of possible high attrition during the study. One couple was lost from both the intervention and control groups, resulting in a sample of 40 couples (80 participants). The analysis of data and results are provided in Research Example 11.6.

RESEARCH EXAMPLE 11.6

ANOVA

Research Study Excerpt

Data Analysis

The study data were gathered by the researcher's assistant who was not informed about the intervention before, immediately after, and one month after the end of the intervention. Demographic information and marital conflict questionnaires were also completed with cooperation of the researcher's assistant. Demographic information included age, sex, and education level... The data were entered into SPSS statistical software... and analyzed using independent and paired t-test*, Chi-square test, Pearson's correlation coefficient, and repeated measures ANOVAs test. Besides,* $p < .05$ *was considered as statistically significant...*

Results

Conflict

The study results revealed no statistically significant differences between the study groups regarding the total marital conflict scores ($t = 2.8$, $p = .93$*)... before the intervention (*$p > .05$*) (Table 3). However, a significant difference was observed between the two groups in this regard immediately and one month after the intervention (*$p < .05$*) (Table 3).*

Repeated measures [ANOVA] test was used to investigate the changes in the couples' mean scores of conflict in three successive stages. The results demonstrated a significant difference between the intervention and control groups regarding the conflict scores... during the three study periods and groups ($p < .001$*) (Table 3). Thus, the results supported the study hypothesis.* (Yektatalab et al., 2017, p. 257)

TABLE 3 Comparison of Couples' Mean Marital Conflict Score[a]

Marital	MEAN ± *SD*			RM-ANOVA, *F, p*		
Conflict	**Pretest**	**Posttest**	**Follow-Up**	**Time**	**Group**	**Time-Group**
Intervention	126.40 (5.79)	106.55 (11.12)	103.17 (12.48)	$F = 45.78$	$F = 45.03$	$F = 79.43$
Control	126.55 (5.75)	128.45 (7.68)	130.25 (7.40)	$p < 0.001$	$p < 0.001$	$p < 0.001$
p Value	$p = 0.930$	$p < 0.001$	$p < 0.001$			
t-Test[b]	$t = 2.80$	$t = 0.86$	$t = 0.75$			

[a]Before, after, and 1 month after the end of the intervention in both groups and between the groups under testing.
[b]Independent *t*-test.
RM-ANOVA, Repeated measures of analysis of variance; *SD,* standard deviation.
From Yektatalab, S., Oskouee, S., & Sodani, M. (2017). Efficacy of Bowen theory on marital conflict in the family nursing practice: A randomized controlled trial. *Issues in Mental Health Nursing, 38*(3), 258.

Critical Appraisal

Yektatalab and colleagues (2017) conducted a longitudinal study to determine the differences between the intervention and control groups at three points in time (pretest, posttest, 1-month follow-up). Marital conflict was measured with a Likert scale that had strong reliability in this study. The final sample of 40 couples was strong based on the power analysis results. Attrition was only 5%, losing one couple from each group, which resulted in equal groups for analysis. Data were collected by the research assistant, who was blinded to the intervention. Repeated measures ANOVA is the appropriate analysis technique for two or more study groups, variables measured at least at the interval level, and repeated posttest measures. They clearly presented their ANOVA results in table format and discussed their results in the article. In summary, this study had a strong design, sample size, and data collection process, with significant results that support the effectiveness of the counseling intervention on marital conflict. These researchers recommended additional studies with larger samples and longer follow-up periods. The implications for practice include ensuring that couples with marital conflict obtain family counseling.

Analysis of Covariance

Analysis of covariance (ANCOVA) allows the researcher to examine the effect of a treatment apart from the effect of one or more potentially confounding variables (see Chapter 5). Potentially confounding variables that are generally of concern include pretest scores, age, education, social class, and anxiety level. If the confounding variables are measured, their effects on study variables can be statistically removed by performing regression analysis before the ANOVA is carried out. Once this effect is removed, the effect of the treatment can be examined more precisely. This technique sometimes is used as a method of statistical control when it is not possible to design the study so that potentially confounding variables are controlled. However, control through careful planning of the design is more effective than statistical control.

ANCOVA may be used in pretest-posttest designs in which differences occur in groups on the pretest. For example, people who achieve low scores on a pretest tend to have lower scores on the posttest than those whose pretest scores were higher, even if the treatment had a significant effect on posttest scores. Conversely, if a person achieves a high pretest score, it is doubtful that the posttest will indicate a strong change as a result of the treatment. ANCOVA maximizes the capability to detect differences in such cases (Plichta & Kelvin, 2013). This information will help you understand why ANCOVA is conducted and can help identify the confounding variables in a study.

INTERPRETING RESEARCH OUTCOMES

Interpreting research outcomes involves examining the entire research process for strengths and weaknesses, organizing the meaning of the results, and forecasting the usefulness of the findings for evidence-based nursing practice (Gray et al., 2017; Melnyk, Gallagher-Ford, & Fineout-Overholt, 2017). The outcomes in research include the following elements: findings, significance of the findings, limitations, conclusions, generalization of findings, implications for nursing, and recommendations for further studies. These elements are included in the final section of studies, entitled "Discussion."

Types of Results

Interpretation of results from quasi-experimental and experimental studies has been traditionally based on decision theory, with five possible results: (1) significant results that agree with those predicted by the researcher; (2) nonsignificant results; (3) significant results that are opposite from those predicted by the researcher; (4) mixed results; and (5) unexpected results (Gray et al., 2017; Shadish et al., 2002). In critically appraising a study, you need to identify which types of results are presented in the study.

Significant and Predicted Results

Significant results agree with those predicted by the researcher and support the logical links developed by the researcher among the framework, purpose, study questions, hypotheses, variables, and measurement tools. In examining the results, however, you must consider the possibility of alternative explanations for the positive findings. What other elements could possibly have led to the significant results?

Nonsignificant Results

Nonsignificant (or inconclusive) **results,** often referred to as "negative" results, may be a true reflection of reality. In that case, the reasoning of the researcher or the theory used by the researcher to develop the hypothesis is in error. If it is, the negative findings are an important addition to the body of knowledge. However, the results also may stem from a Type II error resulting from inappropriate methodology, a biased or small sample, threats to design validity (see Chapter 8), inadequate measurement methods, weak statistical techniques, or faulty analysis. In such cases, the reported results could introduce faulty information into the body of knowledge (Angell, 1989). Negative results do not mean that no relationships exist among the variables. Negative results indicate only that the study failed to find any. Nonsignificant results provide no evidence of the truth or falsity of the hypothesis.

Significant and Unpredicted Results

Significant and unpredicted results are the opposite of those predicted by the researcher and indicate that flaws are present in the logic of the researcher and theory being tested. If the results are valid, however, they constitute an important addition to the body of knowledge. For example, a researcher may propose that social support and ego strength are positively correlated. If the relevant study shows instead that high social support is correlated with low ego strength, the result is the opposite of that predicted.

Mixed Results

Mixed results are probably the most common outcomes of studies. In this case, one variable may uphold predicted characteristics, whereas another does not, or two dependent measures of the same variable may show different results. These differences may be caused by methodology problems, such as differing reliability or sensitivity of two methods of measuring variables. The mixed results may also indicate that existing theory should be modified.

Unexpected Results

Unexpected results usually are relationships found between variables that were not hypothesized and not predicted from the study framework. Most researchers examine as many elements of data as possible in addition to those directed by the questions. These findings can be useful in the modification of existing theory and in the development of new theories and later studies. In addition, unexpected or serendipitous results are important evidence for developing the implications of the study. However, serendipitous results must be interpreted carefully because the study was not designed to examine these results.

Findings

Results in a study are translated and interpreted to become study findings. Although much of the process of developing findings from results occurs in the mind of the researcher, evidence of these thought processes can be found in published research reports.

Exploring the Significance of Findings

The significance of a study's findings is associated with its importance in contributing to nursing's body of knowledge. The significance of study findings is not a dichotomous characteristic (significant or nonsignificant) because studies contribute in varying degrees to the body of knowledge. The study findings' significance may be associated with the amount of variance explained, the degree of control in the study design to eliminate unexplained variance, and/or the ability to detect statistically significant differences or relationships. To the extent possible at the time the study is reported, researchers are expected to clarify the significance of the study findings.

The true importance of a particular study may not become apparent for years after publication. Certain characteristics, however, are associated with the significance of studies; significant studies make an important difference in people's lives. It is possible to generalize the findings far beyond the study sample so that the findings have the potential of affecting large numbers of people. The implications of significant studies go beyond concrete facts to abstractions and lead to the generation of theory or revisions of existing theory (Chinn & Kramer, 2015). A very significant study has implications for one or more disciplines in addition to nursing. The study is accepted by others in the discipline and is referenced frequently in the literature. Over time, the significance of a study is measured by the number of other studies that it generates. For example, the Braden Scale for Predicting Pressure Ulcer Risk has been the focus of extensive research and is currently implemented by many nurses to prevent and manage ulcers in clinical practice.

Clinical Importance of Findings

The strongest findings of a study are those that have both statistical significance and clinical importance. Clinical importance is related to the practical relevance of the findings. There is no common agreement in nursing about how to evaluate the clinical importance of a finding, but the effect size has been relevant in determining clinical importance. For example, one group of patients may have a body temperature 0.1° F higher than that of another group. Data analysis may indicate that the two groups are statistically significantly different, but the findings have no clinical importance. The effect size or differences between two groups is not sufficiently important to warrant changing patient care. In many studies, however, it is difficult to judge how much change would constitute clinical importance (Straus, Glasziou, Richardson, & Haynes, 2011). In studies testing the effectiveness of an intervention, clinical importance may be demonstrated by the proportion of study participants who showed improvement or the extent to which study participants returned to normal functioning. But how much improvement must they demonstrate for the findings to be considered clinically important? Questions also arise regarding who should judge clinical importance—patients and their families, clinicians, researchers, or society at large. At this point in the development of nursing knowledge, clinical importance or relevance is ultimately a value judgment (Gray et al., 2017; LeFort, 1993).

Limitations

Limitations are restrictions or problems in a study that may decrease the generalizability of the findings. Study limitations often include a combination of theoretical and methodological weaknesses. Theoretical weaknesses in a study might include a poorly developed or linked study framework and unclear conceptual definitions of variables. The limited conceptual definitions of the variables might decrease the validity of the operationalization or measurement of the study variables. Methodological limitations result from factors such as nonrepresentative samples, weak designs, single setting, limited control over treatment (intervention) implementation, instruments with limited reliability and validity, limited control over data collection, and improper use of statistical analyses. Study limitations can limit the credibility of the findings and conclusions and restrict the population to which the findings can be generalized. Most researchers identify the limitations of their study and indicate how these might have affected the study findings and conclusions. Identifying study limitations is necessary but, if these limitations are severe and multiple, the credibility of the findings needs to be questioned.

Conclusions

Conclusions are a synthesis of the findings. In forming conclusions, the researcher uses logical reasoning, creates a meaningful whole from pieces of information obtained through data analysis and findings from previous studies, and considers alternative explanations of the data. One of the risks in developing conclusions is going beyond the study results or forming conclusions that are not warranted by the findings.

Generalizing the Findings

Generalization extends the implications of the findings from the sample studied to a larger population (see earlier section on Inference and Generalization). For example, if the study had been conducted on patients with osteoarthritis, it may be possible to generalize the findings from the sample to the larger target population of patients with osteoarthritis or other types of arthritis.

Implications for Nursing

Implications for nursing are the meanings of conclusions from scientific research for the body of nursing knowledge, theory, and practice (Chinn & Kramer, 2015; Melnyk et al., 2017). Implications are based on but are more specific than conclusions; they provide specific suggestions for implementing the findings in nursing. For example, a researcher may suggest how nursing practice should be modified. If a study indicates that a specific solution is effective in decreasing pressure ulcers in hospitalized older patients, the implications will state how the care of older patients needs to be modified to prevent pressure ulcers. Interventions with extensive research support provide the basis for developing evidence-based practice (EBP) guidelines and ensuring quality, safe nursing practice (see Chapter 13).

Recommendations for Further Studies

In every study, the researcher gains knowledge and experience that can be used to design a better study next time. Therefore researchers often make suggestions for further study that emerge logically from the present study. Recommendations for further study may include replications or repeating the design with a different or larger sample, using different measurement methods, or testing a modified or new intervention. Recommendations may also include the formation of hypotheses to further test the framework in use. This section provides other researchers with ideas for further study to develop the knowledge needed for EBP (Brown, 2018; Melnyk et al., 2017).

CRITICAL APPRAISAL GUIDELINES

Research Outcomes

When critically appraising the outcomes of a study, you need to examine the discussion section of the research report and address the following questions:

1. What were the study findings and were they appropriate, considering the statistical results?
2. Were the study findings linked to previous research findings? Was the significance of the findings addressed?
3. Were the findings clinically important?
4. What study limitations were identified by the researchers? What other limitations may be present? How might the study limitations have affected the study conclusions?
5. Were the conclusions appropriate based on the study results, findings, and limitations?
6. To what population(s) did the researchers generalize the study findings? Were the generalizations appropriate?
7. What implications for nursing knowledge, theory, and practice were identified?
8. Were the implications for nursing practice appropriate based on the study findings and conclusions?
9. Did the researchers make recommendations for further studies? Were these recommendations based on the study results, findings, limitations, and conclusions?

The research outcomes from the Valiee and colleagues' (2017) study, introduced earlier, are presented and critically appraised in Research Example 11.7. The purpose of this study was to determine the effectiveness of a psychoeducation program (PEP) on QOL for patients with CHD. The following study excerpt includes information from the discussion section of this study; the key elements of this section are identified in brackets.

RESEARCH EXAMPLE 11.7

Research Outcomes

Research Study Excerpt

Discussion

The findings of this study showed that the PEP improved quality of life across all dimensions for patients with CHD, including emotional health, physical health, and social functioning [findings]. These findings were consistent with the results of Martina-Carrasco et al., who reported that PEP training increased the quality of life for Alzheimer patients and their families (Martina-Carrasco et al., 2009).... Omranifard, Esmailinejad, Maracy, and Jazi (2009) also found that PEP training was an effective, positive factor in the QOL scores of bipolar patients... Some studies, including D'Souza et al. (2010), also used psychological training and stated that this method was effective not only in reducing the severity of anxiety and depressive symptoms but also in decreasing the rate of recurrence of diseases... Another study also reported that PEP improved physical function, general health, and self-care in the control and reduction of the angina pain of heart disease [link to previous studies' findings, significance of findings, clinical importance]...

However, some studies that used PEPs did not find any positive significant effects (Lenz & Perkins, 2000; Tofighian et al., 2009). Those results could be attributed to differences in the content and techniques used, or to differences in the methods and timelines of the sessions. For example, various studies implemented psychological training methods through telephone contact, email, or CDs.... PEPs had a significant, positive impact on patient's quality of life, particularly if PEPs were applied in a face-to-face approach and were tailored to the individual's culture and lifestyle.

Continued

RESEARCH EXAMPLE 11-7—cont'd

In general, PEP changed patients' mental frameworks, increased their awareness of the present moment, and improved their cognitive and information-processing systems. Moreover, group-session PEPs showed additional benefits in facilitating the treatment process, because they allowed patients to gather together in one place to discuss their problems and support one another.... Therefore, PEP programs worked best in conjunction with group treatments [conclusions].

Limitations and Suggestions

This study had some limitations, including its non-blind design and a short follow-up period. Moreover, the psychological status of the patients when answering the questionnaire, and the level of information or support they received from sources other than the investigators, which could affect the results of the study, were not under the researchers' control [limitations]. Further studies are suggested, using larger sample sizes and longer or different follow-up periods at various time-intervals. Studies are also suggested that explore the barriers to PEP implementation and the facilitators who use PEP in practice [recommendations for further studies]...

Conclusion

Based on these findings, PEPs improved the quality of life for CHD patients [conclusion]. Cardiac nurses should consider this cognitive–educational method as routine patient support and follow-up care for CHD patients with an emphasis on improving patients' quality of life. In addition, considering CHD patients' needs for improved quality of life assistance, PEP interventions should be added to the nursing education curricula and routinely integrated into cardiac care plans [nursing implications]. (Valiee et al., 2017, pp. 39–40)

Critical Appraisal

Valiee and colleagues (2017) concisely presented their significant findings, which were consistent with their study results. The findings were also consistent with those of several other studies that included varied patient populations with chronic illnesses. Two studies did not find the PEPs had a significant effect on patients QOL, but Valiee et al. (2017) provided a rationale for why these studies findings were nonsignificant. The findings are clinically important because the PEP intervention was effective in improving QOL of patients with CHD and was best delivered as group sessions.

Valiee et al. (2017) identified their study limitations that could have limited the generalization of findings. However, they did not limit the generalization of their findings and recommended that they be implemented in nursing education curricula, which seems beyond the findings of this study. The integration of PEPs into cardiac care plans seems appropriate, with the conduct of additional research on the effectiveness of this intervention in different practice settings. The researchers suggested relevant additional studies to strengthen the knowledge regarding the PEP intervention.

Valiee et al. (2017) provided specific conclusions for their study at the end of their research report that were consistent with their study results, findings, and limitations. The researchers' conclusions provided a basis for the implications for nursing practice and recommendations for further research. However, the researchers did extend the generalization of their findings to nursing education curricula, which seemed beyond the focus of this study.

KEY POINTS

- Understanding statistical theories and relevant concepts will assist you in appraising the results of quantitative studies.
- Probability theory is used to explain a relationship, the probability of an event occurring in a given situation, or the probability of accurately predicting an event.
- Decision theory assumes that all the groups in a study used to test a particular hypothesis are components of the same population in relation to the study variables.

- A Type I error occurs when the null hypothesis is rejected, although it is true. The researchers conclude that significant results exist in a study, when in reality they do not. The risk of a Type I error is indicated by the level of significance (α).
- A Type II error occurs when the null hypothesis is accepted when it is actually false. The researchers conclude that the study results are nonsignificant when the results are significant. Type II errors often occur because of flaws in the research methods, and their risk can be examined using power analysis.
- Quantitative data analysis includes the following steps: (1) management of missing data; (2) description of the study sample; (3) examination of the reliability of measurement methods; (4) performance of exploratory analyses of the data; and (5) conduct of inferential analyses guided by the hypotheses, questions, or objectives.
- Descriptive or summary statistics covered in this text include frequency distributions, percentages, measures of central tendency, measures of dispersion, and scatterplot.
- Statistical analyses conducted to examine relationships that are covered in this text include Pearson product-moment correlation and factor analysis.
- Regression analysis is conducted to predict the value of one dependent variable using one or more independent variables.
- Statistical analyses conducted to examine group differences and determine causality included in this text are the chi-square test, *t*-test, ANOVA, and ANCOVA.
- Interpretation of results from quasi-experimental and experimental studies is traditionally based on decision theory, with five possible results: (1) significant results predicted by the researcher; (2) nonsignificant results; (3) significant results that are opposite from those predicted by the researcher; (4) mixed results; and (5) unexpected results.
- Research outcomes usually include findings, significance of findings, limitations, conclusions, generalization of findings, implications for nursing, and recommendations for further studies.
- In critically appraising a study, you should evaluate the appropriateness and completeness of the researchers' results and discussion sections.

REFERENCES

American Psychological Association (APA). (2010). *Publication manual of the American Psychological Association* (6th ed.). Washington, D.C.: Author.

Angell, M. (1989). Negative studies. *New England Journal of Medicine, 321*(7), 464–466.

Brown, S. J. (2018). *Evidence-based nursing: The research-practice connection* (4th ed.). Sudbury, MA: Jones & Bartlett.

Chinn, P. L., & Kramer, M. K. (2015). *Integrated theory and knowledge development in nursing* (9th ed.). St. Louis, MO: Elsevier Mosby.

Cohen, J. (1988). *Statistical power analysis for the behavioral sciences* (2nd ed.). New York, NY: Academic Press.

D'Souza, R., Piskulic, D., & Sundram, S. (2010). A brief dyadic group based on psychoeducation program: A pilot randomized controlled trial. *Journal of Affective Disorders, 120*(1-3), 272–276.

Gray, J. R., Grove, S. K., & Sutherland, S. (2017). *The practice of nursing research: Appraisal, synthesis, and generation of evidence* (8th ed.). St. Louis, MO: Elsevier Saunders.

Grove, S. K., & Cipher, D. J. (2017). *Statistics for nursing research: A workbook for evidence-based practice* (2nd ed.). St. Louis, MO: Elsevier.

Hoare, Z., & Hoe, J. (2013). Understanding quantitative research: Part 2. *Nursing Standard (Royal College of Nursing [Great Britain]), 27*(18), 48–55.

Hoe, J., & Hoare, Z. (2012). Understanding quantitative research: Part 1. *Nursing Standard (Royal College of Nursing [Great Britain]), 27*(15–17), 52–57.

Infusion Nurses Society. (2006). Infusion nursing standards of practice. *Journal of Infusion Nursing, 29*(supp), S1–S92.

Juniper, E. F., Guyatt, G. H., Feeny, D. H., Ferrie, P. J., Griffith, L. E., & Townsend, M. (1996). Measuring quality of life in children with asthma. *Quality of Life Research, 5*(1), 35–46.

Lenz, E. R., & Perkins, S. (2000). Coronary artery bypass graft surgery patients and their family member caregivers: Outcomes of a family-focused staged psychoeducation intervention. *Applied Nursing Research, 13*(3), 142–150.

LeFort, S. M. (1993). The statistical versus clinical significance debate. *Image—The Journal of Nursing Scholarship, 25*(1), 57–62.

Martina-Carrasco, M., Martin, M. F., Valero, C. P., Millan, P. R., Garcia, C. I., Montalban, S. R., et al. (2009). Effectiveness of a psychoeducational intervention program in the reduction of caregiver burden in Alzheimer's disease patients' caregivers. *International Journal of Geriatric Psychiatry, 24*(5), 489–499.

McKee, C., Long, L., Southward, L. H., Walker, B., & McCown, J. (2016). The role of parental misperception of child's body weight in childhood obesity. *Journal of Pediatric Nursing, 31*(2), 196–203.

Melnyk, B. M., Gallagher-Ford, E., & Fineout-Overholt, E. (2017). *Implementing evidence-based practice competencies in healthcare: A practical guide for improving quality, safety, & outcomes.* Indianapolis, IN: Sigma Theta Tau International.

Omranifard, V., Esmailinejad, Y., Maracy, M. R., & Jazi, A. H. D. (2009). The effects of modified family psychoeducation on the relative's quality of life and family burden in patients with bipolar type 1 disorder. *Journal of Isfahan Medical School, 27*(100), 563–574.

Park, S. M., Jeong, I. S., Kim, K. L., Park, K. J., Jung, M. J., & Jun, S. S. (2016). The effect of intravenous infiltration management program for hospitalized children. *Journal of Pediatric Nursing, 31*(2), 172–178.

Plichta, S. B., & Kelvin, E. (2013). *Munro's statistical methods for health care research* (6th ed.). Philadelphia, PA: Lippincott Williams & Wilkins.

Polit, D. F. (2010). *Statistics and data analysis for nursing research* (2nd ed.). Boston, MA: Pearson.

Polit, D. F., & Yang, F. M. (2016). *Measurement and the measurement of change.* Philadelphia, PA: Wolters Kluwer.

Shadish, W. R., Cook, T. D., & Campbell, D. T. (2002). *Experimental and quasi-experimental designs for generalized causal inference.* Chicago, IL: Rand McNally.

Slakter, M. J., Wu, Y. B., & Suzaki-Slakter, N. S. (1991). *, **, and ***: Statistical nonsense at the .00000 level. *Nursing Research, 40*(4), 248–249.

Straus, S. E., Glasziou, P., Richardson, W. S., & Haynes, R. B. (2011). *Evidence-based medicine: How to practice and teach it.* Edinburgh: Churchill Livingstone Elsevier.

Tofighian, T., Najjar, L., Akabery, A., & Nakhaee, M. R. S. (2009). Effect of individual counseling on quality of life in patients with myocardial infarction. *Journal of Sabzevar University of Medical Sciences, 16*(4), 206–212.

Valiee, S., Razavi, N. S., Aghajani, M., & Bashiri, Z. (2017). Effectiveness of a psychoeducation program on the quality of life in patients with coronary heart disease: A clinical trial. *Applied Nursing Research, 33*(1), 36–42.

Walker, V. G. (2017). Exploration of the influence of factors identified in the literature on school-aged children's emotional responses to asthma. *Journal of Pediatric Nursing, 33*(1), 54–62.

Waltz, C. F., Strickland, O. L., & Lenz, E. R. (2017). *Measurement in nursing and health research* (5th ed.). New York, NY: Springer Publishing Company.

Yektatalab, S., Oskouee, S., & Sodani, M. (2017). Efficacy of Bowen theory on marital conflict in the family nursing practice: A randomized controlled trial. *Issues in Mental Health Nursing, 38*(3), 253–260.

Because of funding changes, the Agency for Healthcare Research and Quality (AHRQ) National Guideline Clearinghouse website was scheduled for decommissioning as of July 16, 2018. For more information, go to https://www.ahrq.gov/.

CHAPTER

12

Critical Appraisal of Quantitative and Qualitative Research for Nursing Practice

Christy J. Bomer-Norton

CHAPTER OVERVIEW

LEARNING OUTCOMES

After completing this chapter, you should be able to:

1. Describe the purpose of intellectual critical appraisals of studies in nursing.
2. Describe the three steps for critically appraising a study: (1) identifying the steps or elements of the research process in the study; (2) determining study strengths and weaknesses; and (3) evaluating the credibility and meaning of the study findings.
3. Conduct a critical appraisal of a quantitative research report and a qualitative research report.

The nursing profession continually strives for evidence-based practice (EBP), which includes critically appraising studies, synthesizing the findings, applying the scientific evidence in practice, and determining the practice outcomes (Brown, 2018; Melnyk, Gallagher-Ford, & Fineout-Overholt, 2017; Moorhead, Johnson, Maas, & Swanson, 2013). Critically appraising studies is an essential step toward basing your practice on current research findings. The term *critical appraisal* or critique is an examination of the quality of a study to determine the credibility and meaning of the findings for nursing. Critique is often associated with criticize, a word that is frequently viewed as negative. In the arts and sciences, however, critique is associated with critical thinking and evaluation—tasks requiring carefully developed intellectual skills. This type of critique is referred to as an intellectual critical appraisal. An intellectual critical appraisal is directed at the product that is created, such as a study, rather than at the creator, and involves the evaluation of the quality of the product.

The idea of the intellectual critical appraisal of research was introduced earlier in this text and has been woven throughout the chapters. As each step of the research process was introduced, guidelines were provided to direct the critical appraisal of that aspect of a research report. This chapter summarizes and builds on previous critical appraisal content and provides direction for conducting critical appraisals of quantitative and qualitative studies. The background provided by this chapter serves as a foundation for the critical appraisal of research syntheses (systematic reviews, meta-analyses, meta-syntheses, and mixed-methods systematic reviews) presented in Chapter 13.

The critical appraisals implemented in nursing by students, practicing nurses, nurse educators, and researchers are discussed. The key principles for implementing intellectual critical appraisals of quantitative and qualitative studies are described to provide an overview of the critical appraisal process. The steps for critical appraisal of quantitative and qualitative studies, focused on rigor, quality, and meaning of findings, are detailed. Examples of critical appraisals of published quantitative and qualitative studies are provided.

PURPOSE OF CONDUCTING CRITICAL APPRAISALS OF STUDIES IN NURSING

An **intellectual critical appraisal of a study** involves a careful and complete examination of a study to judge its strengths, weaknesses, credibility, meaning, and significance for practice. A high-quality study focuses on a significant problem, demonstrates sound methodology, produces credible findings, indicates implications for practice, and provides a basis for additional studies (Gray, Grove, & Sutherland, 2017; Hoare & Hoe, 2013; Hoe & Hoare, 2012). Ultimately, the findings from several quality studies can be synthesized to provide empirical evidence for use in practice (O'Mathúna & Fineout-Overholt, 2015). Performing a critical appraisal of a study involves the following three steps, which are detailed in this chapter: (1) identifying the steps or elements of the study; (2) determining the study strengths and limitations; and (3) evaluating the credibility and meaning of the study findings. By critically appraising studies, you will expand your analytic skills, strengthen your knowledge base, and increase your use of research evidence in practice.

In general, studies are critically appraised to broaden understanding, summarize knowledge for practice, provide a knowledge base for future research, and determine the research evidence ready for use in practice. In addition, critical appraisals are often conducted for a class project, after verbal presentations of studies, after a published research report, for selection of abstracts when studies are presented at conferences, for article selection for publication, and for evaluation of research proposals for implementation or funding. Therefore nursing students, practicing nurses, nurse educators, and nurse researchers are all involved in the critical appraisal of studies.

Students' Critical Appraisal of Studies

One aspect of learning the research process is being able to read and comprehend published research reports. However, because conducting a critical appraisal of a study is not a basic skill, the content presented in previous chapters is essential for implementing this process. Students usually acquire basic knowledge of the research process and critical appraisal process in their baccalaureate program. Striving for EBP is one of the competencies identified for associate degree and baccalaureate degree (prelicensure) students by the Quality and Safety Education for Nurses (QSEN, 2018) project, and EBP requires a critical appraisal and synthesis of study findings for practice (Sherwood & Barnsteiner, 2017). More advanced analytic skills are often taught at the master's and doctoral levels. Therefore critical appraisal of studies is an important part of your education and your practice as a nurse.

Critical Appraisal of Studies by Practicing Nurses, Nurse Educators, and Researchers

Practicing nurses need to appraise studies critically so that their practice is based on current research evidence and not on tradition or trial and error (Brown, 2018; Craig & Smyth, 2012). Nursing actions need to be updated in response to current evidence that is generated through research and theory development. It is important for practicing nurses to develop strategies to remain current in their practice areas. Reading research journals and posting or emailing current studies at work can increase nurses' awareness of study findings but are not sufficient for critical appraisal to occur. Nurses need to question the quality of the studies, credibility of the findings, and meaning of the findings for practice. For example, nurses might form a research journal club in which studies are presented and critically appraised by members of the group (Gloeckner & Robinson, 2010). Skills in critical appraisal of research enable practicing nurses to synthesize the most credible, significant, and appropriate evidence for use in their practice. EBP is essential in agencies that are seeking or maintaining Magnet status (American Nurses Credentialing Center [ANCC], 2017).

Your faculty members and nurse educators in clinical settings critically appraise research to expand their clinical knowledge base and to develop and refine the nursing educational process. The careful analysis of current nursing studies provides a basis for updating curriculum content for use in clinical and classroom settings. Faculty serve as role models for their students by examining new studies, evaluating the information obtained from research, and indicating which research evidence to use in practice. For example, nursing instructors might critically appraise and present the most current evidence about caring for people with hypertension in class and role-model the management of patients with hypertension in clinical settings (James et al., 2013).

Nurse researchers critically appraise previous research to plan and implement their next study. Many researchers have a program of research in a selected area, and they update their knowledge base by critically appraising new studies in that selected area. For example, a team of nurse researchers might have a program of research to identify effective interventions for assisting patients in managing their hypertension and reducing their cardiovascular risk factors. As new studies are published on hypertension prevention and management, the researchers appraise the studies and consider the effect of the findings for their own research.

Critical Appraisal of Research Following Presentation and Publication

When nurses attend research conferences, they note that critical appraisals and questions often follow presentations of studies. These critical appraisals assist researchers in identifying the strengths and weaknesses of their studies and generating ideas for further research. Participants listening to critiques of studies might gain insight into the conduct of research. In addition, experiencing the critical appraisal process may increase the conference participants' ability to evaluate studies and judge the usefulness of the research evidence for practice.

Critical appraisals have been published following some studies in research journals. For example, the research journals *Scholarly Inquiry for Nursing Practice: An International Journal* and *Western Journal of Nursing Research* include commentaries after the research articles. In these commentaries, other researchers critically appraise the authors' studies, and the authors have a chance to respond to these comments. Published research critical appraisals often increase the reader's understanding of the study and the quality of the study findings (American Psychological Association [APA], 2010). A more informal critical appraisal of a published study might appear in the form of a letter to the editor, in which a reader comments on the strengths and weaknesses of published studies by writing to the journal editor.

Critical Appraisal of Research for Presentation and Publication

Planners of professional conferences often invite researchers to submit an abstract of a study they are conducting or have completed for potential presentation at the conference. The amount of information available is usually limited because many abstracts are restricted to 100 to 250 words. Nevertheless, reviewers must select the best-designed studies with the most significant outcomes for presentation at nursing conferences. This process requires an experienced researcher who needs few cues to determine the quality of a study. Critical appraisal of an abstract usually addresses the following criteria: (1) appropriateness of the study for the conference program; (2) completeness of the research project; (3) overall quality of the study problem, purpose, methodology, and results; (4) contribution of the study to the nursing knowledge base; (5) contribution of the study to nursing theory; (6) originality of the work (not previously published); (7) implication of the study findings for practice; and (8) clarity, conciseness, and completeness of the abstract (APA, 2010; Gray et al., 2017).

Some nurse researchers serve as peer reviewers for professional journals to evaluate the quality of research papers submitted for publication. The role of these scientists is to ensure that the studies accepted for publication are well designed and contribute to the body of knowledge. Journals that have their articles critically appraised by expert peer reviews are called peer-reviewed journals or **referred journals** (Pyrczak, 2008). The reviewers' comments or summaries of their comments are sent to the researchers to direct their revision of the manuscripts for publication. Referred journals usually have studies and articles of higher quality and provide excellent studies for your review for practice.

Critical Appraisal of Research Proposals

Critical appraisals of research proposals are conducted to approve student research projects; permit data collection in an institution; and select the best studies for funding by local, state, national, and international organizations and agencies. You might be involved in a proposal review if you are participating in collecting data as part of a class project or studies done in your clinical agency.

Research proposals are reviewed for funding from selected government agencies, corporations, and foundations. Corporations and foundations develop their own format for reviewing and funding research projects (Gray et al., 2017). The peer review process in federal funding agencies involves an extremely complex critical appraisal. Nurses are involved in this level of research review through national funding agencies such as the National Institute of Nursing Research (NINR, 2017) and the Agency for Healthcare Research and Quality (AHRQ, 2017).

KEY PRINCIPLES FOR CONDUCTING INTELLECTUAL CRITICAL APPRAISALS OF QUANTITATIVE AND QUALITATIVE STUDIES

Because the major focus of this chapter is conducting critical appraisals of quantitative and qualitative studies, key principles for conducting intellectual critical appraisals of these studies are presented in Box 12.1. All studies have weaknesses or flaws; if every flawed study were discarded, no scientific evidence would be available for use in practice. In fact, science itself is flawed. Science does not completely or perfectly describe, explain, predict, or control reality. However, improved understanding and an increased ability to predict and control phenomena depend on recognizing the flaws in studies and science. Additional studies can then be planned to minimize the weaknesses of earlier studies. You also need to recognize a study's strengths to determine the quality of a study and credibility of its findings. When identifying a study's strengths and weaknesses, you need to provide examples and rationale for your judgments that are documented with current literature.

In addition to the 10 principles provided in Box 12.1, three steps are followed for critically appraising both quantitative and qualitative studies and serve as the outline for the more detailed guidelines found in boxes later in this chapter. These guidelines stress the importance of examining the expertise of the authors, reviewing the entire study, addressing the study's strengths and weaknesses, and evaluating the credibility of the study findings (Fawcett & Garity, 2009; O'Mathúna & Fineout-Overholt, 2015; Powers, 2015). The detailed questions in the boxes are specific to the type of study and provide the criteria for a final evaluation to determine the credibility of the study findings, any implications for practice, and ideas for further research. Adding together the strong points from multiple studies slowly builds a solid base of evidence for practice. These guidelines provide a basis for the critical appraisal process of quantitative research discussed in the next section and for qualitative research discussed later.

BOX 12.1 KEY PRINCIPLES FOR CRITICALLY APPRAISING QUANTITATIVE AND QUALITATIVE STUDIES

1. ***Read and critically appraise the entire study.*** A research critical appraisal involves examining the quality of all aspects of the research report.
2. ***Examine the organization and presentation of the research report.*** A well-prepared report is complete, concise, clearly presented, and logically organized. It does not include excessive jargon that is difficult for you to read. The references need to be current, complete, and presented in a consistent format.
3. ***Examine the significance of the problem studied for nursing practice.*** The focus of nursing studies needs to be on significant practice problems if a sound knowledge base is to be developed for evidence-based nursing practice.
4. ***Indicate the type of study conducted and identify the steps or elements of the study.*** This might be done as an initial critical appraisal of a study; it indicates your knowledge of the different types of quantitative and qualitative studies and the steps or elements included in these studies.
5. ***Identify the strengths and weaknesses of a study.*** All studies have strengths and weaknesses, so attention must be given to all aspects of the study.
6. ***Be objective and realistic in identifying the study's strengths and weaknesses.*** Be balanced in your critical appraisal of a study. Try not to be overly critical in identifying a study's weaknesses or overly flattering in identifying the strengths.
7. ***Provide specific examples of the strengths and weaknesses of a study.*** Examples provide evidence for your critical appraisal of the strengths and weaknesses of a study.
8. ***Provide a rationale for your critical appraisal comments.*** Include justifications for your critical appraisal, and document your ideas with sources from the current literature. This strengthens the quality of your critical appraisal and documents the use of critical thinking skills.
9. ***Evaluate the quality of the study.*** Describe the credibility of the findings, consistency of the findings with those from other studies, and quality of the study conclusions.
10. ***Discuss the usefulness of the findings for practice.*** The findings from the study need to be linked to the findings of previous studies and examined for use in clinical practice.

UNDERSTANDING THE QUANTITATIVE RESEARCH CRITICAL APPRAISAL PROCESS

The quantitative research critical appraisal process includes three basic steps: (1) identifying the steps of the research process in studies; (2) determining study strengths and weaknesses; and (3) evaluating the credibility and meaning of study findings. These three steps are presented together with the detailed questions for critical appraisal of quantitative research in Box 12.2. Because you are new to critical appraisal of research, you will probably be focusing on step 1 of identifying the steps of the research process. As you gain critical appraisal experience, you might perform two or three steps of this process simultaneously.

BOX 12.2 CRITICAL APPRAISAL GUIDELINES

Quantitative Study

Step 1: Identifying the Steps or Elements of the Study; and Step 2: Determining the Study Strengths and Limitations

1. Writing quality
   a. Was the writing style of the report clear and concise with relevant terms defined?
2. Title
   a. Is the title clearly focused?
   b. Does the title include key study variables and population?
   c. Does the title indicate the type of study conducted—descriptive, correlational, quasi-experimental, or experimental—and the variables (Gray et al., 2017; Shadish, Cook, & Campbell, 2002)?
3. Authors
   a. Do the authors have credentials such as a doctor of philosophy (PhD) that qualified them to conduct the presented study?
   b. Do the authors have previous research or clinical experience that qualified them to conduct the presented study?
   c. Do any of the authors have a conflict of interest related to the study, such as financial interest in the company that produced the intervention implemented in the study?
4. Abstract
   a. Was the abstract clearly presented?
   b. Does the abstract include purpose, design highlights, sample, intervention (if applicable), and key results (APA, 2010).
5. Research problem (see Chapter 5)
   a. Is a problem statement provided? If a problem statement is not provided, can you infer the problem or gap in the literature?
   b. Is the problem significant to nursing and clinical practice (Brown, 2018)?
6. Purpose
   a. State the purpose of the study.
   b. Does the purpose narrow and clarify the focus of the study (Fawcett & Garity, 2009; O'Mathúna & Fineout-Overholt, 2015)?
7. Literature review (see Chapter 6)
   a. Examine the literature review.
   b. Are most references peer-reviewed primary sources? Do the authors justify references that are not peer-reviewed primary sources?

c. Are most of the references current (number and percentages of sources published in the last 5 and 10 years)? Are references older than 10 years, measurement or theoretical sources, landmark, seminal, or replication studies?
d. Is the content directly related to the study concepts or variables? Are the types of sources and disciplines of the source authors appropriate for the study concepts or variables?
e. Are the studies critically appraised and synthesized (Gray et al., 2017; Hart, 2009)? Is a clear concise summary presented of the current empirical and theoretical knowledge in the area of the study, including identifying what is known and not known (O'Mathúna & Fineout-Overholt, 2015)? Does the study address a gap in the knowledge identified in the literature review?

8. Framework or theoretical perspective (see Chapter 7)
    a. Is the framework explicitly expressed, or must you extract the framework from statements in the introduction, literature review, or other section(s) of the study?
    b. Does the framework identify, define, and describe the relationships among the concepts of interest? If a model or conceptual map of the framework is present, is it adequate to explain the phenomenon of concern (Gray et al., 2017)?
    c. How is the framework related to nursing's body of knowledge (Alligood, 2014; Smith & Liehr, 2014)?
    d. If a proposition from a theory is to be tested, is the proposition clearly identified and linked to the study hypotheses (Fawcett & Garity, 2009; Smith & Liehr, 2014)?
9. Research objectives, questions, or hypotheses (see Chapter 5)
    a. List any research objectives, questions, or hypotheses.
    b. Are the objectives, questions, or hypotheses clearly expressed and logically linked to the research purpose?
    c. Are the objectives, questions, or hypotheses logically linked to the concepts and relationships (propositions) in the framework (Chinn & Kramer, 2015; O'Mathúna & Fineout-Overholt, 2015; Smith & Liehr, 2014)?
    d. Are hypotheses stated to direct the conduct of quasi-experimental and experimental research (Shadish et al., 2002)?
10. Variables (see Chapter 5)
    a. Identify the study variables or concepts. Attribute or demographic variables should be provided. A study usually includes independent and dependent variables or research variables, but not all three types of variables.
        i. Demographic variables
        ii. Independent variables
        iii. Dependent variables
        iv. Research variables or concepts
    b. Identify the conceptual and operational definitions for independent and dependent variables.
    c. Are the variables clearly defined (conceptually and operationally) and based on previous research or theories (Chinn & Kramer, 2015; Gray et al., 2017; Smith & Liehr, 2014)?
    d. Are the variables reflective of the concepts identified in the framework?
11. Research design (see Chapter 8).
    a. Identify the specific design of the study.
    b. Does the design provide a means to examine all the objectives, questions, and hypotheses?
    c. Is the design used in the study the most appropriate design to obtain the required data (Gray et al., 2017)?
    d. Treatment
        i. Does the study include a treatment or intervention?
        ii. Is the treatment clearly described (Eymard & Altmiller, 2016)?

Continued

BOX 12.2 CRITICAL APPRAISAL GUIDELINES—cont'd

iii. Is the treatment appropriate for examining the study purpose and hypotheses?
iv. Was a protocol developed to promote consistent implementation of the treatment to ensure intervention fidelity (Eymard & Altmiller, 2016)?
v. Did the researcher monitor implementation of the treatment to ensure consistency?
vi. If the treatment was not consistently implemented, what might be the impact on the findings?

e. Groups
i. Did the study have more than one group?
ii. If the study had more than one group, how were study participants assigned to groups?
iii. If a treatment was implemented with more than one group, were the participants randomly assigned to the treatment group or were the treatment and comparison groups matched? Were the treatment and comparison group assignments appropriate for the purpose of the study?
iv. If more than one group was used, did the groups appear equivalent?

f. Were pilot study findings used to design this study? If yes, briefly discuss the pilot and the changes made in this study based on the pilot (Gray et al., 2017; Shadish et al., 2002).

g. Did the researcher identify the threats to design validity (statistical conclusion validity, internal validity, construct validity, and external validity) and minimize them as much as possible (Gray et al., 2017; Shadish et al., 2002)?

12. Sample (see Chapter 9).
a. Is the sampling method probability or nonprobability? Is the specific sampling method used in the study to obtain the sample identified and appropriate (Gray et al., 2017)?
b. What are the sampling inclusion criteria and sampling exclusion criteria, and were both clearly identified and appropriate for the study (O'Mathúna & Fineout-Overholt, 2015)?
c. Is the sample size identified (Aberson, 2010)?
d. Is the refusal or acceptance rate identified? Is the sample attrition or retention rate addressed? Are reasons provided for the refusal and attrition rates?
e. Is a power analysis reported? Was the sample size appropriate, as indicated by the power analysis? If groups were included in the study, is the sample size for each group equal and appropriate (Grove & Cipher, 2017)?
f. Is the sampling process adequate to achieve a representative sample? Is the sample representative of the accessible and target populations?
g. Did the researchers define the target and accessible populations for the study?
h. How was informed consent/assent obtained?
i. Was the process used for informed consent/assent appropriate for the study population?

13. Setting (see Chapter 9)
a. What is the study setting?
b. Is the setting appropriate for the study purpose?

14. Measurement (see Chapter 10)
a. Complete Table 12.1 to cover essential measurement content for a study (Waltz, Strickland, & Lenz, 2017).
i. Identify each study variable that was measured.
ii. Identify the name and author of each measurement strategy.
iii. Identify the type of each measurement strategy (e.g., Likert scale, visual analog scale, physiological measure, or existing database).
iv. Identify the level of measurement (e.g., nominal, ordinal, interval, or ratio) achieved by each measurement method used in the study (Grove & Cipher, 2017).
v. Describe the reliability of each scale for previous studies and this study. Identify the precision of each physiological measure (Bialocerkowski, Klupp, & Bragge, 2010; DeVon et al., 2007).
vi. Identify the validity of each scale and the accuracy of physiological measures (DeVon et al., 2007; Ryan-Wenger, 2017).

TABLE 12.1 Measurement Strategies

Variable Measured	Name of Measurement Method (author)	Type of Measurement Method	Level of Measurement	Reliability or Precision	Validity or Accuracy

b. Scales and questionnaires
   i. Are the instruments clearly described?
   ii. Are techniques to complete and score the instruments provided?
   iii. Did the researcher re-examine the validity and reliability of the instruments for the present sample?
   iv. If the instrument was developed for the study, is the instrument development process described (Gray et al., 2017; Waltz et al., 2017)?
c. Observation
   i. Is what is to be observed clearly identified and defined?
   ii. Are the techniques for recording observations described (Waltz et al., 2017)?
   iii. Is interrater reliability described?
d. Interviews
   i. Do the interview questions address concerns expressed in the research problem?
   ii. Are the interview questions relevant for the research purpose and objectives, questions, or hypotheses (Gray et al., 2017; Waltz et al., 2017)?
e. Physiological measures
   i. Are the physiological measures or instruments clearly described (Ryan-Wenger, 2017)? If appropriate, are the brand names of the instruments identified?
   ii. Are the accuracy, precision, and error of the physiological instruments discussed (Ryan-Wenger, 2017)?
   iii. Are the physiological measures appropriate for the research purpose and objectives, questions, or hypotheses?
   iv. Are the methods for recording data from the physiological measures clearly described? Is the recording of data consistent?
f. Do the measurement methods selected for the study adequately measure the study variables? Should additional measurement methods have been used to improve the quality of the study outcomes (Waltz et al., 2017)?
g. Do the measurement methods used in the study have adequate validity and reliability? What additional reliability or validity testing is needed to improve the quality of the measurement methods (Bialocerkowski et al., 2010; DeVon et al., 2007; Waltz et al., 2017)?

15. Data collection (see Chapter 10)
   a. Is the data collection process clearly described (Fawcett & Garity, 2009; Gray et al., 2017)?
   b. Do the data collected address the research objectives, questions, or hypotheses?
   c. How did the research ensure that the data collection process was conducted in an accurate and consistent manner?
      i. Who collected the study data?
      ii. Is the training of data collectors clearly described and adequate?
      iii. Were methods of standardization such as standardized forms or computerized data used?
   d. Was IRB approval obtained before data collection?
   e. Were the data collection methods ethical?
   f. Did any adverse events occur during data collection, and were these appropriately managed?

Continued

BOX 12.2 CRITICAL APPRAISAL GUIDELINES—cont'd

16. Data analyses (see Chapter 11)
    a. Complete Table 12.2 with the analysis techniques conducted in the study (Gray et al., 2017; Grove & Cipher, 2017; Hoare & Hoe, 2013; Plichta & Kelvin, 2013).
        i. Identify the purpose (description, relationships, or differences) for each analysis technique.
        ii. List the statistical analysis technique performed.
        iii. List the statistic.
        iv. Provide the specific results.
        v. Identify the probability (*p*) of the statistical significance achieved by the result.

TABLE 12.2 Statistical Analyses and Results

Purpose of Analysis	Analysis Technique	Statistic	Results	Probability (*p*)

    b. Are data analysis procedures clearly described?
    c. Do the data analysis techniques address the study purpose and the research objectives, questions, or hypotheses (Gray et al., 2017; Grove & Cipher, 2017)?
    d. Are data analysis procedures appropriate for the type of data collected (Grove & Cipher, 2017; Plichta & Kelvin, 2013)?
    e. Did the researcher address any problem with missing data and explain how this problem was managed?
    f. Statistical significance.
        i. Was the level of significance or alpha identified? If yes, what was the level of significance (0.05, 0.01, or 0.001)?
        ii. Is the sample size sufficient to detect significant differences if they are present?
        iii. Was a power analysis conducted for nonsignificant results (Aberson, 2010)?
    g. Are the results presented in an understandable way by narrative, tables, figures, or a combination of methods (APA, 2010; Grove & Cipher, 2017)?
    h. Are the results interpreted appropriately?

Step 3: Evaluating the Credibility and Meaning of the Study Findings

17. Interpretation of findings
    a. Are the findings consistent with previous research findings (Gray et al., 2017; O'Mathúna & Fineout-Overholt, 2015)?
    b. Are findings discussed in relation to each objective, question, or hypothesis?
    c. Are various explanations for significant and nonsignificant findings examined?
    d. Are the findings clinically important (O'Mathúna & Fineout-Overholt, 2015)?
    e. Are the findings linked to the study framework (Smith & Liehr, 2014)? If so, do the findings support the study framework?
    f. What questions emerge from the findings, and does the researcher identify them?
18. Limitations
    a. What study limitations did the researcher identify?
    b. Does the study have limitations not identified by the researcher?
    c. Could the limitations of the study have been prevented or controlled by the researcher?
19. Conclusions
    a. What conclusions did the researchers identify based on their interpretation of the study findings?
    b. Do the conclusions fit the findings from this study and previous studies?
    c. How did the researcher generalize the findings? Did the researcher generalize the findings appropriately?

20. Nursing implications
    a. What implications do the findings have for nursing practice (Melnyk et al., 2017; O'Mathúna & Fineout-Overholt, 2015)?
    b. Were the identified implications for practice appropriate based on the study findings and on the findings from previous research (Melnyk & Fineout-Overholt, 2015)?
21. Future research
    a. What suggestions for further study were identified?
    b. Were quality suggestions made for future research (O'Mathúna & Fineout-Overholt, 2015)?
    c. Is the description of the study sufficiently clear for replication?
    d. Did money, commitment, the researchers' expertise, availability of subjects, facilities, equipment, and/or ethics make the study unfeasible to conduct (Gray et al., 2017)?
22. Critique summary
    a. Review the components of the critique you just conducted. Consider the following to formulate your critique summary.
        i. Were all relevant components covered with adequate detail and clarity?
        ii. What were the study's greatest strengths and greatest weaknesses?
        iii. Were the rights of human subjects protected (Creswell, 2014; Gray et al., 2017)?
        iv. Do you believe the study findings are valid? How much confidence can be placed in the study findings?
        v. The evaluation of a research report should also include a final discussion of the quality of the report. This discussion should include an expert opinion of the study's quality and contribution to nursing knowledge and practice (Melnyk et al., 2017; O'Mathúna & Fineout-Overholt, 2015).

Step 1: Identifying the Steps of the Research Process in Studies

Initial attempts to comprehend research articles are often frustrating because the terminology and stylized manner of the report are unfamiliar. **Identifying the steps of the research process** in a quantitative study is the first step in critical appraisal. It involves understanding the terms and concepts in the report, as well as identifying study elements and grasping the nature, significance, and meaning of these elements.

Begin by reviewing the abstract, reading the study from beginning to end, and highlighting or underlining the steps of the quantitative research process that were identified previously. An overview of these steps is presented in Chapter 2. Reread the article, underline the terms you do not understand, and determine their meaning from the glossary at the end of this text. After reading and comprehending the content of the study, you are ready to write your initial critical appraisal of the study. To write a critical appraisal, you need to identify each step of the research process concisely and respond briefly to the guidelines and questions in Box 12.2.

Step 2: Determining the Strengths and Weaknesses in Studies

The second step in critically appraising studies requires **determining strengths and weaknesses in the studies**. To do this, you must have knowledge of what each step of the research process should be like from expert sources such as this textbook and other research sources (Creswell, 2014; Gray et al., 2017; Grove & Cipher, 2017; Hoare & Hoe, 2013; Hoe & Hoare, 2012; O'Mathúna & Fineout-Overholt, 2015; Waltz, Strickland, & Lenz, 2017). The ideal ways to conduct the steps of the research process are then compared with the actual study steps. During this comparison, you examine the extent to which the researcher followed the rules for an ideal study, and the study elements are examined for strengths and weaknesses.

You also need to examine the logical links or flow of the steps in the study being appraised. For example, the problem needs to provide background and direction for the statement of the purpose.

The variables identified in the study purpose need to be consistent with the variables identified in the research objectives, questions, or hypotheses. The variables identified in the research objectives, questions, or hypotheses need to be conceptually defined in light of the study framework. The conceptual definitions should provide the basis for the development of operational definitions. The study design and analyses need to be appropriate for the investigation of the study purpose, as well as for the specific objectives, questions, or hypotheses. Examining the quality and logical links among the study steps will enable you to determine which steps are strengths and which steps are weaknesses.

The questions in Box 12.2 help you explore the strengths and weaknesses of the steps of the research process and the logical links among these steps. In particular, the abstract, problem, purpose, literature review, framework, methodology, results, and discussion elements of the article are critically appraised. Read the questions and then make judgments about the steps in the study (see Box 12.2). You need to provide a rationale for your decisions and document from relevant research sources, such as those listed previously in this section and in the references at the end of this chapter. For example, you might decide that the study purpose is a strength because it addresses the study problem, clarifies the focus of the study, and is feasible to investigate (Fawcett & Garity, 2009; Gray et al., 2017; O'Mathúna & Fineout-Overholt, 2015).

Step 3: Evaluating the Credibility and Meaning of Study Findings

Evaluating the credibility and meaning of study findings involves determining the validity, significance, and meaning of the study by examining the relationships among the steps of the study, study findings, and previous studies. The steps of the study are evaluated in light of previous studies, such as an evaluation of present hypotheses based on previous hypotheses, present design based on previous designs, and present methods of measuring variables based on previous methods of measurement (Waltz et al., 2017). The findings of the present study are also examined in light of the findings of previous studies. An evaluation builds on the conclusions reached during the first two stages of the critical appraisal so the credibility, validity, and meaning of the study findings can be determined.

You need to re-examine the findings, conclusions, and implications sections of the study and the researchers' suggestions for further study. Use the credibility and meaning of the study section of the critique appraisal guide presented in Box 12.2 as a guide to summarize your evaluation.

EXAMPLE OF A CRITICAL APPRAISAL OF A QUANTITATIVE STUDY

A critical appraisal was conducted of the quasi-experimental study by Whitaker-Brown, Woods, Cornelius, Southard, & Gulati (2017) and is presented as an example in this section. The research report, "Improving quality of life and decreasing readmissions in heart failure patients in a multidisciplinary transition-to-care clinic," is included in this section. This study is followed by the three steps for critically appraising a quantitative study:

- Step 1: Identifying the steps of the research process
- Step 2: Determining study strengths and weaknesses
- Step 3: Evaluating the credibility and meaning of study findings

Nursing students and practicing nurses usually conduct critical appraisals that are focused on identifying the steps of the research process in a study. This type of critical appraisal may be written in outline format, with headings identifying the steps of the research process. A more in-depth critical appraisal includes not only this step but also determines study strengths and weaknesses and evaluates the study findings' credibility and meaning. We encourage you to read the Whitaker-Brown et al. (2017) study in Research Example 12.1, and conduct a comprehensive critical appraisal using the guidelines presented in Box 12.2. Compare your ideas with the critical appraisal presented in this section. The numbers used in the example critique correspond to those in the critical appraisal guidelines (see Box 12.2).

Quantitative Study

Heart & Lung 46 (2017) 79–84

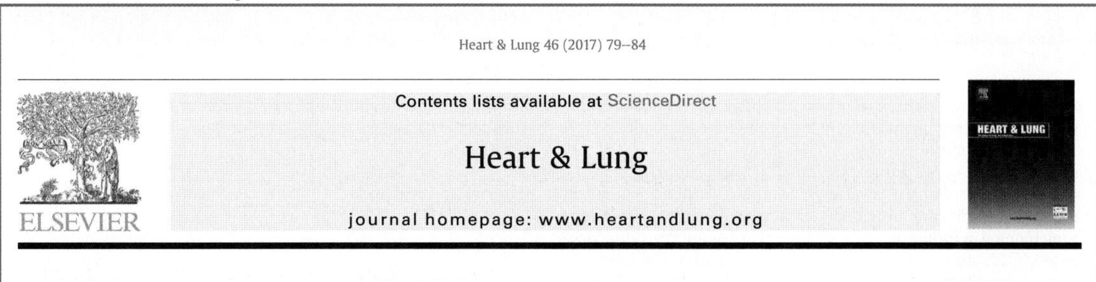

Improving quality of life and decreasing readmissions in heart failure patients in a multidisciplinary transition-to-care clinic

Charlene D. Whitaker-Brown, DNP, MSN, FNP-C[a,b,*], Stephanie J. Woods, PhD, RN[a], Judith B. Cornelius, PhD, MS, RN[a], Erik Southard, DNP, FNP-BC[c], Sanjeev K. Gulati, MD, FACC[b]

[a] University of North Carolina at Charlotte, School of Nursing, College of Health and Human Services, 9201 University City Blvd., Charlotte, NC 28223, USA
[b] Sanger Heart & Vascular Institute's Heart Success Clinic, Carolinas Medical Center-Main, 1000 Blythe Blvd., Charlotte, NC 28203, USA
[c] Indiana State University, College of Nursing, Health, & Human Services, Landsbaum Center 217, 200 North Seventh Street, Terre Haute, IN 47809, USA

ARTICLE INFO

Article history:
Received 20 November 2015
Received in revised form
1 November 2016
Accepted 11 November 2016
Available online 27 December 2016

Keywords:
Heart failure
Transition-to-care
Quality of life
Readmissions
Hospitalization

ABSTRACT

Objectives: The purpose was to pilot the feasibility and impact of a 4-week transition-to-care program on quality of life for heart failure patients.
Background: The transition from the acute care to the outpatient setting has been shown to be a critical time with heart failure patients.
Methods: A pre- and post-test design was used. Quality of Life, measured by the Minnesota Living with Heart Failure Questionnaire, and hospital readmissions were the outcomes. A convenience sample of 50 persons was recruited into a multidisciplinary transition-to-care program for heart failure patients following hospitalization. Thirty-six (72%) completed the study.
Results: There was a significant improvement in quality of life. Men reported greater improvement in physical symptoms and less emotional distress when compared to women. Only 2 participants were readmitted within 30 days.
Conclusions: Study findings support improved quality of life and decreased readmission rates following a multidisciplinary transition-to care program for heart failure patients.

Introduction

The incidence and prevalence of heart failure (HF) has increased dramatically in the past three decades. HF now affects approximately 5.7 million people in the United States and is the cause of more than 55,000 deaths a year; one in five people die within one year of diagnosis from HF syndrome.[1–3] It has been estimated that HF affects 10 per 1000 individuals after 65 years of age, and 1 in 5 will develop it after 40 years of age.[4–6] The most common risk factor of HF is coronary heart disease which is also considered the most costly medical condition in the United States.[1,2,7] Common symptoms of HF are: shortness of breath during daily activities; trouble breathing when lying down; weight gain with swelling in the legs, ankles, or lower back; and general fatigue and weakness.[1,2,8] The Heart Failure Society of America defines HF as a syndrome characterized by high mortality, frequent hospitalization, reduced quality of life (QOL), and a complex therapeutic regimen.[1,2,8,9]

Approximately, 20% of patients hospitalized nationally with HF are readmitted within 30 days.[10–13] All hospital readmissions are expensive with HF considered one of the most expensive diagnosis costing approximately $32 billion annually.[6,10,11,14,15] Further it is the leading cause of hospital admissions and readmissions in persons older than 65 years.[6,16,17] More than 2.5 million Medicare beneficiaries were hospitalized for HF from 2001 to 2005, and 1 in 10 died within 30 days of hospitalization.[6,7] Since HF is one of the most costly diagnosis for Medicare, the Centers for Medicare and Medicaid Services (CMS) began tracking 30-day readmission rates in 2009 as part of the Hospital Readmission Reduction Program of the Affordable Care Act.[6,18,19] The data for readmissions has been utilized to assess penalties to underperforming hospitals through the reduction of Medicare-based reimbursements by 1% in 2013, 2% in 2014 and up to 3% in 2015.[6,19]

Previous literature has shown that HF patients often lack support from healthcare teams especially when transitioning from hospital to home.[6,20] The transition from the acute care to the

* Corresponding author. University of North Carolina at Charlotte, School of Nursing, College of Health and Human Services 444-A, 9201 University City Blvd, Charlotte, NC 28223, USA.
E-mail address: cdwhitak@uncc.edu (C.D. Whitaker-Brown).

0147-9563/$ – see front matter © 2016 Elsevier Inc. All rights reserved.
http://dx.doi.org/10.1016/j.hrtlng.2016.11.003

Continued

RESEARCH EXAMPLE 12.1—cont'd

outpatient setting has been shown to be a critical time; patients are at high risk during this phase and are prone to exacerbations. Patients with chronic diseases such as HF and multiple comorbidities are particularly at risk for readmission.[20–22] To address this problem for patients with HF, a variety of outpatient HF management and transitional care programs of varying lengths have been implemented nationally.[1–3,6,9,11–13,17–31] The American Geriatrics Society[23] identifies transitional care as the "actions designed to ensure coordination and continuity of healthcare as patients transfer between different locations." CMS has addressed this vital area of care management by adding Transition Care Management Codes (TCMs). These TCMs CPT 99495 and 99496 are intended to both reimburse for, and assist in, tracking follow-up care provided for patients following discharge from an acute care facility to their community setting.[32]

It is recommended that transitional care begin during admission and continued through discharge. Transitional care programs have been designed to ensure continuity of care, contribute to clinical stability, improve patient outcomes, and reduce rates of hospital readmissions and related health care costs.[20,23] Most transitional programs include the nurses' role in coordinating multidisciplinary referrals based on patients' needs, communication among the inpatient team, communication with homecare providers and developing and implementing care plans to include patient and family education, medication management/titration, and increasing patient's physical activity levels and functional capacity.[20,24,33]

The hallmark of transitional care is that it is a time limited patient-oriented service. It helps to ensure continuity of care, reduces the risk of poor outcomes, and facilitates safety when transferring between healthcare settings.[25,31] The transitional care goal is to complement, not to replace primary care, disease management, discharge planning or case management, by educating patients with chronic disease and their caregivers.[25,31] Much research on transition-to-care programs focus on reducing medication errors, decreasing re-hospitalizations and length of stay, cutting overall costs, and lowering mortality.[22,24,26–28,33]

In addition to hospital readmissions, quality of life and symptom management are important outcomes associated with transitional care programs.[6,20,25,29,31] Despite optimal medical management, patients with HF experience a myriad of physical symptoms, emotional concerns, and may still have major impairment of functioning upon discharge.[6,34–37] Transitional care programs have generally focused exclusively on hospital readmission. However, little research has examined the impact of these programs on managing the physical and emotional symptoms of patients with HF or on their quality of life.

There is some evidence to support the value of transitional care programs on quality of life in HF patients.[6,20,25,29,31] Moreover, those who participated in transitional care had a better understanding of their illness, increased knowledge of medications[20,29,33] and a reduction in the number of readmissions.[6,20,25,27,29,31] Conversely, several studies of transitional care programs failed to document a significant impact on quality of life.[30] Seto and colleagues[37] identified from their research that some persons needed more time to master the complexities of HF self-management than was offered in the transitional care program, that is, patients, as with all people, learn at their own pace and at times need additional follow-up to understand what is needed for self-care.

Learning from these studies, and guided by the Stetler Model of research utilization to facilitate evidence-base practice,[38] we anticipate that an intensive, individualized, time-limited intervention has the potential to improve the quality of life in patients with HF. Stetler posits that linking research use and research-related actions forms a foundation for evidence-informed practice. The purpose of this study was to examine the feasibility and effects of a 4-week transition-to-care program on quality of life in patients with HF.

Material and methods

Design

A prospective one group pre- and post-test design was used to address the study purposes. In this study participants completed the pre-test prior to beginning the 4-week transition-to-care intervention. The post-test was administered at the end of the transition program.

Sample

A convenience sample of 50 participants was recruited from a major Southern Healthcare System which had initiated a 4-week pilot transition-to-care program for HF patients following inpatient hospitalization. Inclusion criteria were 45 years of age and older, male or female, not pregnant, and with a primary diagnosis of HF. Exclusion criteria were 44 years of age and younger, pregnant, and a primary diagnosis other than HF.

Intervention

This 4-week, multidisciplinary, transitional program was specifically designed to provide weekly education and support to HF patients (see Fig. 1). The HF inpatient coordinator/navigator initiated the discharge protocol and collected data relevant to the appropriate HF measures. The patient was discharged to the outpatient transition clinic within 1–3 days where they began receiving comprehensive and individualized HF management. This program included weekly clinic visits with a multidisciplinary team consisting of a nurse practitioner or physician assistant, nurse navigator, pharmacist, social worker and dietician. At the first visit, the transition clinic personnel initiated a risk assessment, confirmed guideline management, determined if the patient was compensated or decompensated (managed this according to guidelines), and contacted the primary care doctor with a patient update.

The patient attended weekly sessions for 4 weeks. Each visit consisted of a physical assessment and evaluation which included vital signs, weight, assessment of volume overload by checking for lower leg edema, abdominal distention, and jugular venous distention, and assessment of heart and lung sounds by a nurse practitioner. Additionally, medication reconciliation was performed collaboratively between the nurse practitioner, pharmacist, and clinic nurse. The nurse practitioner had the patient provide a 24–48 h recall of their oral intake including food and liquids and reviewed logs of daily weights and blood pressure. The initial visit was 1 h and follow-up visits were 30 min. The clinic provider also initiated the following referrals as needed: rehabilitation, home care, hospice and/or palliative care.

All visits were grounded in evidence-based interventions aimed at HF management and focused on patient education, medication management (e.g. titration of beta blockers and diuretics), and assistance with coordination and delivery of care as needed per living arrangements. Patients also had access to phone triage Monday through Friday during office hours. The telehealth connection consisted of ongoing phone call follow-up for 3 weeks post transition clinic. After attending 4 weeks in the transition clinic the patient's care was coordinated and they were scheduled for follow-up with their primary care provider and or referred to cardiology or the HF Clinic for longitudinal care. This study was

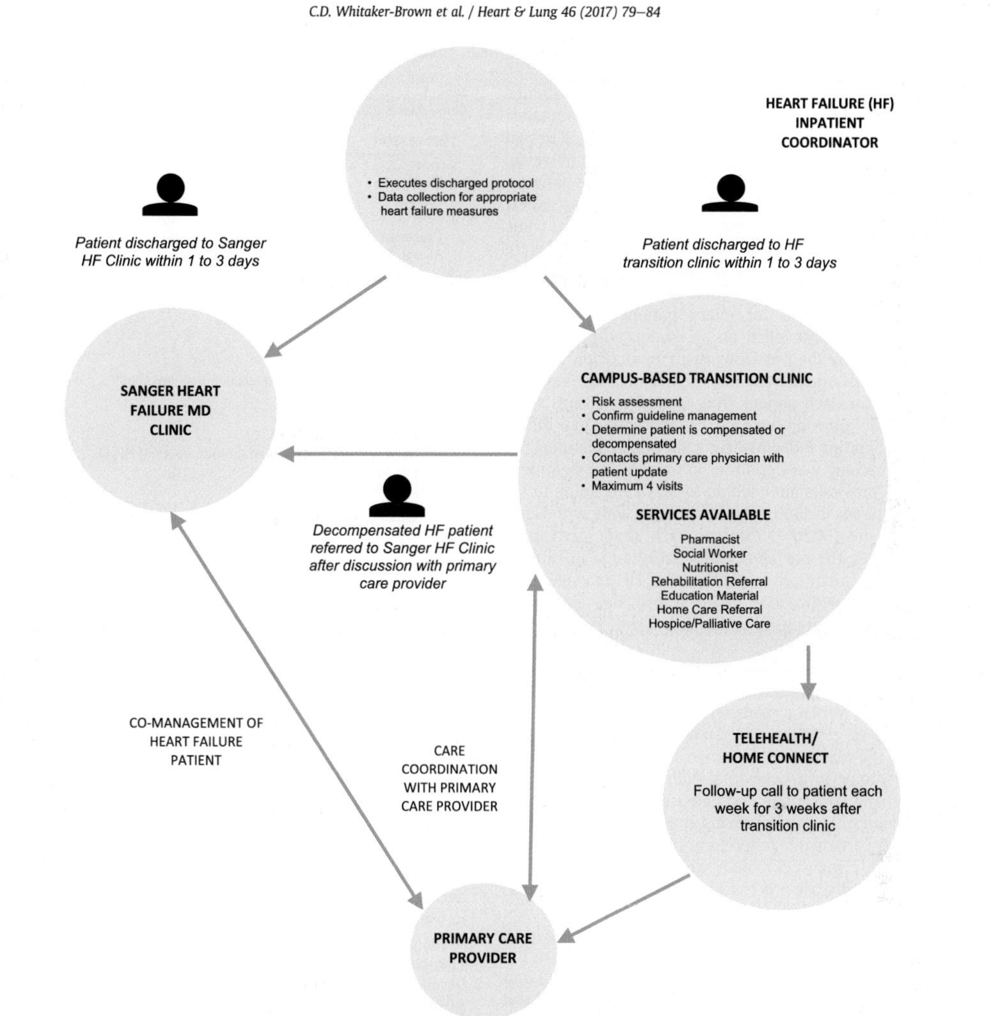

Fig. 1. Heart success transition model. http://www.carolinashealthcare.org/heart-success; re-printed with permission.

approved by the Institutional Review Board of the clinical agency and informed consent was obtained by the principal investigator.

Measures

Demographic data were collected through chart review and using the nurse navigator's patient assessment notes. This included age, gender, race/ethnicity and ejection fraction. Health-related quality of life (QOL) was assessed using the Minnesota Living with Heart Failure Questionnaire (MLHFQ), a 21 item, 6-point Likert scale that reflected the most frequent and important ways heart HF failure affects patient's lives.[39,40] Using this Likert scale, answers were given by choosing a score between 0 (no impairment) and 5 (very much impaired), resulting in a total score variation from 0 to 105, with lower scores indicating improved quality of life. There is a summed overall QOL score as well as two dimension subscale scores that assess physical symptoms and emotional distress. Internal consistency of the MLHFQ has been demonstrated in research with chronically ill persons with a Cronbach's alpha of .92, and test-retest/reproducibility of $r = .87$.[39,40] In this study, the Cronbach alpha for the overall MLHFQ, physical symptoms dimension, and emotional distress dimension were .92, .96, and .93, respectively. Hospital readmissions at 30 days were based on data obtained from the hospital records of the participants. Additionally, retrospective chart review was conducted to examine admission data 6 months and 12 months prior to the current hospitalization. Feasibility was measured by the number of HF patients recruited and the number who completed the transition clinic intervention in 4 weeks and MLHFQ instrument.

Feasibility/treatment fidelity

The fidelity of this intervention was examined following the best practice recommendations from the Behavior Change Consortium.[41] The concept of fidelity refers to the consistency with

Continued

RESEARCH EXAMPLE 12.1—cont'd

which the investigators applied the intervention to all patients. Several treatment fidelity strategies to monitor and enhance behavioral interventions were used in this study. The overall design of the treatment plan was the same for all the patients; however, the plan was tailored to meet the individual needs of the patients. Each weekly clinic visit consisted of all patients receiving expert consultations by the nurse practitioner, pharmacist and the clinic nurse (See Fig. 1). Moreover, clinical notes/dictations were completed by the nurse practitioner and pharmacist for each patient encounter. To ensure equivalency the same level of information and content was used for every patient.[41] The nurse practitioner and pharmacist relied on an evidenced-based algorithm recommended by the American Heart Association and the Heart Failure Society of America to guide them in making treatment recommendations for each patient. This helped to ensure standardized care while allowing for each patients individual differences, thereby facilitating individualized patient care planning.

Standardized training was important in maintaining treatment fidelity. All study providers attended an in-service training to review research materials including the Minnesota Living with Heart Failure Questionnaire (MLHFQ) measure each study participant completed. Moreover, the providers had a background in cardiology and used a standardized algorithm for HF management, including managing medications. Drift in provider skills was minimized by weekly meetings to update providers.

Even though the 4-week program was standardized, each person was treated as an individual with his or her own unique needs. For example, the medication titrations conducted at each visit were different per patient. When a medication dose was adjusted the patient was asked to verbalize understanding of the medication adjustments and the reason for the change. Furthermore, ensuring participant ability to perform behavioral skills was achieved by the participants verbally confirming competence. Treatment fidelity strategies for monitoring and improving the receipt of treatment included ensuring participant comprehension as demonstrated by the patient's weekly homework of daily weight and blood pressure logs, verbalization of disease process and symptoms, and articulation of understanding of treatment regimen.

Finally, strategies for monitoring and improving enactment of treatment skills were achieved by the use of self-report regarding goal achievement and completion of the MLHFQ during week 1 and week 4 of the intervention. Printed materials on living with HF and low sodium recipes as well as an optional monthly support group were available for patients and families in addition to the 4-week intervention. Additionally, patients were encouraged to call the providers with questions anytime.

Analysis

Statistical analysis was performed using Statistical Package for Social Sciences (SPSS), Windows Version, SPSS Inc. Los Angeles, USA. A comparison between the pre- and post-test measure of the MLHFQ and subscales were completed using *t*-tests analysis. Descriptive statistics were used to assess for readmissions.

Results

A total of 50 patients who met eligibility were admitted during the study period; all individuals approached consented to participate (see Table 1 for demographic data). However, only 36 persons (72%) completed the 4-week program, including the pre- and post-test, attendance at all clinic visits, and maintaining a log of daily weights and blood pressure. Attrition was related to voluntary withdrawal ($n = 1$ or 2%) and 13 participants not completing the post-test. Of these 13 people, 7 missed or rescheduled their clinic appointment outside of the 4-week timeframe and 6 patients did not complete the exit questionnaire. The high attrition rate in large part was due to the patient's need for an intervention lasting longer than 4 weeks. The final sample consisted of 21 women and 15 men. The mean age of the sample was 70.1 years (*SD* 11.7). Six persons (16.7%) were African-American and 30 (83.3%) were Caucasian. Hospital readmissions 6 months prior to the intervention had a mean of 1.83 (*SD* 1.16). Compared to the mean 12 months prior to the intervention of .5 (*SD* 1.16). Systolic and diastolic HF ejection fractions for the sample are noted in Table 1. Six percent had both systolic and diastolic HF. The overall numbers of readmissions were greater 6 months prior to the intervention when compared to 12 months prior.

The mean baseline QOL score on the MLHFQ was 55.03 ($SD = 26.07$) and the post-test score was 37.28 ($SD = 26.51$). This decrease in the mean MLHFQ indicated a significant improvement in overall quality of life, ($t = 4.50$, $p < .05$). There was a significant improvement in physical symptoms over time ($t = 5.80$, $p < .001$). The participants also experienced less emotional distress from baseline to the end of the program ($t = 3.66$, $p < .001$) (See Table 2). Although emotional distress was statistically significant, on close inspection of the data, 28% of the participants experienced increased emotional distress, and another 16% had no change following completion of the intervention. Men reported greater improvement in physical symptoms ($t = 2.35$, $p = .03$) and less emotional distress ($t = 2.22$, $p = .03$) when compared to women. There were no differences based on age ($t = 1.56$, $p = .15$) and race ($t = .94$, $p = .35$).

Only 2 participants were readmitted within 30 days of hospital discharge. Neither of these readmissions was related to HF. One

Table 1
Demographic data.

Demographic	Frequency	Percent
Gender		
Male	15	42%
Female	21	58%
Race		
Caucasian	30	83%
African American	6	17%
Marital status		
Single	3	8%
Married	18	50%
Divorce	2	6%[a]
Separated	1	3%[a]
Widowed	12	33%
Systolic heart failure (Reduced ejection fraction) HFrEF		
Moderate 30–40%	7	19%
Moderate Severe 20–30%	3	8%
Severe < 20	4	11%
Diastolic heart failure (Preserved ejection fraction) HFpEF		
Normal 55–65%	15	42%[a]
Mild 40–55%	7	19%

[a] The denotes that this number is a result of rounding.

Table 2
Quality of life status as Assessed by the disease specific questionnaire "The Minnesota Living with Heart Failure Questionnaire" (MLHFQ) with scores ranging from 0 to 105. Baseline values and changes between baseline and week 4 of the transition-to-care clinic ($N = 36$).

	Baseline mean (*SD*)	Week 4 follow-up mean (*SD*)	*t* (df), *p*
Total minnesota living with heart failure questionnaire score	55.03 (26.07)	37.28 (26.51)	4.50 (35), $p < .05$
Physical dimension	25.33 (12.01)	16.17 (11.84)	5.80 (35), $p < .0001$
Emotional dimension	23.35 (26.35)	8.61 (7.0)	3.66 (35), $p < .0001$

person was admitted as a result of metabolic encephalopathy and the other was readmitted because of complete heart block which transitioned into the patient needing a pacemaker.

Discussion

This study examined quality of life and readmission in persons with HF who participated in a multidisciplinary 4-week transition-to-care program following hospitalization. Findings from this study suggest that successful completion of a transitional care program may enhance quality of life and help decrease hospital readmissions for HF patients. These findings are consistent with other research.[6,42] Dunderdale and colleagues[42] reported that the management of chronic HF led to improved life expectancy, functioning, and health-related quality of life. The current study findings are also consistent with Stamp et al's[6] integrative review which reported improvement in a HF patient's quality of life with transitions of care programs.

Transitional care programs ensure coordination and continuity of care as well as meeting specific needs of the HF patient while transitioning from hospital to home.[23] Patients have the opportunity to learn and practice self-management of their care under close supervision and begin a new way of conducting daily activities. It has been observed that patients with increased understanding about their disease processes and medication regimen, and with adequate social support, generally sustain lifestyle changes, and have an enhanced sense of worth and wellbeing and improved quality of life.[3,20,25,33] In this study some of the patients needed the intervention longer than the 4-week period; therefore, they scheduled outside of the study parameters. One could argue that the root cause of the scheduling was related to problems within the clinic structure which could then be viewed as lack of fidelity to the intervention versus person issues with the patient. However, as a new clinic patients had access to available appointments daily. While treatment fidelity was shown in this study by enactment of the HF patients, fidelity can be increased by providing more consistent follow-up once the patient begins the transitional care program, assessing health literacy upon entry into the program, and checking to ensure adequate transportation.

Emotions can influence a person's ability to manage their care and symptoms, their recovery, and possibly future illness events. The scores on the quality of life instrument indicated that there was a general decrease in emotional distress for the entire group from entry to completion of the 4-week transition-to-care program, yet 28% of the participants experienced increased emotional distress. HF patients often experience a wide array of emotions including feeling alone, anxious/scared, and or depressed. Prevalence of depression in patients with HF has been reported as ranging from 15 to 36%, which is above the lifetime prevalence of 13% for major depression in the general population.[43–48] Yet, depressive symptoms are often under-diagnosed in HF patients.[47] Depression has been associated with the risk of hospital readmissions in persons with HF at 3 months and at 1 year, with a 1 year mortality rate independent of age, the New York Heart Association classification, baseline ejection fraction, or ischemic origin of HF.[47,48] In addition to a 4-week transition-to-care program for patients with HF, individuals may benefit from continued monthly support groups meetings to ensure adequate emotional support, protocol modification to include a depression screening to identify the patients earlier and in a future study consider ongoing assessment of emotional status.

Further, in addition to their own emotions, HF patients often worry about their long-term prognosis, finances, ability to independently meet their own daily living needs, transportation to future appointments, and burdening their loved ones. Family caregivers also have their own fears, anxieties, and fatigue. As a result, more effective collaboration is needed between family caregivers and healthcare providers to enhance transition-to-care. Family caregivers, with the support of nurse practitioners, can play an integral role in helping to increase quality of life and decrease hospital readmissions by making important contributions to ensure quality care.[49]

This study was limited to short-term follow-up (4 weeks) and lacked a control group, therefore we were unable to examine longer-term outcomes or definitively say that the positive changes were caused by the intervention. Also, our sample consisted of a small group from one geographic location, and the results cannot be generalized to other geographic areas. The small sample size of this feasibility study may have prevented detection of longitudinal changes and associations with interactive effects. Thus, the results of this study have to be interpreted with caution. Cost data are important facts related to the feasibility of this intervention. Though not addressed in this study, the cost of the clinician's time should be considered for a larger study. Future research is suggested to address both cost of care, down-stream revenue from referrals to the laboratory and other testing as well as the impact on expensive resources such as hospitalizations, emergency room visits. It is noted in this study that some patients had multiple hospitalizations prior to the project. It is a strength of this study that there were only 2 all cause readmissions within 30 days non HF related. Despite its limitations this feasibility study adds to an emerging body of literature on transitional care programs for HF patients.

Conclusions

Findings from this study provide support for the feasibility of a 4-week multidisciplinary, transition-to-care program for HF patients in enhancing quality of life and decreasing 30-day readmissions. Future research is needed using a larger sample size, a randomized design and controlling for the effect of comorbidities and chronic disease like diabetes and COPD, functional class, length of time with HF (e.g., first episode vs. one of many), and depression on study outcomes. Additional research is needed to examine the impact of the intervention on other important outcomes such as adherence to exercise programs, diet and other self-management behaviors. Future studies should include strategies for retention including having providers initiates a 24 h follow-up phone call after each visit. Lastly, the research pertaining to cost information and data were beyond the scope of this study and should be included and explored in a larger study. Despite these limitations, findings from this study support the feasibility of a multidisciplinary 4-week transition-to-care program following hospitalization for HF patients and the potential impact that this type of program can have on quality of life and hospital readmissions. This team based, patient specific and collaborative approach is an effective practice based strategy to improve HF outcomes.

Acknowledgements

This publication was supported by the University of Maryland Online Dissemination and Implementation Institute funded by the University of Maryland and the John A. Hartford Foundation. We would like to thank the subjects who participated in this study. Special thanks to Debbie Fenner, Amanda Thompson, Meghan Emig, Laura Aggabao, Cheryl Boger, Bryan Robinette and Kelli Lanier of Sanger Heart and Vascular Institute for their contributions to this project. Special thanks to Josephine A. Appiah for her assistance with data analysis.

Continued

RESEARCH EXAMPLE 12.1—cont'd

84 C.D. Whitaker-Brown et al. / Heart & Lung 46 (2017) 79–84

References

1. Centers for Disease Control. *Hospitalization for Congestive Heart Failure: United States, 2000–2010*. Available at: http://www.cdc.gov/nchs/data/databriefs/db108; 2011. Accessed 15 October 2012.
2. Centers for Disease Control. Heart Failure Fact Sheet. Available at: http://www.cdc.gov/dhdsp/data_statistics/fact_sheets/fs_heart_failure.htm; Accessed 10 July 2016.
3. Grady KL, Dracup K, Kennedy G, et al. Team management of patients with heart failure: A statement for healthcare professionals from the Cardiovascular Nursing Council of the American Heart Association. *Circulation*. 2000;102(19):2443–2456.
4. American Heart Association. *Target: HF Taking the Failure Out of Heart Failure*. Available at: http://www.heart.org/HEARTORG/HealthcareResearch/GetWithTheGuidelinesHFStrokeResus/Get-With-The-Guidelines—-HFStroke_UCM_001099_SubHomePage.jsp; 2012. Accessed 06 September 2012.
5. Roger VL, Go AS, Lloyd-Jones DM, et al. Heart disease and stroke statistics—2012 update: a report from the American Heart Association. *Circulation*. 2012;125(1):e2–e220.
6. Stamp KD, Machado MA, Allen NA. Transitional care programs improve outcomes for heart failure patients. *J Cardiovasc Nurs*. 2014;29(2):140–154.
7. Agency for Healthcare Research and Quality. *The National Hospital Bill: The Most Expensive Conditions by Payer, 2008*, http://www.hcup-us.ahrq.gov/reports/statbriefs/sb107.pdf; 2011. Accessed 16 March 2012.
8. Heart Failure Society of America. *The 2010 Heart Failure Society of America Comprehensive Heart Failure Practice Guideline*, http://www.hfsa.org/heart-failure-guidelines-2; 2011. Accessed 16 March 2012.
9. Hines P, Yu K, Randall M. Preventing heart failure readmissions: is your organization prepared. *Nurs Econ*. 2010;28(2):74–86.
10. Kociol RD, Peterson ED, Hammill BG, et al. National survey of hospital strategies to reduce heart failure readmissions: findings from the get with the guidelines-heart failure registry. *Circulation*. 2012;5:680–687.
11. Hernandez AF, Greiner MA, Fonarow GC, et al. Relationship between early physician follow-up and 30-day readmission among Medicare beneficiaries hospitalized for heart failure. *JAMA*. 2010;303(17):1716–1722.
12. Bueno H, Ross JS, Wang Y, et al. Trends in length of stay and short-term outcomes among Medicare patients hospitalized for heart failure, 1993–2006. *JAMA*. 2010;303:2141–2147.
13. Jencks SF, Williams MV, Coleman EA. Rehospitalizations among patients in the Medicare fee-for-service program. *N Engl J Med*. 2009;360:1418–1428.
14. National Heart Lung and Blood Institute. What is heart failure? Available at: http://www.nhlbi.nih.gov/health/health-topics/topics/hf/; Accessed 30 March 2014.
15. Heidenreich PA, Trogdon JG, Khavjou OA, et al. Forecasting the future of cardiovascular disease in the United States: a policy statement from the American Heart Association. *Circulation*. 2011;123(8):933–944.
16. Lindenfeld J, Albert NM, Boehmer JP, et al. HFSA 2010 comprehensive heart failure practice guideline. *J Card Fail*. 2010;16(6):e1–e194.
17. Crowder BF. Improved symptom management through enrollment in an outpatient congestive heart failure clinic. *Medsurg Nurs*. 2006;15(1):27–35.
18. Bhalla R, Kalkut G. Could Medicare readmission policy ex-acerbate health care system inequity? *Ann Intern Med*. 2010;152(2):114–117.
19. Kocher RP, Adashi EY. Hospital readmissions and the Affordable Care Act: paying for coordinated quality care. *JAMA*. 2011;306(16):1794–1795.
20. Naylor MD, Aiken LH, Kurtzman ET, et al. The care span: the importance of transitional care in achieving health reform. *Health Aff*. 2011;30(4):746–754.
21. Wijeysundera HC, Trubiani G, Wang X, et al. A population-based study to evaluate the effectiveness of multidisciplinary heart failure clinics and identify important service components. *Circ Heart Fail*. 2013;6(1):68–75.
22. Corbett C, Setter S, Daratha K, et al. Nurse identified hospital to home medication discrepancies: implications for improving transitional care. *Geriatr Nurs*. 2010;31(3):188–196.
23. Coleman EA, Boult C. American geriatrics society health care systems: Improving the quality of transitional care for persons with complex care needs. *J Am Geriatr Soc*. 2003;51(4):556–557.
24. Colandrea M, Murphy-Gustavson J. Patient care heart failure model: The hospitalization to home plan of care. *Home Healthc Nurse*. 2012;30(6):337–344.
25. Naylor MD, Brooten DA, Campbell RL, et al. Transitional care of older adults hospitalized with heart failure: A randomized, controlled trial. *J Am Geriatr Soc*. 2004;52(5):675–684.
26. Harrison MB, Browne GB, Roberts J, et al. Quality of life of individuals with heart failure: A randomized trial of the effectiveness of two models of hospital-to-home transition. *Med Care*. 2002;40(4):271–282.
27. Stewart S, Marley JE, Horowitz JD. Effects of a multidisciplinary, home-based intervention on unplanned readmissions and survival among patients with chronic congestive heart failure: a randomized controlled study. *Lancet*. 1999;354(9184):1077–1083.
28. Daley C. A hybrid transitional care program. *Crit Pathw Cardiol*. 2010;9(4):231–234.
29. Raghu KV, Srinivas V, Kishore Babu AV, Monhanta GP, Uma Rani R. A study on quality of life in patients with heart failure. *Ind J Pharm Pract*. 2010;3(3):33–39.
30. Nucifora G, Albanese MC, De Biaggio P, et al. Lack of improvement of clinical outcomes by a low-cost, hospital-based heart failure management programme. *J Cardiovasc Med*. 2006;7(8):614–622.
31. Naylor MD, Bowles KH, McCauley KM, et al. High-value transitional care: translation of research into practice. *J Eval Clin Pract*. 2013;19:727–733.
32. American College of Physicians. What practices need to know about transition care management codes. Available at: https://www.acponline.org/running_practice/payment_coding/coding/tcm_codes.htm; Accessed on 06 September 2015.
33. Foust J, Naylor M, Bixby B, et al. Medication problems occurring at hospital discharge among older adults with heart failure. *Res Gerontol Nurs*. 2012;5(1):25–33. 2012.
34. Calvert MJ, Freemantle N, Cleland JG. The impact of chronic heart failure on health-related quality of life data acquired in the baseline phase of the CARE-HF study. *Eur J Heart Fail*. 2005;7(2):243–251.
35. de Leon CF, Grady KL, Eaton C, et al. Quality of life in a diverse population of patients with heart failure: baseline findings from the Heart Failure Adherence and Retention Trial (HART). *J Cardiopulm Rehabil*. 2009;29(3):171–178.
36. Juenger J, Schellberg D, Kraemer S, et al. Health related quality of life in patients with congestive heart failure: comparison with other chronic diseases and relation to functional variables. *Heart*. 2002;87(3):235–241.
37. Seto E, Leonard KJ, Cafazzo JA, et al. Self-care and quality of life of heart failure patients at a multidisciplinary heart function clinic. *J Cardiovasc Nurs*. 2011;26(5):377–385.
38. National Collaborating Centre for Methods and Tools (2011). *Stetler Model of Evidence-based Practice*. Hamilton, ON: McMaster University. Retrieved from, http://www.nccmt.ca/resources/search/83; Updated 18 March, 2011. Accessed on 06 September 2015.
39. Minnesota Living with Heart Failure Questionnaire. Available at: http://www.license.umn.edu/Products/Minnesota-Living-With-Heart-Failure- Questionnaire__Z94019.aspx; Accessed on 15 April 2012.
40. Rector TS, Kubo SH, Cohn JN. Patients' self-assessment of their congestive heart failure-part 2: content, reliability and validity of a new measure, the Minnesota living with heart failure questionnaire. *Heart Fail*; 1987:3198–3208.
41. Bellg AJ, Borrelli B, Resnick B, et al. Enhancing treatment fidelity in health behavior change studies: best practices and recommendations from the behavior change consortium. *Health Psychol*. 2004;23(5):452–456.
42. Dunderdale K, Thompson DR, Miles JN, et al. Quality-of-life measurement in chronic heart failure: do we take account of the patient perspective? *Eur J Heart Fail*. 2005;7(4):572–582. http://dx.doi.org/10.1016/j.ejheart.2004.06.006 [Review].
43. Maricle RA, Hosenpud JD, Norman DJ, et al. Depression in patients being evaluated for heart transplantation. *Gen Hosp Psychiatry*. 1989;11(6):418–424.
44. Freedland KE, Carney RM, Rich MW, et al. Depression in elderly patients with congestive heart failure. *J Geriatr Psychiatry*. 1991;24(1):59–71.
45. Koenig HG. Depression in hospitalized older patients with congestive heart failure. *Gen Hosp Psychiatry*. 1998;20(1):29–43.
46. Havranek EP, Ware MG, Lowes BD. Prevalence of depression in congestive heart failure. *Am J Cardiol*. 1999;84(3):348–350.
47. Scherer M, Himmel W, Stanske B, et al. Psychological distress in primary care patients with heart failure: a longitudinal study. *Br J Gen Pract*. 2007;57:801–807.
48. Jiang W, Alexander J, Christopher E, et al. Relationship of depression to increased risk of mortality and rehospitalization in patients with congestive heart failure. *Arch Intern Med*. 2001;161(15):1849–1856.
49. Coleman EA, Williams MV. Executing high quality care transitions: a call to do it right. *J Hosp Med*. 2007;2(5):287–290.

Critical Appraisal

Step 1: Identifying the Steps of the Research Process in the Study; and Step 2: Determining Study Strengths and Weaknesses

1. **Writing Quality:** Overall, the writing quality was adequate. Improvements in writing flow and use of greater detail in some sections would promote clarity. Additionally, key terms such as quality of life should have been clearly defined early in the article.
2. **Title:** The title, "Improving quality of life and decreasing readmissions in heart failure [HF] patients in a multidisciplinary transition-to-care clinic" identified the patient population and the key variables, quality of life and readmissions. From the title, the multidisciplinary transition-to-care clinic could be confused as the setting instead of the study intervention. The type of study conducted was not mentioned in the title but you might infer that this was a quasi-experimental study.
3. **Authors:** Dr. Whitaker-Brown is a family nurse practitioner with a doctorate of nurse practice (DNP) degree who has both clinical and research experience in the area of heart failure (HF) (University of North Carolina at Charlotte, 2017). Dr. Woods and Dr. Cornelius, two of the coauthors, are PhD-prepared nurses with university-based faculty positions. Whitaker-Brown and colleagues (2017) identified their funding sources in the acknowledgments section but did not explicitly state if they had any conflicts of interest related to the study.
4. **Abstract:** The clearly written study abstract included the study problem, purpose, design, sample size, significant results, and conclusions.
5. **Research Problem:** From the literature discussed, the research problem could be inferred as: published studies have not examined "the feasibility and impact of a 4-week transition-to-care program on quality of life in patients with HF" (Whitaker-Brown et al., 2017, p. 80). The researchers provided evidence that the problem was significant to nursing by discussing the burden of HF and the issues of transition to home following hospitalization, including the risk of readmission.
6. **Purpose:** The researchers clearly stated the purpose in the abstract objectives and at the end of the literature review. "The purpose of this study was to examine the feasibility and effects of a 4-week transition-to-care program on quality of life in patients with HF" (Whitaker-Brown et al., 2017, p. 80). The focus of the study was narrowed and clarified by the purpose (Creswell, 2014; O'Mathúna & Fineout-Overholt, 2015). The purpose was supported by the literature review and logically linked to the research design.
7. **Literature Review:** A minimal review of literature was presented in the introduction section of the research report. Most of the references cited by Whitaker-Brown and colleagues (2017) were peer-reviewed, primary sources. Currency of cited sources was a weakness of the literature review. The researchers cited four references with accessed dates but not dates for the actual source, so they could not be assessed for currency. Of the 45 remaining sources, only 8 (18%) were published in the 5 years before publication of this study, and 28 (62%) were published in the previous 10 years. Some of the older sources were for the measurement methods, intervention fidelity, and pathology of HF. The sources cited were appropriate for the study variables and were primarily from the disciplines of medicine and nursing. The researchers described literature on the burden of HF, which supports the intervention and provides a basis for conducting this study. A final summary of what was known and not known about the problem studied would have added clarity to the literature review (Gray et al., 2017).
8. **Framework or Theoretical Perspective:** Whitaker-Brown and colleagues (2017) did not explicitly state the framework used for their study. The Transition to Care Model was the framework that guided the development of the intervention. A detailed diagram of the model, as applied to this patient population, was provided in Figure 1 (in the Whitaker-Brown and colleagues [2017] article). The researchers appeared to use a modified version of the Transition to Care Model to guide their study. A clearer identification of the study's framework would have allowed for critical appraisal of the theory's appropriateness for use with the study.

Continued

RESEARCH EXAMPLE 12.1—cont'd

9. **Research Objectives, Questions, or Hypotheses:** The researchers stated the following hypothesis to direct their study: "we anticipate that an intensive, individualized, time-limited intervention has the potential to improve quality of life in patients with HF" (Whitaker-Brown et al., 2017). A quasi-experimental study to test the effectiveness of an intervention should be guided by a hypothesis (Shadish, Cook, & Campbell, 2002). However, this hypothesis was not clearly linked to the study framework (Smith & Liehr, 2014).
10. **Variables:** Whitaker-Brown and colleagues (2017) presented demographic, independent, and dependent variables. The demographic variables of age, gender, race, marital status, and the incidence of systolic and diastolic HF were described in Table 12.3 and in the results section.
    The independent variable, transition-to-care intervention was conceptually defined by The Heart Success Transition Model provided in Figure 1 of their study (Whitaker-Brown et al., 2017, p.81). The operational definition of the independent variable was a "4-week, multidisciplinary, transitional program… specifically designed to provide weekly education and support to HF patients" (Whitaker-Brown et al., 2017, p. 80).
    Health-related quality of life (QOL) is the main dependent variable, but Whitaker-Brown and colleagues (2017) did not state the conceptual definition for this variable. The phrase *quality of life* was used in the literature review but was not clearly defined. The operational definition or measurement of QOL was clearly described: "Health-related quality of life (QOL) was assessed using the Minnesota Living with Heart Failure Questionnaire (MLHFQ), a 21- item, 6-point Likert scale that reflected the most frequent and important ways HF affects patient's lives" (Whitaker-Brown et al., 2017, p. 81). The operational definitions were linked to the study methodology.
11. **Research Design:** The research design was clearly identified as "a prospective one group pre- and post-test design" (Whitaker-Brown et al., 2017, p. 80). In this type of quasi-experimental design, the subjects serve as their own control. This is a weak design because there was only one group and no separate comparison group to determine if the treatment was effective or if the change from pretest to posttest was caused by extraneous variables (Gray et al., 2017; Shadish et al., 2002).
    The 4-week transition-to-care intervention was appropriate for examining the study purpose and testing the causal hypothesis. The complex intervention was closely representative of clinical practice (see Figure 1 of the Whitaker-Brown and colleagues study [2017]). The researchers clearly defined the transitional program to support patients with HF. However, they needed to provide more detail about how the treatment was implemented, including transparency on the number of providers and characteristics of the providers (Gray et al., 2017).
    Whitaker-Brown and colleagues (2017, p. 81) implemented a protocol to ensure intervention fidelity and provided a detailed description of the study procedures. "Standardized training was important in maintaining treatment fidelity… Moreover, the providers had a background in cardiology and used a standardized algorithm for HF management, including managing medications. Drift in provider skills was minimized by weekly meetings to update providers" (Whitaker-Brown et al., 2017, p. 82). Because the treatment was implemented by more than one person, the training to promote consistency in the administration of treatment needed to be addressed (Eymard & Altmiller, 2016). As described previously, characteristics of the providers were not given, and variations in outcome could have been related to having a provider with 20 years of experience versus a provider with 1 year of experience or a provider with measurable competency in a specific area versus one without that competency.
    The researchers monitored intervention consistency, as indicated by the following quote: "Treatment fidelity strategies for monitoring and improving the receipt of treatment included ensuring patient comprehension as demonstrated by the patient's weekly homework of daily weight and blood pressure logs,

verbalization of disease process and symptoms, and articulation of understanding of treatment regimen" (Whitaker-Brown et al., 2017, p. 82). Consistency is particularly important with a complex intervention because any deviation in the treatment plan or care interaction has the potential to affect the study outcomes (Eymard & Altmiller, 2016; Moorhead et al., 2013).

This study had only one group of 50 participants who served as their own control (Gray et al., 2017). This means that the participants completed the MLHFQ scale as the pretest and then participated in the transition-to-care intervention for 4 weeks, followed by the posttest with the MLHFQ scale. Thus the pretest was considered the control and the posttest was conducted to determine the effect of the treatment. The pretest scores were compared with the posttest scores to determine the effect of the intervention.

This study had many design strengths, such as the quality of the intervention development and implementation, reliability of the MLHFQ, and adequate sample size. However, threats to design validity were also noted, such as lack of a comparison group, no random sample or assignment to groups, use of only one measurement method for the health-related QOL, and high sample attrition. However, this pilot study provided information that could be used to strengthen the design and feasibility of future studies.

12. **Sample:** A nonprobability sample of convenience "was recruited from a major Southern Healthcare System" (Whitaker-Brown et al., 2017, p. 80). Greater potential for sampling error occurs with a nonprobability sample versus a random sample. Sample "inclusion criteria were 45 years of age and older, male or female, not pregnant, and with a primary diagnosis of HF" (Whitaker-Brown et al., 2017, p.80). The following were excluded from the study; "44 years of age and younger, pregnant and a primary diagnosis other than HF" (Whitaker-Brown et al., 2017, p. 80). The researchers provided appropriate sample inclusion criteria, but the exclusion criteria repeated the inclusion criteria and did not limit the potential effects of extraneous variables nor improve the representativeness of the sample (Aberson, 2010).

    The sample size was small for this study (n = 50), but was appropriate for a pilot study. The study had a high attrition rate (28%), with 14 subjects dropping out of the study before the 4 weeks of the treatment were completed. Only 36 (72%) of the participants completed the study. The researchers provided a brief rationale for why the subjects did not complete the study but did not explore the characteristics of those who completed the intervention versus those that did not. Examination of such characteristics through exit interviews might have assisted the researchers in making the intervention more acceptable to this target population in future research.

    No power analysis to determine an adequate sample size for the study was mentioned (Aberson, 2010). However, the study results were significant, indicating that the sample was adequately powered, and no type II error occurred (Gray et al., 2017).

    The target population was determined by the sample inclusion criteria, and the accessible population was evident from the discussion of the study setting. Whitaker-Brown and colleagues (2017) provided minimal demographic information in Table 12.3, which included gender, race, marital status, and type of HF of the study participants. A fairly equal number of males and females participated in the study, but the sample lacked racial and ethnic diversity because 83% of the subjects were white.

    Whitaker-Brown and colleagues (2017, p. 81) noted that "informed consent was obtained by the principal investigator" but the process of informed consent was not described.

13. **Setting:** The setting was a multidisciplinary outpatient transition clinic for patients with HF, which was appropriate for the study. The sample was recruited from a major Southern Healthcare System located in Charlotte, North Carolina.

Continued

RESEARCH EXAMPLE 12.1—cont'd

14. **Measurement:**

TABLE 12.3 Measurement Strategies

Name of Measurement Method (author)	Type of Measurement Method	Level of Measurement	Reliability or Precision	Validity or Accuracy
Minnesota Living with Heart Failure Questionnaire (MLHFQ) (Dr. Thomas Rector)	Likert scale	Interval	"Internal consistency of the MLHFQ has been demonstrated in research with chronically ill persons with a Cronbach's alpha of .92, and test-retest/ reproducibility of $r = .87$. In this study, the Cronbach alpha for the overall MLHFQ, physical symptoms dimension, and emotional distress dimension were .92, .96, and .93, respectively." (Whitaker-Brown et al., 2017, p. 81).	No evidence of validity for the MLHFQ was provided. However, Kelkar et al. (2016) concluded that MLHFQ had evidence of content and construct validity. "The 2 instruments that best fit all of the evaluation criteria and meet the most symptom endpoints are the KCCQ and MLHFQ. These instruments are not only the most commonly used, but they also have been highly rated in systematic reviews" (Kelkar et al., 2016, p.172).

KCCQ, Kansas City Cardiomyopathy Questionnaire.

This table focuses on the dependent variable health-related QOL. The MLHFQ, used to measure the dependent variable health-related QOL, was clearly described and appropriate. The MLHFQ is considered a strong measurement strategy for health-related QOL and has been used in many other studies over the years (see Table 12.3; Kelkar et al., 2016). The scoring for the MLHFQ was clearly described, and scores could range from 0 to 105. They also indicated the meaning for the different scores, with "lower scores indicating improved quality of life" (Whitaker-Brown et al., 2017, p.81). Techniques for MLHFQ completion were not provided. The Cronbach alphas were strong and supported the internal consistency reliability of the MLHFQ in this study (Waltz et al., 2017).

15. **Data Collection:** Overall, data collection could have been described in greater detail. Whitaker-Brown and colleagues (2017) did not indicate specifically who collected the data and how many data collectors were involved. The information provided suggested that the same providers who delivered the intervention

might have also collected the data, which could introduce bias. Because more than one person collected data, the reliability or consistency of the data collection process needed to be addressed (Gray et al., 2017; Eymard & Altmiller, 2016). Training on the MLHFQ was mentioned, but limited information was provided about that process. In addition, specific techniques for data collection standardization were not provided.

Data collection appeared to be ethical. The study was approved by the institutional review board (IRB) of the clinical agency, and "informed consent was obtained by the principal investigator" (Whitaker-Brown et al., 2017, pp. 80–81). IRB approval needed to occur before the start of the study, and the timing of the IRB approval was not specific. Additional information on safeguards of human subjects during data collection would have been useful. However, the researchers did not report any adverse events during data collection.

16. **Data Analyses:** The statistical techniques conducted to analyze data from the MLHFQ scores were clearly identified and appropriate (Table 12.4). The Statistical Package for the Social Sciences, Windows version, was used to perform the statistical analyses. The data analyses addressed the research purpose and hypothesis. The research causal hypothesis was supported by the *t*-test results, indicating that the null hypothesis was rejected (Grove & Cipher, 2017). The analysis techniques (descriptive and inferential) were appropriate for the level of measurement of the variables (Grove & Cipher, 2017; Plichta & Kelvin, 2013). Only the 36 participants who completed the study were included in the analyses. Whitaker-Brown and colleagues (2017) did not explicitly state the level of significance, but it is assumed to be $\alpha \leq 0.05$ because the reported $p \leq .05$ and $p \leq .0001$ were reported as significant. The results of the total scores, physical dimension, and emotional dimension of the MLHFQ at the baseline and 4-week follow-up were clearly and concisely presented in Table 12.4 and the study narrative.

TABLE 12.4 Statistical Analyses and Results

Purpose of Analysis	Analysis Technique	Statistic	Result	Probability
Description of participants' age	Mean	$\bar{X}$	70.1	
Standard deviation (*SD*) of participants' age	*SD*	*SD*	11.7	
Hospital admissions 6 months before study	Mean	$\bar{X}$	1.83	
SD of hospital admissions 6 months before study	*SD*	*SD*	1.16	
Total Minnesota Living with Heart Failure (MLHFQ) score	Baseline (pretest) mean	$\bar{X}$	55.03	
	Week 4 follow-up (posttest) mean	$\bar{X}$	37.28	
MLHFQ scores	Baseline (pretest) *SD*	*SD*	26.07	
	Week 4 follow-up (posttest) *SD*	*SD*	26.51	
Difference between pretest and posttest scores on the MLHFQ	Dependent or paired *t*-test	*t*	4.50	$p \leq .05$

Continued

RESEARCH EXAMPLE 12.1—cont'd

TABLE 12.4 Statistical Analyses and Results—cont'd

Purpose of Analysis	Analysis Technique	Statistic	Result	Probability
MLHFQ: Physical dimension	Baseline (pretest) mean	$\bar{X}$	25.33	
	Week 4 follow-up (posttest) mean	$\bar{X}$	16.17	
	Baseline (pretest) *SD*	*SD*	12.01	
	Week 4 follow-up (posttest) *SD*	*SD*	11.84	
	Dependent or paired *t*-test	*t*	5.80	$p \leq .0001$
MLHFQ: Emotional dimension	Baseline (pretest) mean	$\bar{X}$	23.35	
	Week 4 follow-up (posttest) mean	$\bar{X}$	8.61	
	Baseline (pretest) *SD*	*SD*	26.35	
	Week 4 follow-up (posttest) *SD*	*SD*	7.0	
	Dependent or paired *t*-test	*t*	3.66	$p \leq .0001$

Step 3: Evaluating the Credibility and Meaning of the Study Findings.

17. **Interpretation of Findings:** The findings were as expected, and the statistical and clinical significance of the findings were clearly addressed (Grove & Cipher, 2017; Hoare & Hoe, 2013). The findings were consistent with the study results and with previous research. The study would have been strengthened if the findings had been linked to the heart success transition model (see Figure 1of the Whitaker-Brown and colleagues study [2017]). The researchers identified the study limitations and provided specific and relevant ideas for future studies to overcome the limitations of this study. A randomized clinical trial design was recommended, which would have greatly strengthened the quality of the study and credibility of the findings (Mittlbock, 2008). The researchers did not make recommendations for nursing practice but focused on the need for additional research before making changes in practice.
18. **Limitations:** Whitaker-Brown and colleagues (2017, p. 83) identified the following limitations in their study:

    This study was limited to short-term follow-up (4 weeks) and lacked a control group; therefore we were unable to examine longer-term outcomes or definitively say that the positive changes were caused by the intervention. Also our sample consisted of a small group from one geographic location, and the results cannot be generalized to other geographic areas.

    The high attrition rate of this study was also a limitation that might have altered the study findings and may indicate issues of intervention acceptability in the target population.
19. **Conclusions:** In summary, "Findings from this study provide support for the feasibility of a 4-week multidisciplinary, transition-to-care program for HF patients in enhancing quality of life and decreasing 30-day readmissions" (Whitaker-Brown et al., 2017, p.83). The conclusions fit the study findings and were consistent with previous research. Whitaker-Brown and colleagues (2017, p. 83) noted appropriately that "our sample consisted of a small group from one geographic location, and the results cannot be generalized to other geographic areas... Thus, the results of this study have to be interpreted with caution."

20. **Nursing Implications:** Whitaker-Brown and associates (2017, p. 83) did not include a section on nursing implications but linked the results to patient care in the discussion and conclusions sections: "Despite these limitations, findings from this study support the feasibility of a multidisciplinary 4-week transition-to-care program following hospitalization for HF patients and the potential impact of this type of program can have on quality of life and hospital readmissions."
21. **Future Research:** Whitaker-Brown and associates (2017) provided detailed suggestions for future research that built on their current study. "Future research is needed using a larger sample size, a randomized design and controlling for the effect of comorbidities and chronic disease like COPD [chronic obstructive pulmonary disease] , functional class, length of time with HF (e.g., first episode vs. one of many), and depression on study outcomes" (Whitaker-Brown et al., 2017, p. 83). The researchers also discussed the importance of addressing confounding variables, retention, and cost in future studies. Great detail was provided in some sections, such as feasibility and treatment fidelity. Other parts of the research report lacked sufficient detail to allow for replication of the study. This study was feasible to conduct in terms of researchers' expertise, availability of study participants, and ethical issues.
22. **Critique Summary:** Whitaker-Brown and associates' (2017) study had several strengths, such as the measurement of QOL with the MLHFQ, model of the treatment intervention, and detailed section on treatment fidelity (Gray et al., 2017; Kelkar et al., 2016). The findings from this study were consistent with those of previous researchers and increased our understanding of the link between transition care in HF patients and QOL. Because of the small sample size and other study limitations, the researchers did not recommend generalizing the findings from the sample to the accessible or target populations. Whitaker-Brown and colleagues (2017) provided excellent detailed directions for future studies. They did not recommend using the findings in practice at this time, but emphasized the importance of this area for further research.

UNDERSTANDING THE QUALITATIVE RESEARCH CRITICAL APPRAISAL PROCESS

Nurses in every phase and field of practice need experience in critically appraising qualitative and quantitative studies. Although qualitative studies require a different approach to critical appraisal than quantitative studies (Sandelowski, 2008), appraisal in both cases has a common purpose—determining the rigor with which the methods were applied and the extent to which the conclusions of the study were trustworthy. Critical appraisal of qualitative studies focuses on how the integrity of the design and methods will affect the credibility and meaningfulness of the findings and their usefulness in clinical practice (Roller & Lavrakas, 2015). Different criteria have been used to appraise qualitative studies critically (Burns, 1989; Clissett, 2008; Cohen & Crabtree, 2008; Morse, 1991; Schoe, Høstrop, Lyngsø, Larsen, & Poulsen, 2011). We include a set of criteria synthesized from these published criteria and have organized them into three broad steps, similar to those used for critical appraisal of quantitative studies. Therefore the **qualitative research critical appraisal process** consists of (1) identifying the components of the qualitative research process in studies; (2) determining study strengths and weaknesses; and (3) evaluating the trustworthiness and meaning of study findings.

Each step includes the questions to be addressed to reflect the philosophical orientation of qualitative research. The three steps are presented together in a single guideline for critical appraisal in Box 12.3. This guideline provides relevant questions for each step. These questions have been selected as a means for stimulating the logical reasoning and analysis necessary for conducting a critical appraisal of a study. An individual with critical appraisal experience frequently performs two or three steps of this process simultaneously.

BOX 12.3 CRITICAL APPRAISAL GUIDELINES

Qualitative Study

Step 1: Identifying the Steps of the Research Process in Studies; and Step 2: Determining Study Strengths and Weaknesses

1. Writing quality
   a. Was the writing style of the report clear and concise with relevant terms defined?
2. Title
   a. What is the title?
   b. Is the title clearly focused, and does it include the focus and population of the study? Does the title indicate the type of study conducted—phenomenology, grounded theory, exploratory-descriptive qualitative, and ethnography (Creswell & Poth, 2018; Powers, 2015)?
3. Authors
   a. Do the authors have credentials such as a PhD degree that qualified them to conduct the study?
   b. Do the authors have previous research or clinical experience that qualified them to conduct the study?
   c. Do any of the authors have a conflict of interest, such as a financial interest related to the study?
4. Abstract
   a. Was the abstract clearly presented?
   b. Does the abstract include purpose, specific qualitative methodology, sample, and key results?
5. Research problem
   a. Is a problem statement provided? If a problem statement is not provided, can you infer the problem or gap in nursing's knowledge from the introduction and literature review?
   b. Is the problem significant to nursing and clinical practice (Cohen & Crabtree, 2008)?
6. Purpose
   a. State the purpose.
   b. Does the purpose narrow and clarify the focus of the study (Creswell, 2014; Fawcett & Garity, 2009)?
7. Literature review
   a. Are most references peer-reviewed primary sources? Do the authors justify references that are not peer-reviewed primary sources?
   b. Are the references current (number and percentage of sources in the last 5 and 10 years)? Are references older than 10 years, measurement or theoretical sources, landmark, seminal, or replication studies?
   c. Is the content directly related to the study concepts? Are the types of sources and disciplines of the source authors appropriate for the study concepts?
   d. Are the studies critically appraised and synthesized (Fawcett & Garity, 2009; Gray et al., 2017; Hart, 2009)? Is a clear concise summary presented of the current empirical and theoretical knowledge in the area of the study, including identifying what is known and not known (Gray et al., 2017)?
8. Philosophical orientation or study framework
   a. Was the philosophical orientation of the qualitative approach identified? Was a primary source for the philosophy cited (Creswell & Poth, 2018; Gray et al., 2017; Munhall, 2012)?
   b. If a framework was used, are its major concepts reflected in the questions asked during data collection and in the findings?
   c. Grounded theory
      i. Did the researcher develop a theoretical description or diagram as part of the study findings (Creswell & Poth, 2018)?
      ii. If a framework was developed from the findings (grounded theory study), is it clearly linked to the study findings?
9. Research objectives (aims) or questions
   a. Are the objectives (aims) or questions identified and clearly presented?
   b. List the provided research objectives (aims) or questions, if identified.
   c. Are the objectives or questions linked to the research purpose?

10. Qualitative approach (see Chapter 3)
    a. Identify the qualitative approach used—phenomenology, grounded theory, ethnography, exploratory-descriptive, or unspecified qualitative approach.
    b. Specific qualitative approach not identified.
        i. What aspects of the method, such as natural settings or coding, indicate that a qualitative approach was used (Creswell & Poth, 2018; Hall & Roussel, 2017; Munhall, 2012)?
        ii. Did the researcher provide a rationale for why a qualitative study was conducted (Creswell, 2014; Gray et al., 2017)?
    c. Did the researchers select a qualitative approach that produced data to meet the objectives or answer the research questions?
11. Sample (see Chapter 9)
    a. Is the sampling plan adequate to address the purpose of the study?
        i. If purposive sampling is used, does the researcher provide a rationale for the sample selection process?
        ii. If network or snowball sampling is used, does the researcher identify the networks used to obtain the sample and provide a rationale for their selection?
        iii. If theoretical sampling is used, does the researcher indicate how participants are selected to promote the generation of a theory?
    b. Are the sampling criteria identified and appropriate for the study?
    c. If potential participants refused to participate, or participants did not complete the study, did the researcher acknowledge these issues as limitations?
    d. Does the researcher discuss the quality of the data provided by the study participants?
    e. Were the participants articulate, well informed, and willing to share information relevant to the study topic?
    f. Did the sampling process produce saturation and verification of data in the area of the study?
    g. Is the sample size adequate based on the scope of the study, nature of the topic, quality of the data, and study design?
    h. How was informed consent obtained?
    i. Was the process used for informed consent appropriate for the study population?
12. Setting
    a. What is the study setting?
    b. Is the setting appropriate for the study purpose?
    c. Did the setting in which data were collected protect the confidentiality and promote the comfort of the participants?
13. Data collection
    a. What data collection methods were used—interviews, focus groups, observation, or other sources?
    b. Interviews
        i. Were multiple interviews with the same person conducted, or were data collected once from each participant?
        ii. Were questions used during the interview or focus group relevant to the study's research objectives or questions (Gray et al., 2017; Maxwell, 2013)?
        iii. Did the interviews last long enough for the researcher to gather robust and thorough descriptions of the participants' perspectives?
    c. Focus group
        i. Were the size, composition, and length of the focus group adequate to promote group interaction and produce robust data?
        ii. Were questions used during the interview or focus group relevant to the study's research objectives or questions (Gray et al., 2017; Maxwell, 2013)?

Continued

BOX 12.3 CRITICAL APPRAISAL GUIDELINES—cont'd

d. Observations
    i. Were observations conducted at times and for long enough periods to collect rich data that allowed for a thorough description of the culture, setting, or process of interest (Creswell & Poth, 2018; Wolf, 2012)?
    ii. Did the researcher make field notes or journal entries (Creswell, 2014; Miles, Huberman, & Saldaña, 2014)?
e. How were data recorded during data collection?
f. Was IRB approval obtained before data collection?
g. Did the researcher identify that participants might become upset during the collection of data? If so, what measures were in place to address the safety and emotional needs of the participants (Cowles, 1988; Maxwell, 2013)?
h. Were the data collection methods ethical?

14. Data analysis
    a. How were the data prepared for analysis?
    b. How were the data analyzed? Did the researcher cite a specific method of analysis and provide a primary source?
    c. Was computer-assisted qualitative data management software used during the analysis?
    d. Were the data analysis processes described thoroughly enough to be able to evaluate the logic of the researcher's decisions and support the rigor of the study?
    e. Which methods were used to increase the trustworthiness of the findings e.g., verification of the accuracy of transcripts, immersion in the data, documentation of an **audit trail** [also known as the record of decisions that were made during data collection and analysis], member checking, independent analysis of a portion of the data by another researcher (Cohen & Crabtree, 2008; Hall & Roussel, 2017; Miles et al., 2014; Murphy & Yielder, 2010)?
    f. Were the measures to increase the trustworthiness of the study adequate to give the reader confidence in the findings (Cohen & Crabtree, 2008; Mackey, 2012; Wolf, 2012)?

Step 3: Evaluating the Credibility and Meaning of Study Findings

15. Interpretation of findings
    a. Describe the researcher's interpretation of findings.
    b. Were the findings linked to quotes or specific observations?
    c. Did the researcher address variations in the findings by relevant sample characteristics?
    d. Are the findings related back to the study framework (if applicable)?
    e. Are the findings consistent with previous research findings (Fawcett & Garity, 2009)?
    f. If the findings were unexpected, what explanations were given for why this may have occurred?
16. Limitations
    a. What study limitations did the researcher identify?
    b. Were there study limitations that the researchers did not acknowledge?
    c. Were the study limitations the result of factors under the researcher's control that could have been prevented, or were the limitations external factors over which the researcher had no control (Powers, 2015)?
17. Conclusions
    a. What conclusions did the researchers identify based on their interpretation of the study findings?
    b. Did the conclusions logically flow out of the findings?
    c. Did the researchers identify other settings or populations to whom the findings might be transferable or applied?
18. Nursing implications
    a. What implications for nursing practice were identified?
    b. Does the study expand nurses' understanding of the phenomenon studied? If so, how could the findings be used in nursing practice, theory and education?
    c. How does this study support future knowledge development?

19. Future research
    a. What suggestions were identified for further study?
    b. Did the recommendations for further studies flow out of the findings?
20. Critical appraisal summary
    a. Review the components of the critique you just conducted. Consider the following to formulate your critical appraisal summary.
        i. Were all relevant components covered with adequate detail and clarity?
        ii. What were the study's greatest strengths and greatest weaknesses?
        iii. Were the rights of study participants protected (Creswell, 2014; Gray et al., 2017)?
        iv. Do you believe the study findings are valid? How much confidence can be placed in the study findings (Powers, 2015; Roller & Lavrakas, 2015)?
        v. The evaluation of a research report should also include a final discussion of the quality of the report. This discussion should include an expert opinion of the study's quality and contribution to nursing knowledge and practice (Melnyk & Fineout-Overholt, 2015; Melnyk et al., 2017; Powers, 2015).

Step 1: Identifying the Components of the Qualitative Research Process in Studies

In a qualitative critical appraisal, just like in a quantitative critique, the first step involves reviewing the abstract, reading the study from beginning to end, and highlighting or underlining the elements of the qualitative study. Rereading the article, you might also want to underline the terms that you do not understand and determine their meaning from the glossary at the end of this text. After reading and comprehending the content of the study, you are ready to write your initial critical appraisal of the study.

To write a critical appraisal, you need to identify each element of the qualitative study and concisely respond to the guidelines and questions in Box 12.3. The first step of the critical appraisal process provides you with an overview of the study. As you read the study report in more depth, identify and describe each of the following aspects of the study.

Step 2: Determining the Strengths and Weaknesses in Studies

At this step, the differences in the critical appraisal processes of quantitative and qualitative studies become more obvious. However, the goal of the critical appraisal remains the same—determining the strengths and weaknesses of the study. Knowledge of the different qualitative approaches and data collection processes is needed to answer the questions during this step. You may want to refer to Chapter 3 and supplement your knowledge with additional sources, such as other texts, reference books, and articles (Creswell & Poth, 2018; Fawcett & Garity, 2009; Gray et al., 2017; Miles et al., 2014; Munhall, 2012; Petty, Thomson, & Stew, 2012; Powers, 2015; Sandelowski & Barroso, 2007). The actual methods of the study being appraised are compared with the expectations of qualitative experts, including the original proponents of different qualitative approaches. Because different qualitative experts agree less on the "rules" for implementing qualitative studies, using the guidelines recommended by a specific expert in the method used by the researchers in the study is important. The areas of consistency are strengths of the study, whereas areas of inconsistency may indicate weaknesses of the study. The person conducting the critical appraisal evaluates all aspects of a qualitative study and makes a judgment about its trustworthiness. **Trustworthiness** is a determination that a qualitative study is rigorous and of high quality. Trustworthiness is the extent to which a qualitative study is dependable, confirmable, credible, and transferable.

A thorough report of a qualitative study should include adequate information so that the reader can assess the report's dependability and confirmability (Murphy & Yielder, 2010). Dependability and confirmability are similar to reliability of quantitative studies. **Dependability** is the documentation of steps taken and decisions made during analysis. Remember from Chapter 3 that the researchers' record of the analysis process is called an *audit trail.* **Confirmability** is the extent to which other researchers can review the audit trail and agree that the authors' conclusions are logical (Miles et al., 2014; Murphy & Yielder, 2010). When a study's findings are appraised to be confirmable and dependable, they have more credibility. **Credibility** is the confidence of the reader about the extent to which the researchers have produced results that reflect the views of the participants; this is similar to validity in the critical appraisal of quantitative studies (Murphy & Yielder, 2010). Petty et al. (2012) have explained that qualitative findings are not generalizable but are **transferable** or applicable in other settings with similar participants.

You need to appraise the rigor of the study methods by looking for information about the carefulness of data collection and thoroughness of the data analysis. The questions asked about each component of the study will focus your attention on the rigor of the methods and the logical links among the study elements. Logical links among the study elements are critical to the credibility of the study (Cohen & Crabtree, 2008; Maxwell, 2013). For example:

- Is the purpose of the study consistent with the research questions?
- Are the purpose and research questions appropriate to address the research problem?
- Is the selected qualitative approach the best way to answer the research questions?

Similar to quantitative research, logical inconsistencies and improperly applied methods are common weaknesses of qualitative studies. Because qualitative research has fewer rules, critically appraising qualitative studies can seem daunting. The questions in the critique guidelines in Box 12.3 provide a structure for you to examine the strengths and weaknesses of each aspect of a qualitative study. Remember to consult other references, as needed, to answer the questions.

Step 3: Evaluating the Trustworthiness and Meaning of Study Findings

The final step in the critical appraisal of qualitative studies is based on the information that you have identified and the conclusions that can be made from the first two steps of the process. Evaluating the trustworthiness of a study involves determining the credibility, transferability, dependability, and confirmability of the study findings. Although these terms can be defined individually, strategies used by the researchers to enhance the dependability of the findings directly affect the credibility and confirmability of the findings. Similarly, the findings are transferable (applicable) when the sample is described thoroughly, and the reader has confidence in the credibility, dependability, and confirmability of the findings. The questions in the critique guidelines in Box 12.3 provide a structure to evaluate the trustworthiness and meaning of the study you appraise.

EXAMPLE OF A CRITICAL APPRAISAL OF A QUALITATIVE STUDY

Gorlin, McAlpine, Garwick, & Wieling (2016) conducted a qualitative study about the experiences of family members of children with severe autism, presented in Research Example 12.2. A critical appraisal of the study was performed to demonstrate the application of the critical appraisal guidelines to a published qualitative study. We encourage you to conduct a comprehensive critical appraisal using the guidelines presented in Box 12.3, and compare your ideas with the critical appraisal presented in Research Example 12.2. The numbers used in the example critique correspond to those in the critical appraisal guidelines (see Box 12.3).

RESEARCH EXAMPLE 12.2

Qualitative Study

Journal of Pediatric Nursing (2016) **31**, 580–597

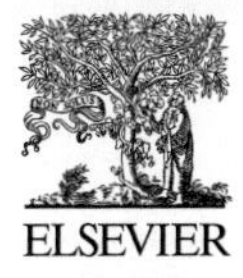

ELSEVIER

Severe Childhood Autism: The Family Lived Experience

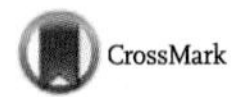

Jocelyn Bessette Gorlin PhD, RN, CPNP [a,*], Cynthia Peden McAlpine PhD, ACNS, BC [b], Ann Garwick PhD, RN, LP, LMFT, FAAN [b], Elizabeth Wieling PhD, LMFT [c]

[a]*Saint Catherine University Department of Nursing, G8H Whitby Hall, 2004 Randolph Avenue, St. Paul, MN*
[b]*University of Minnesota School of Nursing, Weaver-Densford Hall, Minneapolis, MN*
[c]*Family Social Science, University of Minnesota, 293 McNeil Hall, St Paul, MN*

Received 24 March 2016; revised 28 August 2016; accepted 4 September 2016

Key words:
Childhood autism;
Severe autism;
Family;
Phenomenology;
Qualitative research

This research examined the experiences of families living with a child with severe autism. There is limited literature on the experiences of families when a child has severe autism as distinct from milder autism and includes the voices of multiple family members. Van Manen's phenomenological approach was used for data collection and analysis. This approach allowed for the use of innovative data sources, including unstructured individual and family interviews, observations, and family lifelines (a pictorial, temporal picture with comments of the families lives). This study included 29 interviews with 22 participants from 11 families. All data were creatively triangulated and interpreted. Six essential themes were identified. First, families experienced autism as mysterious and complex because it is an invisible and unpredictable condition with diagnostic challenges. Second, families described severe autism behaviors that often caused self-injury, harm to others and damaged homes. Third, profound communication deficits resulted in isolation between the family and child. Fourth, families discussed the unrelenting stress from lack of sleep, managing the child's developmental delays, coordinating and financing services, and concern for the child's future. Fifth, families described consequences of isolation from friends, school, the public, and health providers. Sixth, families portrayed their need for compassionate support and formed 'hybrid families' (nuclear, extended families and friends) to gain support. Study results can be utilized to educate nurses/ other providers about the unique needs of families with children with severe autism and could influence health care policies to improve the care for families caring for children with severe autism.

Background

Autism is the most prevalent developmental disability in the United States, affecting approximately 1 in 68 children (Center for Disease Control (CDC), 2014). Autism is a broad-spectrum neurodevelopmental disability characterized by impairments in social communication and repetitive behaviors or interests, both in varying degrees (American Psychiatric Association (APA), 2013). An example is a child who exhibits limited ability to communicate with others and repetitive behaviors such as hand flapping and/or spinning in circles.

The variability in presentation of autism cannot be underestimated as manifestations can range from mild to very severe. In the past the milder forms of autism were referred to as Asperger's or pervasive developmental disorder-not otherwise specified (PDD-NOS), but currently all degrees of autism are referred to as "autism spectrum disorder" or ASD (APA, 2013; Autism Speaks, 2015). For the remainder of this paper, however, because the focus is only the severe portion of the spectrum, ASD will be referred to simply as "autism."

Approximately one-third of the children with autism are considered to have "severe autism" with significant functional challenges. However this estimate is based on IQ (<70) rather than the child's daily challenges because no functional assessment tool specific to autism has been available (CDC,

* Corresponding author: Jocelyn Bessette Gorlin, PhD, RN, CPNP.
E-mail address: jbgorlin@stkate.edu.

http://dx.doi.org/10.1016/j.pedn.2016.09.002
0882-5963/© 2016 Elsevier Inc. All rights reserved.

Continued

RESEARCH EXAMPLE 12.2—cont'd

Table 1 Autism Functional Challenge Questionnaire

Questions and comments used to assess functional challenges/severity of the child with autism. Developed in collaboration with Michael Reiff, MD (February 2015)

Question	Comment
1. Was there an original diagnosis and severity given? Are there any related conditions such as speech/language and/or intellectual delays?	Usually there are speech and intellectual delays in severe autism, but not always. It is important to assess how "severe" the family perceives the autism is vs. the actual diagnosis e.g., what is severe autism to one family may not be severe autism to another family.
2. Are you aware of any autism testing that has been done: Vineland (functional) and/or IQ?	The children with more severe autism are difficult to test so many may not have had testing and/or families may not remember.
3. How would you describe your child's communication patterns e.g. *words, words together, sentences, any reciprocal communication?*	In severe autism there may be some words, but little to no reciprocal communication.
4. How would you describe your child's autism-related behaviors?	Usually there are significant behaviors that may limit participating in a regular classroom.
5. Can your child accomplish self-care?	Usually there are limited self-care functions such as brushing teeth, bathing, dressing, or feeding self.
6. Is 24 hr. Supervision needed at home?	In severe cases of autism, 24-hour supervision is needed.
7. What type of school does your child attend and what health care-related supports does your child receive both at school and home?	Often the child with more significant challenges will be in full- or part-time autism school (unless not available in their geographic area), a special education class, or receive special services within a regular class, e.g., para-professional time, physical therapy, occupational therapy, speech, adaptive classes
8. What are three functional challenges your child experiences at home and how does this affect your family?	It is important to focus on functional challenges the child experiences within the family versus focusing only on symptoms.

World Health Organization (2001). ICF: International Classification of Functioning, Disability and Health, WHO Library Cataloguing-in-Publication Data, p. 18.
Reiff, MI., & Feldman, HM. (2014). Diagnostic and statistical manual of mental disorders: The solution or the problem?. *Journal of Developmental and Behavioral Pediatrics*, *35*(1), 68–70. 10.1097/DBP.0000000000000017.

2014). Additionally autism severity is difficult to assess because it is subjective and basic autism testing is challenging when children are nonverbal and uncooperative. The American Psychiatric Association's *Diagnostic and Statistical Manual of Mental Disorders* (DSM-5; 5th ed.) defines severe autism (level 3) as children who require substantial support (e.g., 24-hour care), have severe deficits in social communication (e.g., little to no speech), and manifest inflexible repetitive behaviors that are severely limiting (e.g., hand flapping, twirling in circles) (APA, 2013). However this rating also relies more on a list of symptoms than how the child functions in daily life (Reiff & Feldman, 2014).

There has been an effort to clarify autism severity based on a more holistic approach that focuses on the child's daily needs within the context of the family instead of solely on symptoms (Bölte et al., 2014; Gardiner & Iarocci, 2015; Reiff & Feldman, 2014). For example it might be more beneficial to assess autism severity by asking, "What are the daily challenges your child faces and how does this affect your family?" rather than focusing on IQ or a list of autism-related behaviors.

At the time of this study, because there was no tool to assess autism functional severity and few of the children in the study had been given a formal severity diagnosis, the researchers developed the Autism Functional Challenge Questionnaire, which was used for inclusion criterion (Table 1). The questionnaire was developed in collaboration with the medical director of a large urban autism clinic who also reviewed each case individually to assure that the child was qualified as having significant functional challenges or "severe autism."

There has been some exploration in qualitative studies about the experience of families when a child has autism. In many of these studies, however, the severity of the child with autism is not identified (Desai, Divan, Wertz, & Patel, 2012; Dupont, 2009; Farrugia, 2009; Kent, 2011; Lutz, Patterson, & Klein, 2012; Mulligan, MacCulloch, Good, & Nicholas, 2012; Phelps, Hodgson, McCammon, & Lamson, 2009; Safe, Joosten, & Molineux, 2012). In some studies the children are identified as having milder forms of autism such as borderline developmental issues, PPDNOS, or Aspberger's (Bultas & Pohlman, 2014; Dupont, 2009; Hoogsteen & Woodgate, 2013; Kent, 2011; Larson, 2010; Lendenmann, 2010), or the children have a variety of disabilities (Bilgin & Kucuk, 2010; Schaaf, Toth-Cohen, Johnson, Outten, & Benevides, 2011). Only one study of those reviewed included solely children with "severe autism" (Werner DeGrace, 2004).

Additionally, many of the phenomenological studies rely on the response of one family member, usually the mother to portray the family experience (Bilgin & Kucuk, 2010; Bultas & Pohlman, 2014; Larson, 2010; Lutz et al., 2012; Safe et al., 2012). Though fathers are sometimes included in the dialog, extended family members or others considered as family have not been included in the studies reviewed.

This study explored the lived experience of the family when a child has severe autism. During recruitment the parent, usually the mother, was asked to identify who they considered to be family. The mothers included various family members in the nuclear family, but often also included extended family members and friends. Though originally a surprise to the researchers, this was consistent with the definition of family by Poston et al. (2003), "People who think of themselves [as] part of the family, whether related by blood or marriage or not, and who support and care for each other on a regular basis" (p. 319).

This study was based on the premise that it is possible to identify a family lived experience versus that of the individual lived experience. Anderson and Tomlinson (1992) argued that a paradigm shift was needed to provide a theoretical basis for research and practice to discuss the collective family experience, which is often altered by serious illness. They introduced the concept of shared meaning of family experiences. Daly also supported the position that families are groups that construct individual and shared meaning that should be studied using phenomenology (Daly, 1992). Chesla's research program using interpretive phenomenology to study the family living with chronic illness is an example of the construct of the family lived experience (Chesla, 1995; Chesla, 2005; Chesla & Chun, 2005; Gudmundsdottir & Chesla, 2006).

The aim or purpose of this research was to interpret the meaning of the lived experience of families who live with a child who has severe autism. This research simultaneously both narrowed and broadened the focus of previous research studies. It narrowed the focus in that only families of children with severe autism were included in this study and broadened the focus by including all members identified as family and the family unit when possible. A phenomenological approach was used to ask the study question: *What is the lived experience of the family living with a child who has severe autism?*

Literature Review

Since the 1950s, following the dismantling of institutions for children with disabilities, most long-term care has been provided at home by the family. The family has become the primary care provider for children with developmental disabilities such as autism, throughout their lifetime (Cummins, 2001).

The literature on the lived experiences of families caring for a child with autism at home has focused on the stress of these families. Experiences of family stress include: stigma (Dupont, 2009; Farrugia, 2009; Hoogsteen & Woodgate, 2013; Lutz et al., 2012; Safe et al., 2012), autism-related behaviors (Bultas & Pohlman, 2014; Desai et al., 2012; Larson, 2010; Lendenmann, 2010; Lutz et al., 2012), challenges of providing direct care (Bilgin & Kucuk, 2010; Bultas & Pohlman, 2014; Dupont, 2009; Larson, 2010; Mulligan et al., 2012; Safe et al., 2012), social isolation (Bilgin & Kucuk, 2010; Bultas & Pohlman, 2014; Larson, 2010; Luong, Yoder, & Canham, 2009; Lutz et al., 2012; Phelps et al., 2009; Safe et al., 2012; Schaaf et al., 2011), and altered family dynamics (Bilgin & Kucuk, 2010; Bultas & Pohlman, 2014; Dupont, 2009; Farrugia, 2009; Kent, 2011; Phelps et al., 2009; Schaaf et al., 2011; Werner DeGrace, 2004). A number of studies have also reported the positive outcomes that emerge from the experience of living with a child with autism (Bilgin & Kucuk, 2010; Bultas & Pohlman, 2014; Kent, 2011; Lendenmann, 2010; Luong et al., 2009; Phelps et al., 2009; Safe et al., 2012).

One aspect the families perceived as stressful was the stigma or disgrace that they experienced due to the invisible nature of autism and the child's atypical behaviors. Families often felt stigma or shame that they were "bad parents" when the child had tantrums that were misunderstood as poor behavior by the public (Dupont, 2009; Farrugia, 2009; Hoogsteen & Woodgate, 2013; Lutz et al., 2012; Safe et al., 2012).

Autism-related behavior as a source of family stress has been discussed in several studies (Bultas & Pohlman, 2014; Desai et al., 2012; Larson, 2010; Lendenmann, 2010; Lutz et al., 2012). Persistent behaviors associated with autism include crying, lack of sleep, and general agitation (Desai et al., 2012; Lendenmann, 2010; Lutz et al., 2012). Tantrums are most common and self-injurious behaviors are least commonly reported (Lendenmann, 2010). Families spend an exorbitant amount of time dealing with the child's "meltdowns" or tantrum behavior leaving little break time for family members (Larson, 2010). Although these behaviors are referenced, in general they have not been not clearly defined in the literature.

Providing direct care has been another source of family stress (Bilgin & Kucuk, 2010; Bultas & Pohlman, 2014; Desai et al., 2012; Dupont, 2009; Kent, 2011; Larson, 2010; Lutz et al., 2012; Mulligan et al., 2012; Phelps et al., 2009; Safe et al., 2012). Coordinating care is difficult, including balancing the many health care and educational services needed by the child (Bilgin & Kucuk, 2010; Bultas & Pohlman, 2014; Mulligan et al., 2012; Safe et al., 2012). Parents often found it challenging to locate these services and experienced long waiting periods to receive care (Bultas & Pohlman, 2014; Mulligan et al., 2012; Safe et al., 2012). The high cost of care for a child with autism has been noted (Lutz et al., 2012; Phelps et al., 2009; Safe et al., 2012). Concern for the future care of the child when caregivers are no longer alive was also identified as a source of stress (Desai et al., 2012; Kent, 2011; Phelps et al., 2009).

Continued

RESEARCH EXAMPLE 12.2—cont'd

Isolation is another form of stress faced by many families of children with autism as they often feel isolated from extended family who do not fully understand their situation (Bilgin & Kucuk, 2010; Bultas & Pohlman, 2014; Safe et al., 2012), or from friends and the public who do not understand the child's behaviors (Luong et al., 2009; Phelps et al., 2009; Safe et al., 2012). Many families avoid situations outside the home that were uncomfortable for the child and family (Larson, 2010; Lutz et al., 2012; Schaaf et al., 2011).

Challenging family dynamics have been anxiety provoking, specifically the lack of family time spent together as a family (Dupont, 2009; Farrugia, 2009; Kent, 2011; Phelps et al., 2009; Schaaf et al., 2011; Werner DeGrace, 2004). In the study that solely included children with severe autism, it was noted that several families felt "robbed as a family" because their life revolved around autism (Werner DeGrace, 2004, p. 545). Siblings suffered because the family often focused their attention on the child with autism rather than the siblings (Kent, 2011; Phelps et al., 2009; Werner DeGrace, 2004). This resulted in an altered family dynamic where the younger siblings would care for the older child with autism (Kent, 2011). Marital relationships were affected by caring for their child with autism (Bilgin & Kucuk, 2010; Bultas & Pohlman, 2014; Kent, 2011; Phelps et al., 2009). Marital conflicts reported included the father's objection to the time mothers spent caring for the child (Bilgin & Kucuk, 2010) and differences in parenting approaches (Kent, 2011; Phelps et al., 2009).

Several studies discussed positive outcomes related to the experience of raising a child with autism. Families reported that life caring for the child with autism promoted family cohesion (Bilgin & Kucuk, 2010; Kent, 2011; Lendenmann, 2010; Luong et al., 2009; Phelps et al., 2009). Living and learning about autism often resulted in the family uniting to champion for the needs of children with autism (Lendenmann, 2010; Luong et al., 2009). Personal growth includes increased empathy/compassion and less judgment of others (Bultas & Pohlman, 2014; Kent, 2011; Phelps et al., 2009). Personal growth also includes an acceptance of living with the child and an appreciation for the child's unique characteristics (Lendenmann, 2010; Safe et al., 2012).

Design and Method

Max van Manen's philosophical and methodological approach to phenomenology was the basis of this study. Van Manen (2014) describes his approach as hermeneutic phenomenology in which pre-reflexive and reflective experiences are described by those who encounter them and are interpreted for the meaning embedded in these experiences. Ultimately his phenomenological approach focuses on the universal meaning or "essence" of the phenomenon that is conveyed by essential themes based on the particulars of the lived experience (van Manen, 1997; van Manen, 2014).

The goal of phenomenology, according to van Manen, is to identify a phenomenon or situation, in this study, families living with a child with severe autism, and render meaning to this phenomenon. This phenomenological approach was selected for this study because collection of detailed phenomenological interview text and observation results in a description with depth and richness (Pals, 2006; van Manen, 1997; van Manen, 2014). This nuanced data is essential to understand the complex experiences of families of children living with a chronic condition such as severe autism. This approach is also congruent with the use of various types of data collection methods used in this study, including individual and family interviews, observation with field notes, and family lifelines. This approach allows for the assimilation and interpretation of the data sources to portray the lived experience that van Manen describes.

Data Collection

Recruitment

Inclusion criteria were: 1) family members were identified by one parent (who was the primary care giver). Families could include individuals who may or may not be biologically related, but must have ongoing consistent contact and provide care for the child with autism; 2) autism rating of "severe," was evaluated by the researcher by asking the parent to respond to questions on the Autism Functional Challenge Questionnaire and confirmed by consultation; 3) the child with autism was living at home and was 4–13 years old; (4) siblings were at least 6 years of age; and 5) participants were English speaking.

The age for the child with autism was chosen to roughly correlate with school-age for homogeneity of the sample. In addition, school-age children would have been diagnosed with autism and the family would have spent a significant amount of time living with the child. The age for siblings (6 years and above) was selected because those children would be able to articulate their experiences and be capable of providing assent to participate in the study.

Recruitment posters were placed in two urban clinics: one was an autism clinic at a large urban university, and the other was the office of a pediatric psychiatrist located in a large urban public hospital. The poster was also placed in the research studies page of the local Autism Society electronic newsletter. Families interested in participating in the study e-mailed the researcher. Families were called to determine eligibility based on inclusion criteria to participate in the study and to arrange for an interview in their home.

IRB approval for the study was obtained in December 2014. Data collection occurred from February–June 2015. All participants provided written consent/assent prior to any data collection.

Sample

Twenty-two individual family members from 11 families participated in the study. Six families participated in family group interviews (one family had two family group interviews) comprising 29 total interviews from 19 home visits.

Almost half of the mothers (5 out of 11) identified members outside the immediate family and home–such as grandparents, an aunt, or a friend–as part of their "family." Participants included: 11 mothers, 4 fathers, 4 grandmothers, 1 aunt, 1 sibling, and 1 friend. A summary of the families who participated in the study is found in Table 2. Demographic characteristics of the 11 families who participated in the study are found in Table 3. Demographics of the 22 individual family participants are described in Table 4. Demographic data on the children with autism are listed in Table 5.

The sample size of eleven families was used in order to achieve richness in the family interview data. This sample size is also consistent with the recommended number of participants (6–10) for a phenomenological study (Sandelowski, 1995). It was decided that including as many individual family members as possible within those selected families would increase the understanding of the experience of living with a child with autism. Although the qualitative database was large it served the purposes for this study.

Data Sources

Five types of data were utilized in this study: demographic questionnaires, unstructured phenomenological interviews, family/home observations, field notes, and family lifelines.

A demographic questionnaire was used to assess the basic information about the child and family. Information collected about the child included detailed information about their health and healthcare services that were utilized. Family demographic information included family members' level of education and occupation. This questionnaire was given prior to the interview.

Unstructured phenomenological interviews were conducted with each of the 22 family members as well as with six families who were interviewed as a family unit. The basic question, "What is your experience as a family living with a child with autism?" was used to begin conversation and elicit information about the family experience. Additional questions were asked to clarify information. Throughout the interview, the focus was the family versus the individual experience though there was overlap between the two. The average length of the individual interview was 90 minutes; the average length of time of the family unit interview was 60 minutes and all interviews occurred exclusively in the families' homes. Each interview was audio-recorded then transcribed verbatim into written text. All interviews were checked for accuracy against the tapes.

Observations were another method for data collection. Observations were conducted in participants' homes during each individual and family group interviews. Observations included the home environment, the behavior of the child with autism if present, types of interactions between family members, and specifically interactions between the family and child with autism, if the child was present.

Extensive field notes were recorded after each interview, observation and throughout the research process. They included three types of memos: 1) analytic memos were recorded when the researcher interpreted important points during data collection that were incorporated into the analysis e.g., specific observations of the home environment; 2) personal memos were recorded about the subjective experience e.g., feelings such as witnessing children with significant communication challenges in their home; and 3) methodological memos were recorded to document all meetings and discussions among the researchers.

Family lifelines were the fourth form of data collection. The family lifeline was adapted by the primary investigator from the lifeline method described by Gramling and Carr (2004). A lifeline is a visual method used to illustrate a family's life experiences using a timeline that links events: it may include words, dates, or pictures. The participant was given a regular sized paper (8 ½ by 11 inches) that had a horizontal line printed across the bottom. The left of the line was labeled "Birth of Child," on the right was printed "Now." Written on the top of the paper was: "Please draw a picture that describes your family life experiences from before the time your child with special health care needs was born to the present moment. You may draw high points and low points, use pictures and symbols, names and dates-anything that gives a picture of your family's experience." The participant was given colored pencils for use.

Data Analysis

As noted, van Manen's (2014) interpretive approach was used for data analysis in this study. This is a form of hermeneutic analysis in which experiences are interpreted by the researcher to identify essential themes or meanings. The basic phenomenological analysis is reduction, which aims at the insight into the meaning structures (essential themes) of pre-reflexive and reflected experiences.

Treatment of Data

Microsoft Word was chosen to manage the data because it provided an organized, hands-on, approach to data management that allowed the researchers to utilize an iterative analysis to formulate essential themes.

To facilitate identification, each family was assigned a unique color-coded number, each individual within the family and the family interviews was given a letter, and each comment was numbered, with a 'C′ preceding it. For example, 7AC71 is family #7, A is mother, C71 is comment # 71. Thus the focus of the analysis was always on the family experience which was made easier to identify due to the family-coded color.

Each family member unit and corresponding family unit was analyzed independently. The individual family member interviews were analyzed first with an emphasis on their experience as a member of the family rather than their individual experience. The family interviews were then analyzed. Thus the focus of the analysis was always on the family experience.

Continued

RESEARCH EXAMPLE 12.2—cont'd

Table 2 Summary of Family Interviews

Members identified as family	Family members interviewed	Number of individual interviews and number of family interviews	Family living outside the home	Number of home visits
Mother Friend MGM Aunt Son*	Mom Friend MGM Aunt	4 Individual Interviews 2 Family Interviews: • Mom + Friend • Mom, MGM + Aunt	MGM Aunt	3
Mother Father Daughter*	Mother Father	2 individual interviews 1 family interview: • Mom + Dad	None	2
Mother Father Son*	Mother	1 individual interview No family interview	None	1
Mother MGM Son*	Mother MGM	2 individual interviews 1 family interview: • Mother + MGM	MGM	2
Mother Father PGM PGF Son*	Mother Father PGM	3 individual interviews No family Interview	PGM PGF	3
Mother Father Son* Son Son	Mother	1 individual interview No family interviews	None	1
Mother Father Daughter* Daughter* Friend Friend	Mother Father	2 individual interviews 1 family interview: • Mother + Father	Friend Friend	2
Mother Daughter #1 Daughter #2 Son*	Mother Daughter #1	2 individual interviews 1 family interview: • Mother + Daughter	None	1
Mother Father MGM MGF Son*	Mother MGM	2 individual interviews No Family Interviews	Father MGM MGF	2
Mother Father MGM Son*	Mother Father	2 individual interviews 1 family interview: • Mother + Father	None	1
Mother Father Daughter Son*	Mother	1 individual interview No Family Interviews	None	1

* Denotes child with autism.

Table 3 Demographic Characteristics of Family (N = 11)

Variable	Frequency	Percentage
Current relationship status		
Married	7	64%
Separated or divorced	4	36%
Primary care provider		
Mother	9	82%
Mother + Father	1	9%
Mother + Grandmother	1	9%
Children with autism		
Only one child with autism	10	91%
Two children with autism	1	9%
Siblings in family		
None	7	64%
Older	2	18%
Younger	2	18%

Table 4 Demographic Characteristics of Individual Family Participants (N = 22)

Variable	Frequency	%
Relationship to Child **		
Mother	11	50%
Father	4	18%
Grandmother	4	18%
Aunt	1	4%
Friend	1	4%
Sibling	1	4%
Gender		
Male	4	18%
Female	18	82%
Age range		
20–30	2	9%
31–40	7	32%
41–50	7	32%
51–60	2	9%
61–75	4	18%
Race		
White European American	15	68%
African American	3	14%
Southeast Asian	1	4%
Multi-racial	3	14%
Religion		
Practicing Christian	12	54%
Non-practicing Christian	5	23%
No affiliation	3	14%
Agnostic	2	9%
Highest level of education		
High school degree	3	14%
One–two years of college	8	36%
Four year college	7	32%
Graduate degree	4	18%

** Percentage may not equal 100 due to rounding to nearest integer.

A selective approach was used to analyze the interview text in which the text was read several times and statements or phrases that were revealing about the experience were highlighted. As this process continued, themes began to emerge and possible commonalities were gathered. With further review, thematic statements from the text were identified from these commonalities.

This was followed by linguistic transformation, or expanding the meaning of the evolving themes by documenting a summary note about the possible theme. This process was repeated for every interview including the family unit interview that eventually led to identifying themes within and across families, facilitated by the color coding, that ultimately resulted in the essential themes or meaning of the family of living with a child with autism.

As part of the interpretive process family observations and the family lifelines were triangulated during the analysis, which helped to formulate the essential themes. The family observations resulted in information about interactions between family members and the home environment. Particularly rich were the observations of the child with autism who was observed in 8 out of the 11 families. The extensive field notes were integrated into the formation of essential themes.

The family lifelines were also color-coded and interpreted in a similar fashion to the interviews. The family lifelines were evaluated in a two-step process: the first step included analyzing the written information on the lifelines. For example if the family wrote "grieving" on the lifeline this would be added to the evolving theme. The second step included interpreting the entire Family Lifeline for themes or meaning. Like the observations, the lifelines were instrumental in building the composite essential themes that represented the essence of a family living with a child with severe autism.

Two members of the research team were involved in the analysis and when there were questions about the meaning of the analysis or essential theme, there was discussion until consensus was reached. The two researchers discussed themes that emerged in a collaborative manner and would converse about which theme appeared most appropriate in light of the interviews, observations and family lifelines. This insured validity or truthfulness as the actual data were reviewed and interpreted by both researchers. In addition, a third member of the research team, a family therapist and expert in family research, led a process of reflexivity through engaging dialog with the researchers about personal experiences they found challenging, such as observing the difficulties that the families encountered.

Rigor or Appraisal of the Phenomenological Study

Van Manen proposes four criteria for evaluative appraisal of phenomenological studies: orientation, strength, richness, and depth (van Manen, 1997). The first criterion is that the text needs to be centered by the researcher's pedagogic orientation or stance. In this study the focus is pediatric health care with an aim to better understand the experience of families of children with a severe condition such as autism in order to ultimately provide

Continued

RESEARCH EXAMPLE 12.2—cont'd

Table 5 Demographic Characteristics of Child With Severe Autism (N = 12)

Variable	Frequency	%
Gender		
Male	9	75%
Female	3	25%
Age range (mean 8 years)		
4–5	3	25%
6–7	5	41%
8–9	0	0
10–11	2	17%
12–13	2	17%
Age at diagnosis (mean 2.25 years)		
<1 Year	0	0
1–2 Years	8	67%
3–4 Years	4	33%
Time since diagnosis (mean 5 years) **		
2–4 Years	4	33%
5–7 Years	5	43%
8–10 Years	3	25%
Verbal communication		
No words	2	47%
Few words, no sentences	8	66%
Very limited sentences	2	47%
Activities of daily living *		
Requires 24 hour supervision	12	
Cannot complete dress self	7	
Not fully toilet trained	5	
Type of school attending		
Autism school	5	42%
Public school with services	6	50%
Home school	1	8%

* Total does not equal 12 due to multiple listings.
** Percentage may not equal 100 due to rounding to nearest integer.

better health care to these families. Pediatric health and care for families is a core interest of the discipline of nursing and the topic was chosen because of the researchers' orientation in caring for families of children with chronic health needs.

The second criterion is that the research text needs to be strong and based in the researcher's educational experience, with the most rigorous interpretation of the phenomenon. Two of the four researchers have had extensive experience working in pediatrics for over 25 years with families of children with chronic illness. The other two researchers have had extensive experience working with families in practice and qualitative research. The extensive professional background of the investigators gave insight into family experience that assisted with the final interpretation of the phenomenon.

The third criterion is that the text must be rich. Van Manen (1997) states that, "A rich and thick description is concrete, exploring a phenomenon in all its experiential ramifications" (van Manen, p. 152) with anecdotes that capture the experience. In this study all of the five data sources helped to illuminate the experience of families living with severe autism. There were approximately 45 hours of interview tape, 1,500 pages of individual and family interview text from 19 home visits. In addition, there were 20 page of observational field notes and 13 family lifelines.

The fourth criterion for rigor is that the text must be deep: meaning is incorporated beyond what is actually experienced. In this study the meaning of the family lived experience evolved by reviewing and synthesizing all of the data and developing essential themes. In this way essential themes were not merely a recounting of that which was said in the interviews or drawn in the family lifelines, but rather an assimilation and interpretation of the "essence" of the experience of the family living with a child who has severe autism, reflecting van Manen's methodological process.

Results

In this study six essential themes with several subthemes were identified (Table 6).

Family Perception of the Mystery and Complexity of Severe Autism

The first theme identified was that families viewed autism as a mysterious and complex condition. The public's inaccurate stereotypes about autism and the inherent nature of autism added to this mystery. In fact, in one family lifeline the words, "Unsolved Mysteries" was boldly written.

Several families explained that they believe that the public has a stereotype about autism as a mild condition because they are familiar with only milder forms of autism (e.g. Asperger's), or they see movies that portray characters with autism as highly intelligent. Both of these stereotypes were in stark contrast to the family's experience of autism. As a sibling noted:

> My view of what autism looks like started to change completely. It's not like the movies: *Temple Grandin* and *Rain Man*. They can use a toilet and express themselves and earn respect from huge groups of people...They're not the face of autism. Not in my life. Autism is much more painful and degrading and trying and frustrating. Autism isn't genius, it's not "different ability." It **hurts.**
>
> (41BLLC51)

Families also described the stereotype held by others that disabilities are physical, e.g., disabled children would use a wheel chair. Because autism is not a visible physical disability, their child's behavior was misunderstood as "bad behavior" instead of a manifestation of autism. Families subsequently felt shame and constantly needed to educate others about autism.

The mysterious nature of autism also included the abrupt changes that occurred day to day and over time such as the child suddenly losing the ability to talk, typically at about 2 years of age. One grandmother said, "As time went on, one day he was talking...and I remember his dad saying, 'He said "juice," 'He said "juice 'last night.' And the next day...he never talked again" (43BC3). This change may be more striking in severe autism because of the nonverbal nature whereas in milder autism there is usually some verbal ability.

Adding to the uncertainty, the etiology of autism remains unknown and the child faces many diagnostic challenges. The child's behavioral and communication challenges made the child's participation in standardized autism testing almost impossible. In addition the children often faced long wait lists for autism testing; one mother was outraged that there was approximately an 8-month wait list in the state to obtain formal autism assessment.

Dealing with Severe Behavior Challenges

The next essential theme described how the family dealt with the severe behavioral issues of their child. The families shared that, as the child grew, behaviors became more difficult to manage. They discussed a range of significant autism-related behaviors that they encountered each day which included self-injurious behaviors e.g., head banging, biting their own fingers and arms, throwing themselves into furniture, punching themselves in the head, and picking at their own skin, resulting in open lesions.

Most commonly discussed were meltdowns or tantrums, severe sleep issues, and elopement. In reference to sleep, almost all of the children had sleep issues that kept families awake and alert at night. Two families, however, noted that their child did not sleep from birth until about age 4 (39CC32; 41BLL48). One of these mothers noted:

> It was really hard. I ate candy bars, I drank coffee in the middle of the night, and then sometimes he would surprise me and fall asleep, and since I'd had coffee, I'd have to take Nyquil to try to get to sleep so I could be sleeping when he was sleeping. The synergistic effects of Nyquil, coffee, Nyquil, coffee could not have been good for my body. I was just exhausted all the time.
>
> (41AC28)

Families reported how they dealt with elopement of their child. Several families had installed metal bars, alarms, and multiple locks on doors and windows to prevent the child from escaping and running away. Most families often felt safer at home rather than outside the home because of their familiarity with their home's safety features and fear of the chances of the child's running away when in public.

Severe behaviors also included aggression to others, such as pinching, hitting, scratching, biting, head butting, and throwing toys or items. This resulted, among other casualties, in welts and bruises, a teacher's broken nose, and a mother's black eye. One mother said:

> He hits and kicks. He's bit us before. He gets physically aggressive with us.... For instance, [dad] just took him to see relatives and on the way home on the plane he was attacking dad the whole time. [Dad] comes home and he's got scratches down his face and a bloody nose, he's bitten up, because [son] was freaking out on him."
>
> (36AC51 +52)

Another mother explained her son's morning routine, "He'll sit on my head or he'll kick my head if I'm sleeping....and if I don't [get up] within 5 seconds, it's *whap*." (16C49).

Some behaviors caused destruction to their homes and damage to furnishings, such as holes punched in walls, food thrown at walls, feces smeared on furniture, books ripped apart, and light fixtures dismantled. One mother described:

> He just obsesses about an entire roll of toilet paper and he'll unroll the whole thing and put it in the toilet.... He likes to stick things in the drain. He used to flush things down the toilet.... He has a tendency to eat toothpaste.... to the point where he's eaten it and then gone into his room and thrown it all up.
>
> (34AC24 + 25)

Because of this several families created a "minimalist" design to decorating which included few accessories and simple furnishings to decrease the risk of destruction.

As the primary investigator, I observed severe autism-related behavior, home destruction, and austere home decoration through the home visits, which were documented in field notes. I was able to meet several of the children with autism (8 out of 11). I made particular note of one child who shuffled as the child walked across the room and used only groaning sounds for communication. During the interview of her mom, the child pinched my face very hard. The mother's repeated apologies highlighted her own experience of stigma/shame. I observed several homes that had holes in the walls caused by the child with autism throwing toys or other objects. I also observed several homes that were austere, with few to no home decorations to avert home destruction by the child.

Dealing With Significant Communication Challenges

In addition to behavioral challenges, families experienced a significant lack of verbal and nonverbal communication with their child. All of the children had profound communication deficits. A few children were nonverbal and a few could use simple sentences, but the majority had only a few words in their vocabulary and none of the children could carry on meaningful reciprocal conversation. For many there was a delay of several years (e.g., 7–9 years) before they recognized a parent by calling her "mom" and some still had never said it. As one grandmother recounted of her teenage grandson, "No, he doesn't say 'Mom.' It breaks my heart. If he would only say 'Mom,' I would be so happy for my daughter, but he doesn't" (34BC36).

In addition, many of the children with severe autism do not show affection like hugging, but rather used nonverbal

Continued

RESEARCH EXAMPLE 12.2—cont'd

Table 6 Essential Themes and Subthemes

Essential themes	Subthemes
Mystery and complexity of severe autism	Stereotype and stigma • Autism is considered a mild disorder • Invisibility of autism • Constantly teaching others
	Unpredictability of behaviors and communication Diagnosis challenges • Unknown etiology • Testing delay • Testing challenges
Dealing with severe behavior challenges	Child size Specific behaviors • Meltdowns • Repetitive behaviors and strict routine • Sleep issues • Elopement • Destruction and altered home environment
	Aggression to others • Family members + Those outside of family self-injurious behaviors
Dealing with significant communication challenges	Communication patterns Solitary or parallel play What is child thinking? Altered connection • Verbal connection • Non-verbal connection • Delayed connection
Experiencing severe stress	Constant nature of stress Roller coaster experience Child's delayed development Teaching activities of daily living Coordinating services Cost Concern for child's future
Living with severe isolation	Friends • Obstacles to meeting with friends • Friends without children with autism • Friends with children with milder autism
	School • Lack of inclusion + Low expectations • Confrontations
	Public Medical health care providers
A strong dependence on family	Hybrid families: nuclear, extended family and friends Compassion • For the child + For each other • Increase over time

communication such as a head tilt, fist bump or rough play. This grandmother also said:

> He seems to be into fist bumps now. Every time I see him, I'll say, 'Give Grandma a hug!' He'll put his head down, and it's kind of close to your head, and that's as good as you're going to get; that's a hug!"
> (34BC28 + 29)

The lack of communication from the child left families wondering what the child was thinking. The family members worried that they would not be able to help their child if he or she became ill because of the child's inability to communicate basic needs. It was not uncommon that the child could not communicate a toothache or earache which in some cases resulted in severe unresolved pain and medical complications.

Because of the profoundly altered communication, the families often felt disconnected or isolated from their child. One mother said:

> I feel like I haven't had the opportunity to enjoy him as a child. When a baby's born, every mom wants to cuddle with a baby and nurture the baby.... We'll try to play with him and he doesn't engage, so after a while we get tired and frustrated and say, 'Okay, I finally give up.'
> (44A57+59)

During the home visit I observed the communication of several of the children with autism as they interacted with their family members. The child with autism usually had little to no interaction with others and often played alone. One child was precipitously perched on a high couch while I was there and avoided any direct touch from the parents. Another child stood still and repeatedly twirled a ribbon in circles while the family attempted to hug him, while another child aggressively pursued a younger brother and threw toys at the wall. I saw several of the children tilt their head to the side toward the family member in lieu of a hug.

Experiencing Severe Stress

Families discussed the severe and unrelenting stress they experienced because of the child's severe behavioral issues and altered communication. This was evident both in the interviews and the family lifelines. A good illustration of this stress was one father who told me, "I'm glad that someone is doing this kind of research. Certainly it's been a challenge. If you've talked to my wife at all, you've heard that it's been a challenge!" (44BC1) He then placed his head into his hands and began to weep, which was often the case with fathers. This observation of overwhelming emotion was common among all the males interviewed as well as many other family member participants.

Many families described their lives as an unpredictable "roller coaster" because of the daily challenges they experienced caring for their child. One example of the ups and downs of their daily experience was the lack of sleep described by all families because of the child's erratic sleep schedules and the need to maintain vigilance watching the child through the night. One mother exclaimed: "How do I take care of myself? How do I just get breaks?.... I'm to the point where I'm breaking. I can't continue 24/7. I can't do it!"(16C95).

Another mother commented on the dissimilar lives their families led when compared to other families they knew:

> They are children... I'm a mom; but that's where the similarities between me and my children and my friends and their children stops. Beyond that, the way we eat is different, the way we drive is different, the way we dress is different, the way we invite people over is different, the way we decorate is different. The way we shop is different. The way we travel is different. Everything is different.
>
> (39AC38)

Many families shared the frustrations of caring for an older child who acted like an infant because of their delayed development, e.g., they needed to bring a diaper bag on outings. One father described that he and his wife were not able to relax as their child has grown, but rather needed to remain watchful. He said, "I imagine for most people that starts happening at a particular age, that it gets less time-consuming, but that has never happened with us. It's just going to stay. She's 6 and it's always going to be 6" (10CC2).

Families also shared the constant need to reinforce good behavior all day, every day in an effort to model self-care and positive social skills. This involved constantly reminding and patterning behaviors for the child. One aunt recounted, "It's lesson, lesson, lesson" (7BC30).

As the families held the responsibility of primary care provider for the child, they coordinated countless health care providers, which resulted in additional stress. Beginning with the time of diagnosis there was little help in identifying and coordinating services by healthcare providers. The best help came from specialty autism centers, but the centers were often inaccessible because they were generally located in urban areas and families often lived far from them. They reported their frustration about the shortage of autism-related health care services like behavioral therapy, physical therapy (PT), occupational therapy (OT), and speech therapy, each with long waiting lists.

Families recounted the trials of simple visits to the doctor. For these families one trip to a clinic could be exhausting because of the long wait times, child behaviors, and needing to hold the child down to help keep the child calm. As one mother said,

> This is a life-altering experience. It's traumatic every time we go into a clinic or a hospital—or even a place where they're not going to be poked or touched, just the psychologist. This is an event. Like, can I just talk to you over the phone and you can bill for that? Do I really have to be within touching distance?
>
> (39CC43)

The families described the high cost of autism care and the steep out-of-pocket expenses they incurred due to inadequate health care coverage. Some family members held several jobs to make ends meet and several needed to weigh health care coverage in their employment options to procure the best medical insurance coverage.

The stress was constant and the families lived in the present moment, and did not discuss plans for the near future. Although specific plans for the future care of the child were not discussed, a concern echoed by many family members was, "What will happen to my child if I die?" which reflected their concern about who would care for their child if not them.

Overwhelming stress was observed in the home visits as evidenced by the majority of the participants who wept openly during the interview. In addition, anxiety was palpable as family participants often tried to juggle speaking with me while caring for their child, although most had someone helping to care for the child during the interview.

The family lifelines also revealed the extreme degree of distress the family experienced. Although the lifelines were originally printed on standard letter size paper (8 ½ by 11 inches), half of the families printed copies of the lifeline and taped two or three together to obtain more writing space. Family stress was sometimes portrayed in a graph-like representation illustrating the "ups and downs" (Figure 1). In this lifeline, the stress that the family had experienced is evident, particularly when the child was 12–13 years old, during early adolescence. Again, while it might be expected that there would be a general improvement over time, instead there were constant peaks and valleys that continue throughout the child's life. Figure 2 also illustrates the constant anxiety the families experienced; this family lifeline was so chaotic that it was difficult to read.

Families with children who had the most severe functional challenges demonstrated stress on the family lifeline evident from birth (Figure 2). Alternatively, some families experienced a relatively calm period during infancy followed by stress when their child had a sudden onset of symptoms at about 2 years of age. These lifelines showed a different picture with relative calm then anxiety that followed (Figure 3).

Living With Severe Isolation

The fifth theme identified was the extreme isolation related to the child's severe behavioral issues and profound communication challenges. The families discussed not being able to physically leave home because of the child's needs. They described not having the ability to meet with friends

Continued

RESEARCH EXAMPLE 12.2—cont'd

because of their busy schedules and lack of proper childcare. They did not want to socialize with friends who had children who were neuro-typical because they had little in common. Families yearned to meet other parents who had a child as severely affected with autism as their own, although this was a rare occurrence.

Frustration and isolation from school staff was common as their child was often marginalized and taught menial tasks, such as folding towels or drawing, rather than learning educational content like other school children. Families referred to this as "baby sitting" versus "real school." Several families described having altercations with school staff as they advocated for services, with the child ultimately being "kicked out" of the school system. During one family interview, the mother described their school situation: "That's when the principal came down that day and told me, and I quote, 'Get the hell out of my school!'....And then we never went back" (10AC48).

Families were further isolated from the public when their child had behaviors that were misunderstood. One mother recounted a typical experience:

> This is what happens at the grocery store. Someone will say: 'What the hell is wrong with your child?' or 'Get it under control; get *him* out of here! Why do you bring *that* in public?'... The loud speaker will be turned on and someone says: 'What's going on? Maybe if you can't get this under control you should leave!' We have left. Sometimes even with a grocery cart full of groceries–we've left.
> (10AC28+ 29)

There was also isolation from health care providers including, but not limited to gossip about the child's behavior by nursing staff at the hospital, dismissing the diagnosis of autism by a physician, and general lack of patience by health care providers in clinic. These were the very people families depended on and they felt dismissed mainly due to the health provider's lack of knowledge about severe autism.

As previously discussed, families felt isolated from their child relating to the child's developmental delay and lack of communication. Some families described being 'heartbroken' by the fact that they did not know if the child realized that they were not just a child care provider, but rather a dedicated family member called "mom," "dad," "sister," etc. As one mother said,

> When I used to work a lot, it seemed like he didn't even miss me when I was gone. He was 4 when he started to get separation anxiety.... It's different to have a little kid that doesn't seem like they care if you're around or not.... And it's like, I know you like me, but does it matter if it's me or if it's somebody else? It matters because I'm around you more, but is it because I'm mom? You're not requesting mom.
> (43AC83 + 43AC84)

A Strong Dependence on Family and Compassion for Each Other

The last essential theme identified in this research was a strong reliance on hybrid families and compassion learned for others. In an effort to find the necessary physical and emotional support, families cobbled together hybrid families who often consisted of nuclear and extended families, and friends. This was a hybrid support system that seemed to help the families as they navigated through the difficulties associated with severe autism. One mother described the importance of friends:

> Our family here is largely people that we just extremely love like family. There's not a blood connection, but there's a heart connection, so they are our family. So my best friend... she's my sister! Yeah, and then I have another friend .... She's my other

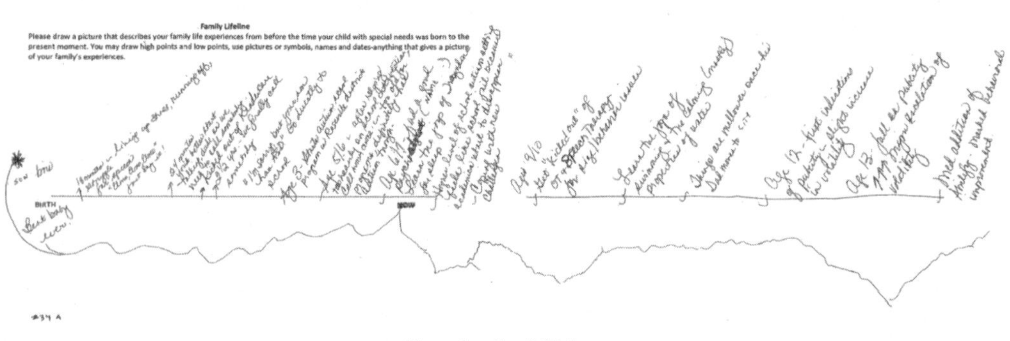

Figure 1 Graph lifeline.

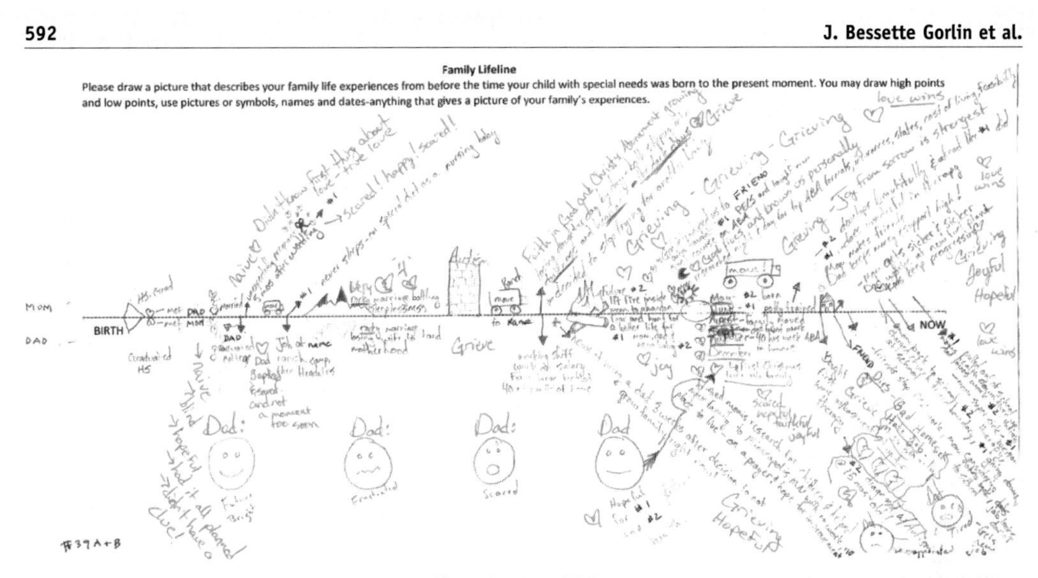

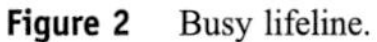
Figure 2 Busy lifeline.

sister. We're all very connected just by crisis or hardship.... There's not a blood tie, but there's something that's just as strong, if not stronger, here. (39AC3)

During this interview this friend came to the family's home to offer the mother assistance to care for the child with autism.

Families demonstrated compassion and empathy between the child and family and compassion for others which appeared to blossom over time. This was evident in one interview when the grandmother said:

So my daughter's goals for him and frustration, I share them, but I have learned in the frustration. He's my darling. There's no shame in my game. I always

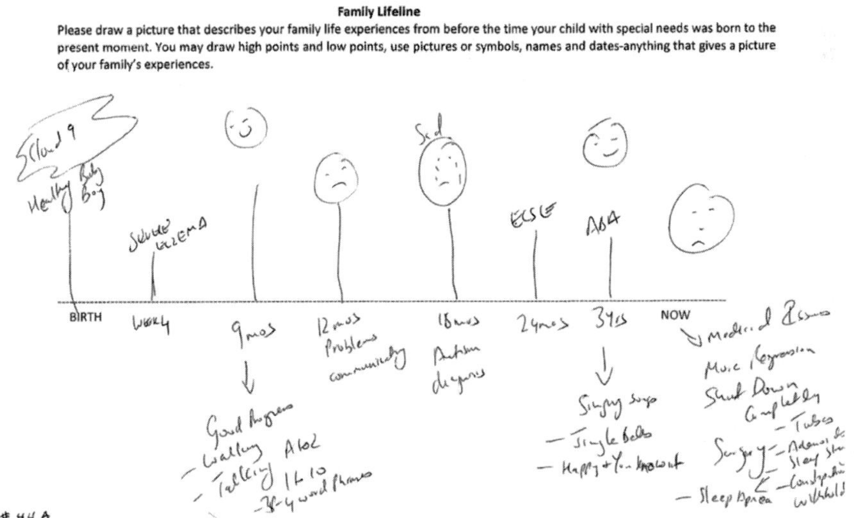

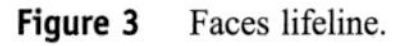
Figure 3 Faces lifeline.

Continued

RESEARCH EXAMPLE 12.2—cont'd

say I only got one little egg and it's cracked. My one little egg and it's cracked. I love him!

(7DC8)

Two family lifelines portrayed family compassion that evolved over time. One example of this is seen in Figure 4. The mother describes their family experience in a progression of the words: "Surface love> Chaos> Stress> Peacefulness again> inner love" with "inner love" being closest to the present time (45LLC67). She described that the family had learned love from caring for the child with autism.

In the second family lifeline (Figure 2), the mother noted early in their family lifeline: "Grieving.... Naive, Didn't know the first thing about love–true love..." Later the mother writes, "Grieving... Joy from sorrow is strongest." At the end of the family lifeline denoting the present time, she draws hearts and writes: "Grieving, joyful, hopeful.... Love wins" (39ALL100).

Discussion

Findings from this study contribute new knowledge that provides unique insight into the experiences of families of children with severe autism. This research included children with only severe autism versus other disabilities or milder forms of autism. It also gave a voice to the family experience from the perspective of multiple family members, including those outside the nuclear family, and the family as a unit versus the parent as the only source of data. The triangulation of several data sources–individual interviews, family interviews, observations and the family lifelines–was also innovative and helped to paint a broad picture of the family lived experience.

The effort to only include children with severe autism was initially a challenge of this study because only one child originally had been given the formal diagnosis of "severe autism" (possibly due in part to the various challenges to severity categorization mentioned previously). Because of this and the lack of a comprehensive assessment tool to assess severity, we developed the Autism Functional Challenge Questionnaire to assess autism severity for inclusion criteria. Including only children with significant functional challenges provided a homogeneity to the family experience since all were all dealing with children who had considerable functional challenges.

The inclusion of family members outside the nuclear family also involved a challenge in the research process and was an iterative process. At the onset of the study, the criteria included only two-parent nuclear families. During recruitment it became apparent that several families were one parent–families, and that their definition of the family extended outside the traditional nuclear family to include extended family and friends. Inclusion of these individuals highlighted the stressful situations the families experienced and their need to reach outside the nuclear family for the physical and emotional support to care for the child with autism. It seemed ironic that these individuals who provided significant support to families were rarely included in the qualitative research studies that had been reviewed.

There was also an effort to include the voices of the families as a unit in family interviews. Family interviews have rarely been conducted by nurses due to the inherent challenges in coordinating and conducting family interviews (Åstedt-Kurki & Hopia, 1996). Individual interviews yield rich data and family interviews often yield information about family interactions (Beitin, 2007; Donalek, 2009). We found this to be the case and appreciated the opportunity to conduct seven family unit interviews with six families, though it was extremely difficult for families to find the time to meet together due to their extensive responsibilities caring for the child with autism.

In this study, the triangulation of the interviews with observations and the family lifelines provided a broad understanding of the family's lived experience. Observations of the home environment, family, and the child with autism (in the majority of cases) were all documented in field notes. Seeing home interiors devoid of decoration to thwart potential destruction by the child with autism; gaping holes in walls caused by toys thrown by the child with autism; and bars and locks on windows and doors, gave a clear snapshot of the severe conditions under which the families were living. Witnessing some of the children with autism not speaking at all or avoiding the touch of family members breathed life into the theme of isolation.

The family lifelines provided yet another piece of the puzzle which was a creative outlet for many families to portray in picture what they might not be able to express in words. Most included a chronologic representation of their family experiences and some included faces, words, and figures which virtually shouted "stress."

In summary, there were six themes that emerged from the use of these research methods that summarized the family experience (see Figure 5). The families found autism mysterious and complex including the yet unknown etiology of autism, challenges in diagnosis and unpredictable nature of the condition. Unlike the study of Hoogsteen and Woodgate (2013), who found that the families of children with autism were surprised to find autism not as severe as they expected, these families found the condition more severe than they expected. One example of this is that the child's behaviors were often unpredictable, and changed often and dramatically throughout their life, such as the child speaking then losing the ability to speak. Similar to other studies (Farrugia, 2009; Hoogsteen & Woodgate, 2013), many families felt stigma or shame related to the invisible nature of autism and the public's misperception that the child's autism-related behavior was reflective of poor parenting versus a disability.

Bultas and Pohlman (2014) and Larson (2010) found fatigue among mothers was due to the erratic sleeping schedule of the child. A few studies mentioned specific stressful behaviors such as crying, sleep issues and general agitation (Desai et al., 2012; Lendenmann, 2010; Lutz et al., 2012). The severe behavioral issues discussed in this study,

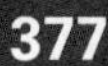

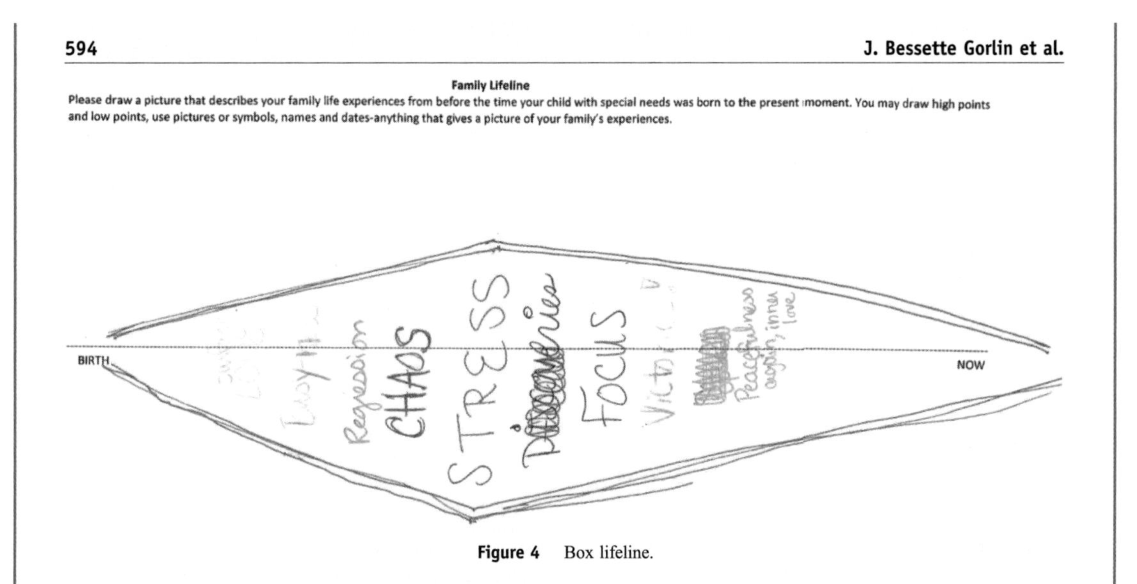

Figure 4 Box lifeline.

however, were numerous and quite severe. The behaviors became more challenging as the child grew in size and included: severe meltdowns or tantrums; severe lack of sleep, often lasting years; harming themselves and others; elopement; and significant destruction of the home.

The families faced profound communication challenges, as most of the children had few words in their vocabulary and most preferred to generally isolate themselves from others. In addition, the children often had delayed verbal and nonverbal connection to the family, such as not acknowledging family members for years and not showing affection. This altered communication resulted in the family experiencing isolation from the child, something not particularly highlighted in previous qualitative research.

Although we framed the review of literature around family stress experienced by families with a child with autism, the synthesis of our data sources revealed more extreme situations than expected. Families described the child's chronic lack of sleep that resulted in severe, and often long-lasting sleep deprivation in family members. Family stress was also related

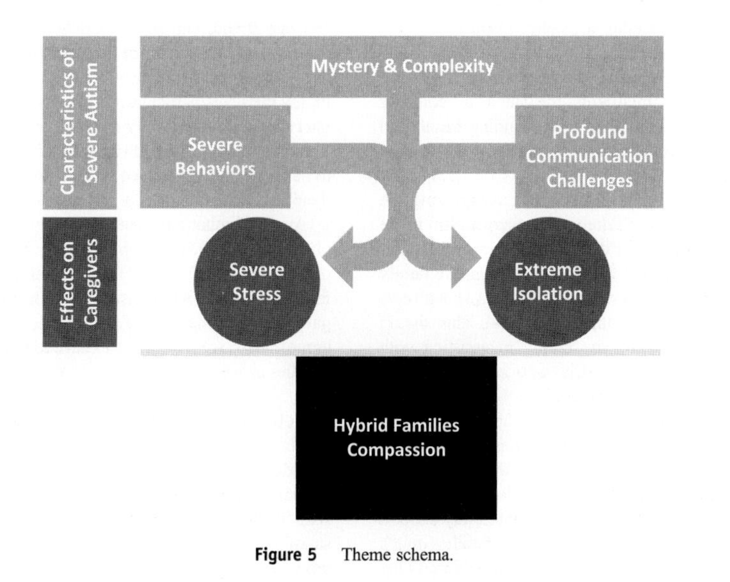

Figure 5 Theme schema.

Continued

RESEARCH EXAMPLE 12.2—cont'd

to caring for a child who was developmentally delayed, and the inordinate amount of time coordinating health care services, educating the child daily, and out-of-pocket expenses.

Families additionally experienced extreme isolation from friends, schools, the public, and health care providers. The previous qualitative literature does support the finding that families of children with autism experienced isolation from friends and the public (Larson, 2010; Luong et al., 2009; Lutz et al., 2012; Phelps et al., 2009; Safe et al., 2012; Schaaf et al., 2011), but isolation from their child has generally not been a focus in the previous research.

The extended family was generally not included in previous study samples though a few studies found that the extended family were in fact unsupportive to the nuclear family who had a child with autism (Bilgin & Kucuk, 2010; Bultas & Pohlman, 2014; Safe et al., 2012). In this study there was evidence of a strong dependence on a network of extended family and friends, with families even forming hybrid families to care for the child with autism.

Lastly, in this research, families experienced a compassion for the child and for each other over time as they cared for their child. This was similar to the positive outcomes reported in other studies that describe empathy and compassion that the families learned from living with a child with autism (Bultas & Pohlman, 2014; Dupont, 2009; Mulligan et al., 2012).

Practice Implications

The findings from this research have implications for health care providers who provide direct care and psychological support to the family who have a child with severe autism. In addition, the findings may be instrumental in laying the groundwork for affecting health care policy change.

Practice implications can be based on the family health system construct discussed by Anderson and Tomlinson (1992). This construct highlights the need to consider the family as a distinct unit when understanding health and illness and when formulating research and healthcare interventions.

Practice implications may include, first, recognizing the unique needs of families of children with severe autism in the health care setting. Because of the behavioral and communication challenges of the child with severe autism, the family may require additional support when the child has a health care visit to a well-child clinic, dentist, or hospital. This should include more staff to support the family in assisting with procedures and healthcare providers who are sensitive to families experiencing significant stress.

Second, there is a need for improved psychological support by health care providers to mitigate family stress and isolation. Psychological support could include individual and family therapy, mentors for family members who have shared experiences, Web-based and in-person parent/family support groups, respite care for children to provide families much needed breaks, and home visits by health care providers. Other supports that may defray family stress could be coordinators or advocates who could assist families in obtaining local health care services (e.g., behavior therapy, PT, etc.) to help navigate complex health care costs. Empathetic healthcare providers who recognize the unique situation of each family would also be beneficial.

The study findings underscore the need to increase the number and/or expand existing autism specialty clinics and services due to the long wait-times families experience to obtain autism testing and receive healthcare services. The development of a comprehensive autism treatment center model might be beneficial. These centers would provide centralized multi-disciplinary health care by autism specialists, e.g., psychologists, physical and occupational therapists, to provide multiple assessments and services at one location. This would improve coordination of care and alleviate the stress for the child and family traveling to various sites.

This research may also provide the catalyst for further research that explores the experiences of families of children with severe autism. Further understanding of family needs and resources may be used ultimately to affect the development of healthcare policy that is sensitive to the needs of the families of children with severe autism.

Study Limitations

The time since diagnosis of autism to the time of the interview varied within the study from 2 to 10 years with the mean of 5 years. This could be considered a limitation of the study because the varied times since diagnosis could result in very different family experiences.

A challenge of the study was that, although the sample was large, the types of family members who participated in the study were limited. For example, only one aunt, one sibling and one friend, and no grandfathers or uncles participated. Having participation from more of these individuals would have broadened the scope of the findings. Additionally, not all family members participated in the individual and family unit interviews and one family did not complete a family lifeline. Though this limited the information gathered, we felt fortunate to have the participation of those who did participate, despite their busy schedules.

Another limitation is that much of the family experience was observed over one day; approximately half of the families had one home visit (5 out of the 11 families) and the other six families had 2–3 home visits. One could argue that one visit gave a limited snapshot of family life, though one could also argue that we were fortunate to have as many contacts with the families as we did.

Conclusion

The aim or purpose of this research was to interpret the experience of families who live with a child with severe autism. The goal of the study was to include only children with severe autism while at the same time broadening the sampling parameters to incorporate all significant people who were considered family. Overall, the results were somewhat surprising. The study findings illuminated the extensive hardships and challenges of families who have a child with severe autism; identified needed resources; and illuminated how families formed hybrid families for additional support. This new knowledge has implications for nursing and health care practitioners which encourages the development of strategies to provide quality care to children with severe autism and their families. This research also provides a foundation for future research that can influence the development of new healthcare policy. Further research is needed to extend our understanding of the unique issues that families of children with severe autism encounter so that overall care to these families can be improved in the future.

Acknowledgments

The authors would like to acknowledge the families that participated in this study. We would also like to acknowledge the assistance of Michael Reiff, MD, LEND Medical Director of the Autism Spectrum and Neurodevelopmental Disorders Clinic at the University of Minnesota, and Elizabeth Reeve, MD, child and adolescent psychiatrist at Regions Hospital in St. Paul, Minnesota. Special thanks to Marguerite Clemens and Arlene Birnbaum.

There are no conflicts of interest. This research was supported by a pre-doctoral fellowship through the University of Minnesota School of Nursing Center for Children with Special Heath Care Needs which was funded by the Maternal Child Health Bureau (MCHB), and the University of Minnesota Leadership Education in Neuro-development and Related Disabilities Fellowship (LEND), also funded by the MCHB.

References

American Psychiatric Association (APA) (2013). Diagnostic and statistical manual of mental disorders (DSM-5). *Autism spectrum disorder diagnostic criteria* (5th ed.). Arlington, VA: American Psychiatric Publishing.

Anderson, KH, & Tomlinson, PS (1992). The family health system as an emerging. *IMAGE: Journal of Nursing Scholarship*, *24*, 57–63.

Åstedt-Kurki, P, & Hopia, H (1996). The family interview: Exploring the experiences of family health and well-being. *Journal of Advanced Nursing*, *24*, 506–511.

Autism Speaks (2015). Facts about autism. Retrieved from www.autismspeaks.org/what-autism/facts-about-autism?

Beitin, B (2007). Qualitative research in marriage and family therapy: Who is in the interview? *Contemporary Family Therapy*, *30*, 48–58.

Bilgin, H, & Kucuk, L (2010). Raising an autistic child: Perspectives from Turkish mothers. *Journal of Child and Psychiatric Nursing*, *23*, 92–99. http://dx.doi.org/10.1111/j.1744-6171.2010.00228.x.

Bölte, S, de Schipper, E, Robison, J, Wong, V, Selb, M, Singhal, N, ... Zwaigenbaum, L (2014). Classification of functioning and impairment: The development of ICF core sets for autism spectrum disorder. *Autism Research*, *7*, 167–172.

Bultas, M, & Pohlman, S (2014). Silver linings. *Journal of Pediatric Nursing*, *29*, 596–605. http://dx.doi.org/10.1016/j.pedn.2014.03.023.

Centers for Disease Control and Prevention (CDC) (2014). Prevalence of autism spectrum disorder among children aged 8 years- Autism and developmental disabilities monitoring network, 11 sites, United States, 2010. *MMWR. Morbidity and Mortality Weekly Report* (Retrieved from http://www.cdc.gov/mmwr/pdf/ss/ss6302.pdf).

Chesla, CA (1995). Hermeneutic phenomenology: An approach to understanding families. *Journal of Family Nursing*, *1*, 68–78.

Chesla, CA (2005). Nursing science and chronic illness: Articulating suffering and possibility in family life. *Journal of Family Nursing*, *11*, 371–387.

Chesla, CA, & Chun, KM (2005). Accommodating type 2 diabetes in the Chinese American family. *Qualitative Health Research*, *15*, 240–255.

Cummins, RA (2001). The subjective well-being of people caring for a family member with a severe disability at home: A review. *Journal of Intellectual and Developmental Disability*, *26*, 83–100.

Daly, K (1992). The fit between qualitative research and characteristics of families. In J. F. Gilgun, K. Daly, & G. Handel (Eds.), *Qualitative methods in family research* (pp. 3–11). Newbury Park, CA: Sage.

Desai, M, Divan, G, Wertz, F, & Patel, V (2012). The discovery of autism: Indian parents' experiences caring for their child with autism spectrum disorder. *Transcultural Psychiatry*, *49*, 613–637. http://dx.doi.org/10.1177/1363461512244713 9.

Donalek, JG (2009). The family research interview. *Nurse Researcher*, *16*, 21–28.

Dupont, M (2009). *An exploration of resilience in families with a child diagnosed with autism spectrum disorder.* (Unpublished doctoral dissertation) Denton, Texas: Texas Women's University.

Farrugia, D (2009). Exploring stigma: Medical knowledge and the stigmatization of parents of children diagnosed with autism spectrum disorder. *Sociology of Health and Illness*, *31*, 1011–1027. http://dx.doi.org/10.1111/j.1467-9566.2009.01174.x.

Gardiner, E, & Iarocci, G (2015). Family quality of life and ASD: The role of child adaptive functioning and behavior problems. *Autism Research*, *8*, 199–213.

Gramling, LF, & Carr, RL (2004). Lifelines: A life history methodology. *Nursing Research*, *53*, 207–210.

Gudmundsdottir, M, & Chesla, CA (2006). Building a new world habits and practices of healing following the death of a child. *Journal of Family Nursing*, *12*, 143–164.

Hoogsteen, L, & Woodgate, R (2013). The lived experience of parenting a child with autism in a rural area; Making the invisible, visible. *Pediatric Nursing*, *39*, 233–237.

Kent, M (2011). *Autism spectrum disorders and the family: a qualitative study.* (Unpublished doctoral dissertation) Berkeley California: Graduate School of Psychology, Wright Institute.

Larson, E (2010). Ever vigilant: Maternal support of participation in daily life for boys with autism. *Physical and Occupational Therapy in Pediatrics*, *30*, 16–27. http://dx.doi.org/10.3109/01942630903297227.

Lendenmann, M (2010). *The lived experience of parents of a preschool age, moderately mentally retarded autistic child.* (Unpublished doctoral dissertation) Washington, D. C.: School of Nursing, Catholic University of America.

Luong, J, Yoder, M, & Canham, D (2009). Southeast Asian parents raising a child with autism: A qualitative investigation of coping styles. *The Journal of School Nursing*, *25*, 222–229. http://dx.doi.org/10.1177/1059840509334365.

Lutz, HR, Patterson, BJ, & Klein, J (2012). Coping with autism: A journey toward adaptation. *Journal of Pediatric Nursing*, *27*, 206–213. http://dx.doi.org/10.1016/j.pedn.2011.03.013.

Mulligan, J, MacCulloch, R, Good, B, & Nicholas, DB (2012). Transparency, hope, and empowerment: A model for partnering with parents of a child with autism spectrum disorder at diagnosis and beyond. *Social Work in Mental Health*, *10*, 311–330. http://dx.doi.org/10.1080/15332985.2012.664487.

Pals, DL (2006). *Eight theories of religion.* New York, NY: Oxford University Press.

Phelps, K, Hodgson, J, McCammon, S, & Lamson, A (2009). Caring for an individual with autism disorder: A qualitative analysis. *Journal of Intellectual and Developmental Disability*, *34*, 27–35. http://dx.doi.org/10.1080/13668250802690930.

Poston, DJ, Turnbull, AP, Park, J, Mannan, H, Marquis, J, & Wang, M (2003). Family quality of life outcomes: A qualitative inquiry launching a long-term research program. *Mental Retardation*, *41*, 313–328.

Continued

RESEARCH EXAMPLE 12.2—cont'd

Reiff, MI, & Feldman, HM (2014). Diagnostic and statistical manual of mental disorders: The solution or the problem? *Journal of Developmental and Behavioral Pediatrics*, *35*, 68–70. http://dx.doi.org/10.1097/DBP.0000000000000017.

Safe, A, Joosten, A, & Molineux, M (2012). The experiences of mothers of children with autism: Managing multiple roles. *Journal of Intellectual and Developmental Disability*, *37*, 294–302. http://dx.doi.org/10.3109/13668250.2012.736644.

Sandelowski, M (1995). Sample size in qualitative research. *Research in Nursing & Health*, *18*, 179–183.

Schaaf, RC, Toth-Cohen, S, Johnson, SL, Outten, G, & Benevides, T (2011). The everyday routines of families of children with autism: Examining the impact of sensory processing difficulties on the family. *Autism*, *15*, 373–389.

Van Manen, M (1997). *Researching lived experience: human science for an action sensitive pedagogy*. Canada: The Althouse Press.

Van Manen, M (2014). *Phenomenology of practice: meaning-giving methods in phenomenological research and writing*. Walnut Creek, CA: Left Coast Press.

Werner DeGrace, B (2004). The everyday occupation of families with children with autism. *The American Journal of Occupational Therapy*, *58*, 543–550.

World Health Organization (2001). *ICF: international classification of functioning*. Disability and Health: WHO Library Cataloguing-in-Publication Data.

Critical Appraisal

Step 1: Identifying the Steps of the Research Process in the Study; and Step 2: Determining Study Strengths and Weaknesses

1. **Writing Quality:** The detailed research report was clear and concise, with a logical flow throughout. Relevant terms such as autism were clearly defined in the background section.
2. **Title:** The title "Severe childhood autism: The family lived experience" indicated that the article was about autism and that families of children with severe autism were the population (Gorlin et al., 2016, p. 580). The title did not directly indicate the type of qualitative approach that was used but phenomenology can be implied by the phrase "lived experience," which researchers typically use in the title of phenomenological studies.
3. **Authors:** The primary author, Dr. Jocelyn Bessette Gorlin, is a PhD-prepared nurse who is a certified pediatric nurse practitioner. The Saint Catherine University website has a record of Dr. Gorlin's scholarly work, which includes peer-reviewed publications on topics related to pediatric nursing (St. Catherine University, 2017). Dr. Gorlin's three coauthors were all PhD-prepared and hold university faculty positions. Gorlin and associates (2016, p. 596) reported no conflicts of interest in the acknowledgments section.
4. **Abstract:** The abstract included the qualitative approach. The purpose of the study and the gap in the current literature that the study addressed were clearly described. The sample size and data collection methods were identified. The six major themes and primary conclusion of the study comprised the remainder of the abstract.
5. **Research Problem:** Gorlin and associates (2016) clearly stated the problem as "There is limited literature on the experiences of families when a child has severe autism as distinct from milder autism and includes the voices of multiple family members" (Gorlin et al., 2016, p. 580).
6. **Purpose:** The purpose was clearly identified the study's focus. "The aim or purpose of this research was to interpret the meaning of the lived experience of families who live with a child who has severe autism" (Gorlin et al., 2016, p. 582). The problem was significant because of the prevalence of the condition and the challenges of meeting the unique healthcare needs of the families affected by severe autism. The research objectives were clearly linked to the study purpose (Creswell & Poth, 2018; Fawcett & Garity, 2009; Maxwell, 2013).
7. **Literature Review:** The literature review was clearly marked with two major headings, background, and literature review (Gorlin et al., 2016, pp. 580–583). Most of the 39 sources that Gorlin and colleagues (2016) cited were peer-reviewed, primary sources. Of the 39 sources Gorlin and associates (2016) cited, 15 (38%) were published within 5 years and 26 (67%) were published within 10 years of the article. Because qualitative researchers often study topics that have been rarely researched, it is not uncommon for the literature they cite to be older. The content in the literature review directly related to the study concepts. Information and background on autism, as well as the method of phenomenology, were included in the review. Sources from multiple disciplines such as nursing, psychology, medicine, and occupational therapy were included in the review and were appropriate for the study. The multidisciplinary review was well organized. The references cited supported the need for the study and appropriateness of the study's methods. Gorlin and associates (2016) did not note strengths or weaknesses of the studies reviewed. Although little information

was provided about the quality of the studies reviewed, the findings of previous studies and information from other references were synthesized and compared with each other. The gap in knowledge addressed by the study was clearly identified.

8. **Philosophical Orientation or Study Framework:** The philosophic orientation of the study was hermeneutic phenomenology. As support for this qualitative approach, Gorlin and colleagues (2016) cited two books by van Manen (1997, 2014) on phenomenology. Although Max van Manen is a commonly cited contemporary expert in hermeneutic phenomenology, the researchers did not cite Heidegger, the originator of hermeneutic phenomenology.
9. **Research Objectives (Aims) or Questions:** The aim and research question were cited in the last paragraph of the background section. "The aim or purpose of this research was to interpret the meaning of the lived experience of families who live with a child who has severe autism" (Gorlin et al., 2016 p. 582). The research question is clearly linked to the research purpose (Creswell & Poth, 2018). "A phenomenological approach was used to ask the study question: *What is the lived experience of the family living with a child who has severe autism?*" (Gorlin et al., 2016, p. 582).
10. **Qualitative Approach:** Interpretive phenomenology was the qualitative approach for this study. Gorlin et al. (2016, p. 583) explained in the design and methods section that van Manen's "phenomenological approach focuses on the universal meaning or essence of the phenomenon that is conveyed by essential themes based on the particulars of the lived experience (van Manen, 1997, 2014)." As mentioned earlier, providing information from Heidegger and citing a primary source would have strengthened the description of the qualitative approach. The qualitative approach was congruent with the study purpose and objectives.
11. **Sample:** The sampling plan was adequate to address the purpose of the study:

    Recruitment posters were placed in two urban clinics: one was an autism clinic in a large urban university, and the other was the office of a pediatric psychiatrist located in a large urban public hospital. The poster was also placed in the research studies page of the local Autism Society electronic newsletter. Families interested in the study e-mailed the researcher. Families were called to determine eligibility based on inclusion criteria to participate in the study and to arrange for an interview in their home. (Gorlin et al., 2016, p. 583)

    Exclusion criteria were not mentioned in the article. However, the sample criteria were clearly identified and appropriate for the study:

    Inclusion criteria were: 1) family members were identified by one parent (who was the primary care giver). Families could include individuals who may or may not be biologically related, but must have ongoing consistent contact and provide care for the child with autism; 2) autism rating of "severe" was evaluated by the researcher by asking the parent to respond to questions on the Autism Functional Challenge Questionnaire and confirmed by consultation; 3) the child with autism was living at home and was 4-13 years old; 4) siblings were at least 6 years of age; and 5) participants were English speaking. (Gorlin et al., 2016, p. 583)

    The researchers did not mention whether any participants refused to participate or did not complete the study. The participants recruited had experience with the research topic and were valuable sources of data. Gorlin and associates (2016) did not discuss reaching saturation with the sample. The sample ($n = 22$), however, was adequate for the study design. "Twenty-two individual family members from 11 families participated in the study. Six families participated in family group interviews (one family had two family group interviews) comprising 29 total interviews from 19 home visits" (Gorlin et al., 2016, p. 583).
    Informed consent was obtained before data collection. The written consent/assent appears to be appropriate for the literacy level of the study population because all 22 participants were reported to have a high school degree or higher. Gorlin and colleagues (2016) did not provide a refusal rate nor did they note whether arrangements were made in advance to address the emotional needs of the participants in case the topic was upsetting to them (Cowles, 1988).
12. **Setting:** The home of participants was the study setting. This setting was appropriate for the study purpose and served to protect the confidentiality and promote the comfort of the participants.

Continued

RESEARCH EXAMPLE 12.2—cont'd

13. **Data Collection:** The researchers appropriately sought IRB approval and received it "in December 2014. Data collection occurred from February–June 2015. All participants provided written consent/assent prior to any data collection" (Gorlin et al., 2016, p. 583). Their data collection methods were ethical. "Five types of data were utilized in this study: demographic questionnaires, unstructured phenomenological interviews, family/home observations, field notes, and family lifelines" (Gorlin et al., 2016, p. 584). The demographic questionnaire provided basic information "about the child and family....The questionnaire was given prior to the interview" (Gorlin et al., 2016, p. 584).

    The unstructured phenomenological interviews were the data collection method that provided the majority of the data and were conducted with each of the 22 family members as well as six families who were interviewed as a family unit. The basic question, "What is your experience as a family living with a child with autism?" was used to begin conversation and elicit information about the family experience. Additional questions were asked to clarify information... all interviews occurred exclusively in the families homes. (Gorlin et al., 2016, p. 583)

    The primary question used in the 29 interviews was relevant to the study's objective and closely mirrored the wording of that objective (Gorlin et al., 2016). Interviews lasted long enough for Gorlin and colleagues (2016) to gather robust and thorough descriptions. The family group interviews could have been labeled focus groups, although Gorlin and associates (2016) did not use the term *focus group.* "Each interview was audio recorded then transcribed verbatim into written text. All interviews were checked for accuracy against the tapes" (Gorlin et al., 2016, p. 584).

    Because the interviews were conducted in the families' homes, the researchers were able to observe the environment and family interactions before and after the interviews. Observations added richness to the data. For example, observations brought depth to the theme "Dealing with Severe Behavior Challenges": "During the interview of her mom, the child pinched my face very hard. The mother's repeated apologies highlighted her own experience of stigma/shame. I observed several homes that had holes in the walls caused by the child with autism throwing toys or other objects" (Gorlin et al., 2016, p. 588).

    Another source of data was field notes "Extensive field notes were recorded after each interview, observation and throughout the research process. They included three types of memos; 1) analytic memos...2) personal memos...3) methodological memos" (Gorlin et al., 2016, p. 583). The lifelines were drawn by the participants on "regular sized paper (8½ by 11 inches) that had a horizontal line printed across the bottom. The left of the line was labeled 'Birth of Child,' on the right was printed 'Now'. Written on top of the paper was: 'Please draw a picture that describes your family life experiences from before the time your child with special needs was born to the present moment. You may draw high points and low points, use pictures and symbols, names and dates - anything that gives a picture of your family's experience.' The participant was given colored pencils for use" (Gorlin et al., 2016, p. 584).

14. **Data Analysis:** As previously stated, the interviews were converted to a written format via word-for-word transcription. The written transcription was then compared back to the original recording to ensure that the transcription was correct. van Manen's (2014) approach was used to analyze the data.

    "This is a form of hermeneutic analysis in which experiences are interpreted by the researcher to identify essential themes or meanings. The basic phenomenological analysis is reduction, which aims at insight into the meaning structures (essential themes) of pre-reflexive and reflected experiences" (Gorlin et al., 2016, p. 584). The data analysis process was described thoroughly enough to be able to evaluate the logic of the researchers' decisions and provided support for the study's rigor.

    "Microsoft Word was chosen to manage the data—Each family member unit and corresponding family unit was analyzed independently" (Gorlin et al., 2016, p. 584).

    Gorlin and colleagues (2016, pp. 586–587) included a section in the article, "Rigor or Appraisal of the Phenomenological Study," in which they described measures taken to evaluate the trustworthiness of the study. Gorlin and colleagues (2016, p. 586) identified aspects of the data collection and analysis that supported "orientation, strength, richness, and depth" which are the four criteria of quality proposed by van Manen (1997). The clearly described measures to increase trustworthiness were adequate to provide confidence in the findings.

Step 3: Evaluating the Credibility and Meaning of the Study Findings.

15. **Interpretation of Findings:** Gorlin and associates (2016) provided detailed interpretation of findings, including the six themes and subthemes. The six themes identified by Gorlin and associates (2016, p. 589) were "Mystery and complexity of severe autism...Dealing with severe behavior challenges... Dealing with significant communication challenges...Experiencing severe stress...Living with severe isolation [and] A strong dependence on family." Their detailed interpretation included quotes to support each theme and subtheme. The participants' quotes and family lifelines added a richness to the data and were clearly reflective of the derived themes. For example, Gorlin and colleagues (2016, pp. 589–590) provided the following narrative and quote as part of the support for the theme "Experiencing severe stress":

    Many families described their lives as an unpredictable 'roller coaster' because of the daily challenges they experienced caring for their child. One example of the ups and downs of their daily experience was the lack of sleep described by all families because of the child's erratic sleep schedules and the need to maintain vigilance watching the child through the night. One mother exclaimed: 'How do I take care of myself? How do I just get breaks?...I'm to the point where I'm breaking. I can't continue 24/7. I can't do it!'

    The weakness of the interpretation was that they did not address variations in findings based on sample characteristics. However, the study findings were clearly linked back to previous research (Gorlin et al., 2016).

16. **Limitations:** The study limitations acknowledged by Gorlin and associates (2016) were minimized as much as possible by the researcher's well-designed study. Gorlin and colleagues (2016, p. 595) acknowledged that the

    ...varied times since diagnosis could result in very different family experiences...the types of family members who participated in the study were limited. For example, only one aunt, one sibling and one friend, and no grandfathers or uncles participated. Having participation from more of these individuals would have broadened the scope of the findings... much of the family experience was observed over one day; approximately half of the families had one home visit (5 out of the 11 families) and the other six families had 2-3 visits. One could argue that one visit gave a limited snapshot of family life...

    An unidentified limitation was that the researchers did not base the sample size on saturation.

17. **Conclusions:** The researchers concluded that:
    The aim or purpose of this research was to interpret the experience of families who live with a child with severe autism. The goal of the study was to include only children with severe autism while at the same time broadening the sampling parameters to incorporate all significant people who were considered family. Overall, the results were somewhat surprising. The study findings illuminated the extensive hardships and challenges of families who have a child with severe autism; identified needed resources; and illuminated how families formed hybrid families for additional support. This new knowledge has implications for nursing and health practitioners, which encourages the development of strategies to provide quality care to children with severe autism and their families. (Gorlin et al., 2016, p. 595)
    The conclusions and recommendations for future studies were logically congruent with the findings. They could have strengthened the conclusions by identifying other settings or populations to whom the findings might be transferable or applied.

Continued

RESEARCH EXAMPLE 12.2—cont'd

18. **Nursing Implications:** Gorlin and associates (2016) clearly discussed implications of the study on nursing practice and what the study contributed to understanding the phenomenon of the lived experience of families of children with severe autism:

    Practice implications may include, first, recognizing the unique needs of families of children with severe autism in the health care setting... the family may require additional support when the child has a health care visit to a well-child clinic, dentist, or hospital...Second, there is a need for improved psychological support by health care providers to mitigate family stress and isolation. (Gorlin et al., 2016, p. 595)

19. **Future Research:** Gorlin and associates (2016, p. 596) noted that "Further research is needed to extend our understanding of the unique issues that families of children with severe autism encounter so that overall care to these families can be improved in the future." Specific recommendations on future study methodology or study variables or concepts were not made.
20. **Critical Appraisal Summary:** Overall, the article was detailed, well organized, and clearly written. The rights of human subjects were protected through the recruitment, data collection, and analysis phases of the study. Gorlin and colleagues (2016) provided a thorough description of each element of this qualitative study sufficient to allow for replication by another researcher. The congruence of the purpose, method, and findings was clearly demonstrated throughout the presentation of the study.
    The trustworthiness of the study was addressed in great detail in the section on "Rigor or Appraisal of the Phenomenological Study" (Gorlin, 2016, p. 586). The use of multiple strategies to enhance trustworthiness increases the reader's confidence in the findings (Cohen & Crabtree, 2008; Murphy & Yielder, 2010). The support provided for the trustworthiness of the study was a major strength of the article. Gorlin and colleagues (2016) conducted a well-designed study that minimized the limitations to a great degree. As a result, the findings provided a credible view of children with severe autism from the perspective of their families. The findings of this study expand current EBP knowledge and can be used to improve the healthcare team's support for these families and better meet the needs of children with severe autism. The study's strengths exceeded its few weaknesses, and it can serve as a strong example of interpretive phenomenology.

KEY POINTS

- An intellectual critical appraisal of research requires careful examination of all aspects of a study to judge its strengths, weaknesses, credibility, meaning, and significance.
- Research is critically appraised to broaden understanding, improve practice, and provide a background for conducting a study.
- All nurses, including students, practicing nurses, nurse educators, and nurse researchers, need expertise in the critical appraisal of research.
- Strong quantitative studies are guided by a clear concise problem and purpose, and by appropriate objectives, questions, and/or hypotheses. The study framework is appropriate; the design is relevant, with limited threats to validity; data analyses address the study objective, questions, or hypotheses; and the study findings are credible and an accurate reflection of reality.
- Strong qualitative studies are based on a philosophical orientation and qualitative approach that are specified. Building on that foundation, the researcher implements data collection and analysis methods that enhance the study's trustworthiness.
- Detailed guidelines for conducting critical appraisals of quantitative and qualitative studies are described. The guidelines are provided for each of the three critical appraisal steps: (1) identifying the steps or elements of the study; (2) determining study strengths and weaknesses; and (3) evaluating the trustworthiness and meaning of the study findings.
- Example critical appraisals are provided for a quantitative study and a qualitative study.

REFERENCES

Aberson, C. L. (2010). *Applied power analysis for the behavioral sciences*. New York: Routledge Taylor & Francis.

Agency for Healthcare Research and Quality (AHRQ). (2017). *AHRQ home*. Retrieved May 5, 2017, from http://www.ahrq.gov.

Alligood, M. R. (2014). *Nursing theory: Utilization & application* (8th ed.). Maryland Heights, MO: Mosby Elsevier.

American Nurses Credentialing Center (ANCC). (2017). *Magnet program overview*. Retrieved November 18, 2017, from http://www.nursecredentialing.org/Magnet/ProgramOverview.

American Psychological Association (APA). (2010). *Publication manual of the American Psychological Association* (6th ed.). Washington, DC: APA.

Bialocerkowski, A., Klupp, N., & Bragge, P. (2010). Research methodology series: How to read and critically appraise a reliability article. *International Journal of Therapy and Rehabilitation, 17*(3), 114–120.

Brown, S. J. (2018). *Evidence-based nursing: The research-practice connection* (4th ed.). Sudbury, MA: Jones & Bartlett.

Burns, N. (1989). Standards for qualitative research. *Nursing Science Quarterly, 2*(1), 44–52.

Chinn, P. L., & Kramer, M. K. (2015). *Integrated theory and knowledge development in nursing* (9th ed.). St. Louis: Elsevier Mosby.

Clissett, P. (2008). Evaluating qualitative research. *Journal of Orthopaedic Nursing, 12*(2), 99–105.

Cohen, D. J., & Crabtree, B. F. (2008). Evaluative criteria for qualitative research in health care: Controversies and recommendations. *Annals of Family Medicine, 6*(4), 331–339.

Cowles, K. (1988). Issues in qualitative research on sensitive topics. *Western Journal of Nursing Research, 10*(2), 163–179.

Craig, J., & Smyth, R. (2012). *The evidence-based practice manual for nurses* (3rd ed.). Edinburgh: Churchill Livingstone Elsevier.

Creswell, J. W. (2014). *Research design: Qualitative, quantitative and mixed methods approaches* (3rd ed.). Thousand Oaks, CA: Sage.

Creswell, J. W., & Poth, C. (2018). *Qualitative inquiry & research design* (4th ed.). Thousand Oaks, CA: Sage.

DeVon, H. A., Block, M. E., Moyle-Wright, P., Ernst, D. M., Hayden, S. J., et al. (2007). A psychometric toolbox for testing validity and reliability. *Journal of Nursing Scholarship, 39*(2), 155–164.

Eymard, A. S., & Altmiller, G. (2016). Teaching nursing students the importance of treatment fidelity in intervention research: Students as interventionists. *Journal of Nursing Education, 55*(5), 288–291.

Fawcett, J., & Garity, J. (2009). *Evaluating research for evidence-based nursing practice*. Philadelphia: F.A. Davis.

Gloeckner, M. B., & Robinson, C. B. (2010). A nursing journal club thrives through shared governance. *Journal for Nurses in Staff Development, 26*(6), 267–270.

Gorlin, J. B., McAlpine, C. P., Garwick, A., & Wieling, E. (2016). Severe childhood autism: The family lived experience. *Journal of Pediatric Nursing, 31*(6), 580–597.

Gray, J. R., Grove, S. K., & Sutherland, S. (2017). *The practice of nursing research: Appraisal, synthesis, and generation of evidence* (8th ed.). St. Louis: Elsevier Saunders.

Grove, S. K., & Cipher, D. J. (2017). *Statistics for nursing research: A workbook for evidence-based practice* (2nd ed.). St. Louis: Elsevier.

Hall, H. R., & Roussel, L. A. (2017). *Evidence-based practice: An integrative approach to research, administration and practice* (2nd ed.). Burlington, MA: Jones & Bartlett.

Hart, C. (2009). *Doing a literature review: Releasing the social science imagination*. Thousand Oaks, CA: Sage Publications.

Hoare, Z., & Hoe, J. (2013). Understanding quantitative research: Part 2. *Nursing Standard (Royal College of Nursing [Great Britain]), 27*(18), 48–55.

Hoe, J., & Hoare, Z. (2012). Understanding quantitative research: Part 1. *Nursing Standard (Royal College of Nursing [Great Britain]), 27*(15-17), 52–57.

James, P. A., Oparil, S., Carter, B. L., Cushman, W. C., Denison-Himmelfard, C., Handler, J., et al. (2013). 2014 evidence-based guidelines for the management of high blood pressure in adults: Report from the panel members appointed to the Eighth Joint National Committee (JNC 8). *Journal of the American Medical Association, 311*(5), 507–520.

Kelkar, A. A., Spertus, J., Pang, P., Pierson, R. F., Cody, R. J., Pina, I. L., et al. (2016). Utility of patient-reported outcome instruments in heart failure. *JACC: Heart Failure, 4*(3), 165–175.

Mackey, M. (2012). Evaluation of qualitative research. In P. L. Munhall (Ed.), *Nursing research: A qualitative perspective* (5th ed.) (pp. 517–531). Sudbury, MA: Jones & Bartlett.

Maxwell, J. (2013). *Qualitative research design: An interactive approach* (3rd ed.). Thousand Oaks, CA: Sage.

Melnyk, B. M. & Fineout-Overholt, E. (Eds.). (2015). *Evidence-based practice in nursing & healthcare: A guide to best practice.* (3rd ed.). Philadelphia: Wolters Kluwer.

Melnyk, B. M., Gallagher-Ford, E., Fineout-Overholt. (2017). *Implementing evidence-based practice competencies in healthcare: A practical guide for improving quality, safety, & outcomes*. Indianapolis, IN: Sigma Theta Tau International.

Miles, M., Huberman, A., & Saldaña, J. (2014). *Qualitative data analysis: A methods sourcebook* (3rd ed.). Thousand Oaks, CA: Sage.

Mittlbock, M. (2008). Critical appraisal of randomized clinical trials: Can we have faith in the conclusions? *Breast Care, 3*(5), 341–346.

Moorhead, S., Johnson, M., Maas, M. L., & Swanson, E. (2013). *Nursing outcomes classification (NOC): Measurement of health outcomes* (5th ed.). St. Louis: Elsevier.

Morse, J. M. (1991). Evaluating qualitative research. *Qualitative Health Research, 1*(3), 283–286.

Munhall, P. L. (2012). *Nursing research: A qualitative perspective* (5th ed.). Sudbury, MA: Jones & Bartlett.

Murphy, F., & Yielder, J. (2010). Establishing rigor in qualitative radiography. *Radiography, 16*(1), 62–67.

National Institute of Nursing Research (NINR). (2017). What is nursing research? Retrieved May 5, 2017, from https://www.ninr.nih.gov.

O'Mathúna, D. P., & Fineout-Overholt, E. (2015). Critically appraising quantitative evidence for clinical decision making. In B. M. Melnyk & E. Fineout-Overholt (Eds.), *Evidence-based practice in nursing & healthcare: A guide to best practice* (2nd ed.) (pp. 87–138). Philadelphia: Lippincott Williams & Wilkins.

Petty, N., Thomson, O., & Stew, G. (2012). Ready for a paradigm shift? Part 2: Introducing qualitative research methodologies and methods. *Manual Therapy, 17*(5), 378–384.

Plichta, S. B., & Kelvin, E. (2013). *Munro's statistical methods for health care research* (6th ed.). Philadelphia: Lippincott Williams & Wilkins.

Powers, B. A. (2015). Critically appraising qualitative evidence for clinical decision making. In B. M. Melnyk & E. Fineout-Overholt (Eds.), *Evidence-based practice in nursing & healthcare: A guide to best practice*. (2nd ed.) (pp. 139–168). Philadelphia: Lippincott Williams & Wilkins.

Pyrczak, F. (2008). *Evaluating research in academic journals: A practical guide to realistic evaluation* (4th ed.). Los Angeles: Pyrczak.

Quality and Safety Education for Nurses (QSEN). (2018). *Pre-licensure knowledge, skills, and attitudes (KSAs)*. Retrieved April 7, 2018, from http://qsen.org/competencies/pre-licensure-ksas.

Roller, M., & Lavrakas, P. (2015). *Applied qualitative research design: A total quality framework approach*. New York: Guilford Press.

Ryan-Wenger, N. A. (2017). Precision, accuracy, and uncertainty of biophysical measurements for clinical research and practice. In C. F. Waltz, O. L. Strickland, & E. R. Lenz (Eds.), *Measurement in nursing and health research* (4th ed.) (pp. 371–383). New York: Springer.

Sandelowski, M. (2008). Justifying qualitative research. *Research in Nursing & Health, 31*(3), 193–195.

Sandelowski, M., & Barroso, J. (2007). *Handbook for synthesizing qualitative research*. New York: Springer.

Schoe, L., Høstrup, H., Lyngsø, E., Larsen, S., & Poulsen, I. (2011). Validation of a new assessment tool for qualitative research articles. *Journal of Advanced Nursing, 68*(9), 2086–2094.

Shadish, W. R., Cook, T. D., & Campbell, D. T. (2002). *Experimental and quasi-experimental designs for generalized causal inference*. Chicago: Rand McNally.

Sherwood, G., & Barnsteiner, J. (2017). *Quality and safety in nursing: A competency approach to improving outcomes* (2nd ed.). Ames, IA: Wiley-Blackwell.

Smith, M. J., & Liehr, P. R. (2014). *Middle range theory for nursing* (3rd ed.). New York: Springer.

St. Catherine University, School of Nursing. (2017). *Jocelyn Bessette Gorlin*. Retrieved May 4, 2017, from https://www.stkate.edu/academics/our-faculty/jocelyn-bessette-gorlin.

University of North Carolina at Charlotte, School of Nursing. (2017). *Charlene Witaker-Brown*. Retrieved May 4, 2017, from http://nursing.uncc.edu/charlene-whitaker-brown.

van Manen, M. (1997). *Researching lived experience: Human science for an action sensitive pedagogy*. Ontario, Canada: Althouse Press.

van Manen, M. (2014). *Phenomenology of practice: Meaning-giving methods in phenomenological research and writing*. Walnut Creek, CA: Left Coast Press.

Waltz, C. F., Strickland, O. L., & Lenz, E. R. (2017). *Measurement in nursing and health research* (5th ed.). New York: Springer.

Whitaker-Brown, C. D., Woods, S. J., Cornelius, J. B., Southard, E., & Gulati, S. K. (2017). Improving quality of life and decreasing readmissions in heart failure patients in a multidisciplinary transition-to-care clinic. *Heart & Lung, 46*(2), 79–84.

Wolf, M. (2012). Ethnography: The method. In P. L. Munhall (Ed.), *Nursing research: A qualitative perspective* (5th ed.) (pp. 285–338). Sudbury, MA: Jones & Bartlett.

Because of funding changes, the Agency for Healthcare Research and Quality (AHRQ) National Guideline Clearinghouse website was scheduled for decommissioning as of July 16, 2018. For more information, go to https://www.ahrq.gov/.

CHAPTER

13

Building an Evidence-Based Nursing Practice

Susan K. Grove

CHAPTER OVERVIEW

LEARNING OUTCOMES

After completing this chapter, you should be able to:

1. Describe the benefits and challenges related to evidence-based practice in nursing.
2. Use the PICO format to formulate clinical questions to identify evidence for use in practice.
3. Implement research-based protocols, algorithms, guidelines, and policies in your practice.
4. Critically appraise systematic reviews, meta-analyses, meta-syntheses, and mixed-methods systematic reviews of research evidence.
5. Describe the models used to promote evidence-based practice in nursing.
6. Apply the Iowa Model of Evidence-Based Practice to make changes in healthcare agencies.
7. Apply the Grove Model to implement national evidence-based guidelines in your practice.
8. Describe the significance of evidence-based practice centers and translational research in developing evidence-based health care.

Research evidence has greatly expanded over the last 30 years as numerous quality studies in nursing and other healthcare disciplines have been conducted and disseminated. These studies are commonly communicated via conferences, journals, and the Internet. The expectations of society and the goals of healthcare systems are the delivery of quality, safe, cost-effective health care to patients, families, and communities (Sherwood & Barnsteiner, 2017; Straus, Glasziou, Richardson, Rosenberg, & Haynes, 2011). To ensure the delivery of quality health care, the care must be based on the current best research evidence available. Over the last 15 years, nursing programs have provided students with knowledge about evidence-based practice (EBP) to encourage graduates to base their practice on current research. The emphasis on EBP in nursing education programs and clinical agencies has improved outcomes for patients and families, nurses, and healthcare agencies (Mackey & Bassendowski, 2017; Melnyk, Gallagher-Ford, & Fineout-Overholt, 2017).

Evidence-based practice (EBP) is an important theme in this text that was defined in Chapter 1 as the integration of the best research evidence with nurses' clinical expertise and patients' circumstances and values in the delivery of quality, safe, and cost-effective health care (Straus et al., 2011). **Best research evidence** is produced by the conduct and synthesis of numerous high-quality studies in a selected health-related area. This chapter builds on previous EBP discussions in this text to provide you with strategies for implementing the best research evidence in your practice and moving the nursing profession toward EBP.

The benefits and challenges associated with EBP are described to increase your understanding of evidence-based nursing practice. A format is provided for developing clinical questions to direct your searches for existing research-based evidence to use in practice. Guidelines are provided for critically appraising research syntheses (systematic reviews, meta-analyses, meta-syntheses, and mixed-methods systematic reviews) to determine the knowledge that is ready for use in practice. Two nursing models that have been developed to facilitate EBP in healthcare agencies are introduced. Expert researchers, clinicians, and consumers—through government agencies, professional organizations, and healthcare agencies—have developed an extensive number of evidence-based guidelines. A framework for reviewing the quality of these evidence-based guidelines and for using them in practice is provided. This chapter concludes with a discussion of the nationally designated EBP centers and translational research implemented to promote evidence-based health care.

BENEFITS AND CHALLENGES RELATED TO EVIDENCE-BASED NURSING PRACTICE

EBP is a goal for the nursing profession and each practicing nurse. At the present time, some nursing interventions are evidence-based, but many interventions require additional research to generate essential knowledge for making changes in practice. Some clinical agencies are supportive of the EBP process, and others are not. This section identifies some of the benefits and challenges associated with implementing evidence-based nursing.

Benefits of Evidence-Based Nursing Practice

The greatest benefits of EBP are improved outcomes for patients, providers, and healthcare agencies (Melnyk et al., 2016; Moorhead, Johnson, Maas, & Swanson, 2013). Agencies and organizations nationally and internationally have promoted the synthesis of the best research evidence in thousands of healthcare areas by teams of expert researchers and clinicians. These research syntheses, such as systematic reviews and meta-analyses, have provided the basis for developing strong evidence-based guidelines for practice. These guidelines identify the best treatment plan, or the gold standard for patient care, in selected areas to improve patient outcomes. Students and clinical nurses have electronic access to numerous evidence-based guidelines to assist them in making the best clinical decisions for their patients. These evidence-based syntheses and guidelines are available nationally and internationally and can be easily accessed online through different institutions, such as the National Guideline Clearinghouse (NGC, 2017a) in the United States, the Cochrane Collaboration (2017) in the United Kingdom, and the Joanna Briggs Institute (2017) in Australia.

Some chief nurse executives (CNEs) and healthcare agencies are highly supportive of EBP, as indicated by their attitudes and provision of resources to support EBP (Melnyk, Fineout-Overholt, Giggleman, & Choy 2017). Leaders in these clinical agencies recognize that EBP promotes quality outcomes, improves nurses' satisfaction, and facilitates achievement of accreditation requirements. In a national study of CNEs, Melnyk et al. (2016) found that an organization with an EBP culture of conducting and using research evidence in practice had substantial improvements in several patient outcomes. The Joint Commission (2017) revised their accreditation criteria to emphasize patient care outcomes achieved through EBP.

Many CNEs and chief nursing officers (CNOs) are trying to obtain or maintain Magnet status, which documents the excellence of nursing care in healthcare agencies. Approval for Magnet status is obtained through the American Nurses Credentialing Center (ANCC), and the national and international healthcare agencies that currently have Magnet status can be viewed online (ANCC, 2017). The Magnet Recognition Program® emphasizes EBP as a way to improve the quality of patient care and revitalize the nursing environment. Clinical agencies seeking or maintaining Magnet status must document research-related outcomes, including nursing studies conducted and professional publications and presentations by nurses. For each study, the title of the study, principal investigator or investigators, role of nurses in the study, and study status need to be documented in Magnet applications and reports (ANCC, 2017).

The Quality and Safety Education for Nurses (QSEN, 2017) project was implemented to improve prelicensure nurses' "knowledge, skills, and attitudes (KSAs) that are necessary to continuously improve the quality and safety of the healthcare systems within which they work." QSEN competencies were developed in six areas essential for students and registered nurses' (RNs) practice: patient-centered care, teamwork and collaboration, EBP, quality improvement (QI), safety, and informatics. EBP is an important area in your prelicensure education, and educators are assisting students in achieving the following EBP competencies:

- Participate effectively in appropriate data collection and other research activities.
- Adhere to institutional review board (IRB) guidelines.
- Base individualized care plan on patient values, clinical expertise, and evidence.
- Read original research and evidence reports related to area of practice.
- Locate evidence reports related to clinical practice topics and guidelines.
- Participate in structuring the work environment to facilitate the integration of new evidence into standards of practice.
- Question rationale for routine approaches to care that result in less than desired outcomes or adverse events.
- Consult with clinical experts before deciding to deviate from evidence-based protocols (QSEN, 2017).

Educators have changed nursing curricula to include EBP content and added courses that have improved students' perceptions and confidence in research and EBP (Keib, Cailor, Kiersma, & Chen, 2017). Warren et al. (2016, p. 15) found that "younger RNs with fewer years in practice were more likely to have positive beliefs toward EBP and embedding it into the organization culture." In working toward EBP, students and practicing RNs are encouraged to embrace the benefits of EBP; critically appraise current research evidence; refine agency protocols, algorithms (clinical decision trees), and policies based on current research; use evidence-based guidelines that are available; and collect data as needed for research projects.

Challenges to Evidence-Based Nursing Practice

Challenges to the EBP movement in nursing have been practical and conceptual. One of the most serious concerns is the limited research evidence available regarding the effectiveness of many nursing interventions. EBP requires synthesizing research evidence from randomized controlled trials (RCTs) and other types of intervention studies, which are still limited in nursing. Systematic reviews and meta-analyses conducted in nursing also are limited when compared with other disciplines, such as medicine and psychology (Cochrane Collaboration, 2017; Gray, Grove, & Sutherland, 2017; NGC, 2017b).

Another challenge is that research evidence is generated based on population data and then is applied in practice to individual patients. Sometimes it is difficult to transfer research knowledge to individual patients, who respond in unique ways or have unique circumstances and values. More work is needed to promote the use of evidence-based guidelines with individual patients. In response to this concern, the National Institutes of Health (NIH, 2017) is supporting translational research (discussed later in this chapter) to improve the use of research evidence with different patient populations in various settings. Patients who have poor outcomes when managed according to an evidence-based guideline need to be reported and, if possible, their circumstances should be published as a case study. Electronic health records (EHRs) make it more feasible to determine patient outcomes of care that have been delivered using EBP guidelines.

Another serious challenge is that some healthcare agencies and administrators do not provide the resources or support necessary for nurses to implement EBP. In their national study, Melnyk and colleagues (2016, p. 9) reported, "Although the CNEs and CNOs stated that their highest priorities were quality and safety, EBP was not listed as a top priority and very little of their budgets were allocated to implementing and sustaining evidence-based care." Lack of support and resources for EBP included: (1) inadequate access to research journals and other sources of synthesized research findings and evidence-based guidelines; (2) inadequate knowledge or mentoring on how to implement evidence-based changes in practice; (3) heavy workload, with limited time to make research-based changes in practice; (4) limited authority to change patient care based on research findings; (5) limited support from nursing administrators or medical staff to make evidence-based changes in practice; (6) limited funds to support research projects and research-based changes in practice; and (7) minimal rewards for providing evidence-based care to patients and families (Eizenberg, 2010; Melnyk et al., 2016; Melnyk et al., 2017; Straka, Brandt, & Brytus, 2013; Warren et al., 2016). The success of EBP is determined by all involved, including healthcare agencies, administrators, nurses, physicians, and other healthcare professionals. The following content was developed to assist students and RNs in facilitating evidence-based nursing practice.

DEVELOPING CLINICAL QUESTIONS TO SEARCH FOR EXISTING RESEARCH-BASED EVIDENCE FOR USE IN PRACTICE

Developing a clinical question in an area of interest and conducting an extensive search of evidence-based sources is an effective way to identify current evidence for use in practice. The clinical question often is developed using the PICO format, which includes the following elements:

P – population or participants of interest in your clinical setting
I – intervention needed for practice
C – comparisons of interventions to determine the best intervention for your practice
O– outcomes needed for practice and ways to measure the outcomes in your practice

The PICO format helps you organize the search for research evidence in a variety of databases and websites. You can identify research syntheses (systematic reviews, meta-analyses, meta-syntheses, and mixed-methods systematic reviews); evidence-based guidelines, protocols, and algorithms; and individual studies through searches of electronic databases, national library sites, and EBP organizations and collections. Some of the key resources for EBP are identified in Table 13.1. At least 2500 new systematic reviews are reported in English and indexed in the Medical Literature Analysis and Retrieval System Online (MEDLINE) each year. The Cochrane Collaboration (2017) library of systematic reviews is an excellent resource, with more than 11,000 entries relevant to nursing and health care. In 2009, the Cochrane Nursing Care (CNC) Field was developed to support the conduct, dissemination, and use of systematic reviews in nursing. The CNC Field produces the *Cochrane Corner* columns (summaries of *Cochrane Reviews* relevant to nursing care) that are regularly published in collaborating nursing care–related journals (CNC, 2017). The Joanna Briggs Institute (2017) also provides resources for locating and conducting research syntheses in nursing. The Nursing Reference Center (NRC) includes evidence-based care sheets for numerous nursing interventions and clinical conditions (see Table 13.1).

TABLE 13.1 EVIDENCE-BASED PRACTICE RESOURCES

RESOURCE	DESCRIPTION
Electronic Databases	
CINAHL (Cumulative Index to Nursing and Allied Health Literature)	CINAHL is an authoritative resource covering the English language journal literature for nursing and allied health. The database was developed in the United States and includes sources published from 1982 to the present.
MEDLINE (PubMed, National Library of Medicine)	MEDLINE was developed by the National Library of Medicine in the United States; it provides access to more than 11 million MEDLINE citations back to the mid-1960s and to additional life science journals.
MEDLINE with MeSH	Also developed by the National Library of Medicine, MEDLINE with MeSH provides authoritative medical information on medicine, nursing, dentistry, veterinary medicine, the healthcare system, preclinical services, and more.
PsycINFO	The American Psychological Association developed this database that includes professional and academic literature for psychology and related disciplines from 1887 to the present.
CANCERLIT	CANCERLIT, containing information on cancer, was developed by the National Cancer Institute in the United States.
National Library Sites	
Cochrane Library	The Cochrane Library provides high-quality evidence for those providing and receiving health care and those involved in research, teaching, funding, and administration of health care at all levels. Included is the Cochrane Collaboration, which has many systematic reviews of research (http://www.cochrane.org/evidence).
National Library of Health (NLH)	The NLH, located in the United Kingdom, provides searchable evidence-based sources at http://www.evidence.nhs.uk.

Continued

TABLE 13.1 EVIDENCE-BASED PRACTICE RESOURCES—cont'd

RESOURCE	DESCRIPTION
Evidence-Based Practice Organizations and Collections	
National Guideline Clearinghouse (NGC)	The Agency for Healthcare Research and Quality (AHRQ) developed the NGC to house the thousands of evidence-based guidelines that have been developed for use in clinical practice; these can be accessed online at http://www.guidelines.gov.
Cochrane Nursing Care (CNC) Field	The Cochrane Collaboration includes over 8000 reviews in 11 different fields; one is the CNC, which supports the conduct, dissemination, and use of systematic reviews in nursing. Most libraries subscribe to the Cochrane Collaboration but free access to abstracts and reviews can be found at http://cncf.cochrane.org.
National Institute for Health and Clinical Excellence (NICE)	The NICE was organized in the United Kingdom to provide access to current evidence-based guidelines, similar to the NGC (http://nice.org.uk).
Joanna Briggs Institute (JBI)	JBI, an international evidence-based organization originating in Australia, has a search website that includes evidence summaries, systematic reviews, systematic review protocols, evidence-based recommendations for practice, best practice information sheets, consumer information sheets, and technical reports; see "Search the Joanna Briggs Institute" (http://www.joannabriggs.org).
Nursing Reference Center (NRC)	The NRC includes a collection of rigorously reviewed, evidence-based care sheets that provide current best practice for over 700 interventions and clinical conditions. This source requires a subscription, so check with your librarian. You can access this resource at http://www.ebscohost.com/nursing.

Evidence Focused on Aspiration During Intramuscular Injections

You might pose a clinical question about whether nurses should aspirate or not when giving intramuscular (IM) injections. Using the PICO format you can identify the evidence needed for practice.

P – populations: infants, toddlers, children, and adults receiving immunizations by the IM route for prophylactic purposes.

I – intervention: IM injection given without aspiration in the right site based on the volume of medication and age of patient (Ogston-Tuck, 2014; Sisson, 2015; Thomas, Mraz, & Rajcan, 2016; Wynaden et al., 2015).

C – comparison intervention: IM injection given with 5 to 10 seconds of aspiration in all sites, regardless of the age of the patient and the volume of medication (Cocoman & Murray, 2008; Nicoll & Hesby, 2002).

O – outcome: IM injection of vaccine without complications.

Older evidence-based guidelines by Nicoll and Hesby (2002) and Cocoman and Murray (2008) recommended aspiration for 5 to 10 seconds with each IM injection to prevent injecting substances directly into a patient's bloodstream. However, a systematic review by Sisson (2015) recommended no aspiration with IM injections given in the deltoid, ventrogluteal, and vastus lateralis sites. Nurses should only aspirate when giving IM injections in the dorsogluteal site because of the close proximity of the gluteal artery. However, researchers recommended that the dorsogluteal site not be used, if possible (Ogston-Tuck, 2014; Sisson, 2015; Wynaden et al., 2015). The current research evidence regarding aspiration during IM injections is summarized in Box 13.1. However, many nurses are

BOX 13.1 CLINICAL PRACTICE GUIDELINE: INTRAMUSCULAR INJECTIONS WITHOUT ASPIRATION

Patient Population
Infants, toddlers, children, and adults receiving immunizations by the IM route for prophylactic purposes

Objective
Administration of IM immunizations to eliminate patient injury and discomfort

Intervention: IM Injection
Site selection based on the age of the patient
(Nicoll & Hesby, 2002; Ogston-Tuck, 2014; Sisson, 2015; Wynaden et al., 2015):
- Infants – vastus lateralis is the preferred site
- Toddlers and children – vastus lateralis or deltoid sites
- Adults – ventrogluteal or deltoid sites

Medication volume
(Nicoll & Hesby, 2002; Sisson, 2015; Wynaden et al., 2015)
- Small volumes of medication (≤2 mL) may be given in the deltoid site for toddlers, children, and adults and in the vastus lateralis for infants.
- Large volumes of medication (2–5 mL) should be given in the ventrogluteal site for adults. Volume must be limited and injected in the vastus lateralis for infants, toddlers, and children.

Injection without and with aspiration
- Cleanse the site with alcohol and allow it to dry.
- Insert the needle into the appropriate site.
  - There should be *no aspiration* with deltoid, ventrogluteal, and vastus lateralis sites (Sisson, 2015; Thomas et al., 2016; Wynaden et al., 2015).
  - Aspirate for 5 to 10 seconds when using the dorsogluteal site because of the proximity to the gluteal artery, but current research recommends not to use this site (Sisson, 2015; Stringer, 2010; Thomas et al., 2016; Wynaden et al., 2015).
- Inject medication slowly.
- Withdraw needle slowly; apply gentle pressure with a dry sponge.

Outcome
- Assess site for complications, immediately and 2 to 4 hours later, if possible.
- Record the number and type of complications: pain, redness, and/or warmth.
- Properly and promptly dispose of all equipment.

IM, Intramuscular.
Adapted from Nicoll, L. H., & Hesby, A. (2002). Intramuscular injections: An integrative research review and guideline for evidence-based practice. *Applied Nursing Research, 16*(2), 149–162; Ogston-Tuck, S. (2014). Intramuscular injection technique: An evidence-based approach. *Nursing Standard, 29*(4), 52–59; Sisson, H. (2015). Aspirating during the intramuscular injection procedure: A systematic literature review. *Journal of Clinical Nursing, 24*(17/18) 2368–2375; Stringer, P. M. (2010). Sciatic nerve injury from intramuscular injections: A persistent and global problem. *International Journal of Clinical Practice, 64*(11), 1573–1579; Thomas, C. M., Mraz, M., & Rajcan, L. (2016). Blood aspiration during IM injection. *Clinical Nursing Research, 25*(5), 549–559; Wynaden, D., Tohotoa, J., Omari, O. A., Happell, B., Heslop, K., Barr, L., & Sourinathan, V. (2015). Administering intramuscular injections: How does research translate into practice over time in the mental health setting? *Nurse Education Today, 35*(1), 620–624.

not using this current research evidence about IM injections in practice. Thomas et al. (2016) found that 74% of the nurses were still aspirating after IM injections 90% of the time. Wynaden et al. (2015) found a higher use of the dorsogluteal site, even though current research recommends use of the ventrogluteal site. Therefore these researchers recommended additional education in nursing programs and continuing education that ensure nurses are knowledgeable about and use the most current research evidence in practice.

CRITICALLY APPRAISING RESEARCH SYNTHESES: SYSTEMATIC REVIEWS AND META-ANALYSES

Research evidence is usually synthesized using systematic review, meta-analysis, meta-synthesis, and mixed-methods systematic review (Whittemore, Chao, Jang, Minges, & Park, 2014). As noted earlier, Sisson (2015) conducted a systematic review to synthesize research related to IM injections and recommended that nurses not aspirate when giving most IM injections (see Box 13.1). Nursing students and RNs must be able to review research syntheses and determine the evidence to use in practice. This section provides guidelines for understanding and critically appraising systematic reviews and meta-analyses.

Critically Appraising Systematic Reviews

A systematic review is a structured, comprehensive synthesis of the research literature to determine the best research evidence available to address a healthcare question or problem. A systematic review involves identifying, locating, appraising, and synthesizing quality research evidence for clinicians to use in practice (Bettany-Saltikov, 2010a, 2010b; Cooper, 2017; Liberati et al., 2009; Moher, Liberati, Tezlaff, Altman, & PRISMA Group, 2009; Setia, 2016). Systematic reviews are often conducted by two or more researchers and/or expert clinicians in a selected healthcare area to determine the best research knowledge in that area.

Systematic reviews should include rigorous research methodology to promote the accuracy of the findings and minimize the reviewers' bias. Table 13.2 provides a checklist for critically appraising the steps or elements of systematic reviews and meta-analyses. These steps are based on the Preferred Reporting Items for Systematic Reviews and Meta-Analyses (PRISMA) statement (Liberati et al., 2009; Moher et al., 2009). The PRISMA statement was developed in 2009 by an international group of expert researchers and clinicians to improve the quality of reporting for systematic reviews and meta-analyses. It includes 27 items, which can be found at http://prisma-statement.org and are detailed in the articles by Liberati et al. (2009) and Moher et al. (2009). These 27 items were consolidated into the checklist in Table 13.2 to assist you in critically appraising systematic reviews and meta-analyses.

The systematic review by Holmen, Wahl, Småstuen, and Ribu (2017), which focused on the use of mobile apps for feedback between patients with diabetes and healthcare professionals, is presented as an example. You can find this systematic review online in the Cumulative Index to Nursing and Allied Health Literature (CINAHL) database (see Table 13.1). We recommend that you read this article and use the guidelines in Table 13.2 to critically appraise this systematic review and compare your findings with the following discussion.

Step 1: Did the title indicate if a systematic review or meta-analysis was conducted?

Holmen et al. (2017, e227) identified the type of research synthesis that they conducted in their report title: "Tailored communication within mobile apps for diabetes self-management: A systematic review."

TABLE 13.2 **CHECKLIST FOR CRITICALLY APPRAISING PUBLISHED SYSTEMATIC REVIEWS AND META-ANALYSES**

SYSTEMATIC REVIEW STEPS OR ELEMENTS	STEP COMPLETE? (YES OR NO)	COMMENTS: QUALITY AND RATIONALE
1. Did the title indicate that a systematic review, meta-analysis, or both were conducted?		
2. Was an abstract included that provided a structured summary of purpose, data sources, study eligibility criteria, study appraisal and synthesis methods, participants, interventions, outcomes, key findings, conclusions, and/or implications for practice?		
3. Was the clinical question clearly expressed and significant? Was the PICOS format (***p***articipants, ***i***ntervention, ***c***omparative interventions, ***o***utcomes, and ***s***tudy design) used to develop the question and focus the systematic review or meta-analysis?		
4. Were the purpose and/or objectives or aims of the research synthesis clearly expressed and used to direct it?		
5. Were the search criteria clearly identified? Were the years covered, language, and publication status of sources identified in the search criteria?		
6. Was a comprehensive, systematic search of the literature conducted using explicit criteria identified in step 5? Were the search strategies clearly reported with examples? Did the search include published studies, grey literature, and unpublished studies?		
7. Was the process for selecting studies for the review clearly identified and consistently implemented? Was the selection process expressed in a flow diagram?		
8. Were the publication biases addressed, such as time lag bias, location bias, duplicate publication bias, citation bias, and language bias?		
9. Were key elements (population, sampling process, design, intervention, outcomes, and results) of each study clearly discussed and presented in a table?		
10. Was a quality critical appraisal of the studies conducted? Were the results related to participants, types of interventions, outcomes, and outcome measurement methods clearly presented in tables and narrative? Were the risks for methodological and outcome reporting biases addressed for the studies?		
11. Was a meta-analysis conducted as part of the systematic review? Was a rationale provided for conducting the meta-analysis? Were the details of the meta-analysis process and results clearly described?		

Continued

TABLE 13.2 CHECKLIST FOR CRITICALLY APPRAISING PUBLISHED SYSTEMATIC REVIEWS AND META-ANALYSES—cont'd

SYSTEMATIC REVIEW STEPS OR ELEMENTS	STEP COMPLETE? (YES OR NO)	COMMENTS: QUALITY AND RATIONALE
12. Were the results of the systematic review or meta-analysis clearly described (i.e., in a narrative and table)? Were details of the study interventions compared and contrasted in a table? Were the outcome variables clearly identified and the quality of the measurement methods addressed?		
13. Did the report conclude with a clear discussion section? a. Were the review findings summarized to identify the current best research evidence? b. Were the limitations of the review and how they might have affected the findings addressed? c. Were the recommendations for further research and practice addressed?		
14. Did the authors of the review develop a clear, concise, quality report for publication? Was the report inclusive of the items identified in the PRISMA statement in this table?		

PRISMA, Preferred Reporting Items for Systematic Reviews and Meta-Analyses.
Adapted from Liberati, A., Altman, D. G., Tetzlaff, J., Mulrow, C., Gotzsche, P. C., Ioannidis, J. P., et al. (2009). The PRISMA Statement for reporting systematic reviews and meta-analyses of studies that evaluate healthcare interventions: Explanation and elaboration. *Annals of Internal Medicine, 151*(4), W-65–W-94; and Moher, D., Liberati, A., Tetzlaff, J., Altman, D. G., & PRISMA Group. (2009). *Preferred Reporting Items for Systematic Reviews and Meta-Analyses: The PRISMA Statement.* http://www.prisma-statement.org.

Step 2: Did the abstract include a structured summary of the research synthesis?

Holmen et al. (2017) provided a clear, concise abstract that was structured by the following headings: background, objective, methods, results, and conclusions of the review.

Step 3: Was a significant, clear clinical question developed to direct the research synthesis?

A systemic review or meta-analysis is best directed by a relevant clinical question that focuses the review process and promotes the development of a quality synthesis of research evidence. The PICOS format is most commonly used to develop clinical questions for research syntheses. The **PICOS format** (similar to the PICO format introduced earlier) is included in the PRISMA Statement (Moher et al., 2009) with the following elements:

P – population or participants of interest (see Chapter 9 on sampling)
I – intervention needed for practice (see Chapter 8 on nursing interventions)
C – comparisons of the intervention with control, placebo, standard care, variations of the same intervention, or different therapies (see Chapter 8)
O – outcomes needed for practice (see Chapter 10 on measurement methods and Chapter 14 on outcomes research)
S – study design (see Chapter 8 on types of study designs)

Holmen et al. (2017) did not provide a clinical question to direct their systematic review but they did provide a strong background for the review. The researchers reported that "About 415 million people have diabetes globally, and management of diabetes and its complications remains a global health emergency that already accounts for 12% of global health expenditures… The mobile health (mHealth) literature indicates that individuals using mobile apps for self-management achieve positive health outcomes" (Holmen et al., 2017, e227.1). The ideas from the report are summarized using the PICOS format:

P – population: patients diagnosed with diabetes
I – intervention: communication and tailored feedback using mobile apps between patients and healthcare professionals
C – comparisons of the intervention with controls and usual care
O – outcomes examined included hemoglobin A1c (HbA1c), blood pressure, satisfaction with mobile app
S – study designs: quasi-experimental and experimental clinical trials

Step 4: Were the purpose and/or the objectives or aims of the review expressed?

Systematic reviews of research might include a purpose or sometimes specific aims or objectives to guide the synthesis process (Bettany-Saltikov, 2010a; Moher et al., 2009; Setia, 2016). Holmen et al. (2017, e227.1) reported:

> *To the best of our knowledge, results based on apps with integrated and tailored communication alone have not been systematically summarized. This review aims to address the knowledge gap by systematically reviewing studies that aimed to evaluate integrated communication within mobile apps for tailored feedback between patient with diabetes and HCP [health care providers] in terms of (1) study characteristics, (2) functions, (3) study outcomes, (4) effects, and (5) methodological quality.*

Step 5: Was the literature search criteria clearly identified?

Research reports of systematic reviews or meta-analyses need to identify the inclusion and exclusion criteria used to direct the literature search (see Table 13.2). The PICOS format might be used to develop the search criteria with more detail being developed for each of the elements. These search criteria might focus on the following: (1) type of research methods, quantitative, qualitative, or mixed methods; (2) population or type of study participants; (3) study designs, such as quasi-experimental and experimental; (4) sampling processes, such as probability or nonprobability sampling methods; (5) intervention and comparison interventions; and (6) specific outcomes to be measured. The search criteria also need to indicate the years for the review, language, and publication status of the studies to be included (Bettany-Saltikov, 2010b; Higgins & Green, 2008).

Holmen et al. (2017) reported specific eligibility criteria for their literature search. The studies included in the review had to test a mobile app with communication between patients with diabetes and their HCPs. The studies had to include a control or usual care group and have a quasi-experimental or experimental design. Studies that focused on primary prevention of diabetes or that included participants with gestational diabetes were excluded.

Step 6: Was a comprehensive, systematic search of the research literature conducted?

The key search terms, different databases searched, and search results should be recorded in the systematic review and meta-analysis publications. Sometimes authors provide a table that identifies the search terms and criteria. The PRISMA statement recommends presenting the full electronic search strategy used for at least one major database, such as CINAHL or MEDLINE (Liberati et al., 2009).

Often, searches are limited to published sources in common databases, which excludes the grey literature from the research synthesis. **Grey literature** refers to studies that have limited distributions, such as theses and dissertations, unpublished research reports, articles in obscure journals, articles in some online journals, conference papers and abstracts, conference proceedings, research reports to funding agencies, and technical reports (Conn, Valentine, Cooper, & Rantz, 2003). Most grey literature is difficult to access through database searches and is often not peer-reviewed, with limited referencing information. These are some of the main reasons why grey literature is not included in systematic reviews and meta-analyses. However, excluding grey literature from any type of research synthesis might result in misleading biased results (Pappas & Williams, 2011).

Holmen et al. (2017) detailed their search strategy for their systematic review that included an extensive number of databases and other sources. They provided an example of the search strategy that was applied in MEDLINE. However, there was no mention of including grey literature in the review, which could have biased the findings. The literature search strategy is briefly presented in the following quote:

> *A systematic literature search was conducted according to the PRISMA guidelines (Moher et al., 2009). Medical literature published from January 2008 was searched in January 2016, with an updated search closed on September 23, 2016, using Medical Literature Analysis and Retrieval System Online (MEDLINE), PubMed, Cumulative Index to Nursing and Allied Health Literature (CINAHL), Excerpta Medica database (EMBASE), ClinicalTrials.gov, and the World Health Organization (WHO) International Clinical Trials Registry Platform. We reviewed reference lists of relevant reviews and studies, and we also conducted hand searches in relevant journals of the field in addition to studies based on tips from colleagues in the field.... we organized a search strategy consisting of the terms mobile applications, cell phones, mobile phones... diabetes mellitus... diabetes mellitus type 2.... We did not set a language limitation; however we did set a limitation on publication year... as we decided technologies prior to 2008 were unlikely to be mobile apps."*
>
> ***Holmen et al., 2017, e227.3***

Step 7: Was the process for selecting the studies for review detailed?

The selection of studies for inclusion in a systematic review or meta-analysis is a complex process that initially involves the review and removal of duplicate sources. The abstracts of the remaining studies are reviewed by two or more authors and sometimes by an external reviewer to ensure that they meet the criteria identified in step 5 (see Table 13.2). The abstracts might be excluded based on the study participants, interventions, outcomes, or design not meeting the search criteria (Bettany-Saltikov, 2010b). The study selection process is best demonstrated by a flow diagram that was developed by the PRISMA Group (Moher et al., 2009). Holmen et al. (2017) provided a detailed description of the process they used to select studies for review. The selection process was documented using a flow diagram that identified the six studies included in the review. The following quote briefly presents the study selection process.

> ***Study Selection***
>
> *Two reviewers (HH and LR [authors]) independently reviewed all the titles and/or abstracts from the search. We applied our inclusion and exclusion criteria set a priori. For possibly eligible*

studies, a full text copy was retrieved and reviewed independently by HH and LR. Discrepancies were resolved by discussion or with the involvement of a third reviewer (AKW)....

A total of 2822 papers were identified during the search (Fig. 1). After the removal of 1694 duplicates, the remaining 1128 citations were screened through title and/or abstract, and we removed 913 citations because they clearly did not meet our inclusion criteria. The full text of the remaining 215 citations was then obtained to clarify their study details, and we contacted 22 authors to clarify that their intervention consisted of an app with integrated and tailored communication... After the termination of the search, 6 citations were included in this review.

Holmen et al., 2017, e227.4–5

Fig. 1 documents the selection process that was used to determine the studies included in Holmen et al.'s (2017) review. This diagram included the four phases identified by the PRIMA Statement (Moher et al., 2009): (1) identification of the sources; (2) screening of the sources based on set criteria; (3) determining if the sources meet eligibility requirements; and (4) identifying the studies included in the review.

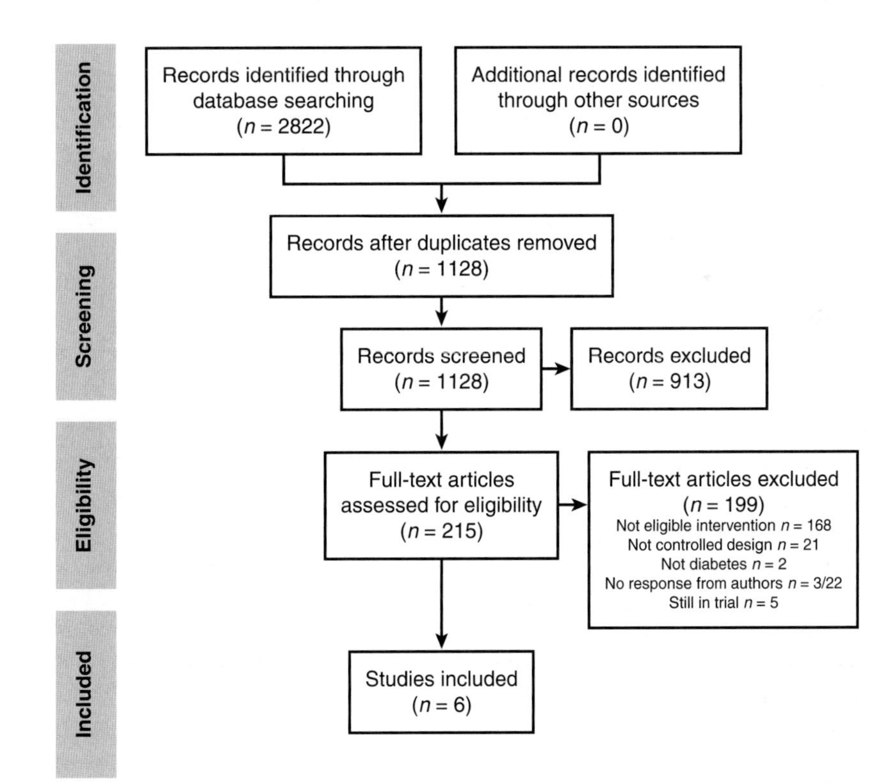

FIG 1 Flowchart. (From Holmen, H., Wahl, A. K., Småstuen, M. C., & Ribu, L. [2017]. Tailored communication within mobile apps for diabetes self-management: A systematic review. *Journal of Medical Internet Research, 19*[6], e227.)

Step 8: Were publication biases addressed?

Even with rigorous literature searches, authors of meta-analyses and systematic reviews are often limited to mainly published studies. The nature of the sources can lead to biases and flawed or inaccurate conclusions in the research syntheses. The common publication biases that can occur in conducting and reporting research syntheses include time lag bias, location bias, duplicate publication bias, citation bias, and language bias. Publication bias occurs because studies with positive results are more likely to be published than studies with negative or inconclusive results. Higgins and Green (2008) found that the odds were four times greater that positive study results would be published versus negative results. **Time lag bias of studies,** a type of publication bias, occurs because studies with negative results are usually published later, sometimes 2 to 3 years later, than studies with positive results. Sometimes, studies with negative results are not published at all, whereas studies with positive results might be published more than once (**duplicate publication bias**). **Location bias of studies** can occur if studies are published in lower impact journals and indexed in less searched databases. A **citation bias** occurs when certain studies are cited more often than others and are more likely to be identified in database searches. **Language bias** can occur if searches focus just on studies in English, and important studies exist in other languages. Holmen et al.'s (2017) systematic review had the potential for publication bias because grey literature was not addressed. However, language was not a limitation of this review, and duplicate abstracts were removed to prevent duplication bias. The time frame of the search was strong based on the topic of mobile apps.

Step 9: Were key elements of the studies presented?

Key elements of studies in systematic reviews and meta-analyses are best identified by constructing a table describing the characteristics of the included studies, such as the purposes of the studies, populations, sampling processes, interventions, outcomes, and results (Bettany-Saltikov, 2010b; Liberati et al., 2009). Holmen et al. (2017) developed three tables to document key information from the six studies they reviewed. One table summarized the study characteristics such as authors, year of publication, country where the study was published, randomization to groups, and attrition of study participants. The studies were from six different countries, and four were RCTs. A second table presented the designs of the studies, and a third table summarized the characteristics of the study participants.

Step 10: Were the studies critically appraised and the risks for biases described?

Two or more experts need to review the studies independently and make judgments about their quality. The critical appraisal of the studies is often difficult because of the differences in types of participants, designs, sampling methods, interventions, outcome variables and measurement methods, and presentation of results. The studies are often rank-ordered based on their quality and contribution to the development of the review (Bettany-Saltikov 2010b; Liberati et al., 2009). Holmen et al. (2017) conducted the Cochrane methodology for risk of systematic bias (ROB) to score each study (Higgins & Green, 2008). The ROB was performed individually by three of the researchers and the scores were discussed to achieve consensus.

Holmen et al. (2017) also provided a detailed discussion and tables to identify the risks for methodological and outcome reporting biases in the studies reviewed. **Methodological bias** is often related to design and data analysis problems in studies. For example, studies might have limitations related to the sample, intervention, outcome measurements, and analysis techniques that result in methodological bias. The following methodological biases were reported for the six studies reviewed by Holmen et al. (2017): (1) varied mobile apps (interventions) implemented; (2) limited blinding of personnel and participants to group assignment; and (3) insufficiently reported randomization procedures. **Outcome reporting bias** occurs when study results are not reported clearly and with complete accuracy. For example, reporting bias occurs when researchers selectively report positive results and not negative results, or positive results might be addressed in detail, with limited discussion of negative results. Holmen et al. (2017) reported incomplete outcome data because of attrition in four of the six studies reviewed. Selective reporting of outcomes was noted in five of the studies.

Step 11: Was a meta-analysis conducted as part of the systematic review?

Some authors conduct a meta-analysis in the synthesis of sources for their systematic review (Liberati et al., 2009). Because a meta-analysis involves the use of statistics to summarize results of different studies, it usually provides strong, objective information about the effectiveness of an intervention or solid knowledge about a clinical problem. For example, a meta-analysis might be conducted on a small group of similar studies to determine the effect of an intervention. The systematic review conducted by Holmen et al. (2017) did not include a meta-analysis because the studies lack rigorous methodological quality to be combined in a meta-analysis.

Step 12: Were the results of the review clearly presented?

The results of a systematic review and meta-analysis should include a description of the study participants, types of interventions implemented in the studies, outcomes measured, and measurement methods. The results of the different types of intervention might be best summarized in a table that includes the following: (1) study source; (2) structure of the intervention (standalone or multifaceted); (3) specific type of intervention (e.g., physiological treatment, education, counseling, behavioral therapy); (4) delivery method (e.g., demonstration and return demonstration, verbal, video, self-administered); (5) length of time the intervention is implemented; and (6) statistical differences between the intervention and control, standard care, placebo, or alternative intervention groups (Liberati et al., 2009).

The systematic review by Holmen et al. (2017) focused on the intervention of communication between patients and HCPs using mobile apps. The six studies reviewed included mobile apps of various forms and functions, which were summarized in a table. The following comments were made about the apps' capabilities: "The feedback used was either automatic or manual… and 4 apps also offered direct messages from the patient in free text… A total of 2 apps had critical alerts sent to the patients if their entered readings were outside present thresholds" (Holmen et al., 2017, e227. 6).

The outcomes, including primary and secondary outcomes, of the reviewed studies are best summarized in a table. This table might include: (1) the study source; (2) outcome variable(s), with an indication as to whether it was a primary or secondary outcome in the study; (3) measurement method used for each study outcome variable; and (4) quality of the measurement methods, such as the reliability and validity of a scale or the precision and accuracy of a physiological measure. Holmen et al. (2017) summarized the primary and secondary outcomes from their review in a table and noted that the primary and secondary outcomes varied for the six studies. The HbA1c was a primary outcome in four studies, and only two studies reported a significant decrease in the HbA1c. Blood pressure (BP) was a primary outcome for three studies, but two trials did not measure BP. Secondary outcomes regarding knowledge of diabetes and usability and satisfaction with mobile apps were inconsistently measured and reported, so no conclusions could be drawn.

Step 13: Did the report conclude with a clear discussion section?

In a systematic review or meta-analysis, the discussion of the findings includes an overall evaluation of the types of interventions implemented and the outcomes measured. You can also expect the methodological issues or limitations of the review to be addressed. Finally, the discussion section needs to provide conclusions and recommendations for further research and practice (Bettany-Saltikov, 2010b; Higgins & Green, 2008; Liberati et al., 2009).

Holmen et al. (2017) provided a discussion of their findings, limitations, and recommendations for research and practice. Overall, the methodological problems of these studies provided varied results and limited conclusive findings about the use of mobile apps that are not ready to guide practice.

> ***Conclusion***
> *The conclusions from this systematic review are limited. The unclear and poor methodological quality of this emerging research field is of major concern, and although 3 studies found that apps with integrated feedback significantly improve the primary outcome, the evidence has limitations because of its poor methodological quality. Mobile apps will be a part of the health care system in the future; therefore, we require robust research in this area to make the right choices for the patient, for the health care system, and for society.*
>
> ***Holmen et al., 2017, e227.11–12***

Step 14: Was a clear and concise report developed for publication?

The systematic review or meta-analysis report needs to include the content discussed in the previous 13 steps. When critically appraising a systematic review, you can use Table 13.2, to indicate if the step is present, and comment about its quality with supporting rationale. In summary, Holmen et al. (2017) developed a quality systematic review following the PRISMA guidelines for publication. The title clearly indicated the type of synthesis conducted. No clinical question was expressed to direct the review but a background was provided so the PICOS format might be developed. A knowledge gap was identified for nursing practice, and the aim of the review focused on this area. The search of the literature might have been more rigorous and might have included additional studies, especially grey literature. The selection of studies for the synthesis was clearly presented in a flow chart and documented with rationale. The studies selected for the systematic review were critically appraised, and the results from these syntheses were clearly presented in tables and narrative. The publication concluded with appropriate findings, limitations, and recommendations for research and practice.

Critically Appraising Meta-Analyses

A meta-analysis is conducted to pool or combine statistically the results from previous studies into a single quantitative analysis that provides one of the highest levels of evidence about the effectiveness of an intervention (Andrel, Keith, & Leiby, 2009; Cooper, 2017; Liberati et al., 2009). This approach has specific objectivity because it includes analysis techniques to determine the effect of an intervention while examining the influences of variations in the studies included in the meta-analysis. Heterogeneity in the studies included in a meta-analysis can lead to different types of methodological and outcome reporting biases previously discussed. Meta-analyses that include more homogeneous (similar) studies have less bias and usually provide more valid findings (Moore, 2012).

Statistically combining data from several studies results in a large sample size, with increased power to determine the true effect of a specific intervention. The ultimate goal of a meta-analysis is to determine if an intervention: (1) significantly improves outcomes; (2) has minimal or no effect on outcomes; or (3) increases the risk of adverse events. Meta-analysis is also an effective way to resolve conflicting study findings and controversies that may have arisen related to a selected intervention (Higgins & Green, 2008).

Strong evidence for using an intervention in practice can be generated from a meta-analysis of multiple quality studies, such as RCTs and other experimental studies. However, the conduct of a meta-analysis depends on the accuracy, clarity, and completeness of information presented in studies. Box 13.2 provides a list of information that needs to be included in a research report to facilitate the conduct of a meta-analysis. You might use this information as a checklist to determine if the reports of RCTs and other interventional studies are complete.

BOX 13.2 RECOMMENDED REPORTING BY RESEARCHERS TO FACILITATE THE CONDUCT OF META-ANALYSES

Demographic Variables Relevant to Population Studied

- Age
- Gender
- Marital status
- Ethnicity
- Education
- Socioeconomic status

Methodological Characteristics

- Sample size (experimental and control groups)
- Type of sampling method
- Sampling refusal rate and attrition rate
- Sample characteristics
- Research design
- Groups included in study—experimental, control, comparison, placebo groups
- Intervention protocol and fidelity discussion
- Data collection techniques
- Outcome measurements
  - Reliability and validity of instruments
  - Precision and accuracy of physiological measures

Data Analysis

- Names of statistical tests
- Sample size for each statistical test
- Degrees of freedom for each statistical test
- Exact value of each statistical test
- Exact *p* value for each test statistic
- One-tailed or two-tailed statistical test
- Measures of central tendency (mean, median, and mode)
- Measures of dispersion (range, standard deviation)
- Post hoc test values for ANOVA (analysis of variance) test of three or more groups

The steps for critically appraising a meta-analysis are similar to those for critically appraising a systematic review (detailed earlier in Table 13.2). The PRISMA statement (Moher et al., 2009), Cochrane Collaboration guidelines for meta-analysis (Higgins & Green, 2008), and other resources (Andrel et al., 2009; Moore, 2012; Setia, 2016; Turlik, 2010) were used in critically appraising a meta-analysis. Conn's (2010) meta-analysis to determine the effect of physical activity (PA) interventions on depressive symptom outcomes in healthy adults is presented as an example.

Clinical Question Directing a Meta-Analysis

The clinical question developed for a meta-analysis is usually clearly focused: "What is the effectiveness of a selected intervention?" The PICOS (***p***articipants or population, ***i***ntervention, ***c***omparative interventions, ***o***utcomes, and ***s***tudy design) format discussed earlier might be used to generate the clinical question (Moher et al., 2009). Conn (2010) reported that only one previous meta-analysis had examined the effect of PAs on depressive symptoms among study participants without clinical depression. The meta-analysis conducted by Conn focused on the following clinical question: "What is the effect of PA on depressive symptoms in healthy adults?"

Purpose and Questions to Direct a Meta-Analysis

Researchers need to identify the purpose of their meta-analysis and the questions or objectives that guide the analysis. Conn (2010) clearly identified the following relevant purpose and research questions to guide her meta-analysis:

> *This meta-analysis synthesized depressive symptom outcomes of supervised and unsupervised PA interventions among healthy adults.... This meta-analysis addressed the following research questions:*
>
> *(1) What are the overall effects of supervised PA and unsupervised PA interventions on depressive symptoms in healthy adults without clinical depression?*
>
> *(2) Do interventions' effects on depressive symptom outcomes vary depending on intervention, sample, and research design characteristics?*
>
> *(3) What are the effects of interventions on depressive symptoms among studies comparing treatment subjects with before versus after interventions?*
>
> ***Conn, 2010, pp. 128–129***

Search Criteria and Strategies for Meta-Analyses

The search criteria are usually more narrowly focused for a meta-analysis than a systematic review to identify the specific studies examining the effect of a particular intervention. Conn (2010) clearly identified her detailed search strategies in the following excerpt. She used **ancestry searches,** which involves the use of citations from relevant studies to identify additional studies.

> ***Primary Study Search Strategies***
>
> *Multiple search strategies were used to ensure a comprehensive search and thus limit bias while moving beyond previous reviews. An expert reference librarian searched 11 computerized databases (e.g., MEDLINE, PsycINFO, EMBASE) using broad search terms (sample MEDLINE intervention terms: adherence, behavior therapy.... PA terms: exercise, physical activity, physical fitness).... Search terms for depressive symptoms were not used to narrow the search because*

> *many PA intervention studies report depressive symptom outcomes but do not consider these the main outcomes of the study and thus papers are not indexed by these terms.... Computerized author searches were completed for project principal investigators located from research registers and for the first three authors on eligible studies. Author searches were completed for dissertation authors to locate published papers. Ancestry searches were conducted on eligible and review papers. Hand searches were completed for 114 journals which frequently report PA intervention research.*
>
> **Conn, 2010, p. 129**

Possible Biases for Meta-Analyses

Publication, methodological, and outcome reporting biases can weaken the validity of the findings from meta-analyses. An analysis method termed the *funnel plot* can be used to assess for biases in a group of studies. This discussion of funnel plots is very brief but will hopefully provide you with some understanding of the funnel plot diagrams included in most meta-analyses.

Funnel plots provide graphic representations of possible effect sizes (ESs) for interventions in selected studies (see Chapter 9 for the calculation of ES). The ES, or strength of an intervention in a study, can be calculated by determining the difference between the experimental and control groups for the outcome variable. The mean difference between the experimental and control groups for several studies is easier to determine if the outcome variable is measured by the same scale or instrument in each study. However, the standardized mean difference (SMD) must be calculated in a meta-analysis when the same outcome, such as depression, is measured by different scales or methods. More details are provided on SMD later in this section.

Fig. 13.1 shows a hypothetical funnel plot of the SMDs from 13 studies. The studies with small sample sizes are toward the bottom of the graph, and the studies with larger samples are toward the top. The SMDs from the studies are fairly symmetrical or are equally divided by the line through the middle of the funnel in the graph. A symmetrical funnel plot indicates limited publication bias. Asymmetry of the funnel plot is mainly the result of publication bias but also of methodological bias, outcome reporting bias, heterogeneity in the studies' sample sizes and interventions, and chance.

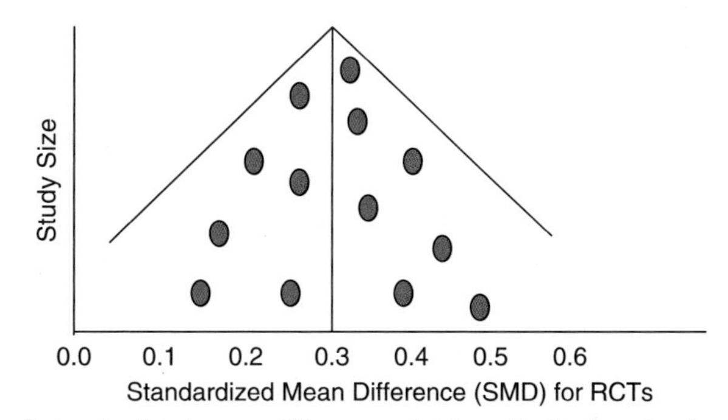

FIG 13.1 Funnel plot of standardized mean differences for hypothetical randomized controlled trials with limited bias. *RCTs*, Randomized controlled trials. (From Gray, J. R., Grove, S. K., & Sutherland, S. [2017]. *The practice of nursing research: Appraisal, synthesis, and generation of evidence* [8th ed.]. St. Louis, MO: Elsevier.)

Conn (2010) provided a quality discussion of her literature search and the bias risks in her meta-analysis. The following quote includes key content related to the search results and the risks of biases:

> *Comprehensive searches yielded 70 reports.... The supervised PA [physical activity] two-group comparison included 1,598 subjects. The unsupervised PA two-group comparison included 1,081 subjects. The treatment single-group comparisons included 1,639 supervised PA and 3,420 unsupervised PA subjects.... Most primary studies were published articles (s = 54), and the remainder were dissertations (s = 14), book chapter (s = 1), and conference presentation materials (s = 1; s indicates the number of reports). Publication bias was evident in the funnel plots for supervised and unsupervised PA two-group outcome comparisons and for treatment group, pre- vs. post-intervention supervised PA and unsupervised PA comparisons.*
>
> ***Conn, 2010, p. 131***

Results of Meta-Analysis

Many nursing studies examine continuous outcomes or outcomes that are measured by methods that produced interval- or ratio-level data. Physiological measures to examine blood pressure produce ratio-level data. Likert scales, such as the Center for Epidemiologic Studies Depression Scale (CES-D), produce interval-level data (see Chapter 10 for a copy of the CES-D). Therefore blood pressure and depression are continuous outcomes. The effect of an intervention on a continuous outcome in a meta-analysis is determined by the mean difference between two groups. The **mean difference** is a standard statistic that identifies the absolute difference between two groups. It is an estimate of the amount of change caused by the intervention (e.g., PA) on the outcome (e.g., depression), on average, compared with the control group. The mean difference is reported in a meta-analysis to identify the effect of an intervention but is appropriate only if the outcome is measured by the same scale in all the studies (Higgins & Green, 2008).

A **standardized mean difference (SMD)**, or *d*, is a summary statistic that is reported in a meta-analysis when the same outcome is measured by different scales or methods. The SMD is also sometimes referred to as the standardized mean effect size. For example, in the meta-analysis by Conn (2010), depression was commonly measured with three different scales—Profile of Mood States, Beck Depression Inventory, and CES-D. Studies that have differences in means in the same proportion to the standard deviations have the same SMD *(d)*, regardless of the scales used to measure the outcome variable. "The differences in the means and standard deviations in the studies are assumed to be the result of the measurement scales and not variability in the outcome" (Higgins & Green, 2008, p. 256).

Conn's (2010) meta-analysis result identified a standardized mean effect size of 0.372 (moderate ES) between the treatment and control groups for the 38 supervised PA studies and an SMD of 0.522 (strong ES) among the 22 unsupervised PA studies. (Chapter 9 provides values for determining small, moderate, and strong ESs.) This meta-analysis documented that supervised and unsupervised PA reduced symptoms of depression in healthy adults or adults without clinical depression. Therefore a decrease in depression is another important reason for encouraging patients to be involved in structured and unstructured PAs.

CRITICALLY APPRAISING META-SYNTHESES

Qualitative research synthesis is the process and product of systematically reviewing, critically appraising, and formally integrating qualitative studies to determine knowledge for practice (Butler, Hall, & Copnell, 2016; Finfgeld-Connett, 2010). The name for a synthesis of qualitative research and the process for conducting it are continuing to evolve in nursing. Various types of qualitative research syntheses have appeared in the literature, such as meta-synthesis, meta-ethnography, meta-study, meta-narrative, qualitative meta-summary, qualitative meta-analysis, and aggregated analysis (Barnett-Page & Thomas, 2009; Butler et al., 2016; Sandelowski & Barroso, 2007; Tong, Flemming, McInnes, Oliver, & Craig, 2012). Despite the lack of consensus, qualitative researchers recognize the importance of summarizing qualitative studies to determine current knowledge that might be used in practice, to direct further research, or for policy development.

Meta-synthesis seems to be the more common name for the process of synthesizing qualitative studies (Butler et al., 2016; Melnyk & Fineout-Overholt, 2015; Sandelowski & Barroso, 2007; Tong et al., 2012). In this text, a **meta-synthesis** is defined as the systematic compilation and integration of qualitative study results to expand understanding and develop a unique interpretation of study findings in a selected area. The focus is on interpretation rather than on combining study results, as with quantitative research synthesis. A meta-synthesis involves the breaking down of findings from different studies to discover essential features and then combining these ideas into a unique, transformed whole. Sandelowski and Barroso (2007) have identified meta-summary as a step in conducting meta-synthesis. A **meta-summary** is the summarizing of findings across qualitative reports to identify knowledge in a selected area.

Tong et al. (2012) developed the Enhancing Transparency in Reporting Synthesis of Qualitative Research (ENTREQ) statement, and Butler et al. (2016) developed guidelines to promote consistency in reporting qualitative syntheses. Merging ideas from different sources, the following questions were developed to guide students and RNs in critically appraising meta-syntheses. A meta-synthesis conducted by Hall, Leach, Brosnan, and Collins (2017) is critically appraised using these questions.

CRITICAL APPRAISAL GUIDELINES

Critically Appraising Meta-Syntheses

A. Introducing and Framing the Meta-Synthesis

1. Did the title of the report identify it as a meta-synthesis?
2. Did the abstract include the background, aim or clinical question addressed, literature search process, methodology for synthesizing the qualitative studies, results, findings, and conclusions?
3. Did the authors clearly identify the aim or objective of their meta-synthesis?
4. Was the meta-synthesis framed to clarify its focus and scope, making it manageable?

B. Searching the Literature and Selecting Sources

5. Did the authors conduct a systematic and comprehensive search for and retrieval of qualitative studies in the target area of the synthesis?
6. Was the process for selecting studies for the meta-synthesis detailed?

C. Critical Appraisal of Studies and Analysis of Data

7. Was the process for critically appraising the studies described?
8. Was the analysis of the qualitative studies' findings detailed and the results clearly presented?

D. Discussion of Meta-Synthesis Findings

9. Did the authors clearly discuss the interpretation of the findings from the qualitative studies?
10. Were the findings from the meta-synthesis clearly presented, including the themes identified and/or a model or map of the overall findings?
11. Was the meta-synthesis report complete and concise? (Butler et al., 2016; Finfgeld-Connett, 2010; Higgins & Green, 2008; Tong et al., 2012)?

Introducing and Framing the Meta-Synthesis

In the title of their article, Hall and colleagues (2017) identified their synthesis of nurses' attitudes toward complementary therapies as a systematic review and meta-synthesis. However, only a meta-synthesis of qualitative studies was included in this article. The researchers provided a quality abstract of their synthesis that included background, aim of the meta-synthesis, search of the literature, ENTREQ process for synthesizing studies, results, discussion of findings, and conclusions.

A meta-synthesis needs to be framed by a clearly stated objective or aim and scope. The aim of the meta-synthesis is usually an important area of interest for the individuals conducting it and is a topic with an adequate body of qualitative studies. The scope of a meta-synthesis is an area of debate, with some qualitative researchers recommending a narrow, precise approach and others recommending a broader, more inclusive approach. However, researchers recognize that framing is essential for making the synthesis process manageable and the findings meaningful and potentially transferable to practice (Butler et al., 2016; Walsh & Downe, 2005).

Hall et al. (2017, p. 48) reported that, "The aim of this meta-synthesis is to review, critically appraise, and synthesize the research to develop a new, more substantial interpretation of nurses' attitudes regarding complementary therapies.... This review is reported according to the Enhancing Transparency in Reporting the Synthesis of Qualitative Research (ENTREQ) guidelines (Tong et al., 2012)."

Searching the Literature and Selecting Sources

Most authors agree that a rigorous search of the literature needs to be conducted. The search needs to include databases, books and book chapters, full reports of theses and dissertations, and conference reports. Researchers often document the specific search strategies they use to locate relevant qualitative studies for their synthesis. The search criteria need to be detailed in the synthesis report, and the years of the search, keywords searched, and language of the sources need to be discussed. Meta-syntheses are usually limited to qualitative studies only and do not include mixed methods studies (Butler et al., 2016; Whittemore et al., 2014). Also, qualitative findings that have not been analyzed or interpreted, such as unanalyzed quotes, field notes, case histories, stories, and poems, are usually excluded (Finfgeld-Connett, 2010). The search process is usually very fluid, with the conduct of additional computerized and hand searches used to identify more studies. Hall et al. (2017) included the following discussion of their search criteria, search strategies, and the selection of studies for synthesis:

> ***Inclusion and exclusion criteria***
> *Published qualitative empirical studies reporting on nurses' attitudes toward complementary therapies were included in this review. Nurses could be employed at any level, in any clinical setting, in any country. For this review, we considered complementary therapies as a broad umbrella term rather than focusing on specific products or practices. Studies involving multiple professional groups were excluded due to the potential difficulty in extracting and interpreting data specific to nursing.*
>
> ***Search strategy***
> *A comprehensive search of relevant articles published in English between January 2000 and December 2015 was conducted using the following electronic databases; MEDLINE, CINAHL, and AMED (Allied and Complementary Medicine Database). A list of the terms used in the search is presented in Table 1. Reference lists of included articles were also hand searched for suitable publications, and opengrey.edu, greylit.com and Google Scholar interrogated for pertinent grey literature.*
>
> **Hall et al., 2017, p. 48**

Hall and colleagues (2017) identified appropriate search criteria and clearly implemented them in their report. The search strategies were detailed, and the inclusion of grey literature reduced the potential for publication bias. The search did have a language bias because only studies in English were reviewed. The key search terms were clearly identified in a table (see Table 1), and the search was strengthened by reviewing the sources from the last 15 years.

TABLE 1 SEARCH TERMS

POPULATION	CONTEXT	OUTCOME
Nurse	Complementary medicine	Attitude
	Complementary therapy	Perception
	Alternative medicine	Decision making
	Alternative therapy	Behavior
	Natural medicine	Communication
	Natural therapy	Experiences
	Herb	Beliefs
	Mind body	
	Acupuncture	

From Hall, H., Leach, M., Brosnan, C., & Collins, M. (2017). Nurses' attitudes towards complementary therapies: A systematic review and meta-synthesis. *International Journal of Nursing Studies, 69*(1), 48.

The final selection of studies to include in a meta-synthesis depends on the focus and scope of the synthesis. Some authors focus on one type of qualitative research, such as ethnography, or on one investigator in a particular area. Others include studies with different qualitative methodologies and investigators in a field or related fields. The search criteria need to be consistently implemented in determining the studies to be included and excluded in the synthesis. Hall et al. (2017) included a detailed flow diagram (see Fig. 1) to document their process for selecting the 15 studies included in their meta-synthesis.

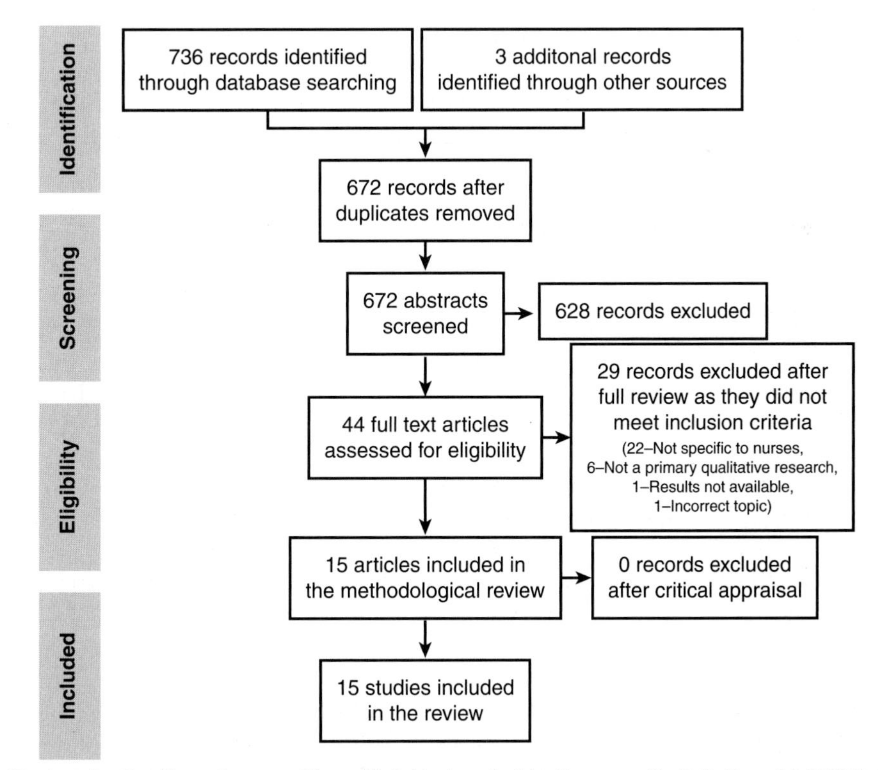

FIG 1 Study selection flow diagram. (From Hall, H., Leach, M., Brosnan, C., & Collins, M. [2017]. Nurses' attitudes towards complementary therapies: A systematic review and meta-synthesis. *International Journal of Nursing Studies, 69*[1], 49.)

Critical Appraisal of Studies and Analysis of Data

The critical appraisal process for qualitative research varies among sources. Usually a table is developed as part of the appraisal process, but this is also an area of debate because tables of studies are more often included in syntheses of quantitative studies. The table headings might include: (1) authors and year of source; (2) aim or goal of the study; (3) methodological orientation; (4) participants; (5) findings; and (6) other key content relevant for comparison. This table provides a display of relevant study elements so that a comparative appraisal might be conducted (Butler et al., 2016; Finfgeld-Connett, 2010). The comparative analysis of studies involves examining methodology and findings across studies for similarities and differences. The frequency of similar findings might be recorded. The differences or contradictions in studies need to be resolved, explained, or both. Varied analysis techniques often are used by the researchers to translate the findings of the different studies into a new or unique description. Tong et al. (2012) present a summary table of the common methodologies used for the synthesis of qualitative studies.

Hall et al. (2017, p. 49) reported that the "findings of this review are based on the five papers from the USA, three papers from Australia, two from both the UK [United Kingdom] and Thailand, and one paper each from Taiwan, Canada, and Israel." These 15 studies were presented in detail in a comparative analysis table that included appropriate headings of authors, year, aim, method, participants, and findings. Two reviewers (HH and MC) independently extracted data from the studies. "Data were analyzed using the thematic synthesis process… In the final stage, the reviewers completed an inductive analysis of the themes to develop an interpretation that went beyond the content of original studies" (Hall et al., 2017, p. 49).

Discussion of Meta-Synthesis Findings

A meta-synthesis report includes findings presented in different formats based on the knowledge developed and the perspective of the authors. A synthesis of qualitative studies in one area might result in the discovery of unique or more refined themes explaining the area of synthesis. The findings from a meta-synthesis might be presented in narrative format or graphically presented in a model or map. Authors should also identify the limitations of the meta-synthesis. The report often concludes with recommendations for further research and implications for practice (Butler et al., 2016; Tong et al., 2012; Walsh & Downe, 2005).

Hall et al. (2017, p. 49) identified the following findings: "Five analytical themes relating to nurses' attitudes towards complementary therapies emerged from the data: the strengths and weaknesses of conventional medicine; complementary therapies as a way to enhance nursing practice; patient empowerment and patient-centeredness; cultural barriers and enablers to integration; and structural barriers and enablers to integration." The meta-analysis report included a discussion of limitations, implications for practice, and conclusions. Hall et al. (2017, p. 47) concluded that "The nursing profession needs to consider how to address current deficiencies in meeting the growing use of complementary therapies by patients."

CRITICALLY APPRAISING MIXED-METHODS SYSTEMATIC REVIEWS

In recent years, nurse researchers have been conducting mixed methods studies that include quantitative and qualitative research methods (Creswell, 2014; Gray et al., 2017) (see Chapter 14 on mixed methods research). Researchers recognize the importance of synthesizing the findings of these studies to determine important knowledge for practice and future research. Creswell (2014) identified the process of combining findings from quantitative and qualitative studies as mixed methods synthesis. Higgins and Green (2008) referred to this synthesis of quantitative, qualitative, and mixed methods studies as a mixed-methods systematic reviews, which is the term we use in this text.

The systematic reviews discussed earlier in this chapter included only studies of a quantitative methodology, such as meta-analyses, RCTs, and quasi-experimental studies, to determine the effectiveness of an intervention. Mixed-methods systematic reviews might include various study designs, such as different types of qualitative research; descriptive, correlational, and quasi-experimental quantitative studies; and/or mixed methods studies (Bettany-Saltikov, 2010b; Higgins & Green, 2008; Liberati et al., 2009; Whittemore et al., 2014).

Higgins and Green (2008) described two types of approaches to integrate the findings from quantitative, qualitative, and mixed methods studies, multilevel synthesis and parallel synthesis. Multilevel synthesis involves synthesizing the findings from quantitative studies separately from qualitative studies and integrating the findings from these two syntheses in the final report. Parallel synthesis involves the separate synthesis of quantitative and qualitative studies, but the findings from the qualitative synthesis are used in interpreting the synthesized quantitative studies.

Further work is needed to develop the methodology for conducting a mixed-methods systematic review. The steps overlap with those of the systematic review and meta-synthesis processes described earlier. The process might be implemented best with a team of researchers with expertise in conducting different types of studies and research syntheses. Guidelines for critically appraising mixed-methods systematic reviews are presented as follows.

CRITICAL APPRAISAL GUIDELINES

Critically Appraising Mixed-Methods Systematic Reviews

A. Introduction of the Mixed-Methods Systematic Review

1. Did the title identify the type of research synthesis that was conducted?
2. Was a clear, concise abstract presented that included the aim of the review, data sources, study selection process, results, findings, and conclusions?
3. Did the aim and/or questions guide the mixed-methods systematic review?

B. Literature Search Methods and Selection of Sources

4. What were the search criteria for identifying quantitative, qualitative, and mixed methods studies?
5. Were the search strategies detailed enough to identify relevant quantitative, qualitative, and mixed methods studies?
6. Was a rigorous search of the literature conducted and detailed in the final report?
7. Was the process for selecting relevant quantitative, qualitative, and mixed methods studies for the synthesis described?

C. Critical Appraisal of Studies and Results

8. Did the authors of the review present a table and narrative that demonstrated a comparative appraisal of the studies was conducted?
9. Were critical appraisals of the studies summarized in the final report, and were the results provided?

D. Findings, Conclusions, and Implications for Research and Practice

10. Was a clear synthesis of study findings presented? Did this synthesis effectively integrate the findings from quantitative, qualitative, and mixed methods studies?
11. Were the implications for research and practice identified and appropriate (Bettany-Saltikov, 2010a, 2010b; Creswell, 2014; Higgins & Green, 2008)?

Introduction of the Mixed-Methods Systematic Review

Karimi and Clark (2016) conducted a mixed-methods systematic review to determine how patients' values influenced the self-care decision-making of patients with heart failure (HF). In their title, they stated that a mixed-methods systematic review was conducted. The title also included the clinical question guiding the review: "How do patients' values influence heart failure self-care decision-making?" (Karimi & Clark, 2016, p. 89). The abstract clearly and concisely covered the background supporting the review, search process, type and number of studies selected for the review, findings, and conclusions. The three objectives or aims of this synthesis were identified early in the review and directed the review process.

Literature Search Methods and Selection of Sources

Karimi and Clark (2016) conducted a comprehensive search of multiple databases and other sources with the assistance of a health sciences librarian. "The search included terms related to three concepts: self-care, values, and HF… The search identified 6467 studies. These were initially screened via title and abstract, resulting in the full-text review of 579 papers (Fig. 1). Of these, 54 met the criteria for inclusion" (Karimi & Clark, 2016, p. 92). As indicated in Fig. 1, the 54 studies reviewed included 30 qualitative studies, 8 mixed methods studies, and 16 quantitative studies. The participants in these studies were 6045 patients, 38 lay caregivers, and 96 healthcare professionals. This mixed-methods systematic review included a strong sample of studies representing the three types of methodologies and included extensive data from numerous patients, caregivers, and health professionals.

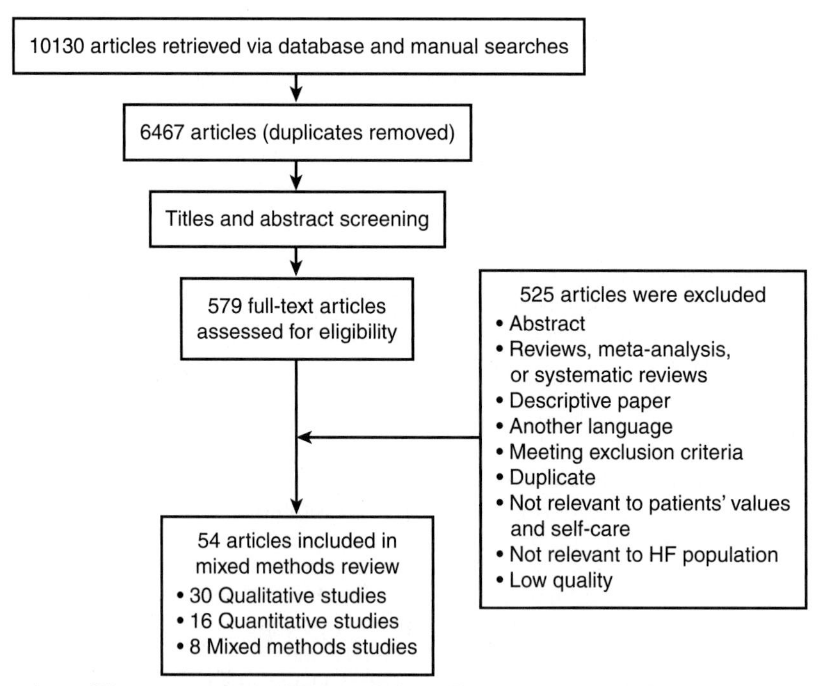

FIG 1 Flow chart of literature review. *HF*, Heart failure. (From Karimi, M., & Clark, A. M. [2016]. How do patients' values influence heart failure self-care decision-making? A mixed-methods systematic review. *International Journal of Nursing Studies, 59*[1], 93.)

Critical Appraisal of Studies and Results

The data from the 54 studies were presented in a comparative table format. The headers in the table included author and year, primary focus, methods, country, data collection methods, sampling, participants, New York Heart Association (NYHA) class, mean age, and a study quality score. A comparative analysis was conducted using the table data that was synthesized in the report. Karimi and Clark (2016, pp. 101–102) recognized the potential for publication bias because "our search was limited to only English language, peer-reviewed journals or dissertations published from the year 2000 and onwards.… The findings were also constrained given the majority of the studies included were conducted in high income countries. Few described the characteristics of those who declined to participate in the study." A serious concern was the lack of studies that explicitly addressed patient values, and the authors had to abstract values' content from the theoretical discussions.

Findings, Conclusions, and Implications for Research and Practice

Karimi and Clark (2016) synthesized their findings into a model of the value-laden, self-care, decision-making process (Fig. 3). The relationships in this model provide direction for practice and should be tested through further research. The authors developed conclusions, implications

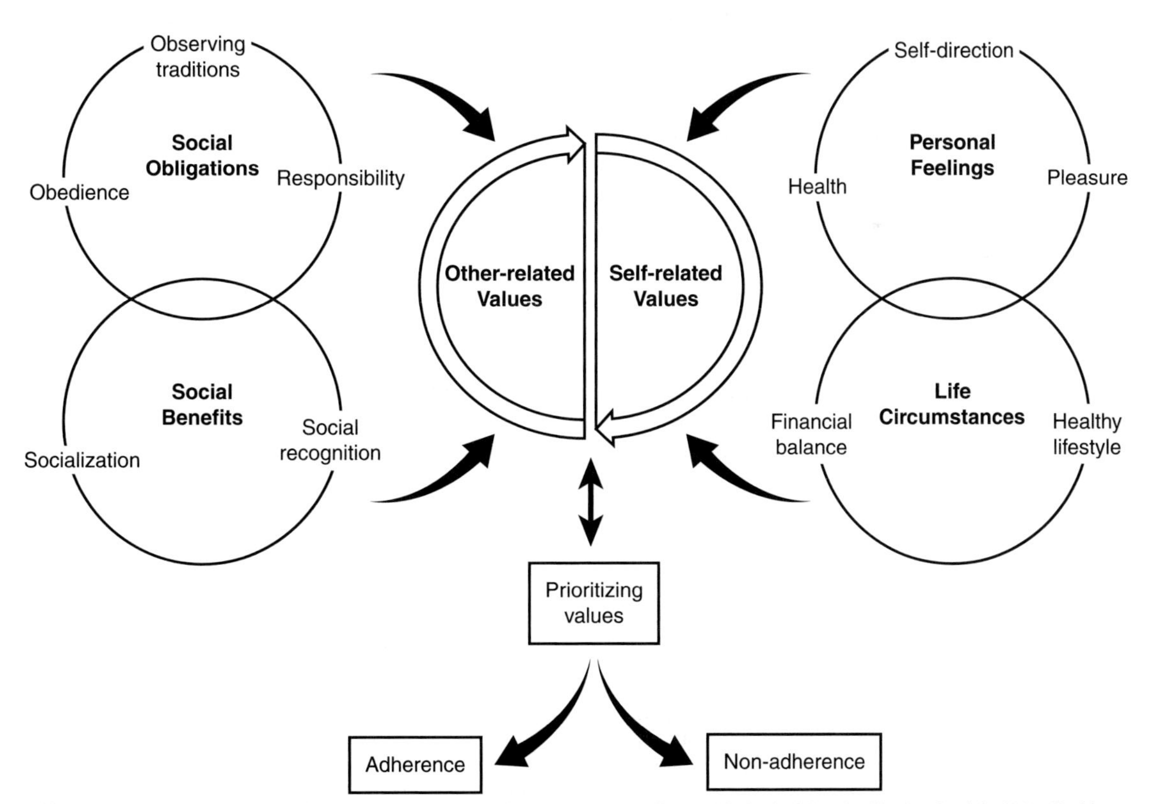

FIG 3 The value-laden, self-care, decision-making process. (From Karimi, M., & Clark, A. M. [2016]. How do patients' values influence heart failure self-care decision-making? A mixed-methods systematic review. *International Journal of Nursing Studies, 59*[1], 99.)

for practice, and directions for further research based on the findings from their mixed-methods systematic review. They reported the following:

> *Values are integral to how patients approach and undertake HF self-care... Values extend to those relating to the self and others and incorporate a notable range of personal, life, and social dimensions [see Fig. 3]. Values cannot be assumed to be fixed, normative or similar to those held by nurses and other health professionals. Future interventions to improve HF self-care must address and respond to the complexity of these values and how they influence patient behavior.*
>
> ***Karimi & Clark, 2016, p. 102***

MODELS TO PROMOTE EVIDENCE-BASED PRACTICE IN NURSING

EBP is a complex phenomenon that requires integration of the best research evidence with clinical expertise, patient circumstances, and patient values in the delivery of quality, safe, cost-effective care. The two models most commonly used in nursing to implement research evidence in practice are the Stetler Model of Research Utilization to Facilitate Evidence-Based Practice (Stetler, 2001) and the Iowa Model of Evidence-Based Practice (Iowa Model Collaborative, 2017). These two models are briefly introduced in this section.

Stetler Model of Research Utilization to Facilitate Evidence-Based Practice

The **Stetler Model of Research Utilization to Facilitate Evidence-Based Practice** (Fig. 13.2) provides a comprehensive framework to enhance the use of research evidence in nursing practice. The research evidence can be used at the institutional or individual level. At the institutional level, study findings are synthesized and the knowledge generated is used to develop or refine policies, algorithms, procedures, protocols, or other formal programs implemented in the institution. Individual nurses, such as RNs, educators, and policy makers, summarize research and use the knowledge to make practice decisions, influence educational programs, and guide political decision making. For example, the evidence-based guideline in Box 13.1 provides knowledge about the age, sites, volume of medication, and aspiration with IM injections that should be implemented by individual nurses to promote quality patient outcomes.

Stetler's model is included in this text to encourage the use of research evidence by individual nurses and healthcare agencies to facilitate the development of evidence-based nursing practice. The five phases of the Stetler (2001) model are briefly described in the following sections: (1) preparation, (2) validation, (3) comparative evaluation and decision making, (4) translation and application, and (5) evaluation.

Phase I: Preparation

The intent of Stetler's (2001) model is to make using research evidence in practice a conscious, critical thinking process that is initiated by the user. Thus **Phase I: Preparation,** involves determining the purpose, focus, and potential outcomes of making an evidence-based change in a clinical agency. Once the agency, individuals, or committee have identified and approved the purpose of the evidence-based project, a detailed search of the literature is conducted to determine the strength of the evidence available for use in practice.

Phase II: Validation

In **Phase II: Validation,** the research reports are critically appraised to determine their scientific soundness (Gray et al., 2017; Grove & Cipher, 2017; Melnyk & Fineout-Overholt, 2015). If the studies are limited in number, weak, or both, the findings and conclusions are considered inadequate

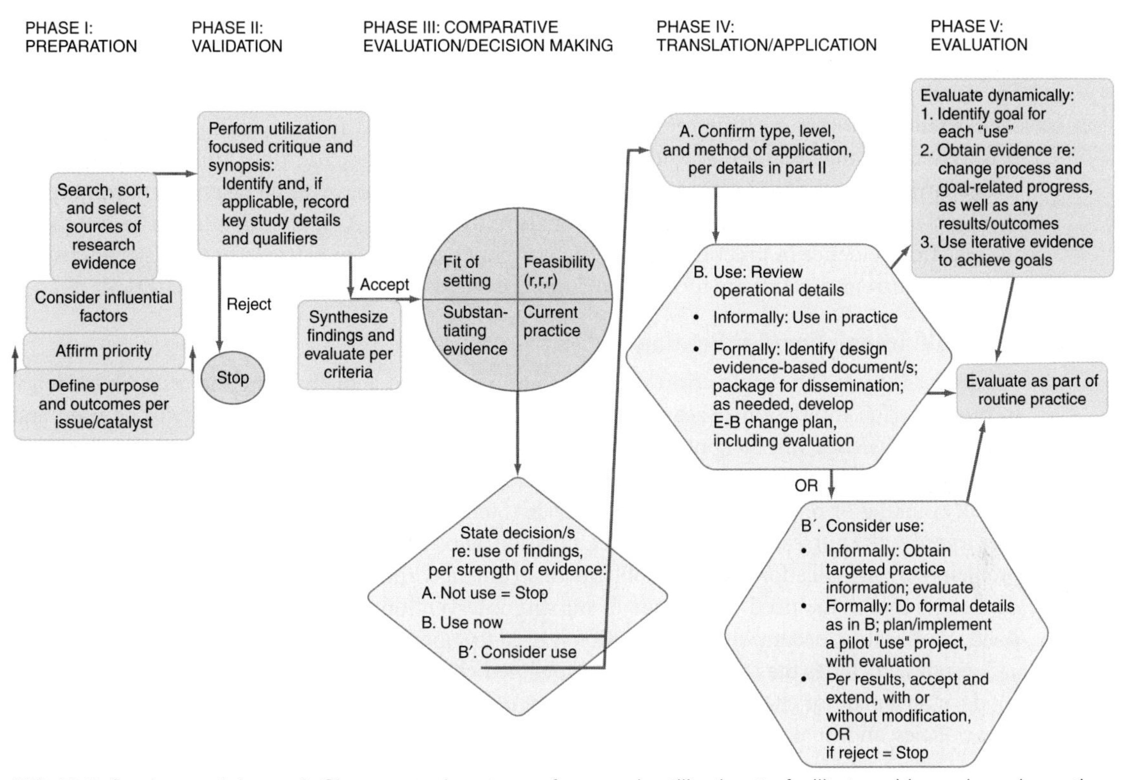

FIG 13.2 Stetler model, part I. Shown are the steps of research utilization to facilitate evidence-based practice. (From Stetler, C. B. [2001]. Updating the Stetler model of research utilization to facilitate evidence-based practice. *Nursing Outlook, 49*[6], 276.)

for use in practice, and the process stops. If a systematic review, meta-analysis, and/or meta-synthesis has been conducted in the area in which you want to make an evidence-based change, this greatly strengthens the quality of the research evidence. If the research knowledge base is strong in the selected area, the clinical agency or individual nurse must make a decision about using the evidence in practice. For example, the guideline related to IM injections (see Box 13.1) can be implemented by individual nurses to improve their practice outcomes.

Phase III: Comparative Evaluation/Decision Making

Phase III: Comparative Evaluation/Decision Making includes four parts: (1) substantiation of the evidence; (2) fit of the evidence with the healthcare setting; (3) feasibility of using research findings; and (4) concerns with current practice (see Fig. 13.2). Substantiating evidence is produced by systematic reviews and meta-analyses of relevant studies. However, individual quasi-experimental and experimental studies also can provide extremely strong evidence for making a change in an agency. To determine the fit of the evidence in the clinical agency, examine the characteristics of the setting to determine the forces that will facilitate or inhibit implementation of the evidence-based change. Stetler (2001) has noted that the feasibility of using research evidence in practice involves examining the three Rs related to making changes in practice: (1) potential *r*isks; (2) *r*esources needed; and (3) *r*eadiness of those involved. By conducting phase III, you can assess the overall benefits and risks of using the research evidence in a practice setting. If the benefits are much greater than the risks for the organization, individual nurse, or both, using the research-based intervention in practice is feasible.

During the decision-making aspect of phase III, three decisions are possible: (1) to use the research evidence; (2) to consider using the evidence; and (3) not to use the research evidence (see Fig. 13.2). The decision to use research knowledge in practice depends mainly on the strength of the evidence. Another decision might be to consider use of the available research evidence in practice. When a change is complex and involves multiple disciplines, additional time is often needed to determine how the evidence might be used and what measures will be taken to coordinate the involvement of different healthcare professionals in the change. A final option might be not to use the research evidence in practice because the current evidence is not strong, or the risks or costs of change in current practice are too high in comparison with the benefits (Stetler, 2001).

Phase IV: Translation/Application

Phase IV: Translation/Application involves planning for and actually using the research evidence in practice. The translation phase involves determining exactly what knowledge will be used and how that knowledge will be applied to practice. The use of the research evidence can be cognitive, instrumental, or symbolic. With cognitive application, the research base is a means of modifying a way of thinking or one's appreciation of an issue (Stetler, 2001). For example, cognitive application may improve the nurse's understanding of a situation, allow analysis of practice dynamics, or improve problem-solving skills for clinical problems. Instrumental application involves using research evidence to support the need for change in nursing interventions or practice protocols. Symbolic or political utilization occurs when information is used to support or change a current policy. The application phase includes the following steps for planned change: (1) assess the situation to be changed; (2) develop a plan for change; and (3) implement the plan. During the application phase, the protocols, policies, and/or algorithms developed with research knowledge are implemented in practice.

Phase V: Evaluation

The final stage, Phase V: Evaluation, is to determine the impact of the research-based change on the healthcare agency, personnel, and patients. The evaluation process can include formal and informal activities conducted by administrators, nurse clinicians, and other health professionals. Informal evaluations might include self-monitoring or discussions with patients, families, peers, and other professionals. Formal evaluations can include case studies, audits, QI projects, and translational or outcomes research projects. In summary, the Stetler (2001) model provides detailed steps to encourage nurses to become change agents to make the necessary improvements in practice based on research evidence.

Iowa Model of Evidence-Based Practice

Nurses have been actively involved in conducting research, synthesizing research evidence, and developing evidence-based guidelines for practice. These activities support their strong commitment to EBP, which has been facilitated by the Iowa Model. The Iowa Model of Evidence-Based Practice promotes the implementation of EBP by nurses in clinical agencies. Recently, the Iowa Model Collaborative (2017) conducted a study to revise and validate the Iowa Model. The most current Iowa Model is presented in Fig. 13.3. In healthcare agencies, there are triggering issues or opportunities that initiate the need for change, with the focus on making changes based on the current, best research evidence. The triggering issues are often problem-focused and evolve from clinical problems and data from risk management, process improvement, benchmarking, and financial reports. The opportunities can be knowledge-focused, such as new research findings, changes in national agencies or organizational standards and guidelines, an expanded philosophy of care, an updated professional model of care (requirement of Magnet recognition), or questions from the

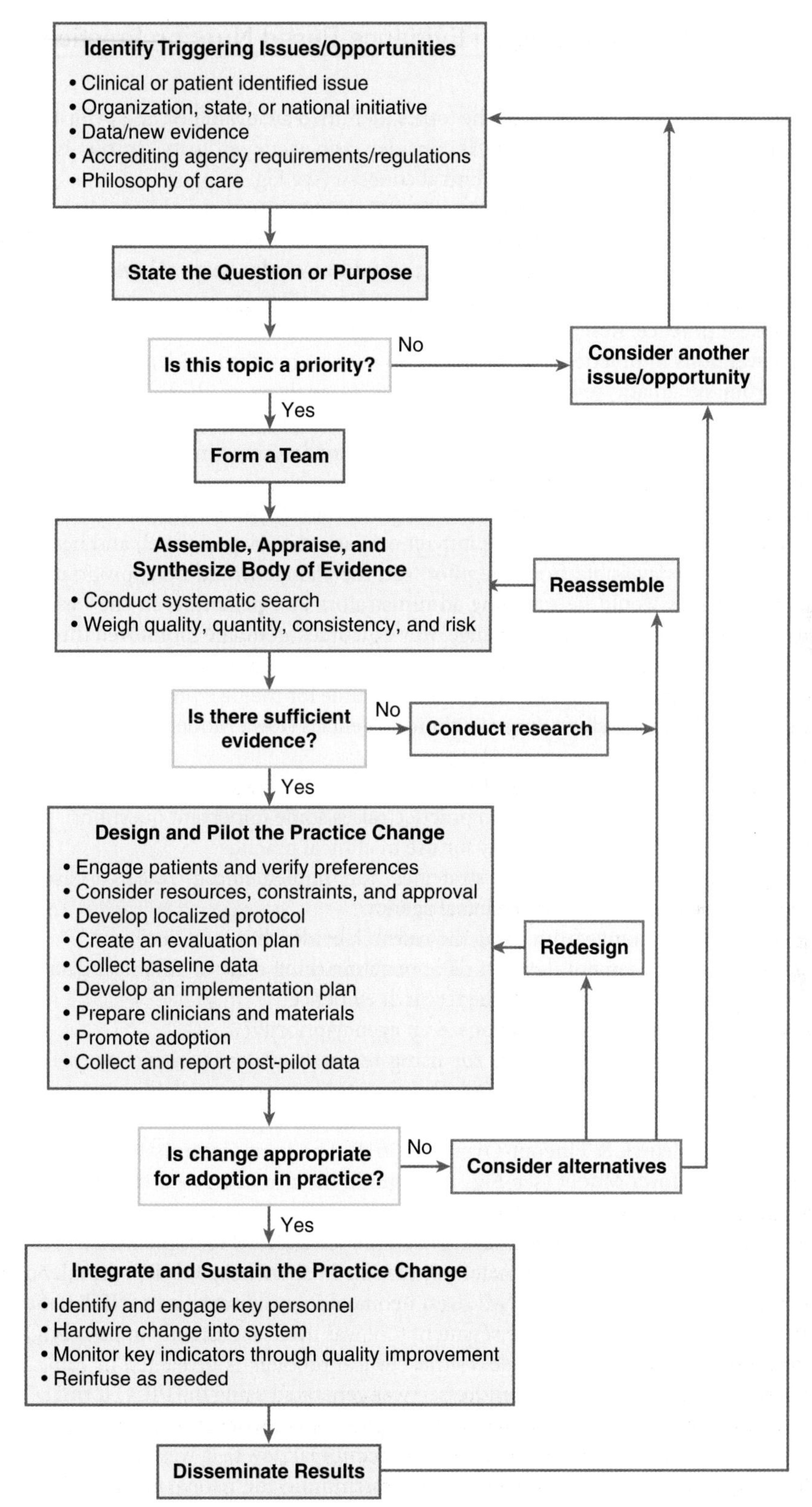

FIG 13.3 The Iowa Model Revised: Evidence-Based Practice to Promote Excellence in Health Care. (From Iowa Model Collaborative. [2017]. Iowa Model of Evidence-Based Practice: Revisions and validation. *Worldviews on Evidence-Based Nursing, 14*[3], 175–182, 178.)

institutional standards' committee. The topics identified are evaluated and prioritized based on the needs of the clinical agency. If a topic is considered an agency priority, a group is formed to search for the best evidence to manage the clinical concern (see Fig. 13.3).

In some situations, the research evidence is inadequate to make changes in practice, and additional studies are needed to strengthen the knowledge base (see Fig. 13.3). Sometimes the research evidence can be combined with other sources of knowledge (e.g., theories, scientific principles, expert opinion, case reports) to provide fairly strong evidence for use in developing research-based protocols for practice. **Research-based protocols** are structured guidelines for implementing nursing interventions in practice that are based on current research evidence. The strongest evidence comes from systematic reviews that include meta-analyses of RCTs. However, meta-syntheses, mixed-methods systematic reviews, and individual studies also provide important evidence for changing practice. The levels of research evidence are described in Chapter 1 (see Fig. 1.3) and are also presented inside the front cover of this text.

The research-based protocols, algorithms, guidelines, or policies developed could be pilot-tested and then evaluated to determine the impact on patient care, personnel, and healthcare agency. If the outcomes are favorable from the pilot test, the change would be appropriate for adoption in practice. Changes would be made by administrators and personnel in the healthcare agency to integrate and sustain the practice change. Key outcomes would be monitored through QI to ensure that the practice change promoted quality, safe, and cost-effective care. The Iowa Model-Revised (see Fig. 13.3) "remains an application-oriented guide for the EBP process" and is a valuable source for implementing research evidence in clinical agencies (Iowa Model Collaborative, 2017, p. 175).

Application of the Iowa Model of Evidence-Based Practice

Preparing to use research evidence in practice raises some important questions:

- Which research findings are ready for use in clinical practice?
- What are the most effective strategies for implementing research-based protocols or evidence-based guidelines in a clinical agency?
- What are the outcomes from using the research evidence in practice?
- Do the risk management data, QI data, benchmarking data, or financial data support making the change in practice based on the research evidence?
- Is the research-based change proposed an agency priority?

We suggest that effective strategies for using research evidence in practice will require a multifaceted approach that takes into consideration the evidence available, attitudes of the practicing nurses, the organization's philosophy, and national organizational standards and guidelines (ANCC, 2017; Melnyk & Fineout-Overholt, 2015; The Joint Commission, 2017). In this section, the steps of the Iowa Model (see Fig. 13.3) guide the use of a research-based intervention in a hospital to facilitate EBP.

Schumacher, Askew, and Otten (2013) used the Iowa Model to implement a pressure ulcer (PU) trigger tool for assessing the neonatal population in their hospital. PU prevalence ranged from 0% to 1% per quarter in this large Midwest neonatal intensive care unit (NICU). Schumacher and colleagues noted that no PU risk assessment tool was used consistently in their NICU. A summary of the application of the Iowa Model to this clinical problem is presented in Table 1 (Schumacher et al., 2013). The clinical question addressed was generated using the PICO format. The population was neonates in the NICU. The intervention to be implemented was a three-question PU trigger tool to assess if the neonates were at risk for skin breakdown. It was compared to the Braden Q tool, the standard care or usual practice of determining the neonates who were at risk for PUs. The outcome measured was the effectiveness of the PU trigger tool as compared to the Braden Q tool in assessing neonates who were at risk for PU. The studies that had examined the effectiveness of different neonatal PU assessment tools were critically appraised. The tools in these studies were judged to be too long for routine clinical use. Schumacher and colleagues (2013) developed a shorter trigger assessment tool based on the research evidence:

> *Trigger Questions for Pressure Ulcer Risk Proposed by the Institute for Clinical Systems Improvement: Is the infant: Moving extremities and/or body appropriately for developmental age? Responding to discomfort in a developmentally appropriate manner? Demonstrating adequate tissue perfusion based on the clinical formula (mean arterial pressure = gestational age and/or capillary refill <3 s)?*
>
> **Schumacher et al., 2013, p. 48**

Schumacher et al. (2013) found that their three-question PU trigger assessment tool was as effective as the Braden Q tool in determining neonatal risk for PUs. Their findings are summarized in the following study excerpt:

> *Following implementation of the trigger questions in 2009, we observed no net increase in the number of WOC [wound, ostomy, and continence] referrals per 1000 patients. Nevertheless, our PU [pressure ulcer] prevalence in the NICU remains low at 0.01 per 1000 patient days. Comparison of results from the 3 trigger questions and the Braden Q scoring by the WOC nurse demonstrated that most infants are correctly identified by the tool, with the exception of those very immature infants who may be at risk for medical device-related ulcers....*
>
> *We implemented a 3-item trigger tool to aid NICU nurses identifying neonates at risk for PU development. While these questions do not quantify risk, we have found that they are an efficient initial screening tool when combined with additional assessment and management in consultation with a WOC nurse.*
>
> **Schumacher et al., 2013, p. 50**

TABLE 1 USE OF THE IOWA MODEL FOR EVIDENCE-BASED PRACTICE PROJECTS TO ESTABLISH A CLINICAL TOOL FOR EVALUATION OF PRESSURE ULCER RISK IN AN NICU

Step	Application
1. Generate the question from either a problem or new knowledge.	For infants in the NICU, does the use of a pressure ulcer trigger tool perform equally as well as the Braden Q to identify an infant at risk? P—Infant in the NICU I—Use of a pressure ulcer trigger tool C—Usual practices of assessing all with Braden Q O—Trigger tool performs equally as well as the Braden Q for risk identification
2. Determine relevance to organizational priorities.	Our hospital is committed to safe and reliable care and ensuring a flawless patient experience. This includes preventing hospital-acquired pressure ulcers—a "never event." Possible impact/outcomes may include: • Potential increase in WOC referrals • Correct triggering of infants requiring further pressure ulcer risk assessment and prevention strategies by nursing • Preservation of nursing time because the trigger tool is a shorter and easier to use tool that indicates for whom full assessment is needed.

Continued

TABLE 1 USE OF THE IOWA MODEL FOR EVIDENCE-BASED PRACTICE PROJECTS TO ESTABLISH A CLINICAL TOOL FOR EVALUATION OF PRESSURE ULCER RISK IN AN NICU—cont'd	
3. Develop a team to gather and appraise evidence.	Team members included a clinical nurse specialist, two WOC nurses, NICU Nursing Practice Council members, and electronic medical records experts. According to IHI, all premature infants are at risk for pressure ulcer development. Although this statement is visionary, it does not assist the bedside nurse to determine for whom to provide interventions. Referrals to the WOC nurse for assessment were based on clinical judgment, and no assessment tools were in place. Risk assessment tools are available for the neonatal population but were judged to be lengthy and time-consuming for every nurse, every shift. A trigger tool was developed, based on IHI pediatric trigger questions to help the nurse determine whom to refer for full assessment.
4. Determine if the evidence answers the question.	Reasonable evidence is present to warrant implementation of this practice. The three IHI trigger questions are based on the concepts of the Braden Q and could trigger those at risk and requiring further assessment and intervention.
5. If there is sufficient evidence, pilot the change in practice.	Prior to implementation, 10 patients were randomly selected to test the feasibility of implementing trigger questions. The three trigger questions were asked of the nurses caring for each patient, and results were compared to a Braden Q score generated by a WOC nurse. We noted that patients with high risk, as defined by the Braden Q, were also identified as at-risk based on the three trigger questions. The three trigger questions were embedded into the electronic medical record. Pressure ulcer data were collected through the surveillance provided by skin team nurses as part of their usual duties.
6. Evaluate structure, process, and outcome data.	The HAPU rate for the NICU remains low and has not changed since the implementation of the trigger tool. The number of WOC nurse consultations has remained stable since implementation of the three trigger questions into NICU nurse practice.
7. Disseminate results.	Results and appropriate feedback have been shared with the NICU nurses via the NICU practice committee.

HAPU, Hospital-acquired pressure ulcer; *IHI,* Institute for Healthcare Improvement; *NICU,* neonatal intensive care unit; *WOC,* wound, ostomy, and continence.
From Schumacher, B., Askew, M., & Otten, K. (2013). Development of a pressure ulcer trigger tool for the neonatal population. *Journal of Wound, Ostomy, and Continence Nursing, 40*(1), 47.

IMPLEMENTING EVIDENCE-BASED GUIDELINES IN PRACTICE

Research knowledge is generated every day and is synthesized to determine the best evidence for use in practice (Cochrane, 2017; Mackey & Bassendowski, 2017: NGC, 2017a). This section addresses the **evidence-based guidelines,** based on current best research evidence, published on national and international websites and in referred professional journals. The Eighth Joint National Committee (JNC 8) evidence-based guideline for the management of high blood pressure in adults is presented as an example (James et al., 2014).

Resources for Evidence-Based Guidelines

Since the 1980s, the Agency for Healthcare Research and Quality (AHRQ) has had a major role in identifying health topics and promoting the development of evidence-based guidelines for these topics (http://www.ahrq.gov). The first evidence-based guidelines were developed by panels of nationally recognized researchers in the topic area, expert clinicians (e.g., physicians, nurses, pharmacists, social workers), healthcare administrators, policy developers, economists, government representatives, and consumers. The panel members designated the scope of the guideline and conducted extensive reviews of the literature, including relevant systematic reviews, meta-analyses, individual studies, and theories. The evidence-based guidelines developed were examined by consultants, other researchers, and additional expert clinicians for their input. Based on the experts' critique, the AHRQ revised and packaged the guidelines for distribution to healthcare professionals.

At present, standardized guideline development ranges from a structured process such as the one just discussed to a less structured process, in which a guideline might be developed by a healthcare organization, healthcare plan, or professional organization. The AHRQ initiated the NGC (NGC, 2017a) in 1998 to store the EBP guidelines. The NGC (2017b) is a publicly available database of evidence-based clinical guidelines and related documents. The NGC is updated weekly with new content that the AHRQ produces in partnership with the American Medical Association and America's Health Insurance Plans. The key components of the NGC and its user-friendly resources can be found on the AHRQ website (http://www.guideline.gov/). Key information provided by the NGC that is relevant to you is as follows:

- Structured abstracts (summaries) about the guideline and its development
- Links to full-text guidelines, where available, and/or ordering information for print copies
- Downloads of the complete NGC summary for all guidelines represented in the database
- Annotated bibliography database in which users can search for citations for publications and resources about guidelines
- *What's New*—enables users to see what guidelines have been added each week; includes an index of all guidelines in the NGC
- The *Glossary*—provides definitions of terms used in the standardized abstracts (summaries)

The NGC provides an easy to use mechanism for obtaining objective and detailed information on clinical practice guidelines. In addition to the evidence-based guidelines, the AHRQ has developed many tools to assess the quality of care provided by the evidence-based guidelines. You can search the AHRQ (2017a) website (http://www.qualitymeasures.ahrq.gov) for an appropriate tool to measure a variable in a research project or evaluate outcomes of care in a clinical agency. Numerous professional organizations, healthcare agencies, universities, and other groups provide evidence syntheses, evidence-based guidelines for practice, and measurement methods for outcomes, which can be found on the websites listed in Box 13.3.

Implementing an Evidence-Based Guideline for Management of Hypertension in Adults

Evidence-based guidelines have become the standards for providing care to patients in the United States and other countries. The 2014 evidence-based guideline for the management of high blood pressure in adults was developed by the JNC 8 panel members, who conducted a systematic review of RCTs to determine the best research evidence. The guideline includes nine revised recommendations for the management of hypertension (HTN) and are available in the article by James et al. (2014, p. 511) or through the NGC (2017a) Guideline Summary NGC-10397. The JNC 8 guideline

BOX 13.3 EVIDENCE-BASED PRACTICE WEBSITES

- Academic Center for Evidence-Based Nursing: http://www.acestar.uthscsa.edu
- Association of Women's Health, Obstetric, and Neonatal Nurses: http://awhonn.org
- Centers for Disease Control Healthcare Providers: http://www.cdc.gov/CDCForYou/healthcare_providers.html
- Centers for Health Evidence: http://www.cche.net
- Guidelines Advisory Committee: http://www.gacguidelines.ca
- Guidelines International Network: http://www.g-i-n.net/
- HerbMed: Evidence-Based Herbal Database, 1998, Alternative Medicine Foundation: http://www.herbmed.org/
- National Association of Neonatal Nurses: http://www.nann.org/
- National Institute for Clinical Excellence (NICE): http://www.nice.org.uk/
- Oncology Nursing Society: http://www.ons.org/
- Primary Care Clinical Practice Guidelines: http://www.medscape.com/pages/editorial/public/pguidelines/index-primarycare
- US Preventive Services Task Force: http://www.uspreventiveservicestaskforce.org

also includes the 2014 Hypertension Guideline Management Algorithm. This algorithm provides clinicians with directions for: (1) implementing lifestyle interventions; (2) setting BP goals; and (3) initiating BP-lowering medication based on age, diabetes, and chronic kidney disease (CKD; James et al., 2014). Nurses and other healthcare providers can use this algorithm to select the most appropriate treatment methods for each individual patient diagnosed with HTN.

Nursing students and RNs need to assess the usefulness and quality of each evidence-based guideline before they implement it in their practice. Fig. 13.4 presents the **Grove Model for Implementing Evidence-Based Guidelines in Practice**. In this model, nurses identify a practice problem, search for the best research evidence to manage the problem in their practice, and identify an evidence-based guideline. Assessing the quality and usefulness of the guideline involves examining the following: (1) the authors of the guideline; (2) the significance of the healthcare problem; (3) the strength of the research evidence; (4) the link to national standards; and (5) the cost-effectiveness of using the guideline in practice. The quality of the JNC 8 guideline is discussed using these five criteria.

Authors of the Guidelines

The panel members of the JNC 8 guideline were specifically selected from more than 400 nominees based on their "expertise in hypertension (n = 14), primary care (n = 6), … pharmacology (n = 2), clinical trials (n = 6), evidence-based medicine (n = 3), epidemiology (n = 1), informatics (n = 4), and the development and implementation of clinical guidelines in systems of care (n = 4)" (James et al., 2014, p. 508). These panel members were specifically selected based on their strong and varied expertise to develop an evidence-based guideline for management of HTN.

Significance of Healthcare Problem

James and colleagues (2014, p. 507) reported that HTN is the most "common condition seen in primary care and leads to myocardial infarction (MI), stroke, renal failure, and death if not detected early and treated appropriately. Patients want to be assured that BP treatment will reduce their disease burden, while clinicians want guidance on HTN management using the best scientific evidence."

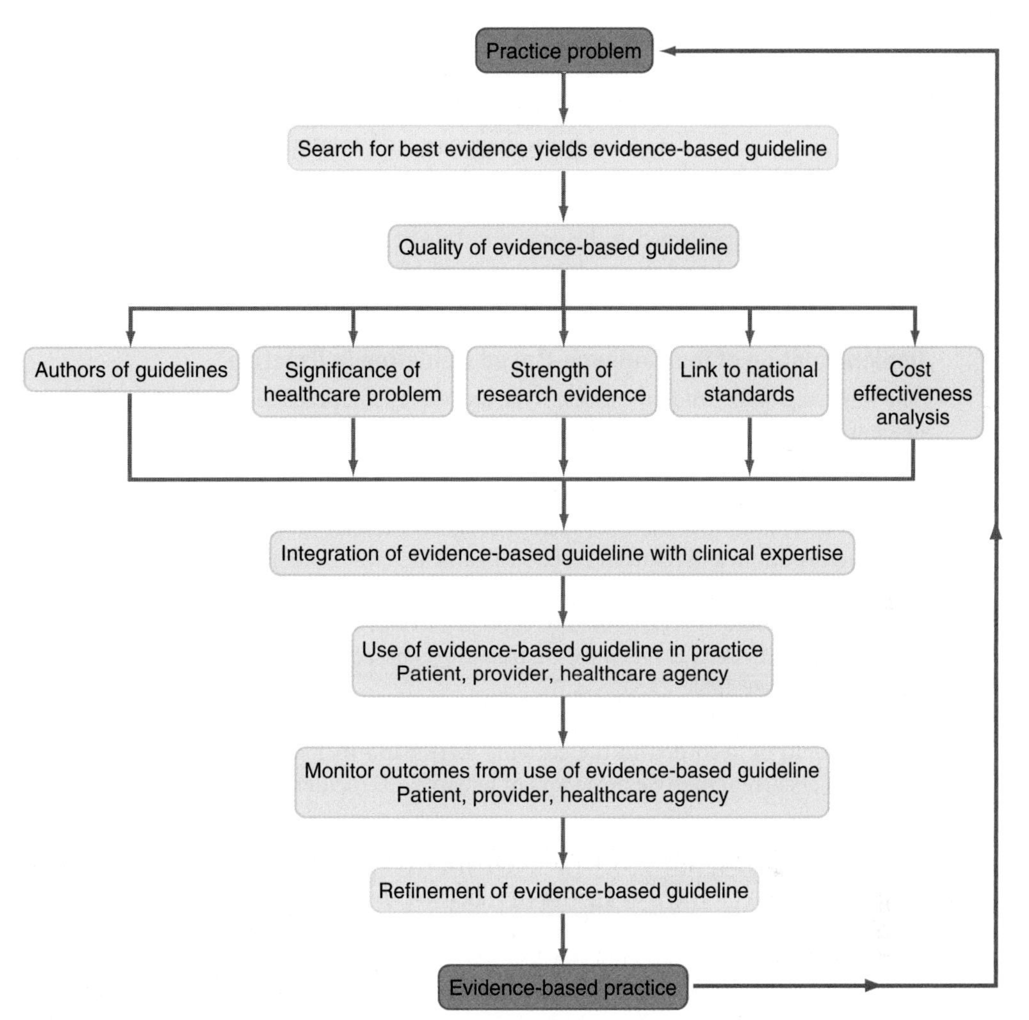

FIG 13.4 Grove Model for Implementing Evidence-Based Guidelines in Practice.

Strength of Research Evidence

James et al. (2014) conducted a systematic review to identify the research evidence for the national guideline for management of HTN. The participants in the studies reviewed were adults aged 18 years and older with HTN. Only the studies with strong sample sizes (>100 participants) and adequate follow-up to yield health-related outcomes (≥1 year) were included in the systematic review. The panel also "limited its evidence review to only randomized controlled trials (RCTs) because they are less subject to bias than other study designs and represent the gold standard for determining efficacy and effectiveness" (James et al., 2014, p. 508).

The JNC 8 panel members had an external methodology team search the literature and summarize the data from selected studies into an evidence table (James et al., 2014). From the evidence review, the panel members developed evidence statements that provided the basis for the nine recommendations for the management of HTN. The research evidence for the development of the JNC 8 guideline for management of HTN was extremely strong.

Link to National Standards and Cost-Effectiveness of Evidence-Based Guideline

Quality evidence-based guidelines should link to national standards and be cost-effective (see Fig. 13.4). The JNC 8 evidence-based guideline for the management of HTN built on the JNC 7 national guideline for the assessment, diagnosis, and treatment of HTN. The recommendations from the JNC 7 have been supported by the Department of Health and Human Services and disseminated through the NIH (NIH, 2003, Publication No. 03-5231). Use of the JNC 8 guideline in practice is projected to be cost-effective because recommendations for the management of HTN should lead to decreased incidences of MI, stroke, CKD, HF, and cardiovascular disease (CVD)–related mortality and should improve health outcomes for adults with HTN.

Implementation of the Evidence-Based Guideline in Practice

The next step is for student nurses, RNs, and advanced practice nurses (APNs) to use the JNC 8 evidence-based guideline in their practice. Student nurses and RNs need to take and record patients' BPs in EHRs accurately, which are part of healthcare agencies' clinical databases (see Table 13.3). RNs and nursing students also need to educate patients and families about the lifestyle modifications needed to improve their BP, such as a regular exercise program, balanced diet, normal weight, smoking cessation, and reduced dietary salt and alcohol. Patients need to know their BP values and the BP goals desired for them. Individuals with high BP readings based on their age and chronic illnesses (e.g., diabetes, CKD) should be reported to APNs and physicians. The APNs and physicians will initiate or revise HTN medication treatments based on the health circumstances and values of their patients (see Table 13.3).

The outcomes for the patient, provider, and healthcare agency need to be examined. The outcomes should be recorded in the patients' EHRs and include the following: (1) BP readings for patients; (2) current lifestyle behaviors of patients; (3) incidence of diagnosis of HTN based on the

TABLE 13.3 EVIDENCED-BASED GUIDELINE FOR ASSESSMENT AND MANAGEMENT OF HIGH BLOOD PRESSURE IN ADULTS

	HIGH BP OR HTN CLASSIFICATION			NURSING STUDENT AND RN INTERVENTIONS		APN AND PHYSICIAN ROLE
AGE (yr)	HTN DIAGNOSIS (mm Hg)	SYSTOLIC BP GOAL (mm Hg)[a]	DIASTOLIC BP GOAL (mm Hg)[a]	LIFESTYLE MODIFICATION EDUCATION[b]	DM OR CKD[c]	PHARMACOLOGICAL MANAGEMENT OF HTN
<60	≥140/90	<140 *and*	<90	Yes	No	Yes
<60	≥140/90	<140 *and*	<90	Yes	Yes	Yes
≥60	≥150/90	<150 *and*	<90	Yes	No	Yes
≥60	≥140/90	<140 *and*	<90	Yes	Yes	Yes

[a]Treatment is determined by the highest BP category, systolic or diastolic.

[b]Lifestyle modifications—balanced diet, regular exercise program, achieving normal weight, smoking cessation, and reduced dietary salt and alcohol; Education should be implemented for all adults with HTN.

[c]Patients with DM or CKD need education about management of these diseases and the link with hypertension.

APN, Advanced practice nurse; *BP,* blood pressure; *CKD,* chronic kidney disease; *DM,* diabetes mellitus; *HTN,* hypertension; *RN,* registered nurse.

Adapted from James, P. A., Oparil, S., Carter, B. L., Cushman, W. C., Denison-Himmelfard, C., Handler, J., et al. (2014). 2014 evidence-based guidelines for the management of high blood pressure in adults: Report from the panel members appointed to the Eighth Joint National Committee (JNC 8). *Journal of the American Medical Association, 311*(5), 507–520.

JNC 8 guidelines; (4) appropriateness of the pharmacological therapies implemented to manage HTN; and (5) incidence of stroke, MI, HF, CKD, and CVD and related mortality over a period of 5, 10, 15, and 20 years. The healthcare agency outcomes include access to care by patients with HTN, patient satisfaction with care, and costs related to diagnosis and management of HTN, in addition to the HTN complications previously mentioned. This EBP guideline will be refined in the future based on clinical outcomes, outcome studies, and new RCTs. The use of this evidence-based guideline and additional guidelines promote EBP for nurses and healthcare agencies (see Fig. 13.4).

INTRODUCTION TO EVIDENCE-BASED PRACTICE CENTERS

The AHRQ launched an initiative to promote EBP by establishing 12 **evidence-based practice centers (EPCs)** in the United States and Canada in 1997. With this program, AHRQ became a "science partner" with public and private organizations to improve the quality, cost-effectiveness, and appropriateness of health care by synthesizing research evidence and facilitating the translation of evidence-based research findings into practice (AHRQ, 2017b).

Through the EPC program, the AHRQ awards 5-year contracts to institutions to serve as EPCs. EPCs review all relevant scientific literature on clinical, behavioral, organizational, and financial topics to produce evidence reports and technology assessments. Topics are nominated by nonfederal partners, such as professional societies, health plans, insurers, employers, and patient groups. The EPC reports are used "to inform and develop coverage decisions, quality measures, educational materials, tools, guidelines, and research agendas" (AHRQ, 2017b). The EPCs also conduct research on the methodology of systematic reviews.

The AHRQ (2017b) website provides the names of the EPCs and the focus of each center. This site also provides a link to the evidence-based reports produced by these centers. These EPCs have had an important role in developing evidence-based syntheses and guidelines for the last 2 decades.

INTRODUCTION TO TRANSLATIONAL RESEARCH

Some challenges to EBP have resulted in the development of a new research methodology, translational research, to improve the application of research evidence in practice. **Translational research** has been termed *bench to bedside research*, which involves the translation of basic scientific discoveries into practical applications (Callard, Rose, & Wykes, 2012). Basic research discoveries from the laboratory setting need to be tested in human studies. Also, the outcomes from human clinical trials need to be adopted and maintained in clinical practice. Translational research is being conducted in nursing and medicine to increase the implementation of evidence-based interventions in practice and determine if these interventions are effective in producing the outcomes desired.

The National Center for Advancing Translation Sciences (NCATS) was developed in 2011 as part of the NIH. To encourage researchers to conduct translational research, the NIH (2017) developed the Clinical and Translational Science Awards (CTSA) consortium. The consortium started with 12 centers located throughout the United States and expanded to 39 centers in April 2009. The program was fully implemented in 2012, with about 60 institutions involved in clinical and translational science. A website has been developed to enhance communication and encourage sharing of information related to translational research projects (see https://ncats.nih.gov/).

The CTSA Consortium is mainly focused on expanding the translation of medical research to practice. Titler (2004, p. S1) defined translational research for the nursing profession as the "Scientific investigation of methods, interventions, and variables that influence adoption of EBPs by individuals and organizations to improve clinical and operational decision making in health care. This includes testing the effect of interventions on and promoting and sustaining the adoption of EBPs." Westra and colleagues (2015, p. 600) developed "a national action plan for sharable and comparable nursing data to support practice and translation research." This plan provides direction for the conduct and use of translation research to change nursing practice.

Translation studies have been appearing more often in the nursing literature. For example, Mello and colleagues (2013) conducted a translation study to promote the use of an alcohol Screening, Brief Intervention, and Referral to Treatment (SBIRT) guideline in pediatric trauma centers. Before the study, only 11% of eligible patients were screened and received an intervention. "After completion of the SBIRT technical assistance activities, all seven participating trauma centers had effectively developed, adopted, and implemented SBIRT policies for injured adolescent inpatients. Furthermore, across all sites, 73% of eligible patients received SBIRT services after both the implementation and maintenance phases" (Mello et al., 2013, p. S301).

We hope that the content in this chapter has increased your understanding of EBP, the critical appraisal of research syntheses, the application of EBP models, and the implementation of EBP guidelines. We encourage you to take an active role in moving nursing toward EBP that improves outcomes for patients, nurses, and healthcare agencies.

KEY POINTS

- Evidence-based practice (EBP) is the conscientious integration of best research evidence with clinical expertise and patient circumstances and values in the delivery of quality, safe, cost-effective health care.
- Best research evidence is produced by the conduct and synthesis of numerous high-quality studies in a health-related area.
- Nurses must be knowledgeable of the benefits and challenges associated with EBP.
- The PICO format is described for generating a clinical question to guide the use of current research evidence in practice.
- Guidelines are provided for critically appraising the research synthesis processes of systematic review, meta-analysis, meta-synthesis, and mixed-methods systematic review.
- A systematic review is a structured comprehensive synthesis of the quantitative research literature to determine the best research evidence available to address a healthcare question.
- A meta-analysis is conducted to pool the results from previous studies statistically into a single quantitative analysis that provides one of the highest levels of evidence about the effectiveness of an intervention.
- A meta-synthesis is defined as the systematic compilation and integration of qualitative studies to expand understanding and develop a unique interpretation of study findings in a selected area.
- Reviews that include syntheses of various quantitative, qualitative, and mixed methods studies are referred to as mixed-methods systematic reviews in this text.
- The Stetler Model of Research Utilization to Facilitate Evidence-Based Practice provides a comprehensive framework to enhance the used of research evidence by nurses in practice.
- The Iowa Model of Evidence-Based Practice presents directions for implementing patient care based on the best research evidence and monitoring changes in practice to ensure quality care.
- The process for developing evidence-based guidelines is described, and an example of the guideline for the assessment, diagnosis, and treatment of hypertension (HTN) is provided.

- The Grove Model for Implementing Evidence-Based Guidelines in Practice is provided to assist nurses in determining the quality of evidence-based guidelines and the steps for using these guidelines in practice.
- Evidence-based practice centers (EPCs), created by the AHRQ, have had an important role in the conduct of research, development of systematic reviews, and formulation of evidence-based guidelines in selected practice areas.
- Translational research is expanding in health care to translate basic scientific discoveries into practical applications.

REFERENCES

Agency for Healthcare Research and Quality (AHRQ). (2017a). *AHRQ's National Quality Measures Clearinghouse (NQMC)*. Retrieved November 28, 2017, from http://qualitymeasures.ahrq.gov.

Agency for Healthcare Research and Quality (AHRQ). (2017b). *Evidence-based Practice Centers (EPCs) evidence-based reports*. Retrieved July 18, 2017, from https://www.ahrq.gov/research/findings/evidence-based-reports/index.html.

American Nurses Credentialing Center (ANCC). (2017). *Find a Magnet hospital: Current number of Magnet facilities*. Retrieved November 29, 2017, from http://www.nursecredentialing.org/Magnet/FindaMagnetFacility.aspx.

Andrel, J. A., Keith, S. W., & Leiby, B. E. (2009). Meta-analysis: A brief introduction. *Clinical and Translational Science, 2*(5), 374–378.

Barnett-Page, E., & Thomas, J. (2009). Methods for the synthesis of qualitative research: A critical review. *BMC Medical Research Methodology, 9*(59). Retrieved March 18, 2018, from https://www.biomedcentral.com/1471-2288/9/59.

Bettany-Saltikov, J. (2010a). Learning how to undertake a systematic review: Part 1. *Nursing Standard, 24*(50), 47–56.

Bettany-Saltikov, J. (2010b). Learning how to undertake a systematic review: Part 2. *Nursing Standard, 24*(51), 47–58.

Butler, A., Hall, H., & Copnell, B. (2016). A guide to writing a qualitative systematic review protocol to enhance evidence-based practice in nursing and health care. *Worldviews on Evidence-Based Nursing, 13*(3), 241–249.

Callard, F., Rose, D., & Wykes, T. (2012). Close to the bench as well as the bedside: Involving service users in all phases of translational research. *Health Expectations, 15*(4), 389–400.

Cochrane Collaboration. (2017). *Cochrane: Our evidence*. Retrieved November 19, 2017, from http://www.cochrane.org/evidence.

Cochrane Nursing Care (CNC). (2017). *Resources*. Retrieved November 30, 2017, from http://nursingcare.cochrane.org/resources.

Cocoman, A., & Murray, J. (2008). Intramuscular injections: A review of best practice for mental health nurses. *Journal of Psychiatric and Mental Health Nursing, 15*(5), 424–434.

Conn, V. S. (2010). Depressive symptom outcomes of physical activity interventions: Meta-analysis findings. *Annals of Behavioral Medicine, 39*(2), 128–138.

Conn, V. S., Valentine, J. C., Cooper, H. M., & Rantz, M. J. (2003). Methods: Grey literature in meta-analyses. *Nursing Research, 52*(4), 256–261.

Cooper, H. (2017). *Research synthesis and meta-analysis: A step-by-step approach* (5th ed.). Los Angeles, CA: Sage.

Creswell, J. W. (2014). *Research design: Qualitative, quantitative and mixed methods approaches* (4th ed.). Thousand Oaks, CA: Sage.

Eizenberg, M. M. (2010). Implementation of evidence-based nursing practice: Nurses' personal and professional factors? *Journal of Advanced Nursing, 67*(1), 33–42.

Finfgeld-Connett, D. (2010). Generalizability and transferability of meta-synthesis research findings. *Journal of Advanced Nursing, 66*(2), 246–254.

Gray, J. R., Grove, S. K., & Sutherland, S. (2017). *The practice of nursing research: Appraisal, synthesis, and generation of evidence* (8th ed.). St. Louis, MO: Elsevier Saunders.

Grove, S. K., & Cipher, D. J. (2017). *Statistics for nursing research: A workbook for evidence-based practice* (2nd ed.). St. Louis, MO: Elsevier.

Hall, H., Leach, M., Brosnan, C., & Collins, M. (2017). Nurses' attitudes towards complementary therapies: A systematic review and meta-synthesis. *International Journal of Nursing Studies, 69*(1), 47–56.

Higgins, J. P. T., & Green, S. (2008). *Cochrane handbook for systematic reviews of interventions*. West Sussex, England: Wiley-Blackwell and The Cochrane Collaboration.

Holmen, H., Wahl, A. K., Småstuen, M. C., & Ribu, L. (2017). Tailored communication within mobile apps for diabetes self-management: A systematic review. *Journal of Medical Internet Research, 19*(6), e227. Retrieved March 18, 2018, from https://www.ncbi.nlm.nih.gov/pmc/articles/PMC5501926/.

Iowa Model Collaborative. (2017). Iowa Model of Evidence-Based Practice: Revisions and validation. *Worldviews on Evidence-Based Nursing, 14*(3), 175–182.

James, P. A., Oparil, S., Carter, B. L., Cushman, W. C., Denison-Himmelfard, C., Handler, J., et al. (2014). 2014 evidence-based guidelines for the management of high blood pressure in adults: Report from the panel members appointed to the Eighth Joint National Committee (JNC 8). *Journal of the American Medical Association, 311*(5), 507–520.

Joanna Briggs Institute. (2017). *Joanna Briggs Institute (JBI): About us.* Retrieved July 19, 2017, from http://www.joannabriggs.org/about.html.

Karimi, M., & Clark, A. M. (2016). How do patients' values influence heart failure self-care decision-making?: A mixed-methods systematic review. *International Journal of Nursing Studies, 59*(1), 89–104.

Keib, C. N., Cailor, S. M., Kiersma, M. E., & Chen, A. M. (2017). Changes in nursing students' perceptions of research and evidence-based practice after completing a research course. *Nurse Education Today, 54*(1), 37–43.

Liberati, A., Altman, D. G., Tetzlaff, J., Mulrow, C., Gotzsche, P. C., Ioannidis, J. P., et al. (2009). The PRISMA Statement for reporting systematic reviews and meta-analyses of studies that evaluate healthcare interventions: Explanation and elaboration. *Annals of Internal Medicine, 151*(4), W-65–W-94.

Mackey, A., & Bassendowski, S. (2017). The history of evidence-based practice in nursing education and practice. *Journal of Professional Nursing, 33*(1), 51–55.

Mello, M. J., Bromberg, J., Baird, J., Nirenberg, T., Chun, T., Lee, C., & Linakis, J. G. (2013). Translation of alcohol screening and brief intervention guidelines to pediatric trauma centers. *Journal of Trauma & Acute Care Surgery, 75*(4), S301–S307.

Melnyk, B. M., & Fineout-Overholt, E. (2015). *Evidence-based practice in nursing and healthcare: A guide to best practice* (3rd ed.). Philadelphia, PA: Lippincott, Williams, & Wilkins.

Melnyk, B. M., Fineout-Overholt, E., Giggleman, M., & Choy, K. (2017). A test of the ARCC© Model improves implementation of evidence-based practice, healthcare culture, and patient outcomes. *Worldviews on Evidence-Based Nursing, 14*(1), 5–9.

Melnyk, B. M., Gallagher-Ford, E., & Fineout-Overholt. E. (2017). *Implementing evidence-based practice competencies in healthcare: A practical guide for improving quality, safety, & outcomes.* Indianapolis, IN: Sigma Theta Tau International.

Melnyk, B. A., Gallagher-Ford, L., Thomas, B. K., Troseth, M., Wyngarden, K., & Szalacha, L. (2016). A study of chief nurse executives indicates low prioritization of evidence-based practice and shortcomings in hospital performance metrics across the United States. *Worldview on Evidence-Based Nursing, 13*(1), 6–14.

Moher, D., Liberati, A., Tetzlaff, J., Altman, D. G., & PRISMA Group. (2009). *Preferred Reporting Items for Systematic Reviews and Meta-Analyses: The PRISMA Statement.* Retrieved July 19, 2017, from http://www.prisma-statement.org.

Moorhead, S., Johnson, M., Maas, M. L., & Swanson, E. (2013). *Nursing outcomes classification (NOC): Measurement of health outcomes* (5th ed.). St. Louis, MO: Elsevier.

Moore, Z. (2012). Meta-analysis in context. *Journal of Clinical Nursing, 21*(19/20), 2798–2807.

National Guideline Clearinghouse (NGC). (2017a). *AHRQ's National Guideline Clearinghouse: Public resource for summaries of evidence-based clinical practice guidelines.* Retrieved December 17, 2017, from https://www.guideline.gov/.

National Guideline Clearinghouse (NGC). (2017b). *National Guideline Clearinghouse: Guideline syntheses.* Retrieved December 19, 2017, from https://www.guideline.gov/syntheses/index.

National Institutes of Health (NIH). (2017). *NIH: National Center for Advancing Translational Science.* Retrieved December 30, 2017, from https://ncats.nih.gov/translation.

National Institutes of Health (NIH). (2003). *Seventh Report of the Joint National Committee on Prevention, Detection, Evaluation, and Treatment of High Blood Pressure (JNC 7).* Retrieved March 18, 2018, from www.nhlbi.nih.gov/files/docs/guidelines/phycard.pdf.

Nicoll, L. H., & Hesby, A. (2002). Intramuscular injections: An integrative research review and guideline for evidence-based practice. *Applied Nursing Research, 16*(2), 149–162.

Ogston-Tuck, S. (2014). Intramuscular injection technique: An evidence-based approach. *Nursing Standard, 29*(4), 52–59.

Pappas, D., & Williams, I. (2011). Grey literature: Its emerging importance. *Journal of Hospital Librarianship, 11*(3), 228–234.

Quality and Safety Education for Nurses (QSEN). (2017). *Pre-licensure knowledge, skills, and attitudes (KSAs)* Retrieved December 23, 2017, from http://qsen.org/competencies/pre-licensure-ksas/.

Sandelowski, M., & Barroso, J. (2007). *Handbook for synthesizing qualitative research*. New York, NY: Springer.

Schumacher, B., Askew, M., & Otten, K. (2013). Development of a pressure ulcer trigger tool for the neonatal population. *Journal of Wound, Ostomy, and Continence Nursing*, *40*(1), 46–50.

Setia, M. S. (2016). Methodology series module 6: Systematic reviews and meta-analysis. *Indian Journal of Dermatology*, *61*(6), 602–607.

Sherwood, G., & Barnsteiner, J. (2017). *Quality and safety in nursing: A competency approach to improving outcomes* (2nd ed.). Ames, IA: Wiley-Blackwell.

Sisson, H. (2015). Aspirating during the intramuscular injection procedure: A systematic literature review. *Journal of Clinical Nursing*, *24*(17/18), 2368–2375.

Stetler, C. B. (2001). Updating the Stetler model of research utilization to facilitate evidence-based practice. *Nursing Outlook*, *49*(6), 272–279.

Straus, S. E., Glasziou, P., Richardson, W. S., Rosenberg, W., & Haynes, R. B. (2011). *Evidence-based medicine: How to practice and teach EBM* (5th ed.). Edinburgh, Scotland: Churchill Livingstone Elsevier.

Straka, K. L., Brandt, P., & Brytus, J. (2013). Brief report: Creating a culture of evidence-based practice and nursing research in a pediatric hospital. *Journal of Pediatric Nursing*, *28*(4), 374–378.

Stringer, P. M. (2010). Sciatic nerve injury from intramuscular injections: A persistent and global problem. *International Journal of Clinical Practice*, *64*(11), 1573–1579.

The Joint Commission. (2017). *About The Joint Commission*. Retrieved December 17, 2017, from https://www.jointcommission.org/about_us/about_the_joint_commission_main.aspx.

Thomas, C. M., Mraz, M., & Rajcan, L. (2016). Blood aspiration during IM injection. *Clinical Nursing Research*, *25*(5), 549–559.

Titler, M. G. (2004). Overview of the U.S. invitational conference "Advancing Quality Care Through Translation Research." *Worldviews on Evidence-Based Nursing*, *1*(1), S1–S5.

Tong, A., Flemming, K., McInnes, E., Oliver, S., & Craig, J. (2012). Enhancing transparency in reporting the synthesis of qualitative research: ENTREQ. *BMC Medical Research Methodology*, *12*(181), 1–8.

Turlik, M. (2010). Evaluating the results of a systematic review/meta-analysis. *Podiatry Management*, *29*(1), 193–198.

Walsh, D., & Downe, S. (2005). Meta-synthesis method for qualitative research: A literature review. *Journal of Advanced Nursing*, *50*(2), 204–211.

Warren, J. I., McLaughin, M., Bardsley, J., Eich, J., Esche, C. A., Kropkowski, L., & Risch, S. (2016). The strengths and challenges of implementing EBP in healthcare systems. *Worldviews on Evidence-Based Nursing*, *13*(1), 15–24.

Westra, B. L., Latimer, G. E., Matney, S. A., Park, J. I., Sensmeier, J., Simpson, R. L., et al. (2015). A national action plan for sharable and comparable nursing data to support practice and translation research for transforming health care. *Journal of American Medical Informatics Association*, *22*(3), 600–607.

Whittemore, R., Chao, A., Jang, M., Minges, K. E., & Park, C. (2014). Methods for knowledge synthesis: An overview. *Heart & Lung*, *43*(5), 453–461.

Wynaden, D., Tohotoa, J., Omari, O. A., Happell, B., Heslop, K., Barr, L., & Sourinathan, V. (2015). Administering intramuscular injections: How does research translate into practice over time in the mental health setting? *Nurse Education Today*, *35*(1), 620–624.

Because of funding changes, the Agency for Healthcare Research and Quality (AHRQ) National Guideline Clearinghouse website was scheduled for decommissioning as of July 16, 2018. For more information, go to https://www.ahrq.gov/.

CHAPTER

14

Introduction to Additional Research Methodologies in Nursing: Mixed Methods and Outcomes Research

Susan K. Grove and Jennifer R. Gray

CHAPTER OVERVIEW

LEARNING OUTCOMES

After completing this chapter, you should be able to:

1. Identify quantitative and qualitative methods in mixed methods studies.
2. Describe mixed methods designs such as concurrent convergent, exploratory sequential, and explanatory sequential.
3. Describe the unique challenges of conducting mixed methods studies.
4. Critically appraise a mixed methods study.
5. Explain the theoretical basis of outcomes research.
6. Discuss the history of outcomes research in nursing.
7. Describe the role of outcomes research in determining the effect of nursing on health outcomes.
8. Differentiate outcomes research from other types of research conducted by nurses.
9. Identify the methodologies used in published outcomes studies.
10. Critically appraise an outcomes study.

This chapter was developed to introduce you to mixed methods and outcomes research methodologies. These types of research have been conducted more frequently in nursing during the last 10 years, and you will find reports of these types of studies in the literature. The content in this chapter was developed to provide you with a background for critically appraising mixed methods and outcomes studies. The first part of the chapter focuses on mixed methods research, followed by a discussion of outcomes research.

MIXED METHODS RESEARCH AND DESIGN

Clinical problems and their related research questions are frequently complex and multidimensional. Some researchers have studied these complex research questions by using quantitative and qualitative methods in the same study, an approach that is called **mixed methods research** (Creswell, 2014, 2015; Leavy, 2017). Mixed methods studies allow researchers to capitalize on the strengths of numbers and words to answer different components or stages of a research question (Creswell, 2015). In this portion of the chapter, you will learn about a philosophical foundation for mixed methods studies, different designs used in mixed methods studies, challenges of mixed methods studies, and how to critically appraise these studies.

Philosophical Foundations of Mixed Methods Designs

The philosophical foundation for mixed methods research is neither purely the objective post-positivistic view of quantitative researchers nor the subjective constructivist view of qualitative researchers. Researchers who use mixed methods designs have exchanged the dichotomy of positivism and constructivism for the middle ground of pragmatism (Yardley & Bishop, 2015). For our purposes, pragmatism is a philosophy that focuses on solving problems by whatever methods fit the problem or question (Leavy, 2017). Pragmatists want to obtain the information that they believe they need to resolve an issue. For example, a nurse manager in a clinic is concerned because patients are missing their follow-up appointments. The manager collaborates with a researcher, and together they plan a mixed methods study to describe facilitators and barriers to keeping clinic appointments. They plan to conduct focus groups with patients (qualitative data) and distribute an exit survey (quantitative data) to develop a deeper understanding of ways to promote adherence to clinic appointments. The mixed methods design was selected because the goal was to obtain the information they needed to improve the attendance rate, a goal that is consistent with a pragmatic approach (Bishop, 2015). With mixed methods designs, the researcher can allow the strengths of one method to compensate for the possible limitations of the other (Creswell, 2015). Stated in a more positive way, mixed methods research allows the strengths of each method to interact in a complementary way with the other method (Leavy, 2017).

Overview of Mixed Methods Designs

When you read an article about a mixed methods study, there are a few questions that you can answer that will help you identify the design:

1. Were the two components of the study, quantitative and qualitative, implemented concurrently or sequentially?
2. If one component preceded the other (sequential design), which was implemented first?
3. How did the researchers combine or interpret the findings of one component in light of the other?

The three questions are displayed as a decision tree in Fig. 14.1. These decisions can result in a wide range of mixed methods designs. Mixed methods designs have been described and categorized in multiple ways. The focus of this chapter will be on the three designs commonly used in nursing and health research and are consistent with Creswell's (2015) three basic designs: (1) convergent concurrent strategy; (2) exploratory sequential strategy; and (3) explanatory sequential strategy. Descriptions, diagrams, and exemplar studies of these three mixed methods approaches are provided to expand your understanding of these designs.

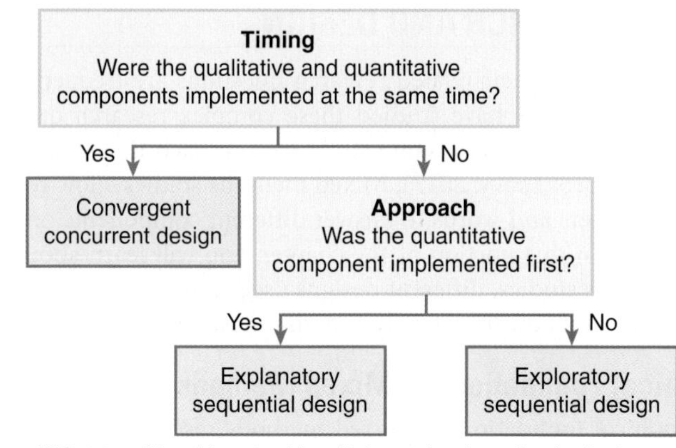

FIG 14.1 Algorithm for identifying mixed methods designs.

Convergent Concurrent Strategy

The convergent concurrent strategy is selected when a researcher wishes to use quantitative and qualitative methods in an attempt to confirm, cross-validate, or corroborate findings using a single sample or two samples from the same population (Leavy, 2017). This design may also be called a *parallel design* because quantitative and qualitative data collection processes are conducted at the same time. This strategy usually integrates the results of the two methods after the data are analyzed and during the interpretation phase. When the findings from the qualitative and quantitative methods yield the same findings, we call this *convergence,* which strengthens the evidence. When the findings from the two parts of the study are different, the researchers may be able to use the different findings to provide a broader description of the problem (Fig. 14.2).

Hagstrom (2017) conducted a convergent concurrent mixed methods study of family stress with parents of children in the pediatric intensive care unit (PICU) for more than 1 week. She clearly stated the research problem to be that "little is known about how families may experience stress as their child's intensive care unit (ICU) stay becomes prolonged" (p. 33). A complex ecological model of living in two worlds was developed from the researcher's clinical experience and the literature as the study's conceptual framework. The framework consisted of multiple factors that affect the parents and children in a family when one child is hospitalized, and the factors helped guide the interview questions. She interviewed nine parents, which represented eight families.

Hagstrom (2017) acknowledged that she emphasized the qualitative component of the study, using the quantitative findings to enrich the description of the families' stress and to compare their quantified stress with their verbal accounts of stress. Qualitative data were collected through an interview, followed by the completion of the two quantitative instruments, the Family Inventory

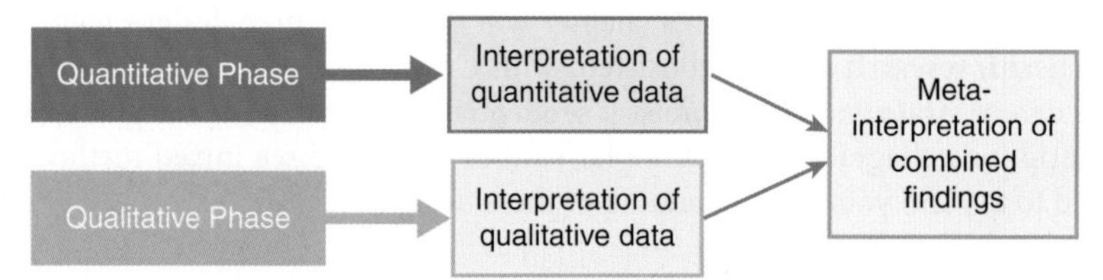

FIG 14.2 Convergent concurrent mixed methods.

of Life Events and Family Systems Stressor-Strength Inventory. The participants completed the instruments after the interview but were encouraged to talk about the reasons for their answers on the inventories as they completed them. The entire interaction with the participant was audio recorded and transcribed for analysis (Hagstrom, 2017). Although the interviews were conducted first, the transcripts were not analyzed before the quantitative phase, and both types of data were collected during one meeting, consistent with a concurrent design.

Because of the small sample size, frequencies and descriptive statistics were the only analyses reported for the quantitative data. Using the demographic data, the families were classified according to their developmental stage as a family, based on the age of the oldest child. The classification allowed the researcher to compare each family's stress scores with national norms for families in the same developmental stage (Hagstrom, 2017). Using this method, only one family was characterized as being a low-stress family. Half of the families lived 50 miles or more from the hospital, and one parent was at the hospital all the time. One family lived 1200 miles away. Some of the children had long histories of illness, with one child having had 21 previous hospitalizations. Two were newborns and were in the PICU following surgery for congenital heart defects. The quantitative analysis provided facts about the families that created the social context for the qualitative phase of the study.

The qualitative analysis revealed three themes, one of which was called *separation*. The theme of separation was comprised of the codes of "being apart," "a constant pull," "family role changes," "leaving the hospital," and "siblings at the hospital." The second theme was called *child's illness and distress*. The future health threats for the child were factors in the parents' stress related to the current illness and the child's distress. *Not knowing*, the last theme, was related to fear about what would happen next as the parents described the roller coaster ride of being in the PICU. One of the stresses was that the healthcare providers also did not know what would happen because of the many factors that affected the progress and prognosis of the child. Despite anticipatory education and guidance, parents felt unprepared for the uncertainty of their child's hospitalization (Hagstrom, 2017).

Hagstrom (2017, p. 35) described the combined analysis of the quantitative and qualitative data as comparing "within and across families to assess how they relate." One of the strengths of the study was the researcher's attention to rigor, including describing the decision trail, sampling until reaching saturation, and other methods used to increase the trustworthiness of the findings. Another strength was the integration of the combined findings with the findings from published studies. The study's contribution to nursing knowledge was the finding that the parents felt unprepared for what occurred during the hospitalization, despite the education and support provided by the healthcare team (Hagstrom, 2017). We noted one ethical concern related to confidentiality, however. In the article, demographic data were summarized for each family. For example, the family who lived 1200 miles from the hospital had a 12-year-old child with diabetes who was in the PICU as a result of having an organ transplant. The unique combination of data reported per family could have made the families identifiable to nurses and other healthcare professionals in the setting where the research took place.

Exploratory Sequential Strategy

The exploratory sequential strategy begins with the collection and analysis of qualitative data, followed by the collection of quantitative data. This strategy is often selected for underresearched topics (Leavy, 2017), with the first phase allowing for exploration of the topic to inform the quantitative phase. The results of the qualitative component may be used to design the quantitative phase (Fig. 14.3). This was the case with the study conducted by Al-Yateem, Docherty, and Rossiter

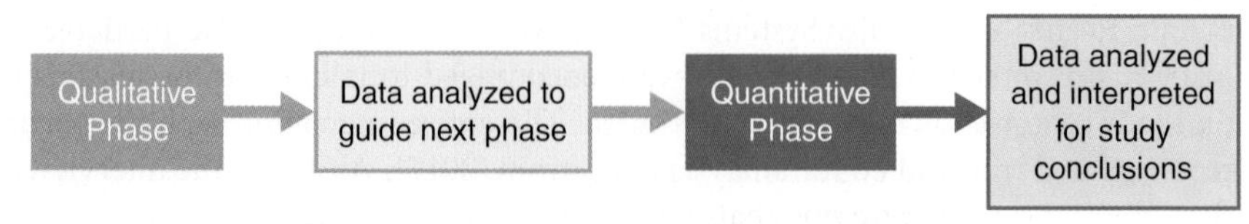

FIG 14.3 Exploratory sequential mixed methods.

(2016). During the first phase of the study, they interviewed 25 adolescents and young adults with cystic fibrosis (CF) to generate perceptions of quality care from this patient population. Using content analysis to analyze the data from the interviews, the researchers identified four determinants of quality of service, the first being "provision of adolescent friendly information related to all aspects of living with CF" (Al-Yateem et al., 2016, p. 259). The remaining three were: "services that facilitate and encourage independence," "services characterized by structure with the capacity to be both dynamic and responsive," and "health care professionals knowledgeable and skilled in adolescent specific issues" (pp. 258–259).

The qualitative findings were used to develop the questionnaire administered during the quantitative phase. The four determinants of quality of service were transformed into items on a questionnaire. "Each proposed healthcare service determinant formed an individual item on the questionnaire" (p. 257). The researchers asked a panel of 10 experts to rate the clarity and relevance of the items, resulting in a high content validity of 0.91 (Waltz, Strickland, & Lenz, 2017). Then, the 24-item questionnaire developed from the interview findings was distributed to a larger group of study participants, who were asked to rank the importance of the determinants of quality to enhance the "validity and transferability of the study results" (Al-Yateem et al., 2016, p. 257).

Recruited from a CF registry, 113 adolescents and young adults completed the questionnaire to prioritize the items. Al-Yateem et al. (2016) identified including only participants who were living with CF as a limitation when the research question more broadly addressed quality of care for children and adolescents with any chronic illness. The researchers also noted that the findings were "disappointingly consistent with the findings of many other studies examining experiences of adolescents and young adults within healthcare systems" (Al-Yateem et al., 2016, p. 261). Similar to previous findings, the findings of their study highlighted the need for services to be informed by the needs of those receiving the services. The participants indicated that healthcare professionals seemed uninformed about the "complexity of adolescent development" (p. 263) and the fact that the professionals' "protocols and checklists… did not match the actual needs" (p. 262) of their adolescent patients.

Al-Yateem and the team (2016) clearly identified the relationship between the two phases of their exploratory sequential design to be corroboration and prioritization. Content validity was reported for the survey, but no reliability information was provided. The team's focus was not on developing a tool for research purposes, but on understanding the population's perspectives on quality care. Their motivation was improving the care for chronically ill children using the four determinants of quality. The comprehensive descriptions of the determinants of quality health care can serve as standards by which adolescent care should be designed and evaluated. The major limitation of the study was that the questionnaire seemed to be developed only for use in the study and would require additional testing before it could be used to evaluate care or test the effects of an intervention.

Researchers have identified additional reasons for using the exploratory sequential design. Unlike the study by Al-Yateem et al. (2016), this mixed method approach is used frequently to develop a rigorous quantitative research tool, provide preliminary information on its psychometric properties, and prepare the tool for use with other samples in the future (Morgan, 2014). Another reason to use the design is to develop research hypotheses for the quantitative phase from the findings of the qualitative phase (Morgan, 2014). The exploratory sequential strategy may also be indicated when a topic has not been studied previously and the researchers want to elicit participants' unbiased perspectives. The concern is that the content of the quantitative instruments may influence the participants' responses. To avoid this, qualitative data are collected and analyzed first, followed by the quantitative instruments.

Explanatory Sequential Strategy

When using an explanatory sequential strategy, the researcher collects and analyzes quantitative data, and then collects and analyzes qualitative data to explain the quantitative findings (Fig. 14.4). A qualitative examination of the phenomenon facilitates a fuller understanding and is well suited to explaining and interpreting relationships.

Lenz and Lancaster (2017) selected an explanatory sequential design to strengthen the validity of their study of the effects of intensive outpatient (IOP) psychological treatment. This intervention was specifically designed for trauma survivors with a diagnosis of posttraumatic stress disorder (PTSD). The IOP format was deemed to be a feasible alternative to inpatient hospitalization when the patient demonstrated no intent to harm self or others, but needed treatment beyond traditional outpatient therapy. Based on the setting and the integration of multiple therapies, the researchers had access to admission and discharge data for persons who had received treatment in the IOP format, but lacked the resources to create a comparison or control group. "...We supplemented quantitative estimates of treatment effects with qualitative data..." to identify "participants' perceptions about which aspects of treatment were helpful for them" (Lenz & Lancaster, 2017, p. 25).

The study had three research questions. The first two questions addressed the magnitude of change in the severity of mental health symptoms and relational health from admission to discharge (Lenz & Lancaster, 2017). Quantitative instruments were used to collect these data. The third question, "What programmatic factors do clients attribute to observed changes," was answered using data from focus groups. The data from the focus groups were analyzed using grounded theory coding and processes (see Chapter 3). Grounded theory was selected as the qualitative methodology because the goal was to "generate a tentative theory to explicate commonalities in clients' experiences" in the program (Lenz & Lancaster, 2017, p. 28).

The sample for the mixed methods study consisted of 30 women and 18 men with a mean age of 43.48 years. From admission to discharge, the quantitative results revealed statistically significant changes in anxiety, depression, hostility, interpersonal sensitivity, and paranoid ideation, with medium to large effect sizes (Lenz & Lancaster, 2017). The participants indicated significant changes also in their relationships with peers and the community.

The theoretical theme of the qualitative data was *reintegration of self* in contrast to the clients' reports of "feeling fragmented and disconnected to themselves and their environment at the outset

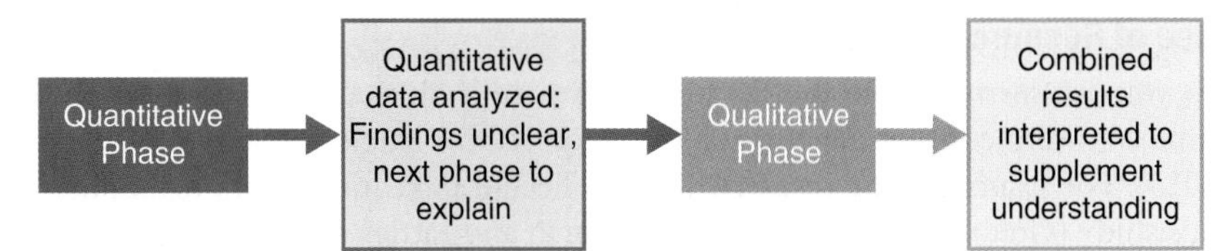

FIG 14.4 Explanatory sequential mixed methods.

of treatment" (Lenz & Lancaster, 2017, p. 29). The changes that they experienced were attributed to "a diverse therapeutic milieu that provided the building blocks of hope and healing" (p. 29). During group therapy, the clients encountered others who had been "similarly fractured by trauma," a commonality that created cohesion in the group (p. 30). Activities such as journaling provided catharsis and helped them better understand the pain that they had experienced and continued to experience. The combination of therapies allowed reintegration to "organically unfold as the clients developed the tools, awareness, and support to tackle their past" (Lenz & Lancaster, 2017, p. 31). From the quantitative phase, the findings were that "participants demonstrated meaningful changes in psychological symptoms and relational health over time"; from the qualitative phase, the findings were that "the human aspects of change and recovery from trauma that extended beyond interpretations of effect sizes" (Lenz & Lancaster, 2017, p. 31).

Lenz and Lancaster (2017, p. 32) appropriately combined two methods to overcome some of the limitations of a single-group quantitative design, which does not "permit causal attributions related to treatment implementation that could be generalized to the larger population…" They acknowledged that maturation was a threat to validity in that participants' symptoms may have improved over time, and recommended that future designs allow for between-group comparisons. Another limitation of the design was that it generated no information about the sustainability of the treatment effects, which could have been overcome by conducting a follow-up assessment a few months after treatment.

Challenges of Mixed Methods Designs

Combining Quantitative and Qualitative Data

Studies must be carefully designed to ensure congruence between the problem, purpose, questions, designs, data collection and analysis, and interpretation of the findings. Congruence of mixed methods studies can be especially challenging because quantitative and qualitative methods were founded within discrepant philosophies. Using pragmatism as an overriding philosophy, the motivation for the study and the desired outcome determine the best way to integrate the data of a mixed methods study (Morgan, 2014). Integration of the results from each component is the critical phase and should be given significant thought during the development of the study (Guetterman, Fetters, & Creswell, 2015). Ideally, plans for integrating the data are part of the research proposal and may include building the second phase of the study on the findings of the first, expanding the view of a phenomenon, or strengthening support by interpreting the findings together.

Some researchers who use mixed methods designs advocate for converting the data from the qualitative phase to the same type of data that was generated by the quantitative phase, or vice versa. When this is done, qualitative codes may be counted and converted into quantitative data, or quantitative data may be converted to conceptual ideas or themes (Leavy, 2017). Other researchers systematically compare and contrast the findings from each arm of the study, demonstrating these relationships in graphs, tables, and figures (Creswell, 2015; Guetterman et al., 2015). The capacity of mixed methods designs to answer the research questions depends on effective methods for integrating the data from each component.

Use of Resources

As you can surmise from the examples provided in this chapter, mixed methods studies require a time commitment that may exceed that required for single-method studies (Wisdom & Creswell, 2013). For example, one research team collected data for 4 years to implement a mixed methods study (Goldman & Little, 2015). Goldman and Little's study of women's empowerment among Maasai tribal groups in Tanzania and Uganda was rigorous and involved individual interviews, group interviews, and ethnographic observation for the qualitative phase and survey data for the quantitative phase. The researchers believed that the effort was worthwhile and ensured a high-quality study by spending extensive time becoming accepted into the communities in which the study was conducted. In sequential designs, the data collection and analysis must be completed for the first phase to develop or revise the second phase. Additional time often translates into a need for greater financial support (van Griensven, Moore, & Hall, 2014).

Funding

Seeking and receiving funding may be needed to ensure that the study is completed. Because of the complexity of concurrent designs, additional personnel are needed to conduct all aspects of quantitative and qualitative research at the same time. Ideally, the research team consists of health professionals with different backgrounds in education and experience (Creswell, 2015). When the research team is multidisciplinary, the team members bring different perspectives, skills, and expertise. Team members may be assigned specific aspects of the study to match their expertise. Additional time may be needed to develop the proposal when working with a multidisciplinary team as it may take longer to come to agreement on the study purpose, design, and methods because of differing philosophical and conceptual beliefs. When mixed methods studies are conducted by individual researchers, they may need additional funding in order to hire a consultant for the component of the study with which they are less familiar.

Critically Appraising Mixed Methods Designs

Agreement is beginning to emerge about the standards by which mixed methods studies should be appraised for quality (Creswell, 2015). Pluye, Gagnon, Griffiths, and Johnson-Lafleur (2009) published a systematic review of the literature to determine whether there was consensus on the quality standards by which to appraise mixed methods designs. The National Institutes of Health (NIH) through its Office of Behavioral and Social Science Research at the NIH convened a panel of experts to develop best practices for mixed methods research (Creswell, Klassen, Clark, & Smith, 2011). Part of the panel's charge was to identify criteria to evaluate mixed methods applications for funding by the NIH. For this text, we have synthesized standards across sources, resulting in a concise set of quality standards for mixed methods research (Table 14.1).

Building on your knowledge of quantitative and qualitative methods, learning how to critique mixed methods studies extends your capabilities as a scholar. The standards of quality displayed in Table 14.1 provide a systematic method for critically appraising mixed methods studies. Using the quality standards proposed, a critical appraisal of a mixed methods study conducted by Giarelli, Denigris, Fisher, Maley, and Nolan (2016) is provided as an example.

Work-related stress (WRS) and compassion fatigue of oncology nurses were the concepts of interest for the study by Giarelli et al. (2016). The study was conducted with a sample of 20 nurses on a hematology-oncology unit and "explored nurses' reports of positive and negative experiences for factors that might be modifiable and could be translated into a responsive prevention program to improve the nurse's satisfaction" (Giarelli et al., 2016, p. E121). The pragmatic reason for conducting this mixed methods study was to develop a program to reduce or prevent WRS and compassion fatigue of nurses.

Significance

The significance of the research question was established to a limited degree. Giarelli et al. (2016) stated that nurses' satisfaction with their work would improve the care provided to patients, but provided minimal evidence to support the statement. The background section included published

TABLE 14.1 CRITERIA FOR CRITICALLY APPRAISING MIXED METHODS STUDIES: QUESTIONS USED TO GUIDE THE APPRAISAL

CRITERION	QUESTION
Significance	1. Were the relevance and significance of the research question convincingly described?
Expertise	2. Did the researcher or research team possess the necessary skills and experience to implement the study rigorously? 3. Were the contributions or expertise of each team member noted?
Appropriateness	4. Was the need to use mixed methods established? 5. Did the mixed methods strategy fulfill the purpose or purposes of the study?
Sampling	6. How was the sample selected and recruited? 7. Was the rationale for selecting the samples for each component of the study provided?
Methods	8. For the quantitative and qualitative components of the study, were the timing, data collection and analysis, interpretation, and integration of findings described in detail? 9. Were the reliability and validity of quantitative methods described? 10. Were the trustworthiness, dependability, and credibility of qualitative methods described? 11. Was protection of human subjects addressed in the study?
Findings	12. Was the integration of quantitative and qualitative results presented in a table, graph, or matrix? 13. Were the study limitations noted? 14. Were the findings consistent with the analysis, interpretation, and integration of the qualitative and quantitative data?
Conclusions and Implications	15. Were the conclusions and implications congruent with the findings of the study?
Contribution to Knowledge	16. Were important benefits of the study noted? 17. Was the study's contribution to knowledge worth the time and resources of a mixed methods study?

Adapted from Creswell, J. W. (2014). *Research design: Qualitative, quantitative, and mixed methods approaches* (4th ed.). Los Angeles, CA: Sage; Creswell, J. W. (2015). *A concise introduction to mixed methods research.* Los Angeles, CA: Sage; and Creswell, J., Klassen, A., Clark, V., Smith, K. (2011). *Best practices for mixed methods research in health sciences.* https://www2.jabsom.hawaii.edu/native/docs/tsudocs/Best_Practices_for_Mixed_Methods_Research_Aug2011.pdf.

research on burnout, compassion fatigue, and WRS, noting some conflicting evidence. The researchers established that these concepts were applicable to healthcare professionals across settings.

Expertise

The research team included three members who were faculty with doctoral degrees, with one having a research doctoral degree, another having a doctor of nursing practice (DNP), and the third a doctor of education degree. Dr. Giarelli had not previously published on the topic of nurses' work stress and satisfaction, but had had several publications on the genetic aspects of cancer published in the same journal. She has also published extensively as an individual and as part of a team in the area of autism spectrum disorder. She has published both quantitative and qualitative studies, but no mixed methods studies were found. Dr. Giarelli was an experienced leader of the research team.

Dr. Fisher had had experience with mixed methods and has had numerous research publications. The remaining team members were a clinic manager of an oncology unit and a student serving as a research assistant (Giarelli et al., 2016). The clinic manager, Ms. Denigris, had had two publications related to the oncology care. Denigris worked with Giarelli to conceptualize the research problem and design of the study, which may indicate concerns about the compassion fatigue of the nurses on her unit. The research team was a highly experienced team. The contributions of each member were clearly noted and appropriate for his or her education.

Appropriateness

This criterion addresses whether the design was appropriate for the study's purpose, beginning with the researchers establishing a need to use mixed methods. The purpose of the study was to "examine factors that influence a nurse's perceived quality of work life and risk for CF" [compassion fatigue] (Giarelli et al., 2016, E121). The need to use a mixed methods design was supported by the researchers noting the complexity and personal nature of the phenomenon. Giarelli et al. (2016, p. E123) also evaluated the literature they reviewed, noting conflicting findings and small sample sizes. The argument was that collecting both quantitative and qualitative data would result in a more comprehensive description of the phenomenon and support the development of a prevention program (Giarelli et al., 2016). They concluded that the ongoing problem of compassion fatigue indicated a need to "expand the understanding and pursue prevention strategies using a highly personal approach, engaging the nurse in the process of thinking about his or her risk, and soliciting recommendations" (Giarelli et al., 2016, p. E123).

Sampling

The study was conducted on a single unit in a hospital that was staffed by 50 registered nurses (RNs) who worked 12-hour shifts. Twenty of the nurses volunteered to participate in the study. The sample was the same for quantitative and qualitative data collections. The unit manager recruited the sample from the unit where she was employed by posting announcements. When nurses expressed an interest, the manager obtained informed consent and provided a packet of research instruments. Inclusion of the unit manager on the team may have had positive or negative effects on whether nurses chose to participate. The nurses in the sample were able to provide the data needed to answer the research questions.

Methods

The researchers labeled their study as a descriptive mixed methods design. Using the questions in Fig. 14.1, the study qualifies as a convergent concurrent design (Giarelli et al., 2016). The researchers used psychometrically sound research instruments, consistent with the logical-positivistic philosophy associated with quantitative research. The reliability and validity of the instruments in previous studies were reported. In-person and telephone interviews were conducted to gather personal qualitative descriptions of WRS and compassion fatigue, consistent with constructivism. Pragmatism was the overriding philosophy of the study, and it guided the interview questions that elicited recommendations about prevention methods.

Sufficient detail was provided for most data collection procedures. As noted, psychometric characteristics of the quantitative instruments were provided, as well as the interview questions (Giarelli et al., 2016). The data analysis procedures were described, but no reliability assessments of the instruments were reported with this sample. The report included insufficient detail for someone to be able to critique how data from the two components were interpreted and integrated. The researchers described the congruence and incongruence of the quantitative and qualitative results

TABLE 14.2 VISUAL DISPLAY OF THE QUANTITATIVE AND QUALITATIVE FINDINGS OF THE MIXED METHODS STUDY OF ONCOLOGY NURSES' WORK-RELATED STRESS AND COMPASSION FATIGUE

VARIABLE OR CONCEPT	INSTRUMENT		
	QUANTITATIVE FINDINGS	QUALITATIVE FINDINGS	SUMMARY
Personal life stress	IES: 14 had none to mild impact and 6 had high impact because of work stress; 19 had none to mild impact on symptoms related to stress. LES: 14 had low to moderate risk and 6 had high risk that stress would affect health.	11 indicated that their work was rewarding and fulfilling; only 3 indicated that work stress affected home life. Almost all had no symptoms of work stress affecting home.	Mixed; quantitative data indicated more stress, whereas qualitative data indicated higher levels of work satisfaction.
Quality of work life	ProQOL: 10 had high compassion satisfaction; 14 had low levels of burnout. None of the nurses reported low compassion satisfaction, high levels of burnout, and STS.	Sources of workplace stress included communication breakdowns, structure of work environment, and care-driven factors, such as demanding families; 75% expected to still be working in oncology in 5 years.	Mixed; qualitative data indicated higher stresses at work, but still found satisfaction in the work.

IES, Impact of events scale; *LES,* life events scale; *ProQOL,* professional quality of life; *STS,* secondary traumatic stress.

in the text, but it was difficult to follow and link to the supporting data. A visual display or table showing the integration of the quantitative and qualitative findings would have been very helpful. Table 14.2 was developed from the study's results to show how the findings might have been integrated.

The protection of human subjects was clear in the study. Giarelli et al. (2016) obtained approval from the university's institutional review board (IRB) and the facility's IRB. Separating identifying information from the coded data of the instruments protected the anonymity of the quantitative data. Having a nonmember of the research team conduct the interviews and having no names on the audiotapes or transcripts protected the confidentiality of the qualitative data.

The quantitative procedures were appropriate for a descriptive nonintervention study. Qualitative procedures were conducted to support trustworthiness, dependability, and credibility of the findings, such as ensuring the accuracy of the interview transcripts (Giarelli et al., 2016). The researchers used peer debriefing to come to a consensus about the themes from the interviews. Quotations from the participants were included in the published report as evidence to support the themes.

Findings

The lack of a table or diagram showing the integration of the results from the quantitative and qualitative design components left integration of the results unclear. Limitations identified by the researchers included the homogeneity of the sample for gender, race, and ethnicity and the unknown impact of 12-hour shifts on WRS. Other limitations include self-selection of the nurses, the unit manager being involved in recruitment, and small sample size for the quantitative arm of the study. Giarelli et al. (2016) noted that the study participants reported minimal WRS stress and compassion fatigue. One explanation may be that some nurses on the unit choose not to participate because of a lack of emotional energy as a result of higher degrees of stress and fatigue.

Conclusions and Implications

Giarelli et al. (2016) concluded that the study supported the social nature of WRS and compassion fatigue. Therefore unit, institution, and interpersonal factors need to be assessed in specific settings before implementing a prevention plan for burnout. The researchers' conclusions and implications for nursing were appropriately cautious based on the study limitations and threats to validity.

Contributions to Knowledge

The investment of time, money, and effort provided helpful information for a specific unit that had physically and psychologically vulnerable patients with high acuity (Giarelli et al, 2016). Because of the conclusion about the specificity of factors influencing WRS and compassion fatigue, the findings have limited generalizability. The researchers did not identify what may have been one of the most important benefits of the study, which might have been providing an opportunity for nurses to verbalize their WRS stress and recommend personal and unit strategies for the prevention of compassion fatigue and burnout.

OUTCOMES RESEARCH

Outcomes research is a rigorous scientific method that is focused on the end results of patient care. More specifically, outcomes research is concerned with the effectiveness of healthcare interventions and health services (Doran, 2011; Kane & Radosevich, 2011). In the context of nursing, outcomes research focuses on how a patient's health status changes as a result of the nursing care received or the nursing services delivered (Moorhead, Johnson, Maas, & Swanson, 2013). According to the Agency for Healthcare Research and Quality (AHRQ), outcomes research is conducted to understand the end results of particular healthcare practices and interventions. End results include effects that people experience and care about, such as a change in their ability to function. In particular, for individuals with chronic conditions, for whom cure is not always possible, end results include quality of life, functioning, symptom management, and mortality. By linking the care people receive to the outcomes that they experience, outcomes research has become the key to developing better ways to monitor and improve quality of care (AHRQ, 2017a).

The momentum propelling outcomes research comes primarily from policy makers, insurers, and the public. They are basing payment for care on the economic efficiency of healthcare systems, especially the public health sector. As a result, there has been a growing demand for data that document the interventions, justify the costs of care, and demonstrate improved patient outcomes. In that regard, nursing-sensitive outcomes have become an issue of increasing interest because of national concerns related to the quality of patient care (Moorhead et al., 2013). Because nurses are at the forefront of care delivery, the demand for professional accountability regarding patient outcomes dictates that we can identify and document outcomes influenced by nursing care.

The first part of this outcomes research section addresses the theoretical basis of outcomes research, provides a brief history of the emerging endeavors to examine outcomes, explains the importance of outcomes research designed to examine nursing practice, and highlights methodologies used in outcomes research. This outcomes research section concludes with an introduction to guidelines that might be used to critically appraise outcomes studies. The movement to outcomes research and the approaches described in this chapter are a worldwide phenomenon (AHRQ, 2017a; Kenner, 2017).

Outcomes research differs significantly from the other types of research addressed in this text. Outcomes studies are more complex in design, population, settings, and data analyses, and the researchers engaged in the studies are often from a mix of disciplines, such as economics and public health, as well as from nursing. The studies use a unique theoretical framework to focus on health outcomes. In keeping with the interprofessional perspective of outcomes research, a broad base of literature from a variety of disciplines was used to develop the content for this chapter.

Theoretical Basis of Outcomes Research

The theorist Avedis Donabedian (1978, 1980, 1987) proposed a theory of quality health care and provided a process for evaluating it. This theory is still the dominating framework for outcomes research. Other theories of outcomes have since been developed, but we will limit our discussion to Donabedian's theory. Although quality is the overriding construct of Donabedian's theory, he never actually defined this concept himself (Mark, 1995). The World Health Organization (WHO; 2017) has defined **quality of care** as the extent to which healthcare services provided to individuals and populations improve desired health outcomes and are consistent with current professional knowledge.

Donabedian (1987) represented the key concepts and relationships in his theory using a cube. The cube shown in Fig. 14.5 helps explain the elements of quality health care. The three dimensions of the cube are health, the subjects of care, and the providers of care. The cube also incorporates

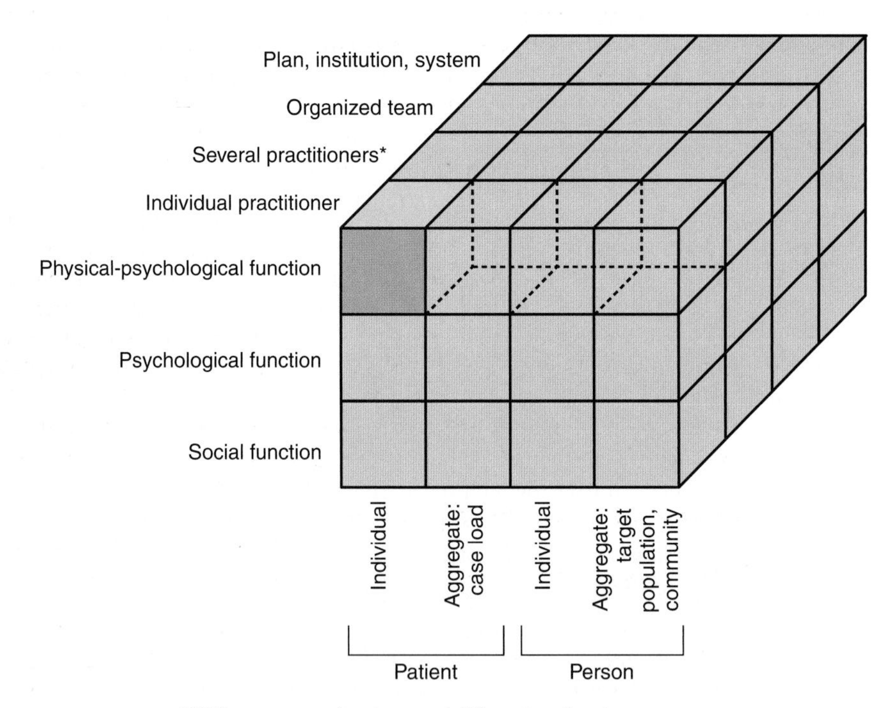

FIG 14.5 Level and scope of concern as factors in the definition of quality. (From Donabedian, A. [1987]. Some basic issues in evaluating the quality of health care. In L. T. Rinke [Ed.], *Outcome measures in home care*. vol. 1 [pp. 3–28]. New York, NY: National League for Nursing.)

three of the many aspects of health—physical function, psychological function, and social function. Donabedian (1987, p. 4) proposed that "the manner in which we conceive of health, and of our responsibility for it, makes a fundamental difference to the concept of quality and, as a result, to the methods that we use to assess and assure the quality of care."

Donabedian (1987, 2005) identified three foci of evaluation in appraising quality—structure (e.g., nursing units, hospitals, home health agencies), process (how care is provided, such as practice style or standard of care), and outcomes (end results of care). Each of these concepts is addressed in this chapter. A complete quality outcomes study requires the simultaneous inclusion of all three and an examination of the relationships among them. However, researchers have had little success in accomplishing this theoretical goal. Studies designed to examine all three concepts would require sufficiently large samples of various structures, each with the various processes being compared, and with large samples of study participants who have experienced the outcomes of those processes. The funding required and cooperation necessary to accomplish this goal have not yet been realized; however, there are examples of nursing research in which two or more aspects of structure, process, and/or outcomes have been examined. Numerous studies conducted by nurses in the United States (Kutney-Lee, Sloane, & Aiken, 2013; Rosenfeld & Glassman, 2016; Staggs, Olds, Cramer, & Shorr, 2017) and internationally (Bakker et al., 2011; Oh, Park, Yin, Piao, & Lee, 2014) have explored the relationships among nursing services, nursing interventions, and patient outcomes. Nursing interventions reflect the care delivered by nurses. A falls risk assessment and pressure ulcer risk assessment are examples of nursing interventions. Nursing services is a general concept referring to the organization and administration of nursing activities. Nursing service variables that have been studied include the skill mix and configuration of nursing personnel; staffing levels; assignment patterns (e.g., primary nursing, functional assignments, team nursing); shift patterns; levels of nursing education, experience, and expertise; ratios of full-time to part-time nurses; level and type of nursing leadership available centrally and on units; cohesion and communication among the nursing staff and between nurses and physicians; implementation of clinical care maps for patients with selected diagnoses; and the interrelationships of these factors (Kane & Radosevich, 2011; Moorhead et al., 2013).

Nursing-Sensitive Outcomes

Nursing-sensitive patient outcomes (NSPOs) are considered sensitive because they are influenced by nursing care decisions and actions. It may not be caused by nursing but is associated with nursing. In various situations, "nursing" might be the individual nurse, nurses as a working group, the approach to nursing practice, the nursing unit or institution that determines the numbers of nurses, their salaries, educational levels of nurses, assignments of nurses, workload of nurses, management of nurses, and policies related to nurses and nursing practice. It might even include the architecture of the nursing unit. In whatever form, nursing actions have a role in the outcome, even though acts of other healthcare professionals, organizational factors, and patient characteristics and behaviors often are involved in the outcome. What patient outcomes can you think of that might be nursing-sensitive? Examples of nursing-sensitive outcomes and their definitions are summarized in Table 14.3 (Doran, 2011; Moorhead et al., 2013).

The Nursing Role Effectiveness Model in Fig. 14.6 was developed to guide conceptualization and research related to nursing-sensitive outcomes. It also provided the theoretical basis for a systematic review of the "state of the science on nursing-sensitive outcomes measurement" (Doran, 2011, p. 15). Irvine, Sidani, and Hall (1998) adapted Donabedian's (1987) theory of quality in their development of the Nursing Role Effectiveness Model. This model has three major components: structure, process (the nurses' roles), and patient and health outcomes.

TABLE 14.3 NURSING-SENSITIVE PATIENT OUTCOMES AND DEFINITIONS

OUTCOME CONCEPT	DEFINITION
Functional status	Functional status is a multidimensional construct that consists of, at least, behavioral (e.g., performance of activities of daily living), psychological (e.g., mood), cognitive (e.g., attention, concentration), and social (e.g., activities associated with roles) components (Doran, 2011; Moorhead et al., 2013).
Self-care	Self-care behavior entails the practice of actions or activities that individuals initiate and perform, within time frames, on their own behalf in the interest of maintaining life, healthy functioning, continued personal development, and well-being (Moorhead et al., 2013; Orem, 2001; Sidani, 2011a).
Symptoms	"Symptoms refer to (a) sensations or experiences reflecting changes in a person's biopsychosocial functions, (b) a patient's perception of an abnormal physical, emotional, or cognitive state, (c) the perceived indicators of change in normal functioning, as experienced by patients, or (d) subjective experience reflecting changes in the biopsychosocial functioning, sensations, or cognition of an individual" (Sidani, 2011b, p. 132).
Pain	Pain has been defined as "the severity of observed or reported adverse cognitive and emotional response to physical pain" (Moorhead et al., 2013, p. 389).
Adverse outcome	An adverse outcome is defined as consequence of injury caused by medical management or complication rather than by the underlying disease itself, and generally includes prolonged health care, a resulting disability, or death at the time of discharge (Doran, 2011).
Psychological distress	Psychological distress has been defined as "the emotional condition that one feels in response to having to cope with situations that are unsettling, frustrating, or perceived as harmful or threatening" (Lazarus & Folkman's work, as cited in Howell, 2011, p. 289).
Patient satisfaction with care	Patient "satisfaction with care outcomes describes an individual's perceptions of the quality and adequacy of health care provided" (Moorhead et al., 2013, p. 49).
Mortality rate	Mortality, in its simplest meaning, reflects death. "When examining death as a quality-of-care outcome, rates of death are examined for specific patient samples or populations" (Tourangeau, 2011, p. 411).
Healthcare utilization	"Healthcare utilization can be thought of as the sum or aggregate of services consumed by patients in their attempts to maintain or regain a level of health status, along with the costs of these services" (Clarke, 2011, p. 441).

Structure in outcomes has three subcomponents—nurse, organization, and patient. Nurse variables that influence the quality of nursing care include factors such as experience level, knowledge, and skill level. Organizational components that can affect the quality of nursing care include staff mix, workload, and assignment patterns. Patient characteristics that can affect the quality of care and outcomes include health status, disease severity, and morbidity.

The process includes the **nurse's role in outcomes,** which has three subcomponents: nurse's independent role functions, nurse's dependent role functions, and nurse's interdependent role

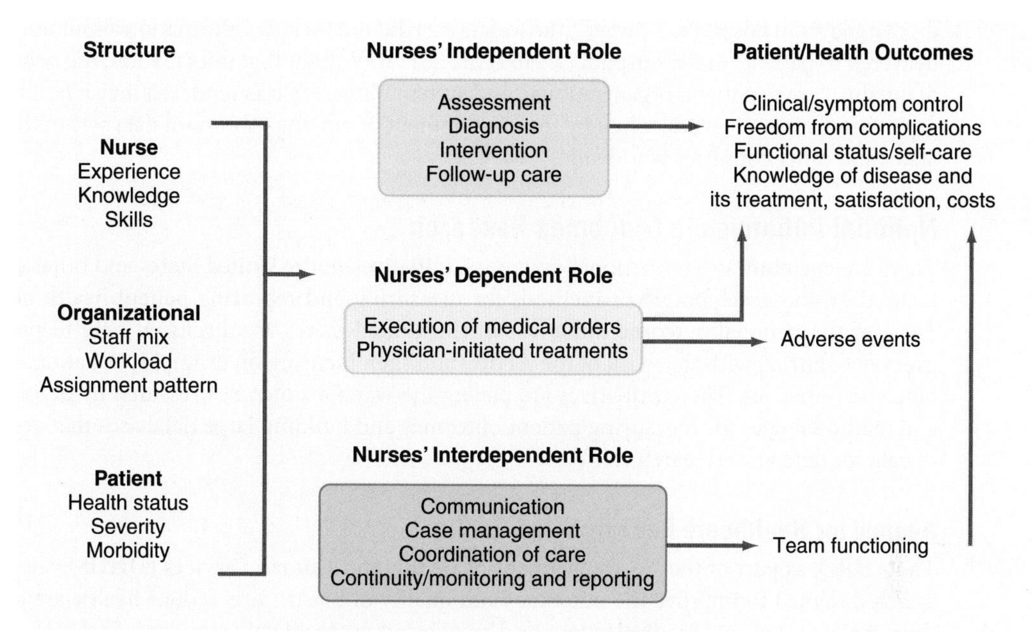

FIG 14.6 Nursing role effectiveness model. (From Irvine, D., Sidani, S., & Hall, L. M. [1998]. Linking outcomes to nurses' roles in health care. *Nursing Economic$, 16*[2], 58–64.)

functions. The nurses' independent role functions include assessment, diagnosis, nurse-initiated interventions, and follow-up care. The patient and health outcomes of the independent role are clinical and symptom control, freedom from complications, functional status and self-care, knowledge of disease and its treatment, satisfaction, and costs (see Fig. 14.7). The nurses' dependent role functions include execution of medical orders and physician-initiated treatments. It is the dependent role functions that can lead to patient and health outcomes of adverse events, such as infection, stroke, or kidney failure. Nurses' interdependent role functions include communication, case management, coordination and continuity of care, monitoring, and reporting. The interdependent role functions result in team functioning and affect the patient and health outcomes of the independent role. Patient and health outcomes are clearly interwoven into the entire care context (Irvine et al., 1998).

Origins of Outcomes and Performance Monitoring

Florence Nightingale has been credited as being the first nurse to collect data to identify nursing's contribution to quality care and conduct research into patient outcomes (Magnello, 2010). However, efforts to collect data systematically to assess outcomes in more modern times did not gain widespread attention in the United States until the late 1970s. At that time, concerns about quality of care prompted the development of the Universal Minimum Health Data Set, which was followed shortly thereafter by the Uniform Hospital Discharge Data Set (Kleib, Sales, Doran, Mallette, & White, 2011). These data sets facilitated consistency in data collection among healthcare organizations by prescribing the data elements to be gathered. The aggregated data were then used to perform an assessment of quality of care in hospitals and provide information on patients discharged from hospitals. However, those data sets did not include information about nursing care delivered to patients in the hospital (Kleib et al., 2011). Without that information, the contribution of nursing care to patient, organizational, and system outcomes was rendered invisible. This major gap in information was addressed by the development of nursing minimum data sets in the United States and other countries worldwide.

National Initiatives in Outcomes Research

There are currently several national outcomes' initiatives in the United States and other countries focused on the development of methods for measuring and reporting patient health outcomes. Some of the national outcome initiatives in the United States are discussed here to provide an overview, starting with the work of the AHRQ and then focusing on examples of national nursing outcome initiatives. These initiatives are paving the way for outcomes research by building tools and methodologies for measuring patient outcomes and building large databases that are sources of data for outcomes research.

Agency for Healthcare Research and Quality

The AHRQ, as part of the US Department of Health and Human Services (DHHS), supports research designed to improve the outcomes and quality of health care, reduce healthcare costs, address patient safety and medical errors, and broaden access to effective services. The AHRQ website (http://www.ahrq.gov) is a valuable source of information about outcomes research, funding opportunities, and results of recently completed research, including nursing research. The AHRQ (2017b) grant announcements focus on "supporting research to improve the quality, effectiveness, accessibility, and cost effectiveness of health care."

Patient-Centered Outcomes Research

One of the most current AHRQ initiatives is comparative effectiveness research. Funding from the American Recovery and Reinvestment Act (Recovery Act), signed into law in 2009, allowed the AHRQ to expand its work in support of comparative effectiveness research, including enhancing the Effective Health Care Program. A total of $473 million was designated for funding patient-centered outcomes research (PCOR) within the PCOR Institute (PCORI). The PCORI (2017) "helps people make informed healthcare decisions, and improves healthcare delivery and outcomes, by producing and promoting high-integrity, evidence-based information that comes from research guided by patients, caregivers, and the broader healthcare community." The number one funding priority for the AHRQ is improving healthcare quality by supporting the implementation of PCOR. The AHRQ has a broad research portfolio that involves almost every aspect of health care, including:

- Clinical practice
- Outcomes and effectiveness of care
- Evidence-based practice (EBP)
- Primary care and care for priority populations
- Healthcare quality
- Patient safety and medical errors
- Organization and delivery of care and use of healthcare resources
- Healthcare costs and financing
- Health information technology
- Knowledge transfer

National Quality Forum

The National Quality Forum (NQF) was created in 1999 as a national standard-setting organization for healthcare performance measures (NQF, 2017a). The NQF portfolio of voluntary consensus standards includes performance measures, serious reportable events, and preferred practices (i.e., safe practices). A complete list of measures included in the NQF portfolio can be found online (http://www.qualityforum.org/Measures_Reports_Tools.aspx). Approximately one-third of the measures in NQF's portfolio are measures of patient outcomes, such as mortality, readmissions, health functioning, depression, and experience of care. The NQF includes several nursing-sensitive measures in its performance measurement portfolio. Those that were submitted by the American Nurses Association (ANA) under the National Database of Nursing Quality Indicators (see later) include the following:

- Nursing staff skill mix
- Nursing care hours per patient day
- Catheter-associated urinary tract infection rate
- Central line–associated bloodstream infection rate
- Fall and injury rates
- Hospital- and unit-acquired pressure ulcer rates
- Nurse turnover rate
- RN practice environment scale
- Ventilator-associated pneumonia rate

These indicators are the first nationally standardized performance measures of nursing-sensitive outcomes in acute care hospitals and have been designed to assess healthcare quality, patient safety, and a professional and safe work environment. Although most of the measures in use focus on the failure to meet expected standards, the NQF believes that quality is as much about influencing positive outcomes as about avoiding negative outcomes. Therefore the NQF is currently developing national standards to evaluate the quality of health care based on how patients feel. It notes that "national quality assessment programs usually measure and reward practices based on improving clinical processes such as re-hospitalization or infection rates. Although this type of information is important and useful to clinicians, it doesn't always take into account what is most important to the patient and families of the patient receiving care, such as the management of long-term symptoms or ability to conduct daily activities" (NQF, 2017b).

National Database of Nursing Quality Indicators

In 1994, the ANA, in collaboration with the American Academy of Nursing Expert Panel on Quality Health Care, launched a plan to identify indicators of quality nursing practice and collect and analyze data using these indicators throughout the United States (Mitchell, Ferketich, & Jennings, 1998). The goal was to identify and/or develop nursing-sensitive quality measures. Donabedian's theory was used as the framework for the project. Together, these indicators were referred to as the ANA **Nursing Care Report Card,** which could facilitate benchmarking or setting a desired standard that would allow comparisons of hospitals in terms of their nursing care quality.

In 1998, the ANA provided funding to develop a national database to house data collected using nursing-sensitive quality indicators. This became the National Database of Nursing Quality Indicators (NDNQI, 2017; Montalvo, 2007). Participation in NDNQI meets requirements for the Magnet Recognition Program®, and 20% of database members participate for that reason. Current research by Richards, Lasater, and McHugh (2017) has linked Magnet hospitals with better outcomes for patients and nurses. Detailed guidelines for data collection, including definitions and decision guides, have been provided by the NDNQI (2017). The NDNQI nursing-sensitive indicators are summarized in Table 14.4.

TABLE 14.4 AMERICAN NURSES ASSOCIATION NATIONAL DATABASE OF NURSING QUALITY INDICATORS

INDICATOR	SUBINDICATOR	MEASURE
1. Nursing care hours per patient day[a,b]	a. Registered nurse (RN) b. Licensed practical nurse, licensed vocational nurse (LPN, LVN) c. Unlicensed assistive personnel (UAP)	Structure
2. Patient falls[a,b]		Process and outcome
3. Patient falls with injury[a,b]	a. Injury level	Process and outcome
4. Pediatric pain assessment, intervention, reassessment cycle		Process
5. Pediatric peripheral intravenous infiltration rate		Outcome
6. Pressure ulcer prevalence	a. Community-acquired b. Hospital-acquired c. Unit-acquired	Process and outcome
7. Psychiatric physical and sexual assault rate		Outcome
8. Restraint prevalence[b]		Outcome
9. RN education and certification		Structure
10. RN satisfaction survey options[a,c]	a. Job satisfaction scales b. Job satisfaction scales short form c. Practice environment scale[b]	Process and outcome
11. Skill mix—percentage of total nursing hours supplied by ANA and National Quality Forum[a,b]	a. RN b. LPN, LVN c. UAP d. Number of total nursing care hours supplied by agency staff (%)	Structure
12. Voluntary nurse turnover[b]		Structure
13. Nurse vacancy rate		Structure
14. Nosocomial infections a. Urinary catheter–associated urinary tract infection[b] b. Central line catheter–associated bloodstream infection[a,b] c. Ventilator-associated pneumonia[b]		Outcome

[a]Original American Nursing Association nursing-sensitive indicator.
[b]National Quality Forum–endorsed nursing-sensitive indicator.
[c]The RN survey is annual, whereas the other indicators are quarterly.
ANA, American Nursing Association.

Other organizations currently involved in efforts to study nursing-sensitive outcomes include the Collaborative Alliance for Nursing Outcomes California Database (CALNOC, 2017a), Centers for Medicare & Medicaid Services (CMS) Hospital Quality Initiative, American Hospital Association, Federation of American Hospitals, and The Joint Commission.

Oncology Nursing Society

The Oncology Nursing Society (ONS, 2017) is a professional organization of more than 35,000 RNs and other healthcare providers dedicated to excellence in patient care, education, research, and administration in oncology nursing. The ONS has taken a leadership role among specialty nursing organizations in developing an EBP resource area on its website (http://www.ons.org/ClinicalResources). The site provides nurses with a guide to identify, critically appraise, and use evidence to solve clinical problems. The ONS website also assists nurses, in particular advanced practice nurses, who are helping others develop EBP protocols. The outcomes resource area is helpful to nurses for achieving desired outcomes for people with cancer by providing outcome measures, resource cards, and evidence tables.

Advanced Practice Nursing Outcomes Research

Demonstrating the value of advanced practice nurses' (APNs) roles within the healthcare system has been the focus of much of the outcomes research in nursing, probably because advanced practice roles are often under threat when healthcare organizations restructure under cost constraints or when new advanced practice roles are first introduced, as was the case with the clinical nurse specialist (CNS) and nurse practitioner (NP) roles. The ANA recognizes four types of APNs—certified registered nurse anesthetists (CRNAs), certified nurse-midwives (CNMs), CNSs, and NPs. Studying APNs requires a determination of what happens during the process of APN care. This care involves a set of activities within, among, and between practitioners and patients and includes technical and interpersonal elements. Thus the process of care for APNs is complex, varied, and individualized. However, clearly describing what occurs during the process is essential to developing a comprehensive understanding of how APNs affect outcomes. Kleinpell's (2013) book provides a detailed discussion of the assessment of outcomes for NPs, CNSs, CRNAs, CNMs, and those with a DNP degree.

Outcomes Research and Nursing Practice

Outcome studies provide rich opportunities to build a stronger scientific underpinning for nursing practice. Nurse researchers have been actively involved in the effort to examine the outcomes of patient care. Ideally, we would like to understand the outcomes of nursing practice within a one-to-one nurse-patient relationship; however, in most cases, the nursing effect is shared because more than one nurse cares for a patient. In addition, nurse managers and nurse administrators have control over the nursing staff and the environment of nursing practice, and this control affects the autonomy of the nurse to implement practice. Consequently, outcomes research must first focus on how nursing care is organized rather than on what nurses do. When that occurs, we may begin to determine how what nurses do influences patient outcomes.

Evaluating Outcomes of Care

In this section, a description of approaches to evaluating outcomes, structural variables, and processes of care is presented. Fig. 14.7 demonstrates the relationship of structure and process that influences healthcare outcomes. The goal of outcomes research is the evaluation of the endpoints of

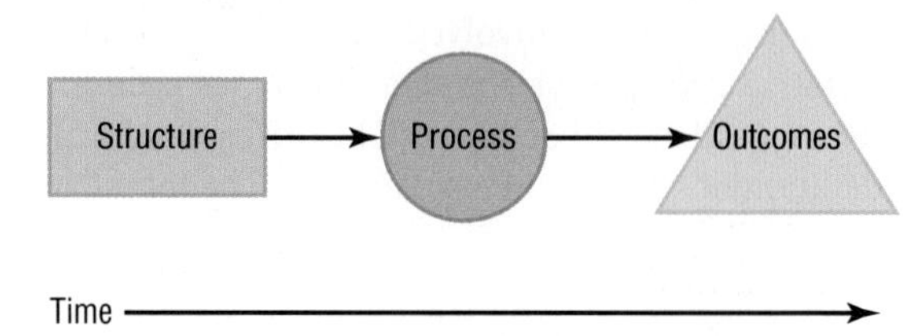

FIG 14.7 Donabedian's theory of quality focused on structure, process, and outcomes. (Adapted from Donabedian, A. [2003]. *An introduction to quality assurance in health care.* Oxford, UK: Oxford University Press.)

care as defined by Donabedian; however, this goal is not as easily realized. Donabedian's (1987) theory requires that identified outcomes be clearly linked with the process that caused the outcome. Researchers need to define the process and justify the causal links with the selected outcomes. The identification of desirable outcomes of care requires dialogue between the recipients and providers of care. Although the providers of care may delineate what is achievable, the recipients of care must clarify what is desirable. A desirable outcome addresses issues of specific concern to patients, such as long-term symptoms or ability to conduct activities of daily living. The outcomes must also be relevant to the goals of the health professionals, the healthcare system of which the professionals are a part, and society.

Outcomes are time-dependent. Some outcomes may not be apparent for a long period after the process that is purported to have caused them, whereas others may be identified immediately (see Fig. 14.8). Some outcomes are temporary, and others are permanent. Therefore an appropriate time frame must be established for determining the selected outcomes.

A final issue in evaluating outcomes is determining attribution. This requires assigning the place and degree of responsibility for the outcomes observed. Many factors other than health care may influence outcomes, and precautions must be taken to hold constant all the significant factors, other than healthcare factors, or to account for their effect if valid conclusions can be drawn from outcomes research. In particular, patient factors such as the pathophysiology of the disease, treatment compliance, genetic predisposition to disease, age, propensity to use resources, high-risk behaviors (e.g., smoking, poor dietary habits, drug abuse), and lifestyle, must be taken into account. Environmental factors such as air quality, public policies related to smoking, and occupational hazards must be included. The responsibility for outcomes may be distributed among the providers, patients, employers, insurers, community, and governmental agencies. Some examples of outcomes studies are presented in Table 14.5.

There is as yet little scientific basis for judging the precise relationship between each of these complicating factors and the selected outcome. Many of the influencing factors may be outside the jurisdiction or influence of the healthcare system or of the providers within it. One way to address this problem of identifying relevant outcomes is to define a set of proximal outcomes specific to the condition for which care is being provided. A **proximal outcome** is an outcome that is close to the delivery of care. An example of a proximal outcome is signs and symptoms of disease (Moorhead et al., 2013; Kane & Radosevich, 2011). A **distal outcome** is removed from proximity to the care or service received and is more influenced by external (nontreatment or nonintervention) factors than a proximal outcome. Quality of life is an example of a distal outcome. Moorhead and colleagues (2013) have developed the Nursing Outcomes Classification (NOC), an important source that identifies proximal and distal nurse-sensitive outcomes for research and practice.

TABLE 14.5 STUDIES INVESTIGATING THE RELATIONSHIPS BETWEEN THE CONCEPTS OF STRUCTURE, PROCESS, AND/OR OUTCOMES

YEAR	STUDY
2017	Richards, M. R., Lasater, K., & McHugh, M. (2017). A race to the top? Competitive pressure and Magnet adoption among U.S. hospitals 1997-2012. *Medical Care, 55*(4), 384–390.
2017	Staggs, V. S., Olds, D. M., Cramer, E., & Shorr, R. I. (2017). Nursing skill mix, nurse staffing level, and physical restraint use in U.S. hospitals: A longitudinal study. *Journal of General Internal Medicine, 32*(1), 35–41
2016	Min, A., & Scott, L. D. (2016). Evaluating nursing hours per patient day as a nurse staffing measure. *Journal of Nursing Management, 24(4),* 439–448.
2016	Rosenfeld, P., & Glassman, K. (2016). The long-term effect of a nurse residency program 2005-2012. *Journal of Nursing Administration, 46*(6), 336–344.
2015	Lasater, K. B., Sloane, D. M., & Aiken, L. H. (2015). Hospital employment of supplemental registered nurses and patients' satisfaction with care. *Journal of Nursing Care Quality, 45*(3), 145–151.
2015	Zivin, K., Yosef, M., Miller, E. M., Valenstein, M., Duffy, S., Kales, H. C., et al. (2015). Associations between depression and all-cause and cause-specific risk of death: A retrospective cohort study in the Veterans Health Administration. *Journal of Psychosomatic Research, 78*(4), 324–331.
2014	Van Bogaert, P., Timmermans, O., Weeks, S. M., van Heusden, D., Wouters, K., & Franck, E. (2014). Nursing unit teams matter: Impact of unit-level nurse practice environment, nurse work characteristics, and burnout on nurse reported job outcomes, and quality of care, and patient adverse events—A cross-sectional survey. *International Journal of Nursing Studies, 51*(8), 1123–1134.
2013	Ausserhofer, D., Schubert, M., Desmedt, M., Blegen, M. A., De Geest, S., & Schwendimann, R. (2013). The association of patient safety climate and nurse-related organizational factors with selected patient outcomes: A cross-sectional survey. *International Journal of Nursing Studies, 50*(2), 240–252.
2013	McHugh, M. D., Kelly, L. A., Smith, H. L., Wu, E. S., Vanak, J. M., & Aiken, L. H. (2013). Lower mortality in Magnet hospitals. *Medical Care, 51*(5), 382–388.
2013	Yoder, L., Xin, W., Norris, K., & Yan, G. (2013). Patient care staffing levels and facility characteristics in US hemodialysis facilities. *American Journal of Kidney Disease, 62*(6), 1130–1140.
2012	Ruesch, C., Mossakowski, J., Forrest, J., Hayes, M., Jahrsdoerfer, M., Comeau, E., & Singleton, M. (2012). Using nursing expertise and telemedicine to increase nursing collaboration and improve patient outcomes. *Telemedicine Journal & E-Health, 18*(8), 591–595.

Outcomes studies being conducted at this time do not examine patient care at the individual nurse or individual patient level, as occurs in many nursing studies; rather, for example, they might examine all the nursing care provided to patients in a particular ICU. Some of the questions researchers might ask in an outcomes study include the following:

- What are the end results of patients' care (all care provided by all care providers)?
- What effect does nursing care (all care by all nurses) have on the end results of a patient's care? Can we measure and thus identify the end results of nursing care?
- Are there some nursing acts that have no effects at all on outcomes or that actually cause harm?

- When do we measure the effects of care, the end results (e.g., change in symptoms, functioning, quality of life)—immediately after the care, when the patient is discharged, or much later?
- How do we distinguish care provided by nurses from care provided by other professionals in examining patient outcomes?

Evaluating Structure of Care

The elements of organization and administration, as well as provider and patient characteristics that guide the processes of care, are referred to as the **structures of care**. We know that the organization of nursing care and nursing leadership have an effect on nursing practice and, in turn, on patient outcomes. These are called **structural variables** in Donabedian's (1987) Theory of Quality. Autonomy in clinical nursing practice is a structural variable, which is recognized as critically important to achieving positive patient outcomes. It is important therefore to identify autonomy-enabling structural variables in the organizational structures of nursing practice. One such structure, determined by a number of nursing studies, is the Magnet hospital designation (Richards et al., 2017). To check the status of a particular hospital regarding its recognition for excellence in nursing care, you can search the American Nurses Credentialing Center (ANCC, 2017) website for the hospital's Magnet status.

The first step in evaluating structure of care is to identify and describe the elements of the structure. Various administration and management theories can be used to identify these elements. They might include leadership, organizational hierarchy, decision-making processes, distribution of power, financial management, and administrative decision-making processes. Nurse researchers investigating the influence of structural variables on quality of care and outcomes have studied factors such as nurse staffing, nursing education, nursing work environment, hospital characteristics, and organization of care delivery. For example, Staggs et al. (2017) conducted an outcomes study to examine the effects of nursing skill mix and nurse staffing level on the use of physical restraints in US hospitals.

The second step is to evaluate the impact of various structural elements on the process of care and on outcomes. This evaluation requires a comparison of different structures that provide the same processes of care. In evaluating structures, the unit of measure is the structure. The evaluation requires access to a sufficiently large sample of "like" structures, with similar processes and outcomes, which can then be compared with a sample of another structure providing the same processes and examining the same outcomes. For example, in nursing research, nurses might want to compare various structures providing primary health care, such as the private physician office, health maintenance organization (HMO), rural health clinic, community-oriented primary care clinic, and nurse-managed center. Alternatively, nurse researchers might examine nursing care provided within the structures of a private outpatient surgical clinic, private hospital, county hospital, and teaching hospital associated with a health science center. In each of these examples, the focus of research would be the impact of structure on the processes and outcomes of care. For example, Lasater, Sloane, and Aiken (2015) examined the effects of hospital employment of supplemental RNs on patients' satisfaction with care. Table 14.5 provides additional examples of outcomes studies.

In the United States, nursing homes, home healthcare agencies, and hospitals are required to collect quality variables that have been defined precisely and measured in specific ways and to report them to the federal government. This mandate was established because of considerable variation in the quality of care in these structures. Various government agencies analyze the quality of these structures so that they can adequately oversee the quality of care provided to the US public. These data are made available to the general public so that individuals can make their own determination of the quality of care provided by various nursing homes, home healthcare agencies, and hospitals. Researchers can also access these data for studies of the quality of various structures. To access these data on the Internet, you can search using the phrases "nursing home compare," "home health compare," and "hospital compare." In addition to being able to select a specific hospital, nursing home, or home healthcare agency, you can access considerable information about quality related to each of these structures of health care.

Evaluating Process of Care

Clinical management or the process of care implemented by nurses has been more of an art than a science until the emphasis on EBP (see Chapter 13). Understanding the process sufficiently to study it must begin with careful reflection, dialogue, and observation. There are multiple components of clinical management, many of which have not yet been clearly defined or tested. Three components of process that are of particular interest are standards of care, practice styles, and costs of care. Standards of care and practice styles are included in the following sections but costs of care are discussed later in this chapter, with the methodologies of evaluation.

Standards of care. A standard of care is a norm on which quality of care is judged. Clinical guidelines, critical paths, and care maps define standards of care for particular situations. In that regard, Donabedian (1982, 1987, 1988) and other researchers have recommended the development of specific criteria to be used as a basis for judging the quality of care. These criteria may take the form of clinical guidelines or care maps based on previous validation that the care contributed to the desired outcomes. The clinical guidelines published by the AHRQ established norms or standards against which the validity of clinical management can be judged. These norms are now established through clinical practice guidelines available through the National Guideline Clearinghouse (NGC, 2017) within the AHRQ (see http://www.guideline.gov). Chapter 13 provides a detailed discussion of the NGC and its resources.

Practice styles, practice patterns, and evidence-based practice. The style of a nurse's practice is another dimension of the process of care that influences quality; however, it is problematic to judge what constitutes goodness in style and to justify the decisions made regarding it. Practice pattern is a concept closely related to practice style. Practice style represents variations in how care is provided, whereas practice pattern represents variations in what care is provided.

EBP is another dimension of the process of care that is considered a critical aspect of professional practice. The ultimate goals of EBP are improved patient health status and quality of care (Graham, Bick, Tetroe, Straus, & Harrison, 2011; Melnyk, Gallagher-Ford, & Fineout-Overholt, 2017). Therefore the impact of EBP should be assessed through the measurement of patient outcomes. Limited empirical studies have examined the impact of evidence-based nursing practice on patient outcomes, suggesting the need for more research in this area.

Methodologies for Outcomes Studies

Outcomes research methodologies have been developed to link the care that people receive with the results that they experience, thereby providing better ways to monitor and improve the quality of care (Clancy & Eisenberg, 1998; Donabedian, 2003, 2005). This section describes some of the current methodologies used in conducting outcomes research, including sampling methods, research strategies or designs, measurement processes, and statistical approaches. These descriptions are not sufficient to guide you in using the approaches described; rather, they provide a broad overview of the variety of methodologies that you will see in outcomes studies. This knowledge will help you understand and critically appraise the methodologies used in published outcomes studies. For additional information, you can refer to the citations in each section and to other sources of outcomes research (Doran, 2011; Gray, Grove, & Sutherland, 2017: Kane & Radosevich, 2011; Moorhead et al., 2013). Outcomes studies cross a variety of disciplines; therefore the emerging methodologies are being enriched by a cross-pollination of ideas, some of which are new to nursing research.

Samples and Sampling

The preferred methods of obtaining samples are different in outcomes studies. Random sampling is seldom used, with the exception of a randomized controlled trial (RCT), when a specific intervention or healthcare service is being evaluated. Usually, heterogeneous samples (with varied types of patients), rather than homogeneous samples (with similar patients), are obtained in outcomes research. Outcome researchers limit sampling criteria in order to obtain large heterogeneous samples that reflects, as much as possible, all patients who would be receiving care in a real healthcare context. For example, samples need to include patients with various comorbidities and patients with varying levels of health status. In addition, individuals should be identified who do not receive nursing or medical treatment for their condition, because they may represent those who refuse treatment or who do not access the healthcare system.

Devising ways to evaluate the representativeness of such samples is problematic. For a sample to be representative, it must be as much like the target population as possible, particularly in relation to the variables being studied (see Chapter 9). Because the target population in outcomes research is often heterogeneous, there are a large number of variables for which sample representativeness needs to be determined. Another challenge in outcomes research is to develop strategies for locating untreated individuals and including them in follow-up studies. The intent is to determine whether outcomes differ between those treated and those untreated. To address some of these challenges, outcomes researchers have used large databases as sample sources in observational research designs.

Large databases as sample sources. One source of samples for outcomes studies is large databases. As illustrated in Fig. 14.8, two broad categories of databases emerge from patient care encounters, clinical databases and administrative databases. **Clinical databases** are created by providers such as hospitals, HMOs, accountable care organizations, and healthcare professionals. The clinical data are generated as a result of routine documentation of care in the electronic health

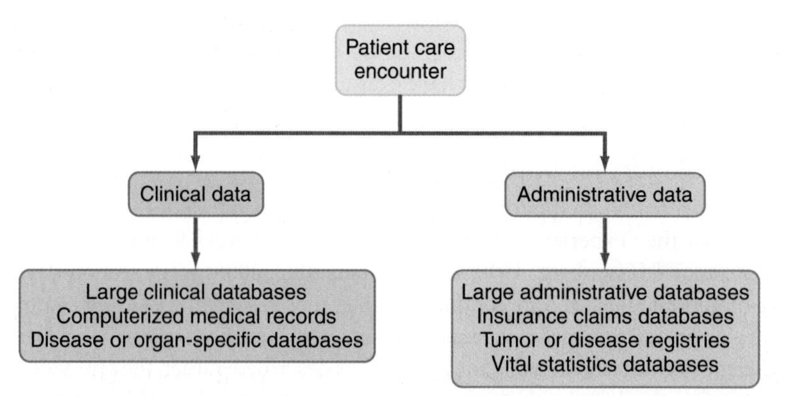

FIG 14.8 Types of databases emanating from patient care encounters. (Grove, S. K., Burns, N., & Gray, J. R. [2013]. *The practice of nursing research: Appraisal, synthesis, and generation of evidence* [7th ed.]. St. Louis, MO: Elsevier Saunders.)

TABLE 14.6 SOME LARGE DATABASE INDICATORS USED TO MONITOR NURSING STRUCTURAL, PROCESS, AND OUTCOME INDICATORS

TYPE OF INDICATOR	INDICATOR	SOURCE
Structural	Nursing (e.g., RN, LPN, UAP) hours per patient day	National Database of Nursing Quality Indicators (NDNQI, 2017); Collaborative Alliance for Nursing Outcomes (CALNOC, 2017a); National Quality Forum (NQF, 2017b)
	Staff mix (RN, LPN, LVN, UAP)	NDNQI (2017);CALNOC (2017a); NQF (2017b)
	Nurse turnover	NDNQI (2017); CALNOC (2017a); NQF (2017b)
	RN practice environment	NDNQI (2017); NQF (2017b)
Process	Risk assessment for pressure ulcers	CALNOC (2017a)
	Physical restraints	NDNQI (2017); CALNOC (2017a)
	Prevention protocols in place	CALNOC (2017a)
	Medication administration accuracy	CALNOC (2017a)
Outcome	Patient falls, injury falls	NDNQI (2017); CALNOC (2017a); NQF (2017b)
	Catheter-associated urinary tract infection rate	NDNQI (2017); NQF (2017b)
	Hospital-acquired pressure ulcer	NDNQI (2017); CALNOC (2017a); NQF (2017b)
	Central line–associated bloodstream infection rate	NDNQI (2017); CALNOC (2017a); NQF (2017b)

LPN, Licensed practical nurse; *LVN*, licensed vocational nurse; *RN*, registered nurse; *UAP*, unlicensed assistive personnel.

record (EHR) or in relation to a research protocol. Some databases are data registries that have been developed to gather data related to a particular disease, such as heart disease or cancer. With a clinical database, you can link observations made by many nurses over long periods of time to patient outcomes (Gray et al., 2017).

Administrative databases are created by insurance companies, government agencies, and others not directly involved in providing patient care. Administrative databases have standardized sets of data for enormous numbers of patients and providers. An example is the Medicare database managed by the CMS. The administrative databases can be used to determine the incidence or prevalence of disease, geographic variations in medical care use, characteristics of medical care, and outcomes of care. Examples of large database indicators used to assess the quality of care are provided in Table 14.6. Initiatives such as CALNOC (2017b) and NDNQI (2017) have been making nursing data more accessible for large database research.

Study Designs

Although RCTs are considered the gold standard for clinical research (see Chapter 8), most outcomes studies use quasi-experimental or observational research designs, which are suitable for addressing questions of effectiveness and efficiency. Like RCTs, outcomes research sometimes seeks to provide evidence about which interventions work best for which types of patients and under what circumstances. However, the "intervention" being evaluated is not limited to medications or new clinical procedures, but may also include the provision of particular services or resources, or even the enforcing of specific policies and regulations, by legislative and financial bodies. Outcomes research often considers additional parameters such as cost, timeliness, convenience, geographic accessibility, and patient preferences. In the next section, common types of designs used in outcomes research are briefly discussed.

Prospective cohort studies. A prospective cohort study uses an epidemiological study design in which the researcher identifies a group of people who are at risk for experiencing a particular event and then follows the group over time to observe whether or not the event occurs. Sample sizes for these studies often must be very large, particularly if only a small portion of the at-risk group will experience the event. The entire group is followed over time to determine the point at which the event occurs, variables associated with the event, and outcomes for those who experienced the event in comparison with those who did not.

Schetter, Niles, Guardino, Khaled, and Kramer (2016) conducted a multicenter prospective cohort study with 5271 pregnant women. These US and Canadian researchers collaborated to determine if demographic, medical, and psychosocial variables were predictors of pregnancy anxiety. The strength of this study is evident in the large sample size, strong outcomes study design, and collaboration of researchers. The abstract from this study is presented as follows:

> ***Background:*** *Pregnancy anxiety is associated with risk of preterm birth and an array of other birth, infant, and childhood outcomes. However, previous research has not helped identify those pregnant women at greatest risk of experiencing this specific, contextually-based affective condition.*
>
> ***Methods:*** *We examined associations between demographic, medical, and psychosocial factors and pregnancy anxiety at 24–26 weeks of gestation in a prospective, multicentre cohort study of 5271 pregnant women in Montreal, Canada.*
>
> ***Results:*** *Multivariate analyses indicated that higher pregnancy anxiety was independently related to having an unintended pregnancy, first birth, higher medical risk, and higher perceived risk of complications. Among psychosocial variables, higher pregnancy anxiety was associated with lower perceived control of pregnancy, lower commitment to the pregnancy, more stressful life events, higher perceived stress, presence of job stress, lower self-esteem and more social support. Pregnancy anxiety was also higher in women who had experienced early income adversity and those who did not speak French as their primary language. Psychosocial variables explained a significant amount of the variance in pregnancy anxiety independently of demographic and medical variables.*
>
> ***Conclusions:*** *Women with pregnancy-related risk factors, stress of various kinds, and other psychosocial factors experienced higher pregnancy anxiety in this large Canadian sample. Some of the unique predictors of pregnancy anxiety match those of earlier U.S. studies, while others point in new directions. Screening for high pregnancy anxiety may be warranted, particularly among women giving birth for the first time and those with high-risk pregnancies.*
>
> ***Schetter et al., 2016, p. 421***

Retrospective cohort studies. A retrospective cohort study includes an epidemiological study design in which the researcher identifies a group of people who have experienced a particular event. This is a common research technique used in the field of epidemiology to study occupational exposure to chemicals. Events of interest to nursing that could be studied in this manner include a procedure, episode of care, nursing intervention, and/or diagnosis. Nurses might use a retrospective cohort study to follow a cohort of women who had undergone mastectomy for breast cancer or for whom a urinary bladder catheter was placed during and after surgery. The cohort is evaluated after the event to determine the occurrence of changes in health status; for example, in nursing, the patients' quality of life and functional status are outcomes of interest. Nurses are also interested in the pattern of recovery after an event or, in the case of catheterization, the incidence of bladder infections in the months after surgery.

On the basis of the study findings, researchers calculate the relative risk of the identified change in health for the group. Relative risk is the probability of the outcome occurring in the exposed group versus that in the unexposed (control) group. For example, if death were the occurrence of interest, the expected number of deaths would be determined. The observed number of deaths divided by the expected number of deaths and multiplied by 100 yields a standardized mortality ratio (SMR), which is regarded as a measure of the relative risk of the studied group to die of a particular condition (Grove & Cipher, 2017). In nursing studies, patients might be followed over time after discharge from a healthcare facility to determine complication rates and the SMR.

In retrospective cohort studies, researchers commonly ask patients to recall information relevant to their previous health status. This information is often used to determine the amount of change occurring before and after an intervention. Recall can easily be distorted, thereby misleading researchers in determining outcomes. Some sources of recall distortion include: (1) the question posed to the study participant may be conceived or expressed incorrectly; (2) the recall process may be in error; and (3) the measurement of recall may result in the recall's appearing to be different from what actually occurred. Therefore recall should be used with caution (Herrmann, 1995).

Chen and Bennett (2016) implemented a retrospective cohort design in their study of a decision tree model for predicting first-time pass-fail rates for the NCLEX-RN® [National Council Licensure Examination-Registered Nurse]. This model successfully classified 92.7% of the students for passing the examination. Additional research is needed on the model because the study included 453 students from one nursing program. The abstract from this study is presented as follows:

> **Background**: *Little evidence shows the use of decision-tree algorithms in identifying predictors and analyzing their associations with pass rates for the NCLEX-RN® in associate degree nursing students. This longitudinal and retrospective cohort study investigated whether a decision-tree algorithm could be used to develop an accurate prediction model for the students' passing or failing the NCLEX-RN.*
>
> **Method**: *This study used archived data from 453 associate degree nursing students in a selected program. The chi-squared automatic interaction detection analysis of the decision trees module was used to examine the effect of the collected predictors on passing/failing the NCLEX-RN.*
>
> **Results**: *The actual percentage scores of Assessment Technologies Institute®'s RN Comprehensive Predictor® accurately identified students at risk of failing. The classification model correctly classified 92.7% of the students for passing.*
>
> **Conclusion**: *This study applied the decision-tree model to analyze a sequence database for developing a prediction model for early remediation in preparation for the NCLEX-RN.*
>
> ***Chen & Bennett, 2016, p. 454***

Population-based studies. Population-based studies are conducted within the context of the patient's community rather than the context of the medical system. With this method, all cases of a condition occurring in the defined population are included, not just the cases treated at a particular healthcare facility. The latter could introduce a selection bias. To avoid selection bias, the researcher might make efforts to include individuals with the condition who had not received treatment.

Community-based norms of tests and survey instruments obtained in this manner provide a clearer picture of the range of values than the limited spectrum of patients seen in specialty clinics. Estimates of instrument sensitivity and specificity are more accurate (see Chapter 10). This method enables researchers to understand the natural history of a condition or the long-term risks and benefits of a particular intervention (Doran, 2011; Kane & Radosevich, 2011).

Economic studies. Many of the problems studied in outcomes research address concerns related to the efficient use of scarce resources and thus to economics. Health economists are concerned with the costs and benefits of alternative treatments or ways of identifying the most efficient means of care. **Economic evaluation** has been defined as a "set of formal, quantitative methods used to compare two or more treatments, programs, or strategies with respect to their resource use and their expected outcomes" (Guyatt, Rennie, Meade, & Cook, 2008, p. 781). An economist defines the term *efficiency* as the least expensive method of achieving a desired end while obtaining the maximum benefit, or outcome, from available resources. If available resources must be shared with other programs or other types of patients, an economic study can determine whether changing the distribution of resources will increase total benefit or welfare.

Measurement Methods

The selection of appropriate outcome variables is critical to the success of an outcomes research study. As in any study, the researcher must evaluate the evidence of validity and reliability of the measurement methods. Outcomes selected for nursing studies should be those most consistent with nursing practice and theory (Moorhead et al., 2013). In some studies, rather than selecting the final outcome of care, which may not occur for months or years, researchers use measures of intermediate endpoints or proximal outcomes. **Intermediate endpoints** are events or markers that act as precursors to the final outcome. It is important, however, to document the validity of the intermediate endpoint in predicting the outcome. In early outcomes studies, researchers selected outcome measures that they could easily obtain, rather than those most desirable for an outcomes study. Later outcome studies selected outcome measures from secondary data sources (e.g., Aiken et al., 2008; Cummings, Midodzi, Wong, & Estabrooks, 2010). This selection involves **secondary analysis,** which is any reanalysis of data or information collected by other researchers, organizations, or agencies (Gray et al., 2017). Outcomes researchers have used secondary data from sources such as the EHR and other minimal clinical data sets collected by hospitals, clinics, and rehabilitation centers. Data collected through NDNQI (2017) or CALNOC (2017b) can also be used in nursing outcomes research.

When critically appraising the approach to measurement in an outcomes study, the reliability, sensitivity, and validity of the measurement tools should be appraised and summarized. Sensitivity to change is an important measurement property to consider in outcomes research because researchers are often interested in evaluating how outcomes change in response to healthcare interventions (Polit & Yang, 2016). As the sensitivity of a measure increases, statistical power increases, allowing smaller sample sizes to detect significant differences. For a full discussion of the reliability and validity of scales and questionnaires, precision and accuracy of physiological measures, and sensitivity and specificity of diagnostic tools, see Chapter 10 of this text and Waltz, Strickland, and Lenz's (2017) text on measurement in nursing and health research.

Statistical Methods for Outcomes Studies

Although outcomes researchers test for the statistical significance of their findings, that evaluation is not considered sufficient to judge the findings as important. Their focus is the clinical importance of study findings (see Chapter 11). In analyzing data, outcomes researchers have moved away from statistical analyses that use the mean to test for group differences. They now place greater importance on analyzing change scores and use exploratory methods for examining the data to identify outliers.

Analysis of Change

With the focus on outcomes studies has come a renewed interest in methods of analyzing change. Harris's (1967) text is the basis for most of the current approaches to analyzing change. However, some new ideas have emerged more recently regarding the analysis of change. Studies by Tracy and colleagues (2006) and Bettger, Coster, Latham, and Keysor (2008) are good references in this regard. For some outcomes, the changes may be nonlinear or may go up and down, rather than always increasing. Therefore it is as important to uncover patterns of change, as it is to test for statistically significant differences at various time points. Some changes may occur in relation to stages of recovery or improvement. These changes may occur over weeks, months, or even years. A more complete picture of the process of recovery is obtained by examining the process in greater detail and over a broader range. With this approach, the examiner can develop a recovery curve, which provides a model of the recovery process that can then be tested.

Analysis of Improvement

In addition to reporting the mean improvement score for all patients treated, it is important to report what percentage of patients improved. Did all patients improve slightly, or is there a divergence among patients, with some improving greatly and others not improving at all? This divergence may best be illustrated by plotting the data. Researchers studying a particular treatment or approach to care might develop a standard or index of varying degrees of improvement that might occur. The index would allow for better comparisons of the effectiveness of various treatments. Characteristics of patients who experience varying degrees of improvement and outliers should be described in the research report. This step requires that the study design include baseline measures of patient status, such as demographic characteristics, functional status, and disease severity measures. An analysis of improvement allows for better judgments to be made about the appropriate use of various treatments (Doran, 2011).

Critical Appraisal of Outcomes Studies

This section discusses approaches for critically appraising outcomes studies. Guyatt and colleagues (2008) outlined the methodology for critically appraising study designs, including those typically used in outcomes research. This guide provides worksheets used to summarize the results of a critical appraisal. The worksheets that are most relevant to outcomes research are those that address studies of economic analysis, retrospective cohort design, health-related quality of life, and prospective cohort design. An example of the types of questions to consider in critically appraising outcome studies of health-related quality of life are provided in the following section.

CRITICAL APPRAISAL GUIDELINES

Outcomes Research

Critical appraisals of outcomes studies are organized by three broad questions: Are the results valid? What are the results? How can I apply the results to patient care?

1. **Are the results valid?**
   a. In a prospective cohort study, did the exposed and unexposed control groups start and finish with the same risk of outcome? How was exposure defined?
   b. In nursing outcome studies, exposure could refer to a particular nursing intervention, staffing model or staff mix, or even healthcare policy.
   c. Three subquestions need to be considered in addressing the original question about the validity of the study results:
      i. Were patients similar for factors or variables known to be associated with the outcome (or was statistical adjustment used to control for differences between the exposed and unexposed control groups)?
      ii. Were the circumstances and methods for detecting the outcome similar? Did the researchers use the same method for measuring the outcome in the exposed and unexposed control groups?
      iii. Was the follow-up sufficiently complete? Ideally, we would like to see approximately 80% follow-up in both control and exposed groups.
   d. In a retrospective cohort study, did the exposed and control groups have the same chance of being exposed in the past? In a retrospective cohort study, the researcher would be interested in determining whether outcomes differ for individuals exposed in the past to a particular health risk, health condition, or health service by following individuals longitudinally after the particular exposure. The following questions need to be addressed in retrospective cohort studies:
      i. Were cases and controls similar with respect to the indication or circumstances that would lead to exposure? For example, were they all equally eligible to receive the particular nursing intervention or receive care under the particular staffing model?
      ii. Were the circumstances and methods for determining exposure similar for cases and controls? In a retrospective cohort study, investigators look back in time to determine exposure to a particular intervention or determine the existence of a particular condition. To answer this question, you would need to determine if the study used the same approach for determining exposure in the control and intervention groups.
2. **What are the results?**
   a. How strong is the association between exposure and outcome? Were the results statistically significant?
   b. How precise was the estimate of effect? Were the confidence intervals for the effect large or small? Small confidence intervals reflect greater precision in the estimate of effect.
   For example, in a study of an outcome such as health-related quality of life (HRQL):
      i. Did the investigators measure aspects of patients' lives that patients consider important? To answer this question, you would need to consider whether the authors described the content of their measure of HRQL in sufficient detail so that it is possible to make a judgment about the relevance of the measure for the particular patient population and/or whether the authors provided direct evidence from their study or indirect evidence from previous studies that the HRQL measure is important to the patient population being investigated.
      ii. Did the HRQL instrument work in the intended way? This question requires an appraisal of the psychometric properties of the HRQL instrument with regard to reliability and validity.
      iii. Were important aspects of HRQL omitted from measurement? This question requires an appraisal of the content validity of the instrument with regard to whether the instrument was complete in its measurement of HRQL.

3. **How can I apply the results to patient care?**
   a. Were the study patients similar to the patients in my practice setting?
   b. Was follow-up sufficiently long to assess an impact on outcome?
   c. Is the exposure (e.g., intervention, staffing model, healthcare policy) similar to what might occur in my practice setting?
   d. What is the magnitude of effect? This question requires you to consider whether the effect was clinically important to make it worthwhile to change practice.
   e. Are there any benefits that are known to be associated with exposure? This question asks you to consider whether the benefits for patients and/or practice settings are sufficiently worthwhile to suggest that you would want to act on the results.

Orwelius and colleagues (2013, p. 229) investigated long-term health-related quality of life (HRQoL or HRQL) after burns. Their study abstract is provided in Research Example 14.1.

RESEARCH EXAMPLE 14.1

Critical Appraisal of an Outcomes Study

Research Study Excerpt

Background: *Health-related quality of life (HRQoL) is reduced after a burn, and is affected by coexisting conditions. The aims of the investigation were to examine and describe effects of coexisting disease on HRQoL, and to quantify the proportion of burned people whose HRQoL was below that of a reference group matched for age, gender, and coexisting conditions.*

Method: *A nationwide study covering 9 years... examined HRQoL 12 and 24 months after the burn with the SF-36 questionnaire. The reference group was from the referral area of one of the hospitals.*

Results: *The HRQoL of the burned patients was below that of the reference group mainly in the mental dimensions, and only single patients were affected in the physical dimensions. The factor that significantly affected most HRQoL dimensions (*n *= 6) after the burn was unemployment, whereas only smaller effects could be attributed directly to the burn.*

Conclusion: *Poor HRQoL was recorded for only a small number of patients, and the declines were mostly in the mental dimensions when compared with a group adjusted for age, gender, and coexisting conditions. Factors other than the burn itself, such as mainly unemployment and pre-existing disease, were most important for the long-term HRQoL experience in these patients.* (Orwelius et al., 2013, p. 229)

Critical Appraisal

The study used a retrospective cohort design. Individuals who experienced a burn were followed for 24 months to determine the impact of the burn, along with other factors, on changes in HRQoL. The exposed group consisted of patients 18 years or older admitted with burns of 10% or more of total body surface area or duration of stay in the burn unit of 7 days or more from 2000 to 2009 (hereafter referred to as the burn cohort). The unexposed cohort was identified from a public health survey, which was completed in 1999 (hereafter referred to as the healthy reference cohort). The two cohorts were not similar for all factors known to be associated with HRQoL. For example, the burn cohort had more males, fewer individuals with higher education, more single individuals, and fewer individuals not employed or retired than the healthy reference cohort. These differences could have influenced HRQoL and, in this study, the investigators accounted for the differences statistically in their analysis. Although the circumstances for detecting the outcome were different for both cohorts, the method of assessment—namely, the SF-36 [Short Form-36] (Ware & Sherbourne, 1992)—was the same. The SF-36 is a well-recognized HRQoL measure, with high reliability and validity established in a representative burn population (Edgar, Dawson, Hankey, Phillips, & Wood, 2010).

Continued

RESEARCH EXAMPLE 14.1—cont'd

Follow-up in the burn cohort was 24 months, a duration that is considered sufficiently long for detecting changes in HRQoL. Of the eligible burn patients, 61% were recruited into the cohort, and follow-up of the sample at 24 months was 48%. Response after two reminders in the healthy reference cohort was 61%. Incomplete follow-up of both cohorts could mean that there are systematic differences (i.e., response bias) between individuals who responded to the survey from those who did not, thus influencing the generalizability of the study findings. There were statistically significant differences in HRQoL between the burn and healthy reference cohorts, primarily in the mental dimension, and the authors reported clinically significant improvements in physical function and role function scores among the burn cohort. The factor that most significantly affected HRQoL after the burn was unemployment, whereas only small effects could be attributed directly to the burn. In conclusion, there were some threats to the validity of the study findings, particularly with regard to differences between the burn and healthy reference cohorts and incomplete follow-up. Some of these differences were accounted for statistically in the analysis. Strengths of the study included use of a reliable and valid measure of HRQoL and statistically and clinically significant effects. Additional research in varied settings would strengthen the translation of these findings to practice.

KEY POINTS

- Mixed methods research combines quantitative and qualitative research methods to answer a research question with a pragmatic focus.
- Data are collected sequentially or concurrently.
- The three mixed methods approaches usually implemented in nursing research are (1) convergent concurrent designs; (2) exploratory sequential designs; and (3) explanatory sequential designs.
- Convergent concurrent designs are used when the research question can be addressed using quantitative and qualitative methods. The researcher collects quantitative and qualitative data at the same time, analyzes each set of data, and integrates the findings.
- Exploratory sequential designs may be used when the researcher wants to expand on what is known about a phenomenon and the researcher does not want the content of the quantitative instruments to bias participants' responses in the qualitative phase. Findings of the qualitative phase are often used to finalize the methods for the quantitative phase.
- Explanatory sequential designs begin with the collection, analysis, and interpretation of quantitative data, followed by a qualitative phase. These studies are most useful in providing answers to "why" and "how" questions that arise from quantitative findings.
- Mixed methods research strategies require a depth and breadth of research knowledge, as well as a significant commitment of time and resources.
- It is critical to determine the method of integration before beginning the study. Integration of the data can be displayed in tables, graphs, or matrices.
- Outcomes research examines the end results of patient care.
- The scientific approaches used in outcomes studies differ in some important ways from those used in traditional nursing research.
- Donabedian (1987, 2005) developed the theory on which outcomes research is based; quality is the overriding construct of the theory.
- The three major concepts of the theory are health, subjects of care, and providers of care.
- Donabedian identified three components of evaluation in appraising quality: structure, process, and outcome.
- The goal of outcomes research is to evaluate outcomes that are clearly linked with the process that caused them.

- Clinical guideline panels were established to incorporate available evidence on health outcomes.
- Outcomes studies provide rich opportunities to build a stronger scientific underpinning for nursing practice.
- A nursing-sensitive patient outcome is "sensitive" because it is influenced by nursing.
- Outcome design strategies tend to have less control than traditional nursing research designs discussed in this text (see Chapter 8).
- Some of the common outcomes studies' methodologies include prospective cohort studies, retrospective cohort studies, population-based studies, and economic analysis.
- Outcomes studies generally use large representative, heterogeneous samples rather than random samples.
- Statistical approaches conducted in outcomes studies focus on examining measurement reliability, analyzing change, and determining health improvement.
- Critical appraisal of outcomes studies focuses on similarity of the exposed cohort and unexposed (control) cohort, adequacy and completeness of follow-up, reliability and validity of the outcome measure(s), and statistical and clinical significance of the study findings.

REFERENCES

Agency for Healthcare Research and Quality (AHRQ). (2017a). *Patient-centered outcomes research (PCOR) at AHRQ*. Retrieved May 30, 2017, from https://www.ahrq.gov/pcor/index.html.

Agency for Healthcare Research and Quality (AHRQ). (2017b). *Funding announcements*. Retrieved May 29, 2017, from https://www.ahrq.gov/funding/fund-opps/index.html.

Aiken, L. H., Clarke, S. P., Sloane, D. M., Lake, E. T., & Cheney, T. (2008). Effects of hospital care environment on patient mortality and nurse outcomes. *Journal of Nursing Administration, 38*(5), 223–229.

Al-Yateem, N., Docherty, C., & Rossiter, R. (2016). Determinants of quality care for adolescents and young adults with chronic illnesses: A mixed methods study. *Journal of Pediatric Nursing, 31*, 255–266.

American Nurses Credentialing Center (ANCC). (2017). *ANCC Magnet Recognition Program*. Retrieved May 14, 2017, from http://nursecredentialing.org/Magnet.aspx.

Ausserhofer, D., Schubert, M., Desmedt, M., Blegen, M. A., De Geest, S., & Schwendimann, R. (2013). The association of patient safety climate and nurse-related organizational factors with selected patient outcomes: A cross-sectional survey. *International Journal of Nursing Studies, 50*(2), 240–252.

Bakker, R., Steegers, E., Biharie, A., Mackenbach, J., Hofman, A., & Jaddoe, V. (2011). Explaining differences in birth outcomes in relation to maternal age: The Generation R Study. *BJOG: An International Journal of Obstetrics and Gynaecology, 118*(4), 500–509.

Bettger, J. A., Coster, W. J., Latham, N. K., & Keysor, J. J. (2008). Analyzing change in recovery patterns in the year after acute hospitalization. *Archives of Physical Medicine & Rehabilitation, 89*(7), 1267–1275.

Bishop, F. (2015). Using mixed methods research designs in health psychology: An illustrative discussion from a pragmatist perspective. *British Journal of Health Psychology, 20*(1), 5–20.

Chen, H., & Bennett, S. (2016). Decision-tree analysis for predicting first-time pass/fail rates for the NCLEX-RN® in associate degree nursing students. *Journal of Nursing Education, 55*(8), 454–457.

Clancy, C. M., & Eisenberg, J. M. (1998). Outcomes research: Measuring the end results of health care. *Science, 282*(5387), 245–246.

Clarke, S. P. (2011). Health care utilization. In D. M. Doran (Ed.), *Nursing outcomes: The state of the science* (2nd ed.) (pp. 439–485). Sudbury, MA: Jones & Bartlett.

Collaborative Alliance for Nursing Outcomes (CALNOC). (2017a). *CALNOC: Home page*. Retrieved May 15, 2017, from http:www.calnoc.org/.

Collaborative Alliance for Nursing Outcomes (CALNOC). (2017b). *Overview*. Retrieved May 15, 2017, from http://www.calnoc.org/?page=A1.

Creswell, J. W. (2014). *Research design: Qualitative, quantitative, and mixed methods approaches* (4th ed.). Los Angeles, CA: Sage.

Creswell, J. W. (2015). *A concise introduction to mixed methods research.* Los Angeles, CA: Sage.

Creswell, J., Klassen, A., Clark, V., & Smith, K. (2011). *Best practices for mixed methods research in health sciences.* Retrieved May 25, 2017, from https://www2.jabsom.hawaii.edu/native/docs/tsudocs/Best_Practices_for_Mixed_Methods_Research_Aug2011.pdf.

Cummings, G. G., Midodzi, W. K., Wong, C. A., & Estabrooks, C. A. (2010). The contribution of hospital nursing leadership styles to 30-day patient mortality. *Nursing Research, 59*(5), 331–339.

Donabedian, A. (1978). *Needed research in quality assessment and monitoring.* Hyattsville, MD: U.S. Department of Health, Education, and Welfare, Public Health Service, National Center for Health Services Research.

Donabedian, A. (1980). *Explorations in quality assessment and monitoring.* Ann Arbor, MI: Health Administration Press.

Donabedian, A. (1982). *The criteria and standards of quality.* Ann Arbor, MI: Health Administration Press.

Donabedian, A. (1987). Some basic issues in evaluating the quality of health care. In L. T. Rinke (Ed.), *Outcome measures in home care: Vol. I* (p. 338). New York, NY: National League for Nursing. (Original work published in 1976.)

Donabedian, A. (1988). The quality of care: How can it be assessed? *Journal of the American Medical Association, 260*(12), 1743–1748.

Donabedian, A. (2003). *An introduction to quality assurance in health care.* Oxford, UK: Oxford University Press.

Donabedian, A. (2005). Evaluating the quality of medical care. *The Milbank Quarterly, 83*(4), 691–729.

Doran, D. M. (Ed.), (2011). *Nursing outcomes: The state of the science* (2nd ed.). Sudbury, MA: Jones & Bartlett.

Edgar, D., Dawson, A., Hankey, G., Phillips, M., & Wood, F. (2010). Demonstration of the validity of the SF-36 for measurement of the temporal recovery of quality of life outcomes in burns survivors. *Burns, 36*(7), 1013–1020.

Giarelli, E., Denigris, J., Fisher, K., Maley, M., & Nolan, E. (2016). Perceived quality of work life and risk for compassion fatigue among oncology nurses: A mixed-methods study. *Oncology Nursing Forum, 43*(3), E121–E131.

Goldman, M., & Little, J. (2015). Innovative grassroots NGOs and the complex processes of women's empowerment: An empirical investigation from northern Tanzania. *World Development, 66*(2), 762–777.

Graham, I. D., Bick, D., Tetroe, J., Straus, S. E., & Harrison, M. B. (2011). Measuring outcomes of evidence-based practice: Distinguishing between knowledge use and its impact. In D. Bick, & I. Graham (Eds.), *Evaluating the impact of implementing evidence-based practice* (pp. 18–37). Oxford, UK: Wiley-Blackwell.

Gray, J. R., Grove, S. K., & Sutherland, S. (2017). *The practice of nursing research: Appraisal, synthesis, and generation of evidence* (8th ed.). St. Louis, MO: Elsevier.

Grove, S. K., & Cipher, D. J. (2017). *Statistics for nursing research: A workbook for evidence-based practice* (2nd ed.). St. Louis, MO: Elsevier.

Guetterman, T., Fetters, M., & Creswell, J. (2015). Integrating quantitative and qualitative results in health science mixed methods research through joint displays. *Annals of Family Medicine, 13*(6), 554–561.

Guyatt, G., Rennie, D., Meade, M. O., & Cook, D. J. (2008). *Users' guides to the medical literature: A manual for evidence-based practice* (2nd ed.). New York, NY: McGraw-Hill Medical.

Hagstrom, S. (2017). Family stress in pediatric critical care. *Journal of Pediatric Nursing, 32*(1), 32–40.

Harris, C. W. (1967). *Problems in measuring change.* Madison, WI: University of Wisconsin Press.

Herrmann, D. (1995). Reporting current, past, and changed health status: What we know about distortion. *Medical Care, 33*(Suppl. 4), AS89–AS94.

Howell, D. (2011). Psychological distress as a nurse-sensitive outcome. In D. M. Doran (Ed.), *Nursing outcomes: The state of the science* (2nd ed.) (pp. 285–358). Sudbury, MA: Jones & Bartlett.

Irvine, D. M., Sidani, S., & Hall, L. M. (1998). Linking outcomes to nurses' roles in health care. *Nursing Economic$, 16*(2), 58–64, 87.

Kane, R. L., & Radosevich, R. M. (2011). *Conducting health outcomes research.* Sudbury, MA: Jones & Bartlett Learning.

Kenner, C. A. (2017). Trends in US nursing research: Links to global healthcare issues. *Journal of Korean Academic Nursing Administration, 23*(1), 1–7.

Kleib, M., Sales, A., Doran, D. M., Malette, C., & White, D. (2011). Nursing minimum data sets. In D. M. Doran (Ed.), *Nursing outcomes: The state of the science* (2nd ed.) (pp. 487–512). Sudbury, MA: Jones & Bartlett.

Kleinpell, R. M. (2013). *Outcome assessment in advanced practice nursing* (3rd ed.). New York, NY: Springer Publishing Company.

Kutney-Lee, A., Sloane, D., & Aiken, L. (2013). Increase in the number of nurses with baccalaureate degrees is linked to lower rates of postsurgery mortality. *Health Affairs, 32*(3), 579–586.

Lasater, K. B., Sloane, D. M., & Aiken, L. H. (2015). Hospital employment of supplemental registered nurses and patients' satisfaction with care. *Journal of Nursing Care Quality, 45*(3), 145–151.

Leavy, P. (2017). *Research design: Quantitative, qualitative, mixed methods, arts-based, and community-based participatory research approaches.* New York, NY: Guilford Press.

Lenz, A., & Lancaster, C. (2017). A mixed-methods evaluation of intensive trauma-focused programming. *Journal of Counseling & Development, 95*(1), 24–34.

Magnello, M. E. (2010). The passionate statistician. In S. Nelson, & A. M. Rafferty (Eds.), *Notes On Nightingale: The influence and legacy of a nursing icon* (pp. 115–129). Ithaca, NY: Cornell University Press.

Mark, B. A. (1995). The black box of patient outcomes research. *Image: Journal of Nursing Scholarship, 27*(1), 42.

McHugh, M. D., Kelly, L. A., Smith, H. L., Wu, E. S., Vanak, J. M., & Aiken, L. H. (2013). Lower mortality in Magnet hospitals. *Medical Care, 51*(5), 382–388.

Melnyk, B. M., Gallagher-Ford, L., & Fineout-Overholt, E. (2017). *Implementing evidence-based practice competencies in healthcare: A practical guide for improving quality, safety, & outcomes.* Indianapolis, IN: Sigma Theta Tau International.

Min, A., & Scott, L. D. (2016). Evaluating nursing hours per patient day as a nurse staffing measure. *Journal of Nursing Management, 24*(4), 439–448.

Mitchell, P. H., Ferketich, S., & Jennings, B. M. (1998). American Academy of Nursing Expert Panel on Quality Health Care: 1998 Quality Health Outcomes Model. *Image—Journal of Nursing Scholarship, 30*(1), 43–46.

Montalvo, I. (2007). *National Database of Nursing Quality Indicators (NDNQI).* Retrieved May 30, 2017, from http://www.nursingworld.org/ojin.

Moorhead, S., Johnson, M., Maas, M. L., & Swanson, E. (2013). *Nursing outcomes classification (NOC): Measurement of health outcomes* (5th ed.). St. Louis, MO: Elsevier Mosby.

Morgan, D. (2014). *Integrating qualitative & quantitative methods: A pragmatic approach.* Los Angeles, CA: Sage.

National Database of Nursing Quality Indicators (NDNQI). (2017). *Nursing quality (NDNQI).* Retrieved May 30, 2017, from http://www.pressganey.com/solutions/clinical-quality/nursing-quality.

National Guideline Clearinghouse (NGC). (2017). *AHRQ's National Guideline Clearinghouse is a public resource for summaries of evidence-based clinical practice guidelines.* Retrieved May 30, 2017, from http://www.guideline.gov.

National Quality Forum (NQF). (2017a). *About NQF.* Retrieved May 15, 2017, from http://www.qualityforum.org/About_NQF/.

National Quality Forum (NQF). (2017b). *NQF's strategic direction 2016-2019: Lead, prioritize, and collaborate for better health measurement.* Retrieved May 15, 2017, from http://www.qualityforum.org/NQF_Strategic_Direction_2016-2019.aspx.

Oh, S. H., Park, E. J., Yin, Y., Piao, J., & Lee, S. (2014). Automatic delirium prediction system in Korean surgical intensive care unit. *Nursing in Critical Care, 19*(6), 281–291.

Oncology Nursing Society (ONS). (2017). *About ONS.* Retrieved May 15, 2017, from http://www.ons.org/about.

Orem, D. (2001). *Nursing concepts of practice* (6th ed.). St Louis, MO: Mosby.

Orwelius, L., Willebrand, M., Gerdin, L., Ekselius, L., Fredrikson, M., & Sjöberg, F. (2013). Long-term health-related quality of life after burns is strongly dependent on pre-existing disease and psychosocial issues and less due to the burn itself. *Burns, 39*(2), 229–235.

Patient-Centered Outcomes Research Institute (PCORI). (2017). *PCORI: About us.* Retrieved August 15, 2017, from http://www.pcori.org/about-us.

Polit, D. F., & Yang, F. M. (2016). *Measurement and the measurement of change.* Philadelphia, PA: Wolters Kluwer.

Pluye, P., Gagnon, M. P., Griffiths, F., & Johnson-Lafleur, J. (2009). A scoring system for appraising mixed methods research, and concomitantly appraising qualitative, quantitative and mixed methods primary studies in mixed studies reviews. *International Journal of Nursing Studies, 46*(4), 529–546.

Richards, M. R., Lasater, K., & McHugh, M. (2017). A race to the top? Competitive pressure and Magnet adoption among U.S. hospitals 1997-2012. *Medical Care, 55*(4), 384–390.

Rosenfeld, P., & Glassman, K. (2016). The long-term effect of a nurse residency program 2005-2012. *Journal of Nursing Administration, 46*(6), 336–344.

Ruesch, C., Mossakowski, J., Forrest, J., Hayes, M., Jahrsdoerfer, M., Comeau, E., & Singleton, M. (2012). Using nursing expertise and telemedicine to increase nursing collaboration and improve patient outcomes. *Telemedicine Journal & E-Health, 18*(8), 591–595.

Schetter, C. D., Niles, A. N., Guardino, C. M., Khaled, M., & Kramer, M. S. (2016). Demographic, medical, and psychosocial predictors of pregnancy anxiety. *Paediatric and Perinatal Epidemiology, 30*(5), 421–429.

Sidani, S. (2011a). Self-care. In D. M. Doran (Ed.), *Nursing outcomes: The state of the science.* (2nd ed.) (pp. 79–130). Sudbury, MA: Jones & Bartlett.

Sidani, S. (2011b). Symptom management. In D. M. Doran (Ed.), *Nursing outcomes: The state of the science* (2nd ed.) (pp. 131–199). Sudbury, MA: Jones & Bartlett.

Staggs, V. S., Olds, D. M., Cramer, E., & Shorr, R. I. (2017). Nursing skill mix, nurse staffing level, and physical restraint use in U.S. hospitals: A longitudinal study. *Journal of General Internal Medicine, 32*(1), 35–41.

Tourangeau, A. E. (2011). Mortality rate: A nursing sensitive outcome. In D. M. Doran (Ed.), *Nursing outcomes: The state of the science* (2nd ed.) (pp. 409–437). Sudbury, MA: Jones & Bartlett.

Tracy, S., Schinco, M. A., Griffen, M. M., Kerwin, A. J., Devin, T., & Tepas, J. J. (2006). Urgent airway intervention: Does outcome change with personnel performing the procedure? *Journal of Trauma, 61*(5), 1162–1165.

Van Bogaert, P., Timmermans, O., Weeks, S. M., van Heusden, D., Wouters, K., & Franck, E. (2014). Nursing unit teams matter: Impact of unit-level nurse practice environment, nurse work characteristics, and burnout on nurse reported job outcomes, and quality of care, and patient adverse events—A cross-sectional survey. *International Journal of Nursing Studies, 51*(8), 1123–1134.

van Griensven, H., Moore, A., & Hall, V. (2014). Mixed methods research – The best of both worlds? *Manual Therapy, 19*(5), 367–371.

Waltz, C. F., Strickland, O. L., & Lenz, E. R. (2017). *Measurement in nursing and health research* (5th ed.). New York, NY: Springer.

Ware, J. R., & Sherbourne, J. E. (1992). The MOS, 36-item short-form health survey (SF-36). I. Conceptual framework and item selection. *Medical Care, 30*(6), 473–483.

Wisdom, J., & Creswell, J. (2013). *Mixed methods: Integrating quantitative and qualitative data collection and analysis while studying patient-centered medical home models.* Rockville, MD: Agency for Healthcare Research and Quality. AHRQ Publication No. 13-0028-EF.

World Health Organization (WHO). (2017). *The conceptual framework for the International Classification for Patient Safety (ICPS).* Retrieved May 15, 2017, from http://www.who.int/patientsafety/implementation/taxonomy/ICPS-report/en/.

Yardley, L., & Bishop, F. (2015). Using mixed methods in health research: Benefits and challenges. *British Journal of Health Psychology, 20*(1), 1–4.

Yoder, L., Xin, W., Norris, K., & Yan, G. (2013). Patient care staffing levels and facility characteristics in US hemodialysis facilities. *American Journal of Kidney Disease, 62*(6), 1130–1140.

Zivin, K., Yosef, M., Miller, E. M., Valenstein, M., Duffy, S., Kales, H. C., et al. (2015). Associations between depression and all-cause and cause-specific risk of death: A retrospective cohort study in the Veterans Health Administration. *Journal of Psychosomatic Research, 78*(4), 324–331.

Because of funding changes, the Agency for Healthcare Research and Quality (AHRQ) National Guideline Clearinghouse website was scheduled for decommissioning as of July 16, 2018. For more information, go to https://www.ahrq.gov/.

GLOSSARY

A

Absolute zero Value of zero indicates the absence of the property being measured; zero weight means the absence of weight.

Abstract (adjective) Idea focuses on a general view of a phenomenon; expressed without reference to any specific instance.

Abstract (noun) Clear, concise summary of a study, usually limited to 100 to 250 words.

Academic journals Periodicals that include research reports and nonresearch articles related to a specific scholarly discipline or research methodology.

Acceptance rate Number and percentage of study participants who agree to take part in a study. The percentage is calculated by dividing the number of participants agreeing to participate by the number approached. For example, if 100 subjects are approached and 90 agree to participate, the acceptance rate is 90%: $(90 \div 100) \times 100\% = 0.90 \times 100\% = 90\%$.

Accessible population Portion of the target population to which the researcher has reasonable access.

Accuracy Closeness of the agreement between the measured value and true value of the quantity being measured.

Accuracy in physiologic measures Term that addresses the extent to which the instrument measures what it is supposed to measure in a study; comparable to validity.

Accuracy of a screening test Screening tests used to confirm a diagnosis are evaluated in terms of their ability to assess the presence or absence of a disease or condition correctly as compared with a gold standard.

Administrative database Resource created by insurance companies, government agencies, and others not directly involved in providing patient care; contains standardized sets of data for enormous numbers of patients and providers.

Algorithm Decision tree that provides a set of rules for solving a particular practice problem. Its development usually is based on research evidence and theoretic knowledge.

Alpha (α) Level of significance or cutoff point used to determine whether the study samples are members of the same population (nonsignificant) or of different populations (significant); alpha is commonly set at 0.05, 0.01, or 0.001. Alpha is also the probability of making a type I error.

Alternate forms reliability Also referred to as *parallel forms reliability*; a test of equivalence that involves comparing the scores for two versions of the same instrument.

American Nurses Association's Code of Ethics Guidelines developed by nurses to protect the rights of people during nursing practice and research.

Analysis of covariance (ANCOVA) Statistical procedure in which a regression analysis is carried out before performing an analysis of variance (ANOVA); designed to reduce the variance within groups by statistically removing the variance caused by a confounding variable.

Analysis of variance (ANOVA) Statistical test used to examine differences between or among groups by comparing the variability between groups with the variability within each group on some continuous dependent or outcome variable.

Analyzing a research report Critical thinking skill that involves determining the value of a study by breaking the contents of a study report into parts and examining the parts for accuracy, completeness, uniqueness of information, and organization.

Ancestry search Examination of references for relevant studies to identify previous studies that are pertinent to the search; used when conducting research syntheses or an exhaustive literature search for a study.

Anonymity Inability of others, including the researcher, to link a study participant's identity to his or her individual responses.

Applied research Scientific investigation conducted to generate knowledge that has the potential to influence clinical practice directly.

Article Paper about a specific topic published with other articles in a journal, encyclopedia, or edited book.

Assent to participate in research Agreement of a child or adult with diminished autonomy to participate in a study when the parents or guardians have given their permission.

Associative hypothesis Statement of a proposed noncausal relationship between or among variables. The variables in this hypothesis occur or exist together in the real world so that when one variable changes, the other changes, but one variable does not cause another variable to change.

Assumption Statement taken for granted or considered true, even though it has not been scientifically tested.

Attrition rate of a sample Number and percentage of participants who drop out of a study before it is completed, creating a threat to the internal validity of the study. The attrition rate is calculated by dividing the number of participants dropping out of a study by the original sample size. For example, if the sample size was 200, and 20 participants dropped out of the study, then $(20 \div 200) \times 100\% = 10\%$.

Audit trail Record of actions taken during the organization of qualitative data and of decisions made during data analysis and interpretation; increases confidence in the transparency of the study.

Authority Person(s) with expertise and power who is (are) able to influence the opinions and behaviors of others.

Autonomy Freedom of an individual to make decisions and act on those decisions; when applied to research, a person chooses whether to participate without undue influence or coercion.

B

Background for a problem Part of the research problem that indicates what is known or identifies key research publications in the problem area.

Basic (pure) research Scientific investigations for the pursuit of "knowledge for knowledge's sake" or for the pleasure of learning and finding truth.

Belmont Report Statement of ethical principles of research developed in the United States in response to the Tuskegee Syphilis Study; provided guidelines for selecting subjects, such as informing them of risks and benefits and documenting their consent.

Benefit-risk ratio Comparison of the potential benefits (positive outcomes) and risks (negative outcomes) of a study that is used by researchers and reviewers to ensure the ethical conduct of research.

Best research evidence Strongest empiric knowledge available in areas of health promotion, illness prevention, and the assessment, diagnosis, and management of acute and chronic illnesses produced by the conduct and synthesis of numerous, high-quality studies. Evidence-based practice is a combination of best research evidence, clinical expertise, and patient circumstances.

Between-group variance Variation of the group means around the grand mean; determined by conducting an analysis of variance (ANOVA) statistical techniques.

Bias Influence or action in a study that distorts the findings or slants them away from the true or expected.

Bibliographic database Electronically stored compilation of citations relevant to a specific discipline or a broad collection of citations from a variety of disciplines; searchable by authors, titles, journals, keywords, or topic.

Bimodal distribution Spread of scores that has two modes (most frequently occurring scores).

Bivariate analysis Statistical procedures that involve comparison of the same variable measured in two different groups or measurement of two distinct variables within a single group.

Bivariate correlation Measure of the extent of the linear relationship between two variables.

Blinding Withholding group assignment or other study information from data collectors, participants, and their healthcare providers to reduce potential bias.

Bonferroni procedure Post hoc analysis to determine differences among three or more groups without inflating a type I error; when a design involves multiple comparisons, the procedure may be during the planning phase of a study to adjust the significance level so as not to inflate type I error.

Bracket or bracketing Qualitative research technique in which a researcher identifies personal preconceptions and beliefs and consciously sets them aside for the duration of the study.

Breach of confidentiality Intentional or nonintentional action that allows an unauthorized person to have access to a participant's identity and study data.

Broad consent Agreement whereby a study participant gives the researcher permission to store, manage, and use private information and biological specimens without violating confidentiality; this type of consent was included in revisions to the Common Rule.

C

Case study In-depth analysis and systematic description of one patient or a group of similar patients to promote understanding of nursing interventions, problems, or situations. Case studies are one example of the practice-related research conducted in nursing.

Causal hypothesis Relationship between two variables, in which one variable (independent variable) is thought to cause or determine the presence of the other variable (dependent variable). Some causal hypotheses can include more than one independent or dependent variable.

Causality Relationship that includes three conditions: (1) there must be a strong correlation between the proposed cause and effect; (2) the proposed cause must precede the effect in time; and (3) the cause must be present whenever the effect occurs.

Chi-square test of independence Test conducted to analyze nominal data to determine significant differences between observed frequencies within the data and frequencies that were expected.

Citation Act of quoting a source, using it as an example, or presenting it as support for a position taken in a paper or report. A citation should be accompanied by the appropriate reference to its source.

Citation bias Preference that occurs when certain studies are cited more often than others and that are more likely to be identified in database searches.

Clinical database Databases of patient, provider, and healthcare agency information that are developed by healthcare agencies and sometimes by providers to document care delivery and outcomes.

Clinical expertise Knowledge and skills of healthcare professionals providing care. In nursing, clinical expertise is influenced by years of clinical experience, current knowledge of the research and clinical literature, and educational preparation. Evidence-based practice is a combination of best research evidence, clinical expertise, and patient circumstances.

Clinical importance Practical relevance of a positive statistical finding in a study; addresses the question "Will this make a meaningful difference to the patient experience or outcomes?"

Clinical journal Periodical containing research reports and nonresearch articles about practice problems and professional issues in a specific, scholarly discipline.

Cluster sampling Sampling method in which a frame is developed that includes a list of all the locations, institutions, or organizations (clusters) that could be used in a study because individual subjects' identities are unknown; a randomized sample is drawn from this list.

Coding Way of indexing or identifying categories in qualitative data.

Coefficient of determination (r^2) Square of a correlation value (r^2), which represents the percentage of variance shared by two variables.

Coefficient of multiple determination (R^2) Refers to a statistical technique conducted when a study includes multiple independent variables to predict one dependent variable. R^2 is the percentage of the total variation that can be explained by all the variables that the researcher includes in the final prediction equation.

Coercion Overt threat of harm or excessive reward intentionally presented by one person to another to obtain compliance—for example, offering prospective subjects a large sum of money to participate in a dangerous research project.

Common Rule Name given to the similarities among federal departments' chapters in the Code of Federal Regulations; includes the contents of a consent document, processes of obtaining informed consent, maintaining an institutional review board (IRB), levels of IRB review, and protection of vulnerable populations.

Comparative descriptive design Design used to describe differences in a variable's value in two or more groups in a natural setting.

Comparison group Group that is not exposed to the research intervention. In nursing research, the comparison group usually receives standard care so that both groups (intervention and comparison) receive time and attention.

Complex hypothesis Hypothesis that predicts the relationship (associative or causal) among three or more variables; thus, the hypothesis can include two (or more) independent and/or two (or more) dependent variables.

Comprehending a source Process completed by reading and focusing on understanding the main points of an article or other sources.

Comprehending a research report Critical thinking process used in reading a research report in which the focus is on understanding the major concepts and logical flow of ideas in a study.

Concept Term that abstractly describes and names an object or phenomenon, thus providing it with a separate identity or meaning.

Conceptual definition Definition that provides a variable or concept with connotative (abstract, comprehensive, theoretic) meaning; may be established through concept analysis, concept derivation, or concept synthesis. A variable's conceptual definition is developed from the study framework and provides a link between the framework and the variable's operational definition.

Conceptual model Set of highly abstract, related constructs that broadly explain phenomena of interest, expresses assumptions; usually reflects a philosophical stance.

Conclusion Statement near the end of a literature review that reflects the synthesis of the knowledge in a particular topic area and includes what is known and not known; in a research report, statements that summarize a study's findings, their meaning, and contribution to knowledge.

Concrete Refers to terms or thinking that is (are) oriented toward and limited by tangible things or events observed and experienced in reality.

Concurrent validity Extent to which an individual's score on a scale can be used to estimate his or her present or concurrent performance on another variable or criterion; type of criterion validity.

Conference proceedings Collection of papers presented at a meeting of major professional organizations, which are later published.

Confidence interval Probability of including the value of the population between higher and lower interval estimates; usually calculated for 95% or 99% intervals.

Confidentiality Management of data during a study in such a way that only the researcher knows participants' identities and can link them to their responses.

Confirmability Extent to which other researchers can review the audit trail of a qualitative study and agree that the authors' conclusions are logical.

Confounding variables Type of extraneous variable that is embedded in the study design and cannot be controlled.

Consent form Written or otherwise recorded documentation of a person's agreement to participate in a study.

Construct Concept at a very high level of abstraction that has a general meaning.

Construct validity Degree to which an instrument actually measures the theoretic construct that it purports to measure; this involves examining the fit between the conceptual and operational definitions of a study variable.

Content validity Extent to which items on a scale include the major elements relevant to the construct being measured. Evidence for content validity includes (1) how well the scale's items reflect the concept's description in the literature (or face validity); (2) experts' evaluation of the relevance of items that may be reported as an index; and (3) the study participants' responses to scale items.

Control In research, the imposing of rules by the researcher to decrease the possibility of error and increase the probability that the study's findings are an accurate reflection of reality.

Control group Group of elements or subjects not exposed to the experimental treatment in a study. The term *control group* is used when study participants are randomly assigned to the group.

Convenience sampling Nonprobability sampling technique in which subjects are included in the study who happened to be in the right place at the right time, with the addition of available subjects, until the desired sample size is reached; also referred to as *accidental sampling.*

Convergent concurrent strategy Mixed methods research design in which qualitative and quantitative data are collected at the same time but analyzed separately. The findings of each component are integrated during the interpretation phase.

Convergent validity Type of measurement validity obtained by using two instruments to measure the same variable, such as depression, and correlating the results from these instruments; evidence of convergence validity is a moderate or strong positive correlation between the two measurements.

Correlational analysis Statistical procedure conducted to determine the direction (positive or negative) and magnitude (or strength) of the relationship between two variables.

Correlational coefficient Indicates the degree of relationship between two variables; coefficients range in value from +1 (perfect positive relationship) to −1.00 (perfect negative or inverse relationship).

Correlational study designs Variety of study designs developed to examine relationships between or among variables.

Correlational research Systematic investigation of relationships between (among) two or more variables to explain the nature of relationships in the world; does not examine cause and effect.

Covert data collection Information about research participants that is collected without their knowledge or awareness.

Credibility Confidence of the reader about the extent to which qualitative researchers have produced results that reflect the views of the participants; similar to validity in the critical appraisal of quantitative studies.

Criterion-related validity Extent to which scores on an instrument can be used to predict another variable or score; criterion-related validity includes predictive and concurrent validity.

Critical appraisal of research Examination of the strengths, weaknesses, meaning, credibility, and significance of nursing studies in generating knowledge.

Critical ethnography Qualitative study that focuses on the sociological and political factors of a culture

Cross-sectional design Types of strategies used to examine groups of participants in various stages of a process simultaneously, with the intent of inferring trends over time. For example, participants might be in various stages of development, severity of illness, or stages of recovery and are described across stages.

Current sources References cited in a research report that have been published within 5 years of the date at which that the manuscript of the report was accepted for publication.

D

Data (plural) Pieces of information collected during a study (singular is datum).

Data analyses Techniques conducted to reduce, organize, and give meaning to data.

Data-based literature Consists of research reports, both published reports in print and online journals and books and unpublished reports such as theses and dissertations.

Data collection Precise, systematic gathering of information (data) relevant to the research purpose or the specific objectives, questions, or hypotheses of a study.

Data saturation See *saturation.*

Deception Misinforming participants about the intent of a study or data collection for research purposes; requires that participants be debriefed or informed of the true purpose and outcomes once their participation has ended.

Decision theory Statistical theory based on the assumptions of the theoretic normal curve; used to test whether differences exist between groups; underlying expectation is that all groups are members of the same population, is expressed as a null hypothesis. The level of significance (alpha) is often set at 0.05 before data collection.

Declaration of Helsinki Statement of ethical principles that followed the Nuremberg Code; specified the differences in therapeutic and nontherapeutic research, with researchers responsible for protecting the dignity, privacy, and health of participants.

Deductive reasoning Reasoning from the general to the specific or from a general premise to a particular situation.

Degrees of freedom (*df*) Freedom of a score's value to vary, given the values of other existing scores and the established sum of these scores; the number of values that are truly independent (formula varies according to statistical test).

Demographic characteristics See *sample characteristics.*

Demographic variables Specific attribute variables of study participants that are collected to describe the sample, such as age, gender, race, and ethnicity.

Dependability Documentation of steps taken and decisions made during qualitative analysis.

Dependent groups See *paired groups.*

Dependent (response or outcome) variable Response, behavior, or outcome that is predicted or explained in research. In a study focused on testing an intervention, changes in the dependent variable are presumed to be caused by the independent variable.

Description Involves identifying and understanding the nature and attributes of nursing phenomena and sometimes the relationships among these phenomena.

Descriptive correlational design Type of design implemented to describe variables and examine relationships that exist in a situation.

Descriptive design Type of quantitative study design conducted to determine the prevalence of a variable and its characteristics in a data set.

Descriptive phenomenological research Research study in which a researcher sets aside her or his own perception, experiences, and values related a phenomenon to describe the lived experience of participants; qualitative method promoted by Husserl (German philosopher who established the school of phenomenology).

Descriptive research Research that provides an accurate portrayal or account of the characteristics of a particular person, event, or group in a real-life situation; research that is conducted to discover new meaning, describe what exists, determine the frequency with which something occurs, and categorize information.

Descriptive statistics Analyses done to summarize and organize data in ways that give meaning and facilitate insight, such as frequency distributions and measures of central tendency and dispersion.

Design validity Probability that the study findings are an accurate reflection of reality. Its four components are construct validity, internal validity, external validity, and statistical conclusion validity.

Determining strengths and weaknesses in studies Second step in the critical appraisal of studies to determine their quality. To complete this step, the researcher must have knowledge of what each step of the research process should be like from expert sources, such as this text and other research sources, and compare the study steps with these sources.

Digital object identifiers (DOIs) Unique series of numbers and letters linked to a specific article or report; DOIs are promoted by the International Standards Organization (http://www.doi.org/), but have not yet received universal support.

Diminished autonomy Condition of subjects whose ability to give informed consent voluntarily is decreased because of legal or mental incompetence, terminal illness, or confinement to an institution.

Direct measurements Measures used for the quantification of simple, concrete variables, such as strategies for measuring height, weight, or temperature.

Directional hypothesis Statement that predicts the direction (positive or negative) of the relationship between (among) two or more variables.

Discomfort and harm Degree of potential and actual risk experienced by a subject participating in a study; risks can be physical, psychological, economic, emotional, or a combination thereof.

Dissemination of research findings Communication of research findings by means of presentations and publications.

Dissertation Extensive, usually original research project completed by a doctoral student as part of the requirements for a doctoral degree.

Distal outcome Outcome removed from proximity to the care or a service received and that is more influenced by external (nontreatment) factors than a proximal outcome.

Distribution In statistics, the relative frequency with which a variable assumes certain values.

Divergent validity Type of measurement validity obtained by using two instruments to measure opposite variables, such as hope and hopelessness; evidence of divergent validity is a moderate or strong negative correlation between the two measurements.

Double-blinding Strategy in which neither subjects nor data collectors are aware of subject assignment to group. Double blinding avoids several threats to construct validity.

Duplicate publication bias Appearance of more research support for a finding than is accurate because a study's findings have been published by the authors in more than one journal, without cross-referencing the other journal.

Dwelling with the data Term in qualitative data analysis used to indicate that the researcher has spent considerable time reading and reflecting on the data.

E

Economic evaluation Analysis and comparison of the costs of implementing, and the expected outcomes, of treatments, strategies, approaches to practice, or other processes of care; desired goal is to identify the least expensive option with the best outcomes.

Effect size Degree to which the phenomenon studied is present in the population or to which the null hypothesis is false. In examining relationships, it is the degree or size of the association between variables; also refers to the effectiveness of an intervention in quasi-experimental and experimental research.

Elements in studies Persons (subjects or participants), events, behaviors, or any other units examined in studies.

Eligibility criteria See *sampling criteria.*

Emic approach Anthropological research approach to studying behaviors from within a culture.

Empirical literature Relevant studies published in journals, books, and online, as well as unpublished studies, such as master's theses and doctoral dissertations.

Encyclopedia Authoritative compilation of information on alphabetized topics that may provide background information and lead to other sources, but is rarely cited in academic papers and publications.

Environmental variables Types of extraneous variables composing the setting in which a study is conducted.

Equivalence reliability Compares two versions of the same instrument or two observers measuring the same event.

Error in physiological measures Inaccuracy of physiological instruments related to the environment, users, study participants, equipment, and interpretation errors.

Ethical principles Standards of appropriate behavior that include giving respect to others, doing good, and treating others fairly; applicable to research.

Ethnographic research Qualitative research methodology for investigating cultures. The research involves the collection, description, and analysis of data to develop a description of a culture.

Ethnonursing research Type of research that emerged from Leininger's Theory of Transcultural Nursing; focuses mainly on observing and documenting how daily life conditions and patterns influence human care, health, and nursing care practices.

Etic approach Anthropological research approach to studying behavior from outside the culture and examining similarities and differences across cultures.

Evaluating the credibility and meaning of the study findings Determining the validity, reliability, significance, and meaning of a quantitative study by examining the links among the study process, study findings, and previous studies.

Evaluating the trustworthiness and meaning of the study findings Determining the credibility, transferability, dependability, and confirmability of the findings of a qualitative study.

Evidence-based guidelines See *evidence-based practice guidelines.*

Evidence-based practice (EBP) Method of practice that involves the conscientious integration of best research evidence with clinical expertise and patients' circumstances and values to produce quality health outcomes.

Evidence-based practice centers (EPCs) Universities and healthcare agencies identified by the Agency for Healthcare Research and Quality as centers for the conduct, communication, and synthesis of research knowledge in selected areas to promote evidence-based health care.

Evidence-based practice guidelines Rigorous, explicit clinical guidelines based on the best research evidence available (e.g., findings from systematic reviews, metaanalyses, mixed-methods systematic reviews, metasyntheses, and extensive clinical trials); supported by consensus from recognized national experts and affirmed by outcomes obtained by clinicians.

Evidence of validity from contrasting groups Tested by identifying groups that are expected to have vastly different scores on an instrument; also called *known groups validity.*

Evidence of validity from convergence See *convergent validity.*

Evidence of validity from divergence See *divergent validity.*

Exclusion sample criteria Characteristics that can result in a person or element being excluded from the target population because the characteristic has a potential to introduce error into the study.

Exempt from review Designation given to studies that have no apparent risks for the research subjects or collect data not linked to a living person; an institutional review board (IRB) representative must designate that the study meets the criteria to be exempt, and no further IRB review is required.

Expedited institutional review board (IRB) review Institutional review process for studies with no apparent risks or minimal risks, such as those encountered in daily life or during routine physical or psychological examinations; may be delegated to representatives of the IRB.

Experiment Study that typically includes randomizing subjects into groups, collecting data, and conducting statistical analyses. See *experimental research.*

Experimental designs Types of designs that provide the greatest amount of control possible to examine causality in studies.

Experimental (or treatment) group Study participants who are exposed to the research treatment or intervention in a study.

Experimental research Objective, systematic, controlled investigation to examine causality characterized by the following: (1) researcher-controlled manipulations of the independent variable; (2) presence of a distinct control group; and (3) random assignment of subjects to either the experiment or the control condition.

Experimenter expectancy Threat to construct validity, characterized by a belief of the person collecting the data that may encourage certain responses from subjects either in support of those beliefs or opposing them.

Explained variance Amount of variation in values explained by the relationship between the two variables.

Explanation Clarification of relationships among variables and identification of reasons why certain events occur.

Exploratory analysis Examining quantitative data descriptively to identify outliers and skewness; allows researcher to become familiar with the data.

Exploratory-descriptive qualitative research Studies that do not identify a specific method or philosophical approach; often motivated by a desire to solve a problem; occurs in naturalistic settings.

Exploratory sequential strategy Mixed methods research design in which qualitative data are collected first and analyzed. The qualitative findings are used in planning the quantitative data collection and drawing conclusions.

Explanatory sequential strategy Mixed methods research design in which quantitative data are collected first and analyzed. The quantitative findings are used in planning data collection for the qualitative phase of the study and drawing conclusions.

External validity Concerned with the extent to which study findings can be generalized beyond the sample used in the study.

Extraneous variables Variables that exist in all studies that can affect the measurement of study variables and the relationships among these variables.

F

Fabrication in research Form of scientific misconduct in research that involves making up data and recording or reporting results that did not occur.

Facilitator See *moderator.*

Factor Hypothetical construct created by factor analysis that represents several separate items or variables; given a name to reflect the focus of the variables associated with each other.

Factor analysis Statistical strategy in which variables or items in an instrument are evaluated for interrelationships to identify closely related variables that share a common idea. Two common types of factor analysis are exploratory and confirmatory.

False-negative (result) Outcome of a diagnostic or screening test indicating that a disease is not present when it is present.

False-positive (result) Outcome of a diagnostic or screening test indicating that a disease is present when it is not present.

Falsification of research Scientific misconduct that involves changing or omitting data, altering equipment, or interfering with a research process; results of the study do not accurately represent reality.

Feasibility of a study Whether or not resources are sufficient for study completion; determined by examining the time and money commitment, researcher's expertise, availability of subjects, facility, and equipment, cooperation of others, and study's ethical considerations.

Field notes Notations recorded by qualitative researchers during or immediate after data collection.

Findings Translated and interpreted results from a study.

Focus groups Refers to a method of collecting qualitative data by soliciting perceptions of participants assembled as a group; facilitator guides discussion and creates a nonthreatening environment.

Focused ethnography Observation and description of a defined, organizational culture conducted in a shorter period of time than a traditional ethnography.

Framework Abstract, logical structure of meaning, such as a portion of a theory, that guides the development of the study, may be tested in the study, and enables the researcher to link the findings to nursing's body of knowledge.

Frequency distribution Statistical procedure that involves listing all possible values of a variable and tallying the number for each value in the data set.

Frequency tables Visual display of the results of a frequency distribution, in which possible values appear in one column of a table and the frequency of each value in the other column.

Full review Institutional review process for studies with risks that are greater than minimal and requires approval from the complete institutional review board; also called *complete review.*

Funnel plots Graphic representations of possible effect sizes *(ESs)* for interventions in selected studies used in meta-analyses.

G

Generalization Extension of the implications of the findings from the sample or situation that was studied to a larger population or situation.

Going native Complication of observation in which the researcher becomes a part of the culture and loses her or his ability to observe clearly.

Gold standard Accepted benchmark for currently assessing and diagnosing a particular patient problem; serves as a basis for comparison with newly developed diagnostic or screening tests; also, a gold standard or benchmark for managing patients' care that is linked to patient outcomes.

Grand nursing theory Abstract, broad-scope theory that encompasses nursing actions and patient responses in multiple settings; initial theories were written by nursing scholars in the 1970s.

Grey literature Research reports that have limited distribution; includes theses and dissertations, unpublished research reports, articles in obscure journals, reports to funding agencies, technical reports, and conference abstracts, papers, and proceedings.

Grounded theory research Qualitative research method based on symbolic interaction theory; conducted to explore and analyze the process that persons use in handling a specific situation or problem. Ideally, the study results in a theoretic description or diagram of the process.

Grouped frequency distribution Visual presentation of a count of variables' values divided into categories. For example, instead of displaying numbers of subjects for every age, ranges of values are considered as groups—for example, ages 20 to 29, 30 to 39.

Grove Model for Implementing Evidence-Based Guidelines in Practice Model developed by one of the textbook authors to promote the use of national, standardized, evidence-based guidelines in clinical practice.

H

Health Insurance Portability and Accountability Act (HIPAA) Federal regulations that protect an individual's health information created during clinical care, electronically stored, and transferred from one entity to another; known as the Privacy Rule; affects health care and research.

Heterogeneous sample Sample in which study participants have a broad range of values being studied; increases the representativeness of the sample and the ability to generalize from the accessible population to the target population.

Highly controlled setting Artificially constructed environment developed for the sole purpose of conducting research, such as a laboratory, research or experimental center, or test unit.

Highly sensitive test Screening or diagnostic test that indicates a true-positive test result for a large proportion of patients with the disease or problem.

Highly specific test Screening or diagnostic test that indicates a true-negative test result for a large proportion of patients without the disease or problem.

History Unplanned event that occurs during a study and may be a threat to internal validity.

Homogeneity reliability See *internal consistency reliability.*

Homogeneous sample Sample in which study participants' scores on selected measurement methods in a study are similar, resulting in a limited or narrow distribution or spread of scores. Use of a homogeneous sample reduces the effect of extraneous variables but limits the potential for generalization because the sample might not be representative of the target population.

Horizontal axis Refers to the *x*-axis in a graph of a regression line or scatter plot that is oriented from left to right across the graph.

Hypothesis Formal statement of the proposed relationship between (among) two or more variables in a specified population.

I

Identifiable private information Documented characteristics of a person and the person's life that can be linked to the person.

Identifying the steps of the research process First step in a critical appraisal. It involves understanding the terms and concepts in the report, as well as identifying study elements and grasping the nature, significance, and meaning of these elements.

Immersed Being in a culture and becoming increasingly familiar with the language, patterns, expression of emotions, and socialization methods of the culture; may also refer to researchers becoming very familiar with qualitative data by spending extensive time reading and re-reading field notes and transcripts and thinking about the meaning of the data. See *dwelling with the data.*

Implications for nursing Meaning of study findings and conclusions for the body of nursing knowledge, theory, and practice.

Implicit framework Conceptual ideas guiding a study but not clearly connected or described as a theory; often included in an introduction or literature review as linkages among variables or findings of previous studies.

Inclusion sample criteria Sampling requirements identified by the researcher that must be present for participants or elements to be considered part of the target population for possible selection to a study sample.

Independent groups Groups in which study participants are assigned to one group or condition or another so that the assignment is unrelated. For example, if participants are randomly assigned to an intervention or control group, the groups are independent.

Independent variable In interventional research, refers to the intervention or treatment that is manipulated or varied by the researcher to cause an effect on the dependent variable. In correlational research, the independent variable(s) are used to predict the occurrence of the dependent variable.

Indirect measures or indicators Quantification of abstract concepts that are measured by the extent to which indicators or attributes of the concepts are present. Scales are examples of indirect measures, such as the use of the FACES Pain Scale to measure pain.

Inductive reasoning Type of reasoning from the specific to the general, in which particular instances are observed and then combined into a larger whole or general statement.

Inference Generalization from a specific case to a general truth, from a part to the whole, from the concrete to the abstract, or from the known to the unknown.

Inferential statistics Analyses conducted to allow inference from the study sample statistic to the population parameter; commonly conducted to test hypotheses and address research questions in studies.

Informed consent Voluntary agreement by a competent potential subject to participate in research after specific and essential information about a study has been disclosed and comprehended.

Institutional review board (IRB) Committee within a university or healthcare organization that reviews research to ensure that the investigator is conducting the research ethically; IRB approval is required before conducting a study in that organization.

Instrumentation Component of measurement that involves the application of specific rules for the development of a measurement device or instrument.

Intellectual critical appraisal of a study Careful examination of all aspects of a study to judge the strengths, weaknesses, meaning, credibility, and significance of the study based on previous research experience and knowledge of the topic.

Intermediate end points Events or markers evaluated for their validity in predicting the outcome and that act as precursors to the final outcome.

Internal consistency reliability Correlation of each item with all other items of a scale to assess the extent to which items are measuring the same concept; higher correlations mean that the scale has consistency; most common measure of internal consistency reliability is called *Cronbach's alpha.*

Internal validity Degree to which measured relationships among variables in a study are a true reflection of reality rather than the result of extraneous variables.

Interpretation Process whereby the researcher places the findings in a larger context; may link different themes or factors in the findings to each other and existing knowledge.

Interpretation of research outcomes Formal process whereby researchers consider the results from data analysis, form conclusions, explore the clinical importance of the findings, consider the implications for nursing knowledge and theory, generalize or transfer the findings, and suggest further studies.

Interpretive phenomenology Study in which a researcher recognizes the influence of her or his own perception, experiences, and values in analyzing the lived experience of participants; qualitative method promoted by Heidigger, a German philosopher, that may also be called hermeneutic phenomenology.

Interrater reliability Degree of consistency between (among) two or more observers or raters who independently assign ratings to variables or elements of interest during a study.

Interval-level measurement Quantification using equal numerical distances between intervals; follows the rules of mutually exclusive categories, exhaustive categories, and rank ordering, such as temperature or scores on scales.

Intervention Treatment or independent variable implemented during the conduct of a study to produce an effect on the dependent or outcome variables.

Intervention fidelity Accuracy, consistency (reliability), and thoroughness with which an intervention is delivered in a study, with adherence to the specified protocol, treatment program, or intervention model; can be affected by the researcher's competence in implementing the treatment.

Intervention group See *experimental group* and *treatment group.*

Interview Structured or unstructured verbal communication between the researcher and study participant during which data are collected for a study.

Intuition Insight or understanding of a situation or event as a whole that usually cannot be explained logically.

Invasion of privacy Sharing private information with others without a person's knowledge or against his or her will.

Iowa Model of Evidence-Based Practice (EBP) Framework for the implementation of EBP that was revised and validated by the Iowa Model Collaborative in 2017. In a healthcare agency, there are triggering issues that initiate the need for change; significant evidence is needed to make the change, the change must be appropriate for practice, and the change needs to be integrated and sustained in practice.

K

Key informant Participant in an ethnographic study with extensive knowledge and influence in a culture with whom a researcher may interact repeatedly to learn about the culture.

Keywords Terms or labels used that are the major concepts, variables, or research methodologies listed near the beginning of a research report; can be used to search bibliographic databases to find articles on a particular topic.

Knowledge Essential content or body of information for a discipline that is acquired through traditions, authority, borrowing, trial and error, personal experience, role modeling and mentorship, intuition, reasoning, and research. Knowledge is expected to be an accurate reflection of reality and is incorporated and used to direct a person's actions.

L

Landmark studies Major research projects generating knowledge that influence a discipline and sometimes society in general.

Language bias Occur if searches for systematic reviews focus only on studies in English, and important studies exist in other languages; studies in other languages are less likely to be included in a systematic review.

Level of statistical significance See *alpha* (α).

Levels of measurement Organized set of rules for assigning numbers to objects so that a hierarchy in measurement from low to high is established. The levels of measurement are nominal, ordinal, interval, and ratio.

Likelihood ratios (LRs) Additional calculations that can help researchers determine the accuracy of diagnostic or screening tests, based on the sensitivity and specificity of results.

Likert scale Type of scale designed to determine the opinions or attitudes of study participants. It contains a number of declarative statements, each of which is followed by a response scale ranging from strongly agree to strongly disagree; other response scale descriptors may be used.

Limitations Aspects or weaknesses of a study that threaten design validity and decrease the generalizability of the findings; examples are nonrepresentative samples, single setting, limited control over intervention, instruments with limited reliability and validity, limited control over data collection, and improper use of statistical analyses.

Line of best fit Best reflection of the values on the scatterplot. The regression line is drawn that best fits all paired variable values.

Literature All written sources relevant to the topic that the researcher has selected, including articles published in periodicals or journals, Internet publications, monographs, encyclopedias, conference papers, theses, dissertations, clinical journals, textbooks, and other books.

Literature review See *review of literature.*

Location bias Occurs when studies are published in lower impact journals and indexed in less searched databases—thus, less likely to be included in a systematic review.

Longitudinal design Noninterventional research that involves collecting data from the same study participants at different points in time to determine change in a variable over time within a defined group; might also be referred to as *repeated measures.*

Low statistical power The power to detect significant relationships and differences is below the acceptable standard of 0.8 needed to conduct a study. Low statistical power increases the likelihood of a type II error.

M

Manipulation Changing the value or aspects of the independent variable to measure its effect on the dependent variable.

Maps (or models) Diagrams that graphically display concepts and relationships of theories or frameworks.

Maturation Threat to internal validity due to normal changes occurring over time during a study that may affect the dependent variable; study participants might become fatigued or wiser over time, resulting in changes in their scores on the dependent variable.

Mean Measure of central tendency conducted with interval- and ratio-level of measurement; the value obtained by summing all the scores and dividing the total by the number of scores.

Mean difference Standard statistic that is calculated to determine the absolute difference between the means of two groups.

Measurement Process of assigning values to objects, events, or situations in accord with some rule.

Measurement error Difference between what exists in reality and what is measured by a research instrument.

Measures of central tendency Statistical analyses to determine the center of a distribution of scores; includes mode, median, and mean.

Measures of dispersion Statistical analyses to determine how scores vary or are dispersed around the mean; these analyses include range, difference scores, sum of squares, variance, and standard deviation.

Median Score at the exact center of the ranked ungrouped frequency distribution; when the number of data points is even, the median value is the average of the two middle values.

Mentor Person who serves as a teacher, sponsor, guide, or exemplar for a novice.

Mentorship In nursing, this is an intense form of role modeling in which an expert nurse serves as a teacher, sponsor, guide, exemplar, and counselor for a novice nurse or mentee.

Meta-analysis Statistical technique conducted to pool data and results from several studies into a single quantitative analysis; provides one of the highest levels of evidence (effect of an intervention or strength of a relationship) for practice. The studies must share a similar design to be included in the analysis.

Metasummary, qualitative Synthesis of multiple primary qualitative studies to develop a description of current knowledge in an area.

Meta-synthesis, qualitative Systematic compilation and integration of qualitative studies to expand understanding and develop a unique interpretation of studies' findings in a selected area.

Methodological bias Occurs when studies selected for a systematic review have weaknesses in their design, interventions, data collection, or data analysis. The influence of the study limitations should be included in the review.

Methodological congruence Consistency among the underlying philosophy, qualitative design being used, and development of the study product.

Methodological limitations See *limitations.*

Middle-range theories Relatively concrete conceptual descriptions with a limited number of concepts and propositions that can be applied in practice, used to guide studies, or tested by research.

Minimal risk See *expedited IRB review.*

Mixed-methods research Research methodology that offers investigators the ability to use the strengths of qualitative and quantitative research designs in a study. Mixed methods research is characterized as research that contains elements of qualitative and quantitative approaches.

Mixed-methods systematic review Synthesis that includes studies with various designs, such as qualitative research and quasi-experimental, correlational, and descriptive quantitative studies to determine the current knowledge in a problem area.

Mixed results Study results that include significant and nonsignificant findings or contradictory findings related to the relationship or intervention examined in the study.

Mode Most frequently occurring value or score in a distribution that does not necessarily indicate the center of the range.

Model testing design Correlational research that measures the proposed relationships within a theoretic model. This design requires concepts relevant to the model to be measured and the relationships among these concepts examined.

Moderator Discussion leader of a focus group, who may or may not be the researcher.

Monographs Books, booklets of conference proceedings, or pamphlets, which may be published once for a specific purpose; may be updated with a new edition, as needed.

Multicausality Recognition that a number of interrelated variables can cause a particular effect.

Multilevel synthesis Conducted during a mixed-methods systematic review that involves synthesizing the findings from quantitative studies separately from qualitative studies and integrating the findings from these two syntheses into the final report.

Multiple regression analysis Statistical technique conducted to predict the dependent variable using more than one independent variable; an extension of simple linear regression.

N

Natural setting Real-life or field setting for conducting research in which the researcher makes no attempts to control extraneous variables. Natural settings include participants' homes, workplace, and school.

Negative likelihood ratio (LR) The ratio of true-negative results to false-negative results; calculated as follows:

$$\text{Negative likelihood ratio} = (100\% - \text{sensitivity}) + \text{specificity}.$$

Negative (inverse) relationship Association in which one variable or concept changes (its value increases or decreases), and the other variable or concept changes in the opposite direction.

Network sampling Nonprobability sampling technique that includes a snowballing technique to take advantage of social networks and the fact that friends tend to hold characteristics in common. Participants meeting the sample criteria are asked to assist in locating others with similar characteristics. Network sampling is synonymous with chain sampling and snowball sampling.

Nominal data Lowest level of data that can only be organized into categories that are exclusive and exhaustive. These data are analyzed with nonparametric statistics.

Nominal-level measurement Lowest level of quantification used when data can be organized into exclusive and exhaustive categories, but the categories cannot be compared or rank-ordered. Variables such as gender, race, marital status, and diagnoses are measured at the nominal level.

Nondirectional hypothesis Type of hypothesis stating that a relationship exists but does not predict the exact nature (positive or negative or strength) of the relationship.

Nonexperimental design Descriptive and correlational design that focuses on examining variables as they naturally occur in an environment, not on the implementation of a treatment by the researcher.

Noninterventional design See *nonexperimental design.*

Nonparametric analysis Statistical technique conducted when data are not normally distributed and measured at the nominal or ordinal levels; data do not meet assumptions of parametric statistics (normal distribution, interval- or ratio-level data).

Nonprobability sampling Nonrandom sampling technique in which not every element of the population has an opportunity for selection, such as convenience sampling, quota sampling, purposive sampling, network sampling, and theoretical sampling.

Nonsignificant results Statistical results that are not strong enough to reach statistical significance; null hypothesis is not rejected; considered to be negative results or unpredicted results; may accurately reflect reality or may be caused by study weaknesses.

Nontherapeutic research Type of research conducted to generate knowledge for a discipline; the results might benefit future patients but will probably not benefit the research participants.

Normal curve Symmetric, unimodal, bell-shaped, theoretical distribution of all possible scores; no real distribution exactly fits the normal curve.

Null hypothesis (H_0) Hypothesis that is the opposite of the research hypothesis, stating there is no significant difference between (among) study groups, or no significant relationships among the variables being studied. The null hypothesis is tested during data analysis and is used for interpreting statistical outcomes.

Nuremberg Code Statements of ethical research conduct that were developed in response to the Nuremberg Trials following World War II.

Nurse's role in outcomes Nurse's role in outcomes of a study has three subcomponents—nurse's independent role, nurse's dependent role, and nurse's interdependent role.

Nurse's dependent role functions Functions that include carrying out medical orders and physician-initiated treatments; evaluated by the absence of adverse outcomes.

Nurse's independent role functions Functions that include assessment, diagnosis, nurse-initiated interventions, and follow-up care; evaluated by the patient outcomes of symptom control, freedom from complications, functional status and self-care, knowledge of disease and its treatment, satisfaction, and costs.

Nurse's interdependent role functions Functions that include communication, case management, coordination and continuity of care, monitoring, and reporting among members of the healthcare team.

Nursing Care Report Card Evaluation of hospital nursing care developed in 1994 by the American Nurses Association and American Academy of Nursing Expert Panel on Quality Health Care for the purpose of identifying and developing nursing-sensitive quality measures using 10 indications—two structure indicators, two process indicators, and six outcome indicators. This report card could facilitate benchmarking or setting a desired standard that would allow comparisons of hospitals in terms of their nursing care quality.

Nursing intervention Deliberate cognitive, physical, or verbal activities planned with or on behalf of individuals and their families that are directed toward accomplishing particular therapeutic objectives related to individuals' health and well-being.

Nursing process Subset of the problem-solving process. Steps include assessment, diagnosis, plan, implementation, evaluation, and modification.

Nursing research Scientific process of inquiry that may generate new knowledge or validate and refine existing knowledge; findings directly and indirectly influence the delivery of evidence-based nursing practice.

Nursing-sensitive outcome See *nursing-sensitive patient outcome.*

Nursing-sensitive patient outcome (NSPO) Patient outcomes that are influenced by or associated with nursing care. These outcomes are sensitive because they are influenced by nursing care decisions and actions.

O

Observation Fundamental method of gathering data for qualitative studies, especially ethnographic studies, by spending time and focusing on communication and actions within a culture.

Observational measurement Use of structured and unstructured observations to measure study variables.

One-tailed test of significance Analysis used with directional hypotheses in which extreme statistical values of interest are hypothesized to occur in a single tail of the normal curve.

Open-ended interview Type of interview used in qualitative research with a defined focus but no fixed sequence of questions. The interview questions may change as the researcher gains insight from previous interviews, and participants are encouraged to raise important issues not addressed by the researcher.

Operational definition Description of how variables or concepts will be measured or manipulated in a study.

Ordinal data Data that can be ranked with intervals between the ranks that are not necessarily equal. Ordinal data are analyzed with nonparametric statistical techniques.

Ordinal-level measurement Method whereby data are assigned to mutually exclusive and exhaustive categories, with one category being judged to be (or is ranked) higher or lower, or better or worse, than another category. The intervals between the ranked data are not necessarily equal, such as ranking pain as mild, moderate, and severe.

Outcome reporting bias Type of bias that occurs when study results are not reported clearly and with complete accuracy.

Outcomes research Scientific methodology developed to examine the end results of patient care. In contrast to traditional scientific endeavors, outcomes research incorporates evaluation research, epidemiology, and economic theory perspectives.

Outliers Extreme scores or values in a data set that seem unlike the rest of the sample; may be due to random variability or errors in measurement redundant or errors in identifying the variables important in explaining the nature of the phenomenon under study.

P

Paired (or dependent) groups Participants or observations selected for data collection are related in some way to the selection of other participants or observations. For example, if study participants serve as their own control by using the pretest as a control group, the measurements (and therefore the groups) are paired.

Parallel synthesis During a mixed-methods systematic review, this involves the separate synthesis of quantitative and qualitative studies, but the findings from the qualitative synthesis are used in interpreting the synthesized quantitative studies.

Parameter Unknown numeric value of a characteristic of a population. Parameters of the population are estimated with statistics.

Parametric statistical analyses Statistical techniques conducted when three assumptions are met: (1) the sample was drawn from a population in which the distribution of scores is expected to be normal or approximately normal; (2) the level of measurement of variables is at the interval or ratio level; and (3) the data can be treated as though they were obtained from random samples; the same techniques can be used for interval or ratio data.

Paraphrasing Clearly and concisely restating the ideas of an author in the researcher's own words.

Partially controlled setting Naturalistic environment that the researcher has manipulated or modified in some way to control for the effects of extraneous variables.

Participants Individuals who voluntarily participate in a study. Qualitative researchers use the term *participants;* quantitative researchers might call them *subjects* or *participants.*

Patient circumstances Individual's clinical state, health goals (e.g., health promotion, illness management, and/or peaceful death), and clinical setting. Evidence-based practice is a combination of best research evidence, clinical expertise, and patient circumstances.

Patient health outcomes Specific outcomes based on the Nursing Role Effectiveness Model. The outcomes of the independent role are clinical and symptom control, freedom from complications, functional status and self-care, and knowledge of the disease and its treatment, satisfaction, and costs.

Pearson product-moment correlation (*r*) Parametric statistical analysis conducted to determine the linear relationship between two variables.

Peer-reviewed Refers to publications that include only articles examined by scholars familiar with the topic and deemed to be accurate, well written, and consistent with the purpose of the journal. If a manuscript is a research report, the experts will also evaluate the rigor of the study. Publications with peer-reviewed articles are sometime called *refereed journals.*

Percentage distributions Data are grouped and percentages calculated for a number of scores falling within a specific group, such as ages 20 to 29 = 20% and 30 to 39 = 12%.

Percentage of variance Amount of variability explained by a linear relationship. The value is obtained by squaring Pearson's correlation coefficient (r). For example, if $r = 0.5$ in a study, the percentage of variance explained is $r^2 = 0.25$, or 25%.

Periodicals Literature sources such as journals that are published a specified number of times each year, continue to be published over time, and are numbered sequentially for the years published.

Permission to participate in research Documentation that a parent(s) or guardian agrees for their child or ward to be in a study.

Personal experience Knowledge gained through participation in rather than observation of functions, including events, situations, or circumstances. Benner (1984) described five levels of experience in the development of clinical nursing knowledge and expertise: (1) novice, (2) advanced beginner, (3) competent, (4) proficient, and (5) expert.

Phase I: Preparation Step that involves determining the purpose, focus, and potential outcomes of making an evidence-based change in a clinical agency; comprises the first step in using the Stetler Model of Research Utilization to Facilitate Evidence-Based Practice.

Phase II: Validation Phase of the Stetler Model of Research Utilization to Facilitate Evidence-Based Practice that involves critically appraising the identified studies to determine their scientific soundness.

Phase III: Comparative Evaluation/Decision Making Phase of the Stetler Model of Research Utilization to Facilitate Evidence-Based Practice that has four parts: (1) substantiation of the evidence; (2) fit of the evidence with the healthcare setting; (3) feasibility of using research findings; and (4) concerns with current practice.

Phase IV: Translation/ Application Phase of the Stetler Model of Research Utilization to Facilitate Evidence-Based Practice that involves planning and determining exactly what knowledge will be used and how that knowledge will be applied to practice. The application may be cognitive, instrumental, or symbolic.

Phase V: Evaluation Final phase of the Stetler Model of Research Utilization to Facilitate Evidence-Based Practice in which the team determines the impact of the research-based change on the healthcare agency, personnel, and patients through formal and informal activities; may include self-monitoring, case studies, audits, QI (quality improvement) projects, and discussions with patients, families, peers, and other professionals.

Phenomenological research Qualitative study focused on the lived experiences of the participants from their perspective.

Phenomenology Philosophy and a group of research methods congruent with the philosophy through which researchers describe and analyze lived experiences from the perspective of those within the experience.

Phenomenon (*pl.,* phenomena) Occurrence or experience of which one is consciously aware and able to observe or describe; may be the focus of a qualitative study.

Philosophies Rational, intellectual explorations of truths; principles of being, knowledge, or conduct.

Physiological measures Techniques and equipment used to measure physiological variables either directly or indirectly, such as techniques to measure blood pressure and heart rate.

PICOS or PICO format Acronym for the population or participants of interest; intervention needed for practice; comparisons of the intervention with control, placebo, standard care, or variations of the same intervention; outcomes needed for practice; and study design. PICOS is one of the most common formats used to delimit a relevant clinical question.

Pilot study Smaller version of a proposed study conducted to develop and refine the methodology, such as the intervention, instruments, or data collection process to be used in the larger study.

Placebo In pharmacology, a substance without discernible effect that is administered to a control group in studies. Broadly, an intervention intended to have no effect.

Plagiarism Using another person's ideas, processes, results, or words without giving appropriate credit; one type of research misconduct.

Population Particular group of elements (people, objects, events, or substances) that is the focus of the study.

Population-based studies Type of outcomes research that involves studying health conditions in the context of the patient's community rather than the context of the medical system. With a population-based study, all cases of a condition occurring in the defined population are included, not just the cases treated at a particular healthcare facility.

Positive likelihood ratio (*LR*) Ratio used to determine the likelihood that a positive test result is a true-positive result. It is calculated by the following:

$$\text{Positive } LR = \text{sensitivity} \div (100\% - \text{specificity})$$

Positive (linear) relationship Numeric association between two variables in which one variable changes (its value increases or decreases), and then the other variable will change in the same direction.

Posthoc analyses Statistical techniques performed to determine which groups are significantly different after the initial test of more than two groups demonstrates significant differences. For example, ANOVA (analysis of variance) indicates significant differences among three groups (intervention, placebo, and control), but the post hoc analyses indicate specifically which groups are different.

Posttest-only control group design Experimental design in which there is no preintervention measurement of the value of the dependent variable in the experimental or control groups.

Posttest-only design with comparison group Quasi-experimental design conducted to examine the difference between the treatment group that receives an intervention and the comparison group that does not; provides poor control of threats to internal validity.

Power Probability that a statistical test will detect a significant difference or relationship if one exists, which is the capacity to reject a null hypothesis correctly.

Power analysis Technique used to determine the risk of a type II error so that the study can be modified to decrease the risk if necessary and ensure that the study has adequate sample size. Conducting a power analysis includes alpha (level of significance), effect size, and standard power of 0.8 to determine the sample size for a study.

Practice pattern Represents variations in what care is provided.

Practice style Represents variations in how care is provided.

Practice theories Very specific middle-range theories designed to describe particular nursing actions and explain patient responses; sometimes called situation-specific theories.

Precision Accuracy with which the population parameters have been estimated in a study; may also be used to describe the accuracy, detail, and order of a research purpose and detailed description of the study design.

Precision of physiological measurement Accuracy and reproducibility of measurements of characteristics or functions of the body, such as weight, blood pressure, and pulse.

Prediction Estimation of the probability of a specific outcome in a given situation that can be achieved through research.

Predictive correlational design Correlational design used to establish strength and direction of relationships between or among variables; design is implemented to predict the value of a dependent variable based on the values obtained for other independent variables; approach to examining causal relationships between or among variables.

Predictive validity Extent to which an individual's score on a scale can accurately predict future performance; one type of criterion-related validity.

Pretest-posttest design with comparison group Quasi-experimental design in which the intervention is applied to the experimental group following the pretest of both the experimental and comparison groups and a posttest after implementation of the intervention; evaluates the effect of the intervention that can be measured—basically, a pretest-posttest design without random assignment to the experimental and comparison groups.

Pretest-posttest design with control group Experimental design with random assignment of participants to the intervention and control groups. Both groups receive pretest and, after the intervention, the posttest; measures effect of the intervention; often called the *classic experimental design*.

Primary data Information or scores collected for a particular study.

Primary source Publication whose author originated or is responsible for generating the ideas published.

Principle of beneficence Ethical principle of doing good and not exposing others to harm. In research, this means to minimize risks, ensure benefits, and maintain the integrity of the study.

Principle of justice Ethical principle of fair treatment; related to studies, opportunities to participate, experience benefits, and be protected from harm are distributed fairly.

Principle of respect for persons Ethical principle of treating people as autonomous agents who may or may not decide to participate in research and to withdraw from a study at any time. Confidentiality and informed consent are based on this principle.

Privacy Freedom to determine the time, extent, and general circumstances under which private information will be shared with or withheld from others.

Probability Likelihood that a given event will occur in a situation; addresses the relative rather than the absolute causality of events. In statistics, it is the percentage chance that the results of the statistical test indicate that the sample actually represents the population from which it was drawn.

Probability sampling Random sampling technique in which every member (element) of the population has a probability higher than zero of being selected for the sample, such as simple random sampling, stratified random sampling, cluster sampling, and systematic sampling.

Probability theory Statistical or mathematical theory that addresses the likelihood of occurrence; in research, the likelihood that the findings from a sample are the same as the population parameters.

Probe Question or open-ended statement of a qualitative researcher during an interview to obtain more information from the participant; may be used to follow up a previous comment or further explore the perspective of the participant.

Problem statement Statement that concludes the discussion of a research problem and indicates the gap in the knowledge needed for practice. The problem statement usually provides a basis for the study purpose.

Process Structured, logical series of actions with a defined goal.

Process of care Construct that includes the actual care delivered by healthcare personnel. The process of care is one of the three components—structure, process, and outcomes of care—of Donabedian's theory of the quality of health care.

Proposition Abstract statement describing relationships between concepts in theories; ranges in scope from general to specific. The latter may lead to hypotheses.

Prospective Looking forward; data collected during a study in real time.

Prospective cohort study Epidemiological study in which the researcher identifies a group of people at risk for experiencing a particular event and then follows them over time to observe whether or not the event occurs.

Protected health information Data generated and collected for research that can be linked to an individual.

Providers of care Individuals responsible for the delivery of care, such as nurses, nurse practitioners, and physicians, who are part of the structure of care of Donabedian's theory of health care.

Proximal outcome Outcome close to the delivery of care.

Publication bias Bias that occurs when studies with positive results are more likely to be published than studies with negative or inconclusive results.

Purposive (or purposeful) sampling Selection of participants who possess certain characteristics, such as having experience or being knowledgeable of the culture or phenomenon for a qualitative study. The researcher selects the participants consciously, making this a nonprobability or nonrandom sampling method.

Q

Qualitative research Scholarly and rigorous methodological approach used to describe life experiences, cultures, and social processes from the perspective of the persons involved.

Qualitative research critical appraisal process Three-part process that consists of the following: (1) identifying the components of the qualitative research process in studies; (2) determining study strengths and weaknesses; and (3) evaluating the trustworthiness, credibility, and meaning of study findings.

Qualitative research process Series of connected actions that begins with the identification of a research problem best addressed from the perspectives of those in the situation. The process may evolve over the course of the study but involves steps to increase the credibility of the findings.

Qualitative research report Written report that includes an introduction, review of literature, methods, results, and discussion of findings for a qualitative study.

Qualitative research synthesis Process and product of systematically reviewing and formally integrating the findings from qualitative studies. *Meta-synthesis* is the term used in this textbook to describe the process of systematically reviewing and integrating qualitative research findings.

Quality and Safety Education for Nurses (QSEN) Initiative focused on identifying the knowledge, skills, and attitudes (KSA) that nurses must have to promote quality and safety in patient care. KSA statements have been developed for each of the competencies for prelicensure and graduate education. One of the competencies is focused on evidence-based practice.

Quality of care Extent to which healthcare services provided to individuals and populations improve desired health outcomes and are consistent with current professional knowledge. Outcomes are examined in the conduct of outcomes research.

Quantitative research Formal, objective, systematic process of research used to describe variables using numbers, test relationships between them, and examine cause and effect interactions among variables.

Quantitative research critical appraisal process Includes three basic steps: (1) identifying the steps of the research process in studies; (2) determining study strengths and weaknesses; and (3) evaluating the credibility and meaning of study findings.

Quantitative research report Written report that includes an introduction, review of literature, methods, results, and discussion of findings for a quantitative study.

Quasi-experimental design Plan for a study developed to determine the effectiveness of interventions when some aspect of an experiment cannot be implemented.

Quasi-experimental research Type of quantitative research conducted to test a cause and effect relationship, but lacks one or more of the three essential elements of experiment research: (1) researcher-controlled manipulation of the independent variable (intervention); (2) traditional control group; and (3) random assignment of study participants to groups.

Questionnaire Self-report form designed to elicit information (data) from participants who respond by selecting from a list of predetermined options or writing textual responses to questions.

Quota sampling Nonprobability convenience sampling technique in which the proportion of identified groups is predetermined by the researcher to increase the sample's representativeness of the population. Quota sampling may be used to ensure the inclusion of study participants who are likely to be underrepresented in the convenience sample, such as women, minority groups, and undereducated persons.

R

Random assignment to groups Procedure used to assign study participants randomly to an intervention or control group. Each study participant should have an equal opportunity of being assigned to either group.

Random measurement error Type of error in which individuals' observed scores vary haphazardly around their true scores.

Random sampling method See *probability sampling method.*

Random variation Normally occurring and expected differences in values that occur when the researcher examines responses or characteristics of the study participants from the same sample.

Randomized controlled trial (RCT) Tightly controlled test of an intervention using a pretest-posttest control group design or another experimental design to produce definitive evidence about the effectiveness of an intervention. An RCT may have a single site or multiple sites.

Range Simplest measure of dispersion. The range is determined by subtracting the lowest score from the highest score (range, 96 – 78 = 18) or just identifying the lowest and highest scores (range, 78 to 96).

Rating scale Method of measurement in which the rater makes a selection, sometimes numeric and sometimes not numeric, from among an ordered set of predefined categories to convey feelings, preferences, and other subjective perceptions. For example, the FACES Pain Scale is a commonly used rating scale to measure pain in pediatric patients.

Ratio data Numerical information based on the real numbers scale; data can be analyzed with parametric statistics. See *ratio level of measurement.*

Ratio level measurement Highest form of measurement meeting all the rules of other levels of measurement—mutually exclusive categories, exhaustive categories, ordered ranks, equally spaced intervals, and continuum of values; also has an absolute zero, such as pulse.

Readability level Degree of difficulty to read and comprehend a text, often applied to a scale or survey instrument; can be determined by counting the length of phrases or sentences and number of syllables in words or by using the assessments available in word processing programs; can influence reliability and validity when used in a study.

Reading a research report Method of reading that includes skimming, comprehending, and analyzing the content of a study to promote understanding.

Reasoning Processing and organizing ideas to reach conclusions; types of reasoning include problematic, operational, dialectic, and logistic.

Recommendations for further research Suggestions provided by researchers for future studies based on their study findings. Recommendations might include replications or repeating the design with a different or larger sample, using different measurement methods, or testing another intervention.

Refereed journals See *peer-reviewed journals.*

Reference Documentation of the origin of a cited quote or paraphrased idea that includes identifying information so that the reader can locate the original material.

Reference group Group of individuals or other elements that constitutes the standard against which individual study participant's scores are compared.

Refusal rate Percentage of potential subjects who declined to participate in the study. The study should include their reasons for not participating. The refusal rate is calculated by dividing the number refusing to participate by the number of potential subjects approached and then multiplied by 100%. For example, if 100 subjects are approached, and 15 refuse to participate, the refusal rate is $(15 \div 100) \times 100\% = 0.15 \times 100\% = 15\%$.

Regression analysis Statistical procedure conducted to predict the value of one variable using known values of one or more other variables. The independent (predictor) variable(s) is (are) analyzed to determine their influence on variation or change in the value of the dependent variable.

Relevant literature Pertinent publications that provide important information needed to synthesize the state of the body of knowledge in a problem area.

Reliability Extent to which an instrument consistently measures a variable or concept. See *reliability testing.*

Reliability testing Method to determine the amount of random error in a measurement method; assesses the following aspects of reliability—stability, equivalence, and internal consistency or homogeneity.

Replication studies Research that reproduces or repeats prior studies to determine whether similar findings will be obtained.

Representativeness of the sample Degree to which the sample is like the population it purportedly represents; also stated as the degree to which the sample, accessible population, and target population are similar or alike.

Research Diligent, systematic inquiry or investigation to validate and refine existing knowledge and generate new knowledge.

Research-based protocol Document providing clearly developed steps for implementing a treatment or intervention in practice that is based on findings from studies.

Research concepts Ideas, experiences, situations, or events that are investigated in qualitative research.

Research design Blueprint for conducting a study; maximizes control over factors that could interfere with the validity of the findings and guides the planning and implementation of a study in a way that is most likely to achieve the intended goal.

Research framework Abstract and logical structure of meaning that guides the development of a study and allows the researcher to link the findings back to the body of knowledge; may be a portion of a theory or variables linked in previous studies.

Research hypothesis Alternative hypothesis to the null hypothesis. It states that a relationship exists between (among) two or more variables or a difference exits between (among) groups.

Research misconduct Intentional deviation from practices commonly accepted within the scientific community for proposing, conducting, or reporting research; may include fabrication, falsification, or plagiarism; does not include honest errors or honest differences in interpretation or judgment of data.

Research objective Clear, concise, declarative statement expressed to direct a study; focuses on identifying and describing variables and relationships among variables.

Research problem Area of concern in which there is a gap in the knowledge base needed for nursing practice. Research is conducted to generate essential knowledge to address the practice concern, with the ultimate goal of providing evidence-based practice. The research problem in a study needs to include significance, background, and problem statement.

Research process Series of connected actions that require an understanding of a unique language; involves rigorous application of a variety of research methods in the conduct of studies.

Research purpose Concise, clear statement of the specific goal or aim of the study. The purpose is the reason for conducting the study and is generated from the problem.

Research question Concise interrogative statement developed to direct a study. Quantitative research questions focus on describing variables, examining relationships among variables, and determining the differences between two or more groups; qualitative research questions identify the major concepts or phenomena to be addressed by the study.

Research report Written description of a completed study designed to communicate the study findings effectively to nurses and other healthcare professionals.

Research setting Site or location for conducting a study. A research setting may be natural, partially controlled, or highly controlled.

Research topics Concepts or broad problem areas that indicate the foci of essential research knowledge needed to provide evidence-based nursing practice. Research topics include numerous potential research problems.

Research variables Qualities, properties, or characteristics identified in the research purpose and objectives or questions that are observed or measured in a study.

Researcher-participant relationship Interaction and shared experience of the researcher and the participant that have effects on the collection and interpretation of data. The researcher creates a respectful relationship with each participant, which includes being honest and open about the purpose and methods of the study.

Results Outcomes from data analysis that are generated for each research objective, question, or hypothesis. Results can be mixed, nonsignificant, significant and not predicted, significant and predicted, or unexpected.

Retention rate Number and percentage of study participants completing the study.

Retrospective Looking backward; when applied to research, using information previously obtained as data in a study.

Retrospective cohort study Epidemiological study in which the researcher identifies a group of people who have experienced a particular event and study their outcomes.

Review of literature Summary of current theoretical and empirical sources to generate a picture of what is known and not known about a particular problem; may lead to the statement of a research problem or identification of knowledge ready to be used in practice.

Review of relevant literature See *review of literature.*

Rigor Excellence in research; attained through the use of discipline, scrupulous adherence to detail, and strict accuracy.

Role modeling Learning by imitating the behavior of an exemplar or role model. For example, in an internship program, novice nurses learn by imitating the behaviors of expert nurses.

S

Sample Subset of the population that is selected for a study.

Sample attrition See *attrition rate of a sample.*

Sample characteristics Data analyzed and summarized to describe the study participants. Common demographic variables measured in nursing studies include age, gender, ethnicity, race, and medical diagnoses.

Sample retention Number of study participants remaining in and completing the study.

Sample size Number of participants, events, behaviors, or situations examined in a study.

Sampling Process of selecting a group of people, events, behaviors, or other elements that are representative of the population being studied.

Sampling, or eligibility, criteria List of the characteristics essential for inclusion or exclusion in the target population.

Sampling frame List of every member of the target population. Sampling criteria are used to define membership in this population.

Sampling method Process of selecting a group of people, events, behaviors, or other elements that meet the sampling criteria. Sampling methods may be random or nonrandom (probability and nonprobability).

Sampling plan Includes proposed strategies to be used to obtain a sample in a study; may include random and nonrandom (probability and nonprobability) sampling methods.

Saturation Point during a qualitative study when additional data collection provides no new information; rather, there is redundancy of previously collected data. Sample size in a qualitative study is determined when saturation of data occurs.

Scale Self-report form of measurement composed of several items designed to measure a construct. The participants respond to each item on the continuum or scale provided, such as a depression scale.

Scatter diagrams or scatter plots Diagrams or figures showing the dispersion of scores on a variable or depicting the relationship of data on one variable with data on another variable. A scatter plot has two scales, horizontal (x-axis) and vertical (y-axis).

Scientific theory Conceptual structure with exhaustive research evidence to support its claims. Concepts are clearly defined and can be measured reliably and with validity to test its propositions; its propositions may be considered laws and principles ready for application in practice.

Secondary analysis Re-analysis of information or data that was previously collected by another researcher or organization. A secondary analysis may involve the use of research or administrative databases.

Secondary data Information collected in clinical practice or for another study prior to the current study; stored electronically in a database.

Secondary source Publication whose author summarizes or quotes content from primary sources.

Seminal studies First research carried out on a particular topic.

Semistructured interview Interaction between a researcher and participant guided by a fixed set of questions and no fixed responses.

Sensitivity Extent to which a physiologic measure can detect small changes. Higher sensitivity means that the measure is more precise.

Sensitivity of a screening or diagnostic test Accuracy of a screening or diagnostic test; proportion of patients with the disease who have a positive test or true-positive result.

Setting See *research setting.*

Significance of a research problem Indicates the importance of the problem to nursing and health care and to the health of individuals, families, and communities.

Significant and unpredicted results Results are opposite to those predicted by the researcher, indicating flaws in the logic of both the researcher and/or the theory being tested.

Significant results Statistically significant results consistent with the researcher's prediction; highly unlikely to have occurred by chance.

Simple hypothesis Statement of a relationship (associative or causal) between two variables.

Simple descriptive design Plan for a study to examine variables in one sample.

Simple linear regression Parametric analysis technique that estimates the value of a dependent variable based on the value of an independent variable.

Simple random sampling Selection of participants or elements at random from a sampling frame for inclusion in a study. Each study participant has a probability greater than zero of being selected for inclusion in the study.

Skimming research reports Quickly reviewing a source to gain a broad overview of the content by reading the title, author's name, abstract or introduction, headings, one or two sentences under each heading, and discussion section.

Snowball sampling See *network sampling.*

Specific propositions Statements found in theories that are at a moderate level of abstraction and provide the basis for the generation of hypotheses to guide a study.

Specificity Extent to which a physiological measure can determine the absence of a disease. Higher specificity means that the measure is more precise.

Specificity of a screening or diagnostic test The proportion of patients without the disease who have a negative test or true-negative result.

Stability reliability Extent to which a measurement produces the same score on repeated administration; often referred to as *test-retest reliability.*

Standard deviation (*SD*) Measure of the amount of dispersion from the mean that characterizes a data set; square root of variance.

Standardized mean difference (SMD) Summary statistic that is reported in a meta-analysis when the same outcome is measured by different scales or methods. The SMD is also referred to as the *d* statistic.

Standardized mortality ratio (SMR) Observed number of deaths divided by the expected number of deaths and multiplied by 100. SMR is regarded as a measure of the relative risk of the studied group to die of a particular condition.

Standardized score Expressing deviations from the mean (difference scores) in terms of standard deviation units, such as *z* scores, with the mean as 0 and the standard deviation as 1.

Standard of care Norm on which the quality of care is judged. Standards of care are based on research findings in conjunction with current practice patterns. According to Donabedian, standard of care is considered one of the processes of care.

Statements Sentences that clarify the existence of concepts, their definitions, and the relationships among them.

Statistical analysis Techniques conducted to examine, reduce, and give meaning to a study's numeric data.

Statistical conclusion validity Degree to which the researcher makes decisions about the proper use of statistics so that the conclusions about relationships and differences drawn from the analyses are an accurate reflection of reality.

Statistical hypothesis See *null hypothesis.*

Statistical significance See *alpha.*

Stetler Model of Research Utilization to Facilitate Evidence-Based Practice Model developed by Stetler that provides a comprehensive framework to enhance the use of research findings by nurses as they implement evidence-based practice.

Stratified random sampling Method used when the researcher knows that some of the variables in the population are critical to achieving representativeness. The sample is divided into strata or groups using these identified variables, and participants are selected randomly from each strata.

Structural variables Factors such as the organization of nursing care and nursing leadership that have effects on nursing practice and, in turn, on patient outcomes.

Structured interview Communication between the researcher and participant during which predetermined questions are asked in the same order for all interviews; can be used to collect quantitative data by assigning numbers to the answer options.

Structured observations Clear identification of which behaviors are of interest and will be translated into data; observations are precisely defined, recorded, and coded.

Structure in outcomes Based on Donabedian's theory, structure of outcomes includes three subcomponents—nurse, organization, and patient.

Structures of care Elements of organization and administration, as well as provider and patient characteristics that guide the processes of care.

Study validity Measure of the truth or accuracy of the findings obtained from a study. The validity of a study's design is central to obtaining quality results and findings from a study.

Subject attrition See *attrition rate.*

Subjects Individuals participating in a study (those being studied), who are sometimes referred to as participants.

Substantive theory Conceptual structure of clearly identified concepts, definitions, and relational statements; can also be called *middle-range theories*; useful as practice guidelines and research frameworks.

Summary statistics See *descriptive statistics.*

Summated scale Various items on the scale that are added together or summed to obtain a single score.

Symbolic interaction theory Principle that explores how interactions among people and the environment create social processes and meanings, resulting in communication and behaviors.

Symmetric Term used to describe the normal curve, with the left side of the curve as a mirror image of the right side.

Synthesis of sources Connecting and summarizing ideas from several sources to promote a new understanding of what is known and not known in an area.

Systematic bias or variation Phenomenon that occurs when selected study participants share various characteristics, making the sample less representative of the population.

Systematic measurement error Nonrandom measurement error that occurs consistently with the same magnitude and in the same direction; for example, a weight scale that inaccurately weighs all participants 3 pounds heavier than their actual weight.

Systematic review Structured, comprehensive synthesis of quantitative studies in a particular healthcare area to determine the best research evidence available for expert clinicians to use to promote evidence-based practice. Systematic reviews are guided by PICOS questions.

Systematic sampling Conducted when an ordered list of all members of the population is available; involves selecting every *k*th (value determined by the researcher) individual on the list, starting with a randomly selected point.

T

Tails of normal curve Extreme ends of the normal curve at which statistically significant values can be found.

Target population All elements (individuals, objectives, or events) that meet the sampling criteria for inclusion in the study and to which the study findings might be generalized.

Tentative theory Newly proposed conceptual structure that has had minimal exposure to critique by scholars in the discipline and has undergone little testing.

Testable hypothesis A hypothesis containing variables that can be measured or manipulated in the real world.

Test-retest reliability Stability of a measurement over time; determined by correlating the scores from repeated measurements.

Textbook Monograph or book regarded as the standard for the study of a particular subject; may serve as a source of information for an academic course.

Theoretical literature Concept analyses, maps, theories, and conceptual frameworks that support a selected research problem and purpose.

Theoretical sampling Method of sampling often used during grounded theory studies; involves recruiting eligible participants on the basis of their ability to advance the emergent theory.

Theory Integrated set of defined concepts, existence statements, and relational statements that present a systematic view of a phenomenon.

Therapeutic research Studies providing a patient with an opportunity to receive an experimental treatment that might have beneficial results.

Thesis Research project completed by a graduate student as part of the requirements for a master's degree.

Threats to design validity Possible problems or conditions in a study that decrease the accuracy or validity of the research results. These threats are organized into four categories—statistical conclusion validity, internal validity, construct validity, and external validity.

Threat to construct validity Design flaw in which the measurement of a variable is not adequate for the concept it represents. A measurement may include not only the concept of interest but also other related concepts.

Threat to external validity Limit to the generalization based on differences between the conditions of participants of the study and the conditions or characteristics of persons or settings to which generalization is considered.

Threat to internal validity In interventional research, a factor that causes changes in the dependent variable in addition to the changes caused by the independent variable. In nonintervention research, a researcher may implement the study with inconsistent methods.

Threat to statistical conclusion validity Factor that produces a false data analysis conclusion, usually due to inadequate sample size or inappropriate use of a statistical test.

Time lag bias of studies Type of publication bias; occurs because studies with negative results are usually published later, sometimes 2 to 3 years later, than studies with positive results. Sometimes, studies with negative results are not published at all.

Total variance Sum of within-group variance and between-group variance determined by an analysis of variance (ANOVA).

Traditions Truths or beliefs based on customs and past trends that are a source of knowledge. Traditions are transferred from nurse to nurse by role modeling and written and oral communication.

Transcripts Verbatim written record created from an audio recording of an interview or focus group.

Transferability Term used to describe qualitative findings as they are applicable in other settings with similar participants when the study has a thorough description of the sample, and the reader has confidence in the credibility, dependability, and confirmability of the findings.

Translational research Evolving concept defined by the National Institutes of Health (NIH) as the translation of basic scientific discoveries into practical applications.

Treatment See *intervention.*

Treatment fidelity See *intervention fidelity.*

Treatment group See *experimental or intervention group.*

Trial and error Approach with unknown outcomes used in an uncertain situation when other sources of knowledge are unavailable.

True measure, or score Score that would be obtained if no measurement error had occurred. Theoretically, some measurement error always occurs when a sample is used to estimate a population parameter.

True-negative (result) Diagnostic or screening test result that accurately indicates the absence of a disease.

True-positive (result) Diagnostic or screening test result that accurately indicates the presence of a disease.

Trustworthiness Strength of a qualitative study as determined by the extent to which the interrelated characteristics of credibility, transferability, dependability, and confirmability of the study findings are evident in the research report.

***t*-Test** Parametric analysis technique used to determine significant differences between measures of two samples. There are two types of *t*-tests: independent samples *t*-test and dependent samples *t*-test. See the definitions for independent samples and paired samples.

Two-tailed test of significance Analysis used to test a nondirectional hypothesis in which the researcher assumes that an extreme score can occur in either tail of the normal curve.

Type I error Occurs when the researcher concludes that a significant difference exists between groups when, in fact, the samples are not significantly different. The null hypothesis is rejected when it is true.

Type II error Occurs when the researcher concludes that no significant difference exists between the samples examined when, in fact, a difference exists. The null hypothesis is regarded as true when it is, in fact, false.

U

Unexpected results Results seen when the researcher finds relationships between variables or differences among groups that were not hypothesized and not predicted from the framework being used.

Unexplained variance Variation between or among two or more variables that is the result of things other than the relationships.

Ungrouped frequency distribution Listing all values of a variable, with a tally of the number of times the value was recorded in the data.

Unstructured interview Communication between the researcher and the participant that begins with a broad question. Participants are encouraged to elaborate on a topic, introduce new topics, and thereby control the content of the interview; commonly used to collect qualitative data.

Unstructured observation Spontaneous observation and recording of what is seen with a minimum of planning; commonly used to collect qualitative data.

V

Validity Extent to which an instrument or measurement method accurately reflects or is able to measure the construct (or concept) being examined.

Variables Concrete or abstract qualities, properties, or characteristics of persons, things, or situations that change or vary and are manipulated or measured in quantitative research.

Variance Measure of dispersion in which a larger variance indicates a larger dispersion of scores. This is calculated as one step in determining standard deviation; also, in a prediction model, the total amount of the dependent variable explained by the independent or predictor variables.

Vertical axis Refers to the y-axis in a graph of a regression line or scatter plot. The vertical axis is oriented in a top to bottom direction across the graph.

Visual analog scale Refers to a 100-mm line, with right angle stops and descriptive words or phrases at each end. Study participants are asked to record the intensity, magnitude, or strength of their symptoms or attitudes on the line.

Voluntary agreement Decision made by a prospective subject to participate in a study of his or her own volition, without coercion or any undue influence.

Vulnerable populations Potential research participants who are more susceptible to undue influence or coercion, such as children, prisoners, and those who are economically disadvantaged.

W

Washout period Amount of time that is required for the effects of an intervention to dissipate and for the study participant to return to baseline.

Websites Internet pages maintained by individuals, organizations, and companies to provide information, which must be evaluated for their accuracy, bias, and relevance prior to citation in a literature review.

Within-group variance Variation of individual scores in a group from the group mean; determined by conducting analysis of variance (ANOVA).

X

***x*-Axis** Horizontal scale of a scatter plot. See *horizontal axis.*

Y

***y*-Axis** Vertical scale of a scatterplot. See *vertical axis.*

***y* intercept** Point at which the regression line crosses (or intercepts) the y-axis. At this point on the regression line, $x = 0$.

Z

***z*-Scores** Standardized scores developed from the normal curve that are equivalent to the standard deviation of the curve.

INDEX

Note: Page numbers followed by "*f*" indicate figures, "*t*" indicate tables, and "*b*" indicate boxes.

D

E

F

O

P

Q

S

T

U

V